DATE DUE

Safety Evaluation of *Medical Devices*

Safety Evaluation of Medical Devices

Second Edition
Revised and Expanded

Shayne Cox Gad
Gad Consulting Services
Cary, North Carolina

MARCEL DEKKER, INC. NEW YORK · BASEL

ISBN: 0-8247-0617-X

This book is printed on acid-free paper.

Headquarters
Marcel Dekker, Inc.
270 Madison Avenue, New York, NY 10016
tel: 212-696-9000; fax: 212-685-4540

Eastern Hemisphere Distribution
Marcel Dekker AG
Hutgasse 4, Postfach 812, CH-4001 Basel, Switzerland
tel: 41-61-261-8482; fax: 41-61-261-8896

World Wide Web
http://www.dekker.com

The publisher offers discounts on this book when ordered in bulk quantities. For more information, write to Special Sales/Professional Marketing at the headquarters address above.

Current printing (last digit):
10 9 8 7 6 5 4 3 2 1

PRINTED IN THE UNITED STATES OF AMERICA

*To Joyce, my wife, partner, and best friend,
for all the light and joy that she has brought
into my world.*

Preface to the Second Edition

The second edition of *Safety Evaluation of Medical Devices* continues to focus on the objective of the first edition—to serve as a single-volume practical guide for those who are responsible for or concerned with ensuring safety in the use and manufacture of medical devices. It benefits from recognition of the limitations and shortcomings of the previous edition, and also reflects the changes in regulations, science, and the marketplace.

Foremost, this new edition has been recast throughout to address the fact that device markets are global, and that their regulation has also become so. Each aspect of safety evaluation is considered in terms of International Standards Organization (ISO), U.S. Food and Drug Admininstration (FDA), European Union (EU), and Japanese Ministry of Health and Welfare (MHW) perspectives. Additionally, the continuing growth of technology has led to both new classes of devices (such as combination products, covered here in a new chapter) and new incorporation of science (particularly in the areas of immunotoxicology and carcinogenicity). Also incorporated are citations and means of access to Internet-based regulatory and scientific sites, reflecting the universal adoption of this technology into our world.

Shayne Cox Gad

Preface to the First Edition

Safety Evaluation of Medical Devices has been written with the sole objective of providing a practical guide for those who are responsible for, or concerned with, ensuring the safety of medical devices for patients, health care providers, and those involved in their manufacture. As such, the basic aspects of device regulation and materials utilized in devices have been addressed. In areas where it was deemed appropriate, the history and underlying science have also been presented to allow the reader to make more informed decisions.

This volume attempts to present a road map for the device and device material safety evaluation process as part of the overall development of new products. It reflects the experience and judgment of the author. It is my hope that it provides a utilitarian yet scientifically valid path through the everyday challenges of safety evaluation for all those involved.

I owe the greatest thanks to Joyce Todd for her help in proofreading this manuscript, as well as assisting me with the word processing. I am also grateful to Roger's Word Service and Janine Maves for decoding my handwriting and turning out excellent first typed drafts of the manuscript, and to the Touchberry Group for producing finished graphics.

Shayne Cox Gad

Contents

Contents

1

Introduction

The medical device industry in the United States and worldwide is immense in its economic impact (sales in 1998 were $138 billion worldwide, and $59 billion in the United States, $34 billion in the European Community, and $23 billion in Japan; in 1998, the U.S. medical equipment trade surplus was $8.7 billion), scope (between 87,000 and 140,000 different devices are produced in the United States by approximately 8200 different manufacturers employing some 311,000 people; it is believed that approximately 1000 of these manufacturers are development-stage companies without products yet on the market), and importance to the health of the world's citizens (Nugent, 1994; the Wilkerson Group, 1999). The assessment of the safety to patients using the multitude of items produced by this industry is dependent on schemes and methods that are largely peculiar to these kinds of products, are not as rigorous as those employed for foods, drugs, and pesticides, and are in a state of flux. Regulation of such devices is, in fact, relatively new. It is only with the Medical Device Amendments (to the Food, Drug and Cosmetic Act) of 1976 that devices have come to be explicitly regulated at all, and with the Safe Medical Devices Act of 1990, the Medical Device Amendments of 1992, and subsequent laws that the regulation of devices for biocompatibility became rigorous. The causes behind this timing are reviewed in the case histories presented in Chapter 17.

For purposes of this book, the safety we are concerned with is that related to the biological and chemical interactions of devices with patients' bodies, and not that due to mechanical or structural malfunction (e.g., as structural failure of heart valves and pacemakers). Such safety, also referred to as biocompatibility,

1

has not been of much concern to the public until recent years, but three cases of perceived significant risk on the part of devices (the Dalkon shield intrauterine device, the silicones in breast implants, and the latex present in gloves and a wide range of other devices) have changed both public and professional perceptions significantly and have led to much greater regulatory (and legal) scrutiny.

I. BIOCOMPATIBILITY

A medical device that is adequately designed for its intended use should be safe for that use. The device should not release any harmful substances into the patient that can lead to adverse effects. Some manufacturers believe that biocompatibility is sufficiently indicated if their devices are made of medical grade material or materials approved by FDA as direct or indirect additives. The term medical grade does not have an accepted legal or regulatory definition and can be misleading without biocompatibility testing.

There is no universally accepted definition for biomaterial and biocompatibility, yet the manufacturer who ultimately markets a device will be required by FDA to demonstrate biocompatibility of the product as part of the assurance of its safety and effectiveness. The manufacturer is responsible for understanding biocompatibility tests and selecting methods that best demonstrate the following:

> The lack of adverse biological response from the biomaterial
> The absence of adverse effects on patients

The diversity of the materials used, types of medical devices, intended uses, exposures, and potential harms present an enormous challenge to design and conduct well-defined biocompatibility testing programs. The experience gained in one application area is not necessarily transferable to another application. The same applies to different or sometimes slightly different (variable) materials. Biodegradation and interaction of materials complicates the issue.

Biocompatibility describes the state of a biomaterial within a physiological environment without the material adversely affecting the tissue or the tissue adversely affecting the material. Biocompatibility is a chemical and physical interaction between the material and the tissue and the biological response to these reactions.

Biocompatibility assays are used to predict and prevent adverse reactions and establish the absence of any harmful effects of the material. Such assays help to determine the potential risk that the material may pose to the patient. The proper use of biocompatibility tests can reject potentially harmful materials while permitting safe materials to be used for manufacturing the device.

Any biocompatibility statement is useful only when it is considered in the proper context. A statement such as ''propylene is biocompatible'' lacks precision and can lead to misunderstanding. Any statement of biocompatibility should include information on the type of device, the intended conditions of use, the degree of patient contact, and the potential of the device to cause harm. Manufacturers should avoid using the term biocompatible without clearly identifying the environment in which it is used and any limitations on such use.

The need for biocompatibility testing and the extent of such testing that should be performed depends on numerous factors, which are presented and considered in Chapter 2. These factors include the type of device, intended use, liability, degree of patient contact, nature of the components, and potential of the device to cause harm. There are no universal tests to satisfy all situations, and there is no single test that can predict biological performance of the material or device and reliably predict the safety of the device. The types and intended uses of medical devices determine the types and number of tests required to establish biocompatibility. Biological tests should be performed under conditions that simulate the actual use of the product or material as closely as possible and should demonstrate the biocompatibility of a material or device for a specific intended use. These tests will be more extensive for a new material than for those materials that have an established history of long and safe uses.

All materials used in the manufacture of a medical device should be considered for an evaluation of their suitability for intended use. Consideration should always be given to the possibility of the release of toxic substances from the base materials, as well as any contaminants that might remain after the manufacturing process or sterilization. The extent of these investigations will vary, depending on previously known information (prior art) and initial screening tests.

A. Fundamentals of Biocompatibility Tests

Biocompatibility is generally demonstrated by tests utilizing toxicological principles that provide information on the potential toxicity of materials in the clinical application. Many classical toxicological tests, however, were developed for a pure chemical agent, and are not applicable to biocompatibility testing of materials. In addition, medical devices are an unusual test subject in toxicity testing. A biomaterial is a complex entity, and the material toxicity is mediated by both physical and chemical properties. Toxicity from biomaterial often comes from leachable components, and the chemical composition of a material is often not known. Toxicological information on the material and its chemical composition is seldom available, and the possible interactions among the components in any given biological test system are seldom known.

Biocompatibility should not be defined by a single test. It is highly unlikely that a single parameter will be able to ensure biocompatibility, therefore it is necessary to test as many biocompatibility parameters as appropriate. It is also important to test as many samples as possible, therefore suitable positive and negative controls should produce a standard response index for repeated tests.

Additionally, the use of exaggerated conditions, such as using higher dose ranges and longer contact durations or multiple insults that are many factors more severe than the actual use condition, is important. Adopting an acceptable clinical exposure level that is multiple factors below the lowest toxic level has been a general practice.

Most of the biocompatibility tests are short-term tests to establish acute toxicity. Data from these short-term tests should not be stretched to cover the areas in which no test results are available.

Biocompatibility testing should be designed to assess the potential adverse effects under actual use conditions or specific conditions close to the actual use conditions. The physical and biological data obtained from biocompatibility tests should be correlated to the device and its use. Accuracy, reproducibility, and interpretability of tests depend on the method and equipment used and the investigator's skill and experience.

There are several toxicological principles that the investigator must consider before planning biocompatibility testing programs. Biocompatibility depends on the tissue that contacts the device. For example, the requirements for a blood-contacting device would be different from those applicable to a urethral catheter. Also, the degree of biocompatibility assurance depends on the involvement and the duration of contact with the human body. Some materials, such as those used in orthopedic implants, are meant to last for a long period in the patient. In this case, a biocompatibility testing program needs to show that the implant does not adversely affect the body during the long period of use. The possibility of biodegradation of material or device should not be ignored. Biodegradation by the body can change an implant's safety and effectiveness. The leachables from plastic used during a hemodialysis procedure may be very low, but the patient who is dialyzed three times a week may be exposed to a total of several grams during his or her lifetime, therefore cumulative effects (chronicity) should be assessed.

Two materials having the same chemical composition but different physical characteristics may not induce the same biological response. Also, past biological experiences with seemingly identical materials have their limits, too. Toxicity may come from leachable components of the material due to differences in formulation and manufacturing procedures.

Empirical correlation between biocompatibility testing results and actual toxic findings in humans and the extrapolation of the quantitative results from short-term in vitro tests to quantitate toxicity at the time of use are controversial. These need careful and scientifically sound interpretation and adjustment. The control of variation in biological susceptibility and resistance to obtain a biological response range for toxic effect and host factors that determine the variability of susceptibility in toxicological response adjustment to susceptibility in the human population also need careful attention.

The challenge of biocompatibility is to create and use knowledge to reduce the degree of unknowns and to help make the best possible decisions. The hazard presented by a substance, with its inherent toxic potential, can only be manifested when fully exposed in a patient. Risk, which is actual or potential harm, is therefore a function of toxic hazard and exposure. The safety of any leachables contained in the device or on the surface can be evaluated by determining the total amount of potentially harmful substance, estimating the amount reaching the patient's tissues, assessing the risk of exposure, and performing the risk versus benefit analysis. When the potential harm from the use of biomaterial is identified from the biocompatibility tests, this potential must be compared against the availability of an alternate material.

II. SCOPE OF DEVICES AND THE MEDICAL DEVICE MARKET

According to section 201(h) of the Food, Drug and Cosmetic Act, a medical device is an instrument, apparatus, implement, machine, contrivance, implant, in vitro reagent, or other similar or related article, including a component, part, or accessory that is

Recognized in the official National Formulary, or the United States Pharmacopoeia (USP, 2000), or any supplement to them.
Intended for use in the diagnosis of disease, in man or other animals
Intended to affect the structure or any function of the body of man or other animals, and that does not achieve any of its primary intended purposes through chemical action within or on the body of man or other animals, and that is not dependent upon being metabolized for the achievement of any of its principal intended purposes (CDRH, 1992)

Under this definition, devices might be considered as belonging to one of eight categories (North American industrial classification): surgical and medical instruments, ophthalmic, dental, lab apparatus, irradiation, specialty devices, medical/surgical supplies, in vitro diagnostics, and electromedical. There are (in 2000) 16,170 companies involved in these sectors—6750 of them manufacturers worldwide. This is a global industry with a $160 billion annual market. The U.S. market is $68 billion, or 42% of this (MDDI, 2000).

The top 20 medical devices by revenues in 1999 were the following:

1. Incontinence supplies
2. Home blood glucose-monitoring products
3. Wound closure products
4. Implantable defibrillators

5. Soft contact lenses
6. Orthopedic fixation devices
7. Pacemakers
8. Examination gloves
9. Interventional cardiovascular coronary stents
10. Arthroscopic accessory instruments
11. Prosthetic knee joint implants
12. Lens care products
13. Prosthetic hip joint implants
14. Multiparameter patient-monitoring equipment
15. Mechanical wound closure
16. Wound suture products
17. Absorbable polymers
18. Hearing aids
19. Wheelchair and scooter/mobility aids
20. Peritoneal dialysis sets

The 10 projected biggest growth device products are (in 2000) as follows:

Rank	Product	Percentage revenue growth rate (ys)	Specialty
1	Fibrin sealants	174.6 (95-02)	Wound care
2	Solid artificial organs	141.2 (95-02)	Transplant/implant
3	Left ventricular assist devices	96.0 (95-02)	Cardiovascular
4	Skin substitute products	63.1 (97-04)	Wound care
5	Refractive surgical devices	54.4 (98-05)	Ophthalmic
6	Gynecologic falloposcopes	49.5 (95-00)	Endoscopic/MIS
7	PTMR products	47.8 (00-04)	Cardiovascular
8	Bone growth substitutes and growth factors	47.0 (97-04)	Orthopedics
9	Growth factor dressings	46.0 (97-04)	Wound care
10	Vascular stent-grafts	46.0 (97-04)	Cardiovascular

Source: Frost & Sullivan, 2000.

III. HISTORY

As has previously been reviewed by Hutt (1989), the regulation of medical devices has followed a different history from that of drugs. Medical devices go back to at least the Egyptians and Etruscans. Problems with fraudulent devices in the United States date back to the late 1700s, though no legislative remedy was attempted until the 1900s. In fact, the legislative history of the 1906 Food and Drug Act contains no references to devices. Devices continued to be regulated under the postal fraud statutes. Such regulation was evidently ineffectual, as fraudulent devices flourished during this period. Starting in 1926, the FDA monitored such devices and assisted the U.S. Postal Service in its regulatory actions. Medical devices were covered in the 1938 act, but only in regard to adulteration and misbranding. Over the intervening years, various committees that examined medical device regulation consistently came to similar conclusions: that the FDA has inadequate authority and resources to regulate the medical device industry. As part of the agreement that resulted in passage of the 1962 amendments, however, all references to medical devices were deleted. The need and demand for increased regulation continued to grow. In 1967, President Lyndon Johnson supported the proposed Medical Device Safety Act, which nevertheless was not well received by Congress. In fact, no legislation pertaining to medical device safety was passed until 1976.

In 1969, at the request of President Richard Nixon, the Department of Health, Education and Welfare (HEW) established a study group in medical devices, also known as the Cooper committee, because it was chaired by the director of the National Heart and Lung Institute, Dr. Theodore Cooper. Its report in 1970 concluded that a different regulatory approach was needed to deal with medical devices. This report initiated the chain of events that culminated in the Medical Device Amendment of 1976. In the interim, the Bureau of Medical Devices and Diagnostic Products was created in 1979. Remarkably, the 1976 amendment retained the essential provisions of the Cooper committee report regarding inventory and classification of all medical devices by class: Class I (general controls), Class II (performance standards), or Class III (premarket approval). These classifications are discussed in greater detail later in this chapter. These remain the essential regulations applicable to medical devices. Both the Drug Price Competition and Patent Restoration Act of 1984 and the Orphan Drug Act of 1983 contained language that made the provisions of the laws applicable to medical devices but did not have provisions unique to medical devices. The recent perceptions, revelations, and controversy surrounding silicone breast implants will probably cause additional changes in the regulation of devices.

As a consequence, 1978 brought guidelines for investigational device exemptions (IDEs, the equivalent of investigational new drug applications (INDAs) for drugs). As shall be seen later, these requirements effectively excluded a wide range of medical devices from regulation by establishing an exemption for those new or modified devices that are equivalent to existing devices. The year 1990 saw the passage of the Safe Medical Devices Act, which made premarketing requirements and postmarketing surveillance more rigorous. The actual current guidelines for testing started with the USP guidance on biocompatibility of plastics. A formal regulatory approach springs from the tripartite agreement, which is a joint intergovernmental agreement between the United Kingdom, Canada, and the United States (with France having joined later). After lengthy consideration, the FDA has announced acceptance of International Standards Organization (ISO) 10993 guidelines for testing (ASTM, 1990; FAO, 1991; MAPI, 1992; O'Grady, 1990; Spizizen, 1992) under the rubric of harmonization. This is the second major trend operative in device regulation: the internationalization of the marketplace with accompanying efforts to harmonize regulations. Under the ICH (International Conference on Harmonization) great strides have been made in this area.

Independent of FDA initiatives, the USP has promulgated test methods and standards for various aspects of establishing the safety of drugs (e.g., the recent standards for inclusion of volatiles in formulated drug products), which were, in effect, regulations affecting the safety of drugs and devices. Most of the actual current guidelines for the conduct of nonclinical safety evaluations of medical devices have evolved from such quasi-agency actions [e.g., the USP's 1965 promulgation of biological tests for plastics and ongoing American National Standards Institute (ANSI) standard promulgation].

Public concern about three specific device safety issues have seemed to increase regulatory scrutiny. The first of these, the Dalkon Shield, was an intrauterine contraceptive device produced by the A. H. Robbins Corporation (Sivin, 1993). Its use was associated with unacceptable rates of pregnancy, pelvic inflammatory disease, and death in women who used it. The device was withdrawn from the market in 1974, and in 1988 Robbins reached a $3.3 billion settlement in response to a class action suit (Nocera, 1995).

The second case is that of silicone-filled breast implants, which have been purported to cause a range of autoimmune and neurologic effects on some women who have them. Although as of this writing (late 2000) the validity of these claims is largely disproven, litigation over them drove the primary manufacturer (Dow Corning) into bankruptcy and led to the removal of this product from the market.

Finally, since the late 1980s concern has grown about allergic responses to latex in devices. Several deaths have been blamed on anaphylactic responses to such effects (Lang, 1996).

IV. NONSPECIFIC REGULATORY CONSIDERATIONS

A broad-scope review of regulatory toxicology is presented in Gad (2001). Some regulations that it is necessary to understand beyond those covered in Chapter 2 require review here, however.

A. Good Laboratory Practices (GLPs)

The original promulgation of GLPs was by the U.S. FDA in 1978 in response to a variety of cases that led the agency to conclude that some of the data that it had obtained in support of product approvals were not trustworthy. Subsequently, other regulatory agencies and authorities in the United States and across the world have either promulgated their own version of similar regulations or required adherence to the set generated by the U.S. FDA or another body. The EEC requirement for compliance with GLPs for safety tests has recently been reinforced in a modification of directive 75/318/EEC (Regulatory Affairs Focus, 1996; ISO, 1990; European Community, 1991). The FDA last revised the GLP regulations in 1989 (FDA, 1989).

The GLPs require that all pivotal preclinical safety studies—that is, those that are used and regulatorily required to make decisions as to the safety of the product (in our case, a device)—be conducted under a well-defined protocol utilizing procedures set forth in written standard operating procedures by trained (as established by documentation) personnel under the direction of a study director. All work must be reviewed by an independent quality assurance unit (QAU). The regulations require rigorous attention to record keeping, but do not dictate how actual studies are designed or conducted in a technical sense (Gad and Taulbee, 1996).

B. Animal Welfare Act (AWA)

Gone are the days when the biomedical scientist could conduct whatever procedures or studies that were desired using experimental animals. The AWA (APHIS, 1989) (and its analogues in other countries) rightfully requires careful consideration of animal usage to ensure that research and testing uses as few animals as possible in as humane a manner as possible. As a start, all protocols must be reviewed by an institutional animal care and use committee. Such review takes time, but should not serve to hinder good science. When designing a study or developing a new procedure or technique, the following points should be kept in mind:

1. Will the number of animals used be sufficient to provide the required data, yet not constitute excessive use? (It ultimately does not reduce animal use to utilize too few animals to begin with and then have to repeat the study.)
2. Are the procedures employed the least invasive and traumatic available? This practice is not only required by regulations, but is also sound scientific practice, since any induced stress will produce a range of responses in test animals that can mask or confound the chemically induced effects. Most recently (September 2000) USDA (which administers the AWA) decided to begin including rodents in all aspects of the AWA's reporting requirements (an issue still in litigation in mid-2001).

TABLE 1.1 Congressional Committees Responsible for FDA Oversight

Authorization	
Senate	All public health service agencies are under the jurisdiction of the Labor and Human Resources Committee.
House	Most public health agencies are under the jurisdiction of the Health and the Environmental Subcommittee of the House Energy and Commerce Committee.
Appropriation	
Senate	Unlike most other public health agencies, the FDA is under the jurisdiction of Agriculture, Rural Development, and Related Agencies Subcommittee of the Senate Appropriations Committee.
House	Under the jurisdiction of the Agriculture, Rural Development, and Related Agencies Subcommittee of the House Appropriations Committee.

C. Regulations Versus Law

A note of caution must be inserted here. The law (the document passed by Congress) and the regulations (the documents written by the regulatory authorities to enforce the laws) are separate documents. The sections in the law do not necessarily have numerical correspondence. For example, the regulations on the product marketing application (PMA) process is described in 21 CFR 312, but the law describing the requirement for a PMA process is in section 515 of the FDLI. Because the regulations rather than the laws themselves have a greater impact on toxicological practice, greater emphasis is placed on regulation in this chapter. For a complete review of FDA law, the reader is referred to the monographs by Food and Drug Law Institute in 1995 (FDLI, 1995).

Laws authorize the activities and responsibilities of the various federal agencies. All proposed laws before the U.S. Congress are referred to committees for review and approval. The committees responsible for FDA oversight are summarized in Table 1.1, which also highlights the fact that authorizations and appropriations (the funding necessary to execute authorizations) are handled by different committees. Figure 2.1 presents the organization of the CDRH. As can be seen by the organizational structure presented in Figure 2.1, the categorization of devices for division review purposes is functionally based.

D. Organizations Regulating Drug and Device Safety in the United States

The agency formally charged with overseeing the safety of drugs and devices in the United States is the FDA. It is headed by a commissioner who reports to the secretary of the Department of Health and Human Services (DHHS) and has a tremendous range of responsibilities. Medical devices are overseen by the CDRH, headed by a director. Drugs are overseen primarily by the Center for Drug Evaluation and Research (CDER) (though some therapeutic or health care entities are considered as biologically derived and therefore regulated by the Center for Biologic Evaluation and Research, or CBER). There are also "combination products" (part drug, part device), which may be regulated by either CDER or CBER or both, or by CDRH, depending on where the expertise is perceived to be in the FDA (CFR, 1992).

Most of the regulatory interaction of a toxicologist involved in assessing the biocompatibility of devices is with the appropriate part of the CDRH, though for combination products the two centers charged with drugs or biologicals may also come into play. Within the CDRH there is a range of groups (called divisions) that focus on specific areas of use for devices (e.g., general and restorative devices; cardiovascular, respiratory, and neurological devices; ophthalmic devices; reproductive, abdominal, ear, nose, and throat, and radiological devices; and clinical laboratory devices). Within each of these there are engineers, chemists, pharmacologists/toxicologists, statisticians, and clinicians.

There is also at least one nongovernmental body that must review and approve various aspects of devices, setting forth significant "guidance" for the evaluation of safety of devices. This is the USP, and its responsibilities and guidelines are presented in Chapter 2.

REFERENCES

APHIS. (1989). Animal and Plant Health Inspection Service, U.S. Department of Agriculture, Fed. Reg., 54(168):36112–36163.

ASTM. (1990). Standardization in Europe: A success story, ASTM Standardiz. News, 38.

CDRH. (1992). Regulatory Requirements for Medical Devices: A Workshop Manual, Center for Device and Radiological Health, HHS publication FDA 92-4165.

CFR. (1992). FDA's policy statement concerning cooperative manufacturing arrangements for licensed biologics, Fed. Reg., 57:55544.

European Committee for Standardization. (1991). CEN annual report 1991, Brussels.

FAO. (1991). Report of the FAO/WHO Conference on Food Standards, Chemicals in Food and Food Trade (in cooperation with GATT), vol. 1, Rome, March 18–27.

FDLI. (1995). Compilation of Food and Drug Laws, vols. I and II, Food and Drug Law Institute, Washington, DC.

FDA. (1989). Good laboratory practice regulations: Final rule, part VI, Fed. Reg., 52 (172).

Gad, S. C. (2001). Regulatory Toxicology, 2nd ed. Taylor & Francis, Philadelphia.

Gad, S. C. and Taulbee, S. (1996). Handbook of Data Recording, Maintenance and Management for the Biomedical Sciences, CRC Press, Boca Raton, FL.

Hutt, P. B. (1989). A history of government regulation and misbranding of medical devices, Food Drug Cosmet. Law J., 44(2):99–117.

ISO. (1990). ISO 9000 International Standards for Quality Management Vision 2000—A Strategy for International Standards' Implementation in the Quality Arena During the 1990s, 2nd ed., compendium, EEC, Brussels.

Lang, L. A. (1996). A review of latex hypersensitivity, Toxic Subst. Mech., 15:1–11.

MAPI. (1992). The European Community's new approach to regulation of product standards and quality assurance (ISO 9000): What it means for U.S. manufacturers, MAPI Economic Report ER-218.

MDDI. (2000). Industry snapshot, Med. Dev. Diag. Ind., Dec.:47–56.

Nocera, J. (1995). Fatal litigation, Fortune, Oct. 16, pp. 60–82.

Nugent, T. N. (1994). Health Care Products and Services Basic Analysis, Standard & Poor's Industry Surveys, New York.

O'Grady, J. (1990). Interview with Charles M. Ludolph, ASTM Standardiz. News, 26.

Regulatory Affairs Focus. (1996). European update, Reg. Aff. Focus, 1(4):8.

Sivin, I. (1993). Another look at the Dalkon shield: Meta-analysis underscores the problems, Contraception, 48:1–12.

Spizizen, G. (1992). The ISO 9000 standards: Creating a level playing field for international quality, Nat. Prod. Rev., summer.

USP. (2000). The United States Pharmacopoeia, XXIV § NF-19, U.S. Pharmacopoeial Convention, Rockville, MD.

The Wilkerson Group (1999). Forces Reshaping the Performance and Contribution of the U.S. Medical Device Industry, Health Industry Manufacturers Association, Washington, DC.

2

Regulatory Aspects and Strategy in Medical Device and Biomaterials Safety Evaluation

As discussed in Chapter 1, according to section 201(h) of the Food, Drug and Cosmetic Act, a medical device is defined in the United States as an instrument, apparatus, implement, machine, contrivance, implant, in vitro reagent, or other similar or related article, including a component, part, or accessory that is

1. Recognized in the official National Formulary, or the *United States Pharmacopoeia* (USP, 2000), or any supplement to them
2. Intended for use in the diagnosis of disease or other condition, or in the cure, mitigation, treatment, or prevention of disease, in man or other animals, or intended to affect the structure or any function of the body of man or other animals, and that does not achieve any of its primary intended purposes through chemical action within or on the body of man or other animals, and that is not dependent upon being metabolized for the achievement of any of its principal intended purposes (CDRH, 1992)

I. REGULATORY BASIS

A. Regulations: General Considerations for the United States

The U.S. regulations for medical devices derive from the following five principal laws:

Federal Food, Drug and Cosmetic Act of 1938
Medical Device Amendments of 1976
Safe Medical Devices Act of 1990
Medical Device Amendments of 1992
FDA Modernization Act of 1997 (Section 204)

The U.S. federal regulations that govern the testing, manufacture, and sale of medical devices are covered in Chapter 1, Title 21 of the Code of Federal Regulations (21 CFR). These comprise nine 6 × 8 inch volumes that each stack 8 inches high. This title also covers foods, veterinary products, medical devices, and cosmetics. As these topics will be discussed elsewhere in this book, here we will briefly review those parts of 21 CFR that are applicable to medical devices (Gad, 2001; Heller, 1999).

Of most interest to a toxicologist working in this arena would be Chapter 1, subchapter A (parts 1–78), which covers general provisions, organization, and so on. The good laboratory practices (GLPs) are codified in 21 CFR 58. The regulations applicable to medical devices are covered in subchapter H, parts 800–895 of 21 CFR. As discussed earlier, the term medical device covers a wide variety of products: contact lenses, hearing aids, intrauterine contraceptive devices, syringes, catheters, drip bags, orthopedic prostheses, and so on. The current structure of the law was established by the Medical Device Amendment of 1976. Products on the market on the day the amendment was passed were assigned to one of three classes (I, II, or III), based on the recommendations of advisory panels. Medical device classification procedure is described in part 860. Class I products (the least risk-laden) were those for which safety and effectiveness could be reasonably assured by general controls. Such devices are available over the counter to the general public. Class II products were those for which a combination of general controls and performance standards were required to reasonably assure safety and effectiveness. Class II devices are available only with a doctor's prescription. Class III products were those for which general controls and performance standards were inadequate; these were required to go through a premarket approval process. All devices commercially distributed after May 28, 1976 ("preamendment Class III devices") that are not determined to be substantially equivalent to an existing marketed device are automatically categorized as Class III and require the submission of a premarket approval (PMA). Please note that these are classifications for regulatory purposes only and are distinct from the classification [Health Industry Manufacturing Association (HIMA)/Pharmaceutical Research and Manufacturers Association (PHRMA)] of product types (e.g., internal versus external) discussed elsewhere in this chapter. Kahan (1995) provides a detailed overview of what comprises general controls, performance standards, and such.

As with the subchapter on drugs, much of the subchapter on medical devices in the regulations concerns categorizations and specifics for a wide variety of devices. For a toxicologist involved in new product development, the parts of greatest interest are 812 and 814. As with drugs, devices must be shown to be safe and effective when used as intended, and data must be provided to demonstrate such claims. In order to conduct the appropriate clinical research to obtain these data, a sponsor applies to the agency for an IDE, as described in 21 CFR 812. As stated in this section, "an approved investigational device exemption (IDE) permits a device that would otherwise be required to comply with a performance standard or to have premarket approval to be shipped lawfully for the purpose of conducting investigations of that device." Given the broad range of products that fall under the category of medical devices, the toxicological concerns are equally broad; testing requirements to support an IDE are vaguely mentioned in the law, even by FDA standards. In this regard, the law simply requires that the IDE application must include a report of prior investigations that "shall include reports of all prior clinical, animal and laboratory testing." There is no absolute requirement for animal testing, only a requirement that such testing must be reported. There are, of course, standards and conventions to be followed in designing a safety package to support an IDE, and these are discussed in a subsequent section of this chapter.

In order to obtain a license to market a device, a sponsor either submits a 510(k) premarket notification or applies for a PMA, as described in 21 CFR 814. Like a new drug application (NDA), a PMA application is a very extensive and detailed document that must include, among other things, a summary of nonclinical laboratory studies submitted in the application 921 CFR 814.20(b)(3)(v)(A), as well as a section containing the results of the nonclinical laboratory studies with the device, including microbiological, toxicological, immunological, biocompatibility, stress, wear, shelf life, and other laboratory or animal tests as appropriate. As with drugs, these tests must be conducted in compliance with the GLP regulations. Under the language of the law, a sponsor submits a PMA, which the FDA then "files." The filing of an application means that "FDA has made a threshold determination that the application is sufficiently complete to permit substantive review." Reasons for refusal to file are listed in 814.44(e), and include items such as an application that is not complete and has insufficient justification for the omission(s) present. The agency has 45 days from receipt of an application to notify the sponsor as to whether or not the application has been filed. The FDA has 180 days after filing of a complete PMA (21 CFR 814.40) to send the applicant an approval order, an "approved" letter or a "not approved" letter, or an order denying approval. An approval order is self-explanatory and is issued if the agency finds no reason (as listed in 814.45) for denying approval. An approved letter, 814.44(e), means the application substantially meets requirements, but some specific additional information is needed. A not approved letter, 814.45(f), means that the application contains false statements of fact, does not comply with labeling guidelines, nonclinical laboratory studies were not conducted according to GLPs, and so on. Essentially, an order denying approval means that the sponsor must do substantially more work and must submit a new application for PMA for the device in question. 510(k) premarket approval submissions are less extensive than PMAs, but must still include appropriate preclinical safety data. 510(k)s are supposed to be approved in 90 days.

Actual review and approval times historically have been much longer than the statutory limits. For 1995, the average total review time for class III products in the United States cleared by 510(k) was 579 days (versus 240 or less in the EU) (the Gray Sheet, 1996a). For fiscal year 1996, overall average 510(k) review times (for an expected 5,875 filings) is projected to be 137 days (with low-risk exempted devices and refusals to file not being included in the totals or average). Average PMA review times are projected to be 250 days (the Gray Sheet, 1996b). See Chapter 1 for a discussion of general regulatory considerations (such as GLPs) that are applicable to all safety evaluation studies.

B. Regulations Versus Law

A note of caution must be inserted here. The law (the document passed by Congress) and the regulations (the documents written by the regulatory authorities to enforce the laws) are separate documents. The sections in the law do not necessarily have numerical correspondence. For example, the regulations on the PMA process are described in 21 CFR 312, but the law describing the requirement for a PMA process is in Section 515 of the FDCA. Because the regulations rather than the laws themselves have a greater impact on toxicological practice, greater emphasis is placed on regulation in this chapter. For a complete review of FDA law, the reader is referred to the monographs by the Food and Drug Law Institute (FDLI) in 1995, 1996, and 1998.

Figure 2.1 presents the organization of the Center for Devices and Radiological Health (CDRH). As can be seen by the organizational structure presented in Figure 2.1, the categorization of devices for division review purposes is functionally based.

C. Organizations Regulating Device Safety in the United States

The agency formally charged with overseeing the safety of drugs and devices in the United States is the FDA. It is headed by a commissioner who reports to the secretary of the Department of Health and Human Services (DHHS) and has a

FIGURE 2.1 Organization of the Office of Device Evaluation (ODE) for the Center for Devices and Radiological Health (CDRH) of the FDA. Current officials (as of 5/1/1996) are identified by name. ODE evaluates submissions for new device approvals.

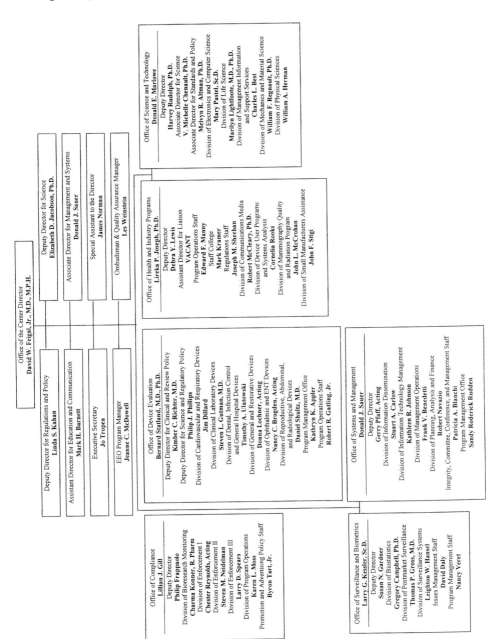

Office of the Center Director
David W. Feigal, Jr., M.D., M.P.H.

Deputy Director for Science
Elizabeth D. Jacobson, Ph.D.

Associate Director for Management and Systems
Donald J. Sauer

Special Assistant to the Director
James Norman

Ombudsman & Quality Assurance Manager
Les Weinstein

Deputy Director for Regulations and Policy
Linda S. Kahan

Assistant Director for Education and Communication
Mark H. Barnett

Executive Secretary
Jo Tropea

EEO Program Manager
Jeanne C. McDowell

Office of Science and Technology
Donald E. Marlowe
Deputy Director
Harvey Rudolph, Ph.D.
Associate Director for Science
V. Michelle Chenault, Ph.D.
Associate Director for Standards and Policy
Melvyn R. Altman, Ph.D.
Division of Electronics and Computer Science
Mary Pastel, Sc.D.
Division of Life Science
Marilyn Lightfoote, M.D., Ph.D.
Division of Management Information
and Support Services
Charles L. Best
Division of Mechanics and Material Science
William F. Regnault, Ph.D.
Division of Physical Sciences
William A. Herman

Office of Health and Industry Programs
Lireka P. Joseph, Ph.D.
Deputy Director
Debra Y. Lewis
Assistant Director for Liaison
VACANT
Program Operations Staff
Edward F. Manny
Staff College
Mark Kramer
Regulations Staff
Joseph M. Sheehan
Division of Communications Media
Robert McCleary, Ph.D.
Division of Device User Programs
and Systems Analysis
Cornelia Rooks
Division of Mammography Quality
and Radiation Program
John L. McCrohan
Division of Small Manufacturers Assistance
John F. Stigi

Office of Device Evaluation
Bernard Statland, M.D., Ph.D.
Deputy Director for Clinical and Review Policy
Kimber C. Richter, M.D.
Deputy Director for Science and Regulatory Policy
Philip J. Phillips
Division of Cardiovascular and Respiratory Devices
Jim Dillard
Division of Clinical Laboratory Devices
Steven L. Gutman, M.D.
Division of Dental, Infection Control
and General Hospital Devices
Timothy A. Ulatowski
Division of General and Restorative Devices
Donna Lochner, Acting
Division of Ophthalmic and ENT Devices
Nancy C. Brogden, Acting
Division of Reproductive, Abdominal,
and Radiological Devices
Daniel Shultz, M.D.
Program Management Office
Kathryn K. Appler
Program Operations Staff
Robert R. Gatling, Jr.

Office of Systems and Management
Donald J. Sauer
Deputy Director
Gerry Pfaff, Acting
Division of Information Dissemination
Stuart A. Carlow
Division of Information Technology Management
Kathleen R. Johnson
Division of Management Operations
Frank V. Benedetti
Division of Planning, Analysis and Finance
Robert Navazio
Integrity, Committee, Conference, and Management Staff
Patricia A. Bianchi
Program Management Office
Sandy Roderick Rudden

Office of Compliance
Lillian J. Gill
Deputy Director
Philip Frappaolo
Division of Bioresearch Monitoring
Charma Konner, R. Pharm
Division of Enforcement I
Chester Reynolds, Acting
Division of Enforcement II
Steven M. Neidelman
Division of Enforcement III
Larry D. Spears
Division of Program Operations
Karen L. Moss
Promotion and Advertising Policy Staff
Byron Tart, Jr.

Office of Surveillance and Biometrics
Larry G. Kessler, Sc.D.
Deputy Director
Susan N. Gardner
Division of Biostatistics
Gregory Campbell, Ph.D.
Division of Postmarket Surveillance
Thomas P. Gross, M.D.
Division of Surveillance Systems
Leighton W. Hansel
Issues Management Staff
David Daly
Program Management Staff
Nancy Veret

tremendous range of responsibilities. Medical devices are overseen by the CDRH, headed by a director. Drugs are overseen primarily by the Center for Drug Evaluation and Research (CDER) (although some therapeutic or health care entities are considered as biologically derived and therefore regulated by the Center for Biologic Evaluation and Research, or CBER). There are also "combination products" (part drug, part device), which may be regulated by either CDER or CBER (or both), and CDRH, depending on where the expertise is perceived to be in the FDA (CFR, 1992), as discussed in Chapter 14.

D. Classification of Devices

In accordance with the 1976 Medical Device Amendments, devices in the United States are categorized as follows:

> Class I—general controls (equivalent to OTC)
> Class II—performance standards and special controls (distribution is physician-controlled)
> Class III—premarket approval (clinical use only)
> Preamendment devices

In Europe, there is a lengthy set of rules in the EC medical device directive (Council Directive, 1993) to place devices in classes I, IIa, IIb, or III. Class I is the minimum grade and class II the maximum. This classification determines the extent of supporting data that are required to obtain marketing approval.

In the United States, the FDA Center for Devices and Radiological Health recognizes three classes of medical devices, and this system is based on whether or not the product was on the market prior to the passage of the 1976 Medical Device Amendments. If a new device is substantially equivalent to a preamendment device, then it will be classified the same as that device. This means that for Class I and II products, no PNA is necessary. Class III products need premarketing approval, and all new devices that are not substantially equivalent to existing products fall automatically into Class III.

Japan (MHW) and Korea have a somewhat different three-class system. Class I includes products that have no body contact and that would not cause any damage to the human body if they failed; for example, X-ray film. These products need to have premarketing approval in terms of medical device regulations, although they may need to be tested under industrial guidelines, such as those of the OECD. Class II products have external contact with the body, Class III have internal contact, and both need additional testing. Figure 2.2 presents the EFC scheme for device classification.

Most of the regulatory interaction of a toxicologist involved in assessing the biocompatibility of devices is with the appropriate part of the CDRH, although for combination products the two centers charged with drugs or biologicals may also

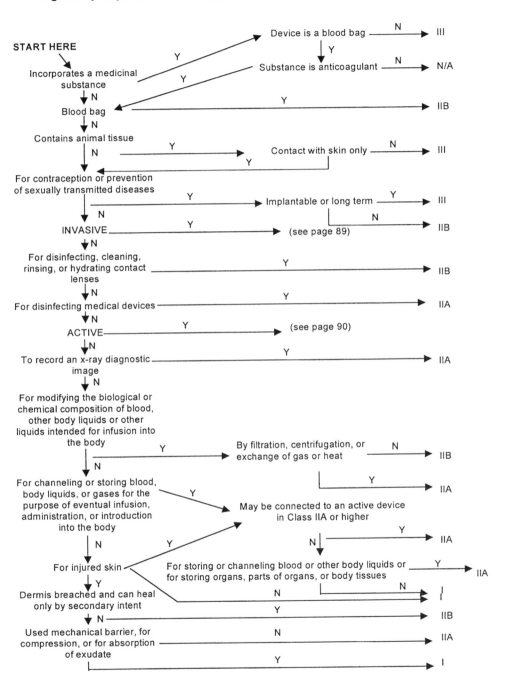

FIGURE 2.2 Medical device classification flowchart.

Invasive with respect to a natural orifice

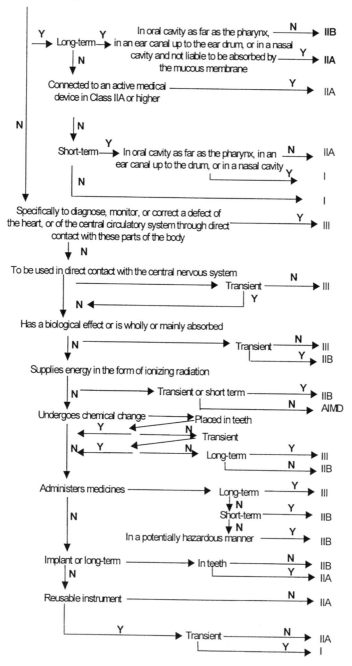

FIGURE 2.2   Continued

come into play. Within the CDRH there is a range of groups (called divisions) that focus on specific areas of use for devices (e.g., general and restorative devices; cardiovascular, respiratory, and neurological devices; ophthalmic devices; reproductive, abdominal, ear, nose, and throat, and radiological devices; and clinical laboratory devices). Within each of these there are engineers, chemists, pharmacologists/toxicologists, statisticians, and clinicians.

There is also at least one nongovernmental body that must review and approve various aspects of devices, setting forth significant "guidance" for the evaluation of safety of devices. This is the United States Pharmacopoeia (USP), and its responsibilities and guidelines are presented later in this chapter.

The other two major regulatory organizations to be considered are the International Standards Organization (ISO), with ISO 10993 standards (ISO, various dates), and the Japanese Ministry of Health and Welfare (MHW) with its guidelines (MHW, 1995).

II. TOXICITY TESTING: MEDICAL DEVICES

In a statutory sense, any item promoted for a medical purpose that does not rely on chemical action to achieve its intended effect is a medical device (as discussed earlier). In vitro diagnostic tests are also regulated as medical devices. The regulation of devices under these definitions has had a different history than that of drugs; it has not been as strict and it has evolved at a slower rate. Also, requirements for safety evaluation of devices have not been as strict as those for drugs. The safety concerns are also somewhat different. Toxicologic safety concerns for devices (as opposed to concerns of mechanical safety, such as disintegration of heart valves) are called biocompatibility concerns.

Medical devices are classified as being in three different classes and are regulated accordingly. Class III devices are subject to the greatest degree of regulation and include devices that are implanted in the body, support life, prevent health impairment, or present an unreasonable risk of illness or injury. These are subject to premarketing approval. Class II and Class I devices are subject to lesser control, required only to comply with general controls and performance standards.

There are several governing schemes for dictating what testing must be done on new Class III devices in the general case, with each developed and proposed by a different regulatory organization at different times over the last few years. International Conference on Harmonization (ICH) has attempted to harmonize these requirements so that different (or duplicate) testing would not need to be performed to gain device approval in different national markets. As discussed in Chapter 17, there are also specialized testing requirements for some device types, such as contact lenses (CDRH, 1995a,b) and tampons (CDRH, 1995c). The ICH/ISO effort has generally been successful. The major differences in requirements are largely matters of test design, with Japan being the primary variant. These differences are highlighted as requirements and designs are presented.

As with drugs, all safety testing for devices must be conducted in conformity with GLPs (FDA, 1987; Fries, 1999; Gad and Taulbee, 1996). Table 2.1 presents the existing FDA/CDRH requirements for device characterization and testing. The exact nature of the test protocols is based on recommendations by USP, ISO, and others. It should be noted that Class I devices, if new, are also subject to the ISO guidelines. It should also be noted that in general FDA now adheres to the ISO guidance on test requirements. (This will be seen later in Tables 2.12 and 2.13.)

Additional concerns with devices are considerations of their processing after production. Recently concerns have risen about the potential for latex components to cause allergies. Concern has grown not only for natural rubber used in devices with systemic exposure (catheters, stoppers on syringes, etc.), but also for devices that have been washed in fluids used to wash other items that contain latex. It is likely that all devices containing latex will soon have to be labeled as such.

Devices that have systemic exposure need to be sterilized. Radiation and heat can be used for some devices, but others cannot be sterilized in these. Ethylene oxide or other chemical sterilants must be used, raising concerns that residual sterilants may present problems. At the same time, devices with exposure to the fluid path must be demonstrated to be neither pyrogenic nor hemolytic in their final manufactured form.

1. The selection of material(s) to be used in device manufacture and its toxicological evaluation should initially take into account full characterization of the material; for example, formulation, known and suspected impurities, and processing.
2. The material(s) of manufacture, the final product, and possible leachable chemicals or degradation products should be considered for their relevance to the overall toxicological evaluation of the device.
3. Tests to be utilized in the toxicological evaluation should take into account the bioavailability of the bioactive material; that is, the nature, degree, frequency, duration, and conditions of exposure of the device to the body. This principle may lead to the categorization of devices, which would facilitate the selection of appropriate tests.
4. Any in vitro or in vivo experiments or tests must be conducted according to recognized GLPs, followed by evaluation by competent, informed persons.
5. Full experimental data, complete to the extent that an independent conclusion could be made, should be available to the reviewing authority, if required.

TABLE 2.1 FDA Device Categories and Suggested Biological Testing (FDA, 1995)

Device categories		Irritation tests	Sensitization assay	Cytotoxicity	Acute systemic toxicity	Hemocompatibility/hemolysis	Pyrogenicity (material-mediated)	Implantation tests	Mutagenicity (carcinogenicity)	Subchronic toxicity	Chronic toxicity	Carcinogenesis bioassay
		Short-term									*Long-Term*	
Body contact duration A—Transient (< 5 minutes) B—Short-term (5 minutes-29 days) C—Long-term (> 30 days)												
Intact surface	A	*	*	*								
	B	*	*	*								
	C	*	*	*	*							
External devices												
Breached or surface comprised	A	*	*	*	*	*						
	B	*	*	*	*	*				*		
	C	*	*	*	*	*			*	*	*	
Intact natural channels	A	*	*	*	*	*	*	*				
	B	*	*	*	*	*	*	*	*	*		
	C	*	*	*	*	*	*	*	*	*	*	*
Externally communicating devices												
Blood path indirect	A	*	*	*	*	*	*	*	*			
	B	*	*	*	*	*	*	*	*	*		
	C	*	*	*	*	*	*	*	*	*	*	*
Blood path direct	A	*	*	*	*	*	*	*	*			
	B	*	*	*	*	*	*	*	*	*		
	C	*	*	*	*	*	*	*	*	*	*	*
Bone	A	*	*	*	*	*	*	*	*			
	B	*	*	*	*	*	*	*	*	*		
	C	*	*	*	*	*	*	*	*	*	*	*
Internal devices												
Tissue and tissue fluids	A	*	*	*	*	*	*	*	*			
	B	*	*	*	*	*	*	*	*	*		
	C	*	*	*	*	*	*	*	*	*	*	*
Blood	A	*	*	*	*	*	*	*	*			
	B	*	*	*	*	*	*	*	*	*		
	C	*	*	*	*	*	*	*	*	*	*	*

1. For these devices with possible leachables or degradation products, e.g., absorbable surfaces, hemostatic agents, etc., testing for pharmacokinetics may be required.
2. Reproductive and developmental toxicity tests may be required for certain materials used for specialized indications.
3. Considerations should be given to long-term biological tests where indicated in the table taking into account the nature and mobility of the ingredients in the materials used to fabricate the device.

6. Any change in chemical composition, manufacturing process, physical configuration, or intended use of the device must be evaluated with respect to possible changes in toxicological effects and the need for additional toxicity testing.

7. The toxicological evaluation performed in accordance with this guid-

ance should be considered in conjunction with other information from other nonclinical tests, clinical studies, and postmarket experiences for an overall safety assessment.

A. Device Categories: Definitions and Examples

I.   Noncontact devices: devices that do not contact the patient's body directly or indirectly; examples include in vitro diagnostic devices.

II. External devices

A.   Intact surfaces.   Devices that contact intact external body surfaces only; examples include electrodes, external prostheses, and monitors of various types.

B.   Breached or compromised surfaces.   Devices that contact breached or otherwise compromised external body surfaces; examples include ulcer, burn and granulation tissue dressings or healing devices, and occlusive patches.

III. Externally communicating devices

A.   Intact natural channels.   Devices communicating with intact natural channels; examples include contact lenses, urinary catheters, intravaginal and intraintestinal devices (sigmoidoscopes, colonoscopes, stomach tubes, gastroscopes), endotracheal tubes, and bronchoscopes.

B.   Blood path, indirect.   Devices that contact the blood path at one point and serve as a conduit for fluid entry into the vascular system; examples include solution administration sets, extension sets, transfer sets, and blood administration sets.

C.   Blood path, direct.   Devices that contact recirculating blood; examples include intravenous catheters, temporary pacemaker electrodes, oxygenators, extracorporeal oxygenator tubing and accessories, and dialyzers, dialysis tubing, and accessories.

IV. Internal devices

A.   Bone.   Devices principally contacting bone; examples include orthopedic pins, plates, replacement joints, bone prostheses, and cements.

B.   Tissue and tissue fluid.   Devices principally contacting tissue and tissue fluid or mucus membranes where contact is prolonged; examples include pacemakers, drug supply devices, neuromuscular sensors and stimulators, replacement tendons, breast implants, cerebrospinal fluid drains, artificial larynx, vas deferens valves, ligation clips, tubal occlusion devices for female sterilization, and intrauterine devices.

C.   Blood.   Devices principally contacting blood; examples include permanent pacemaker electrodes, artificial arteriovenous fistulae, heart valves, vascular grafts, blood monitors, internal drug delivery catheters, and ventricular assist pumps.

B. Biological Tests

Also required to properly utilize the tables is a knowledge of the objectives of the specified biological tests. These can be considered as follows (Gad and Chengelis, 1998; Goering and Galloway, 1989):

Sensitization assay.   Estimates the potential for sensitization of a test material and/or the extracts of a material using it in an animal and/or human. The International Standards Organization (ISO, 1992; 1996) and MHW procedures are contrasted in Table 2.2.

Irritation tests.   Estimates the irritation potential of test materials and their extracts, using appropriate site or implant tissue such as skin and mucous membrane in an animal model and/or human. The International Standards Organization and MHW procedures are contrasted in Table 2.3, and for eye irritation in Table 2.4.

Cytotoxicity.   With the use of cell culture techniques, this test determines the lysis of cells (cell death), the inhibition of cell growth, and other toxic effects on cells caused by test materials and/or extracts from the materials. The International Standards Organization and MHW procedures are contrasted in Table 2.5.

Acute systemic toxicity.   Estimates the harmful effects of either single or multiple exposures to test materials and/or extracts in an animal model

TABLE 2.2   Differences Between Sensitization Test Procedures Required by ISO 10993-10 and the MHW Guidelines

ISO 10993-10	MHW 1995
Sample preparation: Extraction in polar and/or nonpolar solvents.	Two extraction solvents, methanol and acetone, recommended.
Extraction ratio: Extraction ratio is dependent on thickness of device or representative portion.	Specific extraction ratios: 10:1 (volume solvent:weight sample).
Extract used for testing: If extraction is not possible, the adjuvant and patch test can be utilized.	Residue obtained from extraction is redissolved and used for testing. (If residue does not dissolve in DMSO, or a sufficient amount of residue is not obtained, the adjuvant and patch test is recommended.) Sufficient amount of residue: 0.1 to 0.5% (weight residue:weight test material).

TABLE 2.3 Differences in Intracutaneous Reactivity Test Procedures Required by ISO 10993-10 and the MHW Guidelines

ISO 10993-10	MHW
Number of test animals: three rabbits for 1 to 2 extracts	Two rabbits for each extract
Number of test/control injections per extract: five test and five control injections	10 test and five control injections
Evaluation of responses: quantitative comparison of responses of test and control responses	Qualitative comparison of test and control responses

TABLE 2.4 Differences in Eye Irritation Testing Procedures Outlined in ISO 10993-10 and the MHW Guidelines

ISO 10993-10	MHW 1995
Time of exposure: 1 sec	30 sec
Grading scale: classification system for grading ocular lesions	Draize or McDonald–Shadduck scale

TABLE 2.5 Differences Between Cytotoxicity Test Procedures Specified by ISO 10993-5 and the MHW Guidelines

ISO 10993-10	MHW 1995
Number of cells per dish: 0.5–1 million cells	40 to 200 cells per dish
Extraction ratio: 60 cm^2 per 20 ml if thickness 80.5 mm; 120 cm^2 per 20 ml if thickness 70.5 mm; or 4 g per 20 ml	5 cm^2/ml or 1 g/10 ml
Exposure period: typically 24–72 hr (2 hr for filter diffusion test)	6–7 days
Toxicity determination: visual grading and/or quantitative assessments	Quantification of surviving colonies
Positive controls: materials providing a reproducible cytotoxic response (e.g., organo-tin-impregnated polyvinyl chloride)	Segmented polyurethane films containing 0.1% zinc diethyldithiocarbamate and 0.25% zinc dibutyldithiocarbamate

Source: MHW, 1995.

during a period of less than 24 hours. The International Standards Organization and MHW procedures are contrasted in Table 2.6.

Hematocompatibility.   Evaluates any effects of blood contacting materials on hemolysis, thrombosis, plasma proteins, enzymes, and the formed elements using an animal model. Traditionally, hemolysis, which determines the degree of red blood cell lysis and the separation of hemoglobin caused by test materials and/or extracts from the materials in vitro, has been *the* representative test employed. A broader range of primary tests (adding evaluations of thrombosis, coagulation, platelets, and immunology aspects) is currently recommended. The International Standards Organization and MHW procedures for hemolysis are contrasted in Table 2.7.

Pyrogenicity, material mediated.   Evaluates the material mediated pyrogenicity of test materials and/or extracts. The International Standards Organization and MHW procedures are contrasted in Table 2.8.

Implantation *tests*.   Evaluate the local toxic effects on living tissue, at both the gross level and microscopic level, to a sample material that is surgically implanted into an appropriate animal implant site or tissue (e.g., muscle, bone) for 7 to 90 days. The International Standards Organization and MHW procedures are contrasted in Table 2.9.

Mutagenicity (genotoxicity).   The application of mammalian or nonmammalian cell culture techniques for the determination of gene mutations, changes in chromosome structure and number, and other DNA or gene toxicities caused by test materials and/or extracts from materials. Selected tests representing gene mutation tests (Ames or mouse lymphoma), chromosomal aberration tests (CHO), and DNA effects tests (mouse micronucleus and sister chromatid exchange) should generally be employed. The International Standard Organization and MHW procedures are contrasted in Table 2.10.

Subchronic toxicity.   The determination of harmful effects from multiple exposures to test materials and/or extracts during a period of one day to less than 10% of the total life of the test animal (e.g., up to 90 days in rats).

Chronic toxicity.   The determination of harmful effects from multiple exposures to test materials and/or extracts during a period of 10% to the total life of the test animal (e.g., over 90 days in rats).

Carcinogenesis bioassay.   The determination of the tumorigenic potential of test materials and/or extracts from either single or multiple exposures, over a period of the total life (e.g., 2 years for rats, 18 months for mice, or 7 years for dogs).

Pharmacokinetics.   To determine the metabolic processes of absorption,

TABLE 2.6 Comparison of Grading Scales Used to Score Responses of Test Animals to ASTM and ISO/USP Procedures

Response	ASTM		ISO/USP
	Description		
Normal, no symptoms	Mouse exhibits no adverse physical symptoms after injection.		
Slight	Mouse exhibits slight but noticeable symptoms of hypokinesis, dyspnea, or abdominal irritation after injection.		
Moderate	Mouse exhibits definite evidence of abdominal irritation, dyspnea, hypokinesis, ptosis, or diarrhea after injection. (Weight usually drops to between 15 and 17 g.)		
Marked	Mouse exhibits prostration, cyanosis, tremors, or severe symptoms of abdominal irritation, diarrhea, ptosis, or dyspnea after injection. (Extreme weight loss; weight usually less than 15 g.)		

Dead, expired   Mouse dies after injection.

Interpretation: The test is considered negative if none of the animals injected with the test article extracts shows a significantly greater biological reaction than the animals treated with the control article.

If two or more mice show either marked signs of toxicity or die, the test article does not meet the requirements of the test.

If any animals treated with a test article shows slight signs of toxicity, and not more than one animal shows marked signs of toxicity or dies, a repeat test using freshly prepared extract should be conducted using groups of 10 mice each. A substantial decrease in body weight for all animals in the group, even without other symptoms of toxicity, requires a retest using groups of 10 mice each. In the repeat test, the requirements are met if none of the animals injected with the test article shows a substantially greater reaction than that observed in the animals treated with the control article.

Interpretation: The test is considered negative if none of the animals injected with the test article shows a significantly greater biological reaction than the animals treated with the control article.

If two or more mice die, or show signs of toxicity such as convulsions or prostration, or if three or more mice lose more than 2 g of body weight, the test article does not meet the requirements of the test.

If any animal treated with a test article shows only slight signs of biological reaction, and not more than one animal shows gross signs of biological reaction or dies, a repeat test should be conducted using groups of 10 mice. On the repeat test, all 10 animals must not show a significantly greater biological reaction than the animals treated with the control article.

TABLE 2.7 Differences in Hemolysis Test Procedures Recommended by ISO 10993-4 and the MHW Guidelines

ISO 10993-4	MHW 1995
Hemolysis can be assessed by any of several validated methods to assay hemoglobin in plasma.	Hemolytic index is assessed by measuring hemoglobin at 1, 2, and 4 hr by spectrophotometric methods. The hemolysis over this period is expressed as a percentage of the positive control.

distribution, biotransformation, and elimination of toxic leachables and degradation products of test materials and/or extracts.

Reproductive and developmental toxicity. The evaluation of the potential effects of test materials and/or extracts on fertility, reproductive function, and prenatal and early postnatal development.

The tests for leachables such as contaminants, additives, monomers, and degradation products must be conducted by choosing appropriate solvent systems that will yield a maximal extraction of leachable materials to conduct biocompatibility testing. Chapter 3 addresses the issues behind sampling, sample preparation, and solvents.

The effects of sterilization on device materials and potential leachables, as well as toxic by-products as a consequence of sterilization, should be considered. Testing should therefore be performed on the final sterilized product or representative samples of the final sterilized product. Table 2.10 presents the basis for test selection under the tripartite agreement.

TABLE 2.8 Comparison of Pyrogen Test Procedures Required by ISO 10993-11 and the MHW Guidelines

ISO 10993-11	MHW 1995
Number of animals: three rabbits required; comparison of febrile response in test animals to baseline temperature for evaluation of pyrogenicity potential	Three rabbits (test) required; comparison to baseline temperature is evaluated as index of pyrogenicity potential
Test duration: test measurement intervals: every 30 min for 3 hr	Test measurement intervals: every hr for 3 hr
Evaluation: Cutoff for positive febrile response: 0.5°C	Cutoff for positive febrile response: 0.6°C

TABLE 2.9   Differences in ISO 10993-3 and the MHW Guidelines for Assessing the Effects of Device or Material Implantation

ISO 10993-3	MHW 1995
Time point(s) of assessment: sufficient to achieve steady state (e.g., 2, 4, 6, and 12 weeks).	7 days and 4 weeks.
Number of animals: at least three per time period of assessment.	At least four per time period.
Number of samples of evaluation: at least eight per time period for test and control.	No minimum number specified.
Evaluation criteria: comparative evaluation of responses to test and control materials.	If more than two of the four test sites in each animal exhibit a significant response compared to control sites, the test is considered positive.

TABLE 2.10   Differences in Genotoxicity Testing Procedures Required by ISO 10993-3 and the MHW Guidelines

ISO 10993-10	MHW 1995
Extraction vehicles: a physiological medium is used and, where appropriate, a solvent (e.g., dimethylsulfoxide).	Recommends methanol and acetone as extracting vehicles.
Extraction: extract test material and test the extract or dissolve material in solvent and conduct test. The conditions of extraction should maximize the amount of extractable substances, as well as subject the test device or material to the extreme conditions it may be exposed to, without causing significant degradation. Extraction ratio is dependent on thickness of test material.	Extract at room temperature at a ratio of 10:1 (solvent:material) and obtain residue [at least 0.1–0.5% (weight of residue/weight of test material)], redissolve in appropriate solvent and test residue.
	If sufficient residue is unobtainable, extract test material (in ethanol, acetone, or DMSO at 10 g of test material per 20 ml for the Arnes mutagenicity assay, and in cell culture medium at 120 cm^3 or 4 g/20 ml for the chromosomal aberration assay), at 37°C for 48 h and test extract. The Ames mutagenicity assay is conducted with a volume of 200 µl per plate.

C. U.S. Pharmacopoeial Testing

The earliest guidance on what testing was to be done on medical devices was that provided in the USP and other pharmacopoeias. Each of the major national pharmacopoeias offers somewhat different guidance. The test selection system for the USP (presented in Table 2.11), which classified plastics as classes I through VI, is now obsolete and replaced in usage by the other guidelines presented here, but the actual descriptions of test types, as provided in the USP (and presented in the appropriate chapters later in this book) are still very much operative (USP, 1994).

There are British, European, and Japanese pharmacopoeias, of which the latter require the most attention due to some special requirements still being operative if product approval is desired.

D. ISO Testing Requirements

The European Economic Community has adopted a new set of testing guidelines for medical devices under the aegis of ISO (ISO, 1992; the Gray Sheet, 1992). The ISO 10993 guidelines for testing provide a unified basis for international medical device biocompatibility evaluation, both in terms of test selection (as presented in Tables 2.12 and 2.13) and test design and interpretation (Table 2.14). In 1996, the U.S. FDA also announced that it would adhere to ISO 10993 standards for device biocompatibility evaluation.

This international standard specifies methods of biological testing of medical and dental materials and devices and their evaluation in regard to their biocompatibility. Because of the many materials and devices used in these areas, the standard offers a guide for biological testing.

E. MHW Requirements

The Japanese ISO test selection guidelines vary from those of FDA and ISO and are summarized in Table 2.15 (MHW, 1995; Japanese Pharmacopoeia, 1996).

Actual test performance standards also vary, as shown in Tables 2.3–2.10. Committees dealing with materials and devices must decide on tests and test series relevant to the respective materials and devices. It is the responsibility of the product committees to select adequate test methods for products. The standard contains animal tests, but tries to reduce those tests to the justifiable minimum. Relevant international and national regulations must be observed when animals are used.

ISO 10993 is based on existing national and international specifications, regulations, and standards wherever possible. It is open to regular review whenever new research work is presented to improve the state of scientific knowledge. Tables 2.3 and 2.4 provide the test matrices under ISO 10993. Subsequently,

TABLE 2.11 Classification of Plastics

Plastic classes						Tests to be conducted			
I	II	III	IV	V	VI	Test material	Animal	Dose	Procedures
x	x	x	x	x	x	Extract of sample in sodium chloride inspection	Mouse	50 ml/kg	A (iv)
	x	x	x	x	x		Rabbit	0.2 ml/animal at each of 10 sites	B
			x	x	x	Extract of sample in 1 in 20	Mouse	50 ml/kg	A (iv)
			x	x	x	Solution of alcohol in sodium chloride injection	Rabbit	0.2 ml/animal at each of 10 sites	
x	x		x	x	x	Extract of sample in polyethylene glycol 400	Mouse	10 g/kg	A (ip)
	x		x	x	x		Rabbit	0.2 ml/animal at each of 10 sites	
		x	x	x	x	Extract of sample in vegetable oil	Mouse	50 ml/kg	A (ip)
		x	x	x	x		Rabbit	0.2 ml/animal at each of 10 sites	B
				x	x	Implant strips of sample	Rabbit	4 strips/animal	C

Notes: Tests required for each class are indicated by x in appropriate rows. A (ip), systemic injection test (intraperitoneal); A (iv), systemic injection test (intravenous); B, intracutaneous (intracutaneous); C, implantation test (intramuscular implantation). The table lists the biological tests that might be applied in evaluating the safety of medical devices and/or polymers. This does not imply that all the tests listed under each category will be necessary or relevant in all cases. Tests for devices made of metals, ceramics, biological materials, etc., are not included here but are under consideration. Categorization of medical devices is based on body contact and contact duration.

Source: USP XXIII (USP, 1993).

TABLE 2.12 ISO Initial Evaluation Tests

Device categories		Biological tests								
Body contact duration A—Limited exposure B—prolonged or repeated exposure C—permanent contact		Cytotoxicity	Sensitization	Irritation or Intracutaneous	Acute systemic toxicity	Subchronic toxicity	Mutagenicity	Pyrogenicity	Implantation	Hemocompatibility
Surface devices										
Skin	A	x	x	x						
	B	x	x	x						
	C	x	x	x						
Mucous membranes	A	x	x	x						
	B	x	x	x						
	C	x	x	x		x	x			
Breached surface	A	x	x	x						
	B	x	x	x						
	C	x	x	x		x	x			
Externally communicating										
Blood path indirect	A	x	x	x				x		x
	B	x	x	x				x		x
	C	x	x		x	x	x	x		x
Tissue/bone communicating	A	x	x	x						
	B	x	x				x		x	
	C	x	x				x		x	
Internal devices										
Circulating blood	A	x	x	x	x			x		x
	B	x	x	x	x		x	x		x
	C	x	x	x	x	x	x	x		x
Implant devices										
Bone/tissue	A	x	x	x						
	B	x	x				x		x	
	C	x	x				x		x	
Blood	A	x	x	x	x			x	x	x
	B	x	x	x	x		x	x	x	x
	C	x	x	x	x	x	x	x	x	x

specific guidance on individual test designs, conduct, and interpretation has been provided as subparts 2–11 of ISO 10993 (Table 2.14) (AAMI, 1997).

F. Medical Device Directive Guideline

The EEC had adopted its own guidance, council directive 93/42/EEC, for manufacturers of medical devices (the Gray Sheet, 1992; European Committees on Standardization, 1991; Bunger and Tummler, 1994). According to the preamble of the MD Directive, the classification rules are ''based on the vulnerability of

TABLE 2.13 ISO Special Evaluation Tests

Device categories		Biological tests			
Body contact duration A—Limited exposure B—prolonged or repeated exposure C—permanent contact (time limits to added)		Chronic toxicity	Carcinogenicity	Reproductive/developmental	Degradation
Surface devices					
Skin	A				
	B				
	C				
Mucous membranes	A				
	B				
	C				
Breached surface	A				
	B				
	C				
Externally communicating					
Blood path indirect	A				
	B				
	C	x	x		
Tissue/bone communicating	A				
	B				
	C		x		
Internal devices					
Circulating blood	A				
	B				
	C	x	x		
Bone/tissue	A				
	B				
	C	x	x		
Blood	A				
	B				
	C	x	x		

the human body taking account of the potential risks associated with the technical design and Manufacture of the devices.'' The classification rules are presented in Annex IX of the MD directive. Implementation of the MD directive requires that the classification rules are applied in accordance with the intended purpose—or most critical specified use—of a device. Should more than one rule apply, the strictest takes precedence.

Except for the special rules 13–18, which will probably not be combined with the active device rules, the classification rules contained in Annex IX distinguish between two categories of devices: noninvasive and invasive. Both these categories are further divided into four rules. Among noninvasive devices, distinction is made among

TABLE 2.14 ISO/ANSI/AAMI Standards

	ISO designations	Year issued
Guidance on selection of tests	10993-1	1992
Animal welfare requirements	10993-2	1992
Tests for genotoxicity, carcinogenicity, and reproductive toxicity	10993-3	1992
Selection of tests for interactions with blood	10993-4	1992
Tests for cytotoxicity: in vitro methods	10993-5	1992
Tests for local effects after implantation	10993-6	1994
Ethylene oxide sterilization residuals	10993-7	1995
Degradation of materials related to biological testing	10993-9	1994
Tests for irritation and sensitization	10993-10	1995
Tests for systemic toxicity	10993-11	1994

TABLE 2.15 Japanese MHW Test Selection Guidelines

Device category	Body contact	Contact duration	Cytotoxicity	Sensitization	Irritation or intracutaneous	Systemic toxicity (acute)	Subchronic toxicity	Genotoxicity	Pyrogen	Implantation	Hemocompatibility	Chronic Toxicity	Carcinogenicity
Surface Devices	Skin	A	X	X	X								
		B	X	X	X								
		C	X	X	X								
	Mucosal membrane	A	X	X	X								
		B	X	X	X								
		C	X	X	X		X	X					
	Breached/compromised surface	A	X	X	X								
		B	X	X	X								
		C	X	X	X		X	X					
External Communicating Devices	Blood path indirect	A	X	X	X	X			X		X		
		B	X	X	X	X			X		X		
		C	X	X		X	X	X	X		X	X	X
	Tissue/bone dentin communicating	A	X	X	X								
		B	X	X				X		X			
		C	X	X				X		X			X
	Circulating blood	A	X	X	X	X			X		X		
		B	X	X	X	X		X	X		X		
		C	X	X	X	X	X	X	X		X	X	X
Implant Devices	Bone/tissue	A	X	X	X								
		B	X	X				X		X			
		C	X	X				X		X			X
	Blood	A	X	X	X	X			X	X	X		
		B	X	X	X	X		X	X	X	X		
		C	X	X	X	X	X	X	X	X	X	X	X

A = Temporary contact (<24 hours)   B = Short- and medium-term contact (24 hours – 29 days)   C = Long-term contact (>30 days)

Devices for channeling or storing substances for infusion, administration, or introduction into the body
Devices for the biological or chemical modification of liquids for infusion
Devices that come into contact with injured skin
All other noninvasive devices

Invasive devices are divided into those that are introduced into natural body orifices and those that are surgically introduced into the body. Classification criteria of the surgically introduced devices include

Duration (transient, short-term, or long-term use)
Interaction (biological, chemical, or ionizing radiation)
Location (heart, central circulatory, or central nervous systems)

Four additional rules are stated for active medical devices, and within these a distinction is made among

Devices used for therapy
Devices for diagnosis
Devices for the administration and/or removal of substances to and from the body
All other active devices

Classification criteria for medical devices are based on potential hazards, taking into account

Nature, density, and site of energy application
Substance involved
Part of the body concerned
Mode of application or immediate danger to the patient with respect to cardiac performance, respiration, and/or the central nervous system

Reduction of nonactive characteristics: By combining active and nonactive characteristics, the following assumptions regarding active medical devices were made:

Only those nonactive characteristics that would lead to a higher class were considered, therefore all Class I characteristics of rules 1–8 were omitted.
Implantable and long-term surgically invasive devices (rule 8) that are also active should be covered by the active implantable medical device (AIMD) directive, 90/385/EEC (although definitions of ''implantable'' in the AIMD and MD directives are slightly different).
Connection to another active medical device, as described in rules 2 and 5, will not change the class of an active medical device.
Energy supplied in the form of ionizing radiation (rules 6 and 7) is sufficiently covered under rule 10.

Because surgically invasive active devices are not intended to be wholly or mainly absorbed by, or chemically changed in, the body (rules 6 and 7), these characteristics were omitted.

Devices "intended to administer medicines" (rules 6 and 7) are sufficiently covered under rule 11.

Table 2.16 summarizes the classification procedure. Table 2.17 (Bunger and Tummler, 1994) shows the reduced scheme for the combined characteristics.

G. CE Marking of Devices

After June 14, 1998, all medical products distributed in Europe have had to bear the CE mark. ISO 9000 certification supplements and supports an assessment of conformity to the medical devices directive (MDD), which must be performed by a certification body appointed by the EU member states (Haindl, 1997). To qualify for the CE mark, manufacturers of Class IIa, IIb, and III devices must be certified by a notified body (recognized by the national health authorities) to Annex II, V, or VI of the MDD (also known as 93/42/EEC) and comply with the essential requirements of the directive. Manufacturers of active implantables and IVDs have separate directives to contend with. When auditing for compliance, the notified body will check a number of items in addition to a manufacturer's QA system, including technical files, sterility assurance measures, subcontracting procedures, recall and vigilance systems, and declarations of conformity. Depending on the classification and certification route, some devices will also require an EC-type examination or a design review by the notified body.

Manufacturers of Class I products, who require minimal interaction with a notified body, appear to be the clear winners in this scheme, but even they must deal with a number of vague or confusing requirements. (See Table 2.18.) Simply classifying their products according to the dictates of 93/42/EEC, Annex IX, can be a tricky affair, and faulty classification can lead to bigger problems. The simplified flowcharts in Figure 2.1 should help manufacturers determine whether or not their products qualify as Class I devices. For more difficult products, manufacturers may need to refer to a consultant or obtain a suitable software program.

Classification is based on the intended and declared use of a product, not solely on its salient features. The Class I designation usually—but not always—excludes sterile products and measuring devices that measure physiological parameters or require a high degree of accuracy; so, for example, a reusable scalpel is Class I, but a sterile scalpel is Class IIa, a scalpel blade for the reusable device is Class I, but if it is supplied sterile, it is Class IIa, a scalpel blade for the reusable device is Class I, but if it is supplied sterile, it is Class IIa. A stethoscope, a simple graduated syringe (not for injection pumps), and a measuring spoon for administering an expectorant are not considered measuring devices, although a hand-driven blood-pressure gage and a digital thermometer are.

TABLE 2.16 An Overview of the Classification of Medical Devices (Rules 1–12)

Class	(Others)	Noninvasive devices			Invasive devices				Additional rules for active devices			(Others)
		Channeling or storing substances for introduction into the body	Biological or chemical modification of liquids for infusion	Contact with injured skin	Body orifices	Surgically invasive devices			Therapeutic devices for administration or exchange of energy	Diagnostic devices to supply energy, vital physiological processes; radio pharmaceutical imaging	Devices for administration or removal of substances to or from the body	
						Transient use	Short-term use	Long-term use, implantable devices				
I	Regular	Regular		Mechanical barrier; compression; absorption of exudates	Transient use; ENT short-term	Reusable surgical instruments				Illumination of human body in visible spectrum		Regular
IIa	Regular	Body substances; connections to AMD ≥ IIa	Filtration; centrifugation; gas or heat exchange	Regular	Short-term use ENT, long-term connection to AMD ≥ IIa	Regular	Regular	Placed in teeth	Regular	Regular	Regular	
IIb			Regular	Wounds with breached dermis, healing by secondary intent	Long-term use	Ionizing radiation; biological effect; absorbed; potential hazard of medicine delivery system	Ionizing radiation: chemical change (except in teeth); medicine administration	Regular	Potentially hazardous (nature, density, site of energy); class IIb ATD monitor or control development	Immediate danger to heart, respiration, CNS; ionizing radiation including control monitoring	Potentially hazardous (substances, part of body, mode of applications)	
III						Heart; CCS	Heart; CCS; CNS; biological effect; absorbed	Heart; CCS; CNS; biological effect; absorbed; chemical change; medicine administration				
Rule	1	2	3	4	5	6	7	8	9	10	11	12

Note: AMD, active medical device; ATD, active therapeutic device; CCS, central circulatory system; CNS, central nervous system; ENT, ear, nose, and throat.

TABLE 2.17 Reduced Scheme for Combined Characteristics of Active and Nonactive Devices

Class	Noninvasive devices				Invasive devices				Additional rules for active devices			
						Surgically invasive devices						
	Others	Channeling or storing substances for introducing into the body	Biological or chemical modification of liquids for infusion	Contact with injured skin	Body orifices	Transient use	Short-term use	Long-term use, implantable devices	Therapeutic devices for administration of exchange of energy	Diagnostic devices to supply energy, vital physiological processes; radio-pharmaceutical imaging	Devices for administration or removal of substances to or from the body	Others
I										Illumination of human body in visible spectrum		Regular
IIa		Body substances	Filtration; centrifugation; gas or heat exchange	Regular	Short-term use ENT, long-term	Regular	Regular		Regular	Regular	Regular	
IIb			Regular	Wounds with breached dermis, healing by secondary intent	Long-term use	Biological effects			Potentially hazardous (nature, density, site of energy); Class IIb ATD monitor or control development	Immediate danger to heart, respiration, CNS; ionizing radiation, including control monitoring	Potentially hazardous (substances, part of body, mode of applications)	
III						Heart; CCS	Heart; CCS; CNS; biological effects					
Rule	1	2	3	4	5	6	7	8	9	10	11	12

Note: ATD, active therapeutic device; CCS, central circulatory system; CNS, central nervous system; ENT, ear, nose, and throat.

TABLE 2.18   Which Products Are Class I?

The classification of a product refers to its intended use. The following is a simplified listing of Class I products:

Noninvasive (and nonactive) devices that do not modify the biological or chemical composition of blood or liquids intended for infusion; store blood, body liquids, or tissues for administration; or connect to an active medical device.

Dressings intended only as a mechanical barrier or for absorption of exudates.

Invasive products for use in natural body orifices and stomas for no longer than 1 h or in the oral or nasal cavity or ear canal for up to 30 days.

Surgical invasive products if they are reusable instruments and not intended for continuous use of more than 1 hr.

Active devices that administer neither energy nor substances to the body nor are made for diagnosis.

Class I products cannot

Incorporate medicinal products (drugs) or animal tissue.

Be intended for contraception or the prevention of sexually transmitted diseases.

All of the classification rules are included in the directive, but they're not easy to understand. An EC working group has drawn up a separate paper known as MEDDEV 10/93 to explain the rules and provide some practical guidelines. For example, the directive stipulates that reusable surgical instruments belong in the class I designation as long as they are not intended for more than an hour of continuous use. According to this definition, items such as scissors and tweezers, even if they are used in a 6-hour operation, are still considered Class I devices because they are not used continuously during that time.

Even if a Class I product is supplied sterile, the manufacturer must issue a self-declaration of conformity. In this case, the manufacturer need only certify the quality control (QC) system governing those aspects of manufacture concerned with securing and maintaining sterile conditions. If the device is packaged and sterilized by a company that works with a certified process, then the manufacturer must only validate the process for the particular device and submit the results to a notified body. The manufacturer still needs certification by a notified body in regard to the performance aspects relating to sterility and measurement function; the notified body will also want to inspect the manufacturer's facility. Nonetheless, the procedure is far less complicated than a full production audit.

All manufacturers applying for CE marking privileges—including manufacturers of Class I devices—must prepare the proper technical documentation; appoint a ''responsible person'' within the EEC; design product labels and labeling according to 93/42/EEC, Annex I, paragraph 13; and sign a declaration of

TABLE 2.19 Contents of a Device Master File

1. EC declaration of conformity and classification according to Annex IX of the MDD
2. Name and address of the manufacturer's European responsible person
3. Product description, including
   All variants
   Intended clinical use
   Indications/contraindications
   Operating instructions/instructions for use
   Warnings/precautions
   Photographs highlighting the product
   Photographs highlighting the usage
   Brochures, advertising, catalog sheets, marketing claims (if available)
   Product specifications including parts list, list of components
   Specifications of materials used, including data sheets
   List of standards applied
   Details of substance(s) used (in the event of drug-device combination)
   QA specifications (QC specs, in-process controls, etc.) etc.
   Labeling, accompanying documents, package inserts (DIN EN 289, prEN 980)
   Instruction for use (prEN 1041)
   Service manual
   Product verification, including testing data and reports, functionality studies, wet lab or benchtop testing
   Materials certificates/reports on biological tests
   EMC testing and certificates
   Validation of the packaging/aging studies
   Compatibility studies (connection to other devices)
   Risk analysis (DIN EN 1441)
   Clinical experience
4. List of requirements (Annex I) indicating cross-reference with documentation

conformity. The technical dossier should not pose a major problem for manufacturers familiar with device master files. A list of required dossier contents is given in Table 2.19. For biological material testing, Europe uses the ISO 10993 (EN 30993) protocols, but test results according to the tripartite agreement (or USP XXIII) are accepted. Every electrical device must also be proven to comply with the EMC requirements defined in the MDD; suppliers of preassembled electrical components may have the appropriate test results already available. Reformatting an existing device master file is not necessary, only creating an index that cross-references the essential requirements of the directives with the device file contents. The master file is a controlled document, as defined in ISO 9000, and manufacturers would do well to regard it as highly confidential.

The technical dossier is closely linked to the responsible person, a representative in the EEC governed by European law and authorized by the manufacturer to oversee routine regulatory affairs. Specifically, the responsible person must ensure compliance with the European vigilance system, which covers both post-market surveillance and adverse-incident reporting. For example, if a patient were injured by a device, or if a patient would have been injured had the caregiver not intervened, the responsible person would have to investigate the incident together with the device's manufacturer and file a report with the competent authorities. Moreover, the European authorities must be able to obtain the master file in case of trouble; therefore, the manufacturer must either store the file or its abbreviated form with the responsible person or draw up a contractual agreement that gives the agent the right to access the master file without delay if required by the authorities. The agent must be available all year, as the time frame for notification could be as short as 10 days. Ideally, the responsible person should be familiar with the national regulations in all member states.

The simplest way to maintain a European address will be to appoint a distributor as the responsible person, although this course is not without potential problems. The selected distributor does not need certification as long as the manufacturer's name and CE mark are on the product labeling. The name of the responsible person must also appear on the label, package insert, or outer packaging, even if the product is sold by a completely different distributor in another country. There is no official rule or proposal regarding how many responsible persons a manufacturer should have, but each one must appear on the labeling; therefore, appointing more than one is of limited use. The responsible person should be selected with great care; device master files (Table 2.18) must be made available to the responsible person in the event of patient injury or near injury, and many distributors are potential competitors. By nature, Class I devices will rarely lead to patient injury, but manufacturers should still consider labeling issues when choosing a representative. It's easy to change distributors, but changing the responsible person means changing all the product labeling. As an alternative, manufacturers can contract with a professional agency to serve as a representative completely independent from any distribution network.

The issue of labeling is itself a source of contention. Not all countries have decided yet whether or not they will insist on having their own language on device labels. Many countries have rather imprecise rules, dictating that their national language must appear only if necessary. Manufacturers can reduce potential trouble by using the pictograms and symbols defined in the harmonized European standard EN 980. For instructions of use, manufacturers are advised to use all 12 languages used in the European economic area. The requirements for labeling are presented in Annex I, paragraph 13, of the MDD; some devices may be subject to additional requirements outlined in product standards.

Class I products fall under the jurisdiction of local authorities, but who serves as those authorities may differ from country to country. In Germany, for example, there are no clear-cut regulations that define the competence of the local authorities, except in the case of danger to the patient. European product liability laws more or less give the consumer the right to sue anybody in the trade chain. Normally, claims would be filed against the manufacturer, but it is possible that there will be claims against a responsible person. This is a rather new legal situation, and the rules will be determined by court decisions. It is hoped that class I products will not instigate many court actions, but clearly even manufacturers of class I devices will have a host of new concerns under the CE marking scheme.

H. Risk Assessment

The reality is that not all materials used on devices are entirely safe. Generally, if one looks long enough at small enough quantities, some type of risk can be associated with every material. Risk can be defined as the possibility of harm or loss. Health risk, of course, is the possibility of an adverse effect on one's health. Risk is sometimes quantified by multiplying the severity of an event times the probability the event will occur, so that

Risk = severity × probability

While this equation appears useful in theory, in practice it is difficult to apply to the biological safety of medical devices. The process known as health-based risk assessment attempts to provide an alternative strategy for placing health risks in perspective (Stark, 1998; AAMI, 1998).

I. Standards and Guidances

A paradigm for the risk assessment process has been detailed in a publication prepared by the U.S. National Academy of Sciences (Hayes, 1994). Although devised primarily for cancer risk assessment, many of the provisions also apply to the assessment of other health effects. The major components of the paradigm are (1) hazard identification, (2) dosage-response assessment, (3) exposure assessment, and (4) risk characterization (Ecobichon, 1992).

The general approach to risk assessment was adapted to medical devices via the draft CEN standard Risk Analysis, published in 1993,* and more recently via the ISO standard, ISO 14538—Method for the Establishment of Allowable Limits for Residues in Medical Devices Using Health-Based Risk Assessment,

---

* CEN BTS 3/WG 1—Risk Analysis is available through the British Standards Institute.

published in 1996.† At the present time, the FDA is also working to develop a health-based risk assessment protocol adapted to medical devices. Informally called the medical device paradigm, the document is not yet generally available (Brown and Stratmeyer, 1997).‡

Some manufacturers may object that regulators are once again attempting to impose a "drug model" on medical devices. We shall see in the following pages, however, that judicious application of these risk assessment principles can provide a justification for using materials that carry with them some element of risk, and that may, under traditional biocompatibility testing regimes, be difficult to evaluate or be deemed unsuitable for medical device applications.

J. Method

Hazard Identification. The first step in the risk assessment process is to identify the possible hazards that may be presented by a material. This is accomplished by determining whether a compound, an extract of the material, or the material itself produces adverse effects, and by identifying the nature of those effects. Adverse effects are identified either through a review of the literature or through actual biological safety testing.

Dose-Response Assessment. The second step is to determine the dose response of the material; that is, What is the highest weight or concentration of the material that will not cause an effect? This upper limit is called the allowable limit. There are numerous sources in the literature of data from which to determine allowable limits; some will be more applicable than others, and some may require correction factors.

Exposure Assessment. The third step is to determine the exposure assessment by quantifying the available dose of the chemical residues that will be received by the patient. This is readily done by estimating the number of devices to which a patient is likely to be exposed in a sequential period of use (e.g., during a hospital stay) or over a lifetime. For example, a patient might be exposed to 100 skin staples following a surgical procedure, or to two heart valves in a lifetime; thus the amount of residue available on 100 skin staples or two heart valves would be determined.

---

† Available from the Association for the Advancement of Medical Instrumentation, 3330 Washington Blvd., Suite 400, Arlington, VA 22201.

‡ Draft copies of the medical device paradigm may be obtained by contacting Dr. Melvin Stratmeyer, FDA Center for Devices and Radiological Health, HFZ-112, Division of Life Sciences, Office of Science and Technology, FDA, Rockville, MD 20857.

Risk Characterization. Characterizing the risk constitutes the final step of the process. The allowable limit is compared with the estimated exposure: if the allowable limit is greater than the estimated exposure by a comfortable safety margin, the likelihood of an adverse event occurring in an exposed population is small, and the material may be used.

K. Case Studies

We can best get a sense of how these standards work by looking at some actual medical case studies that illustrate the risk assessment process (Stark, 1997).

1. Nitinol Implant

Nitinol is an unusual alloy of nickel and titanium that features the useful property of "shape memory." A nitinol part can be given a particular shape at a high temperature, then cooled to a low temperature and compressed into some other shape; the compressed part will subsequently deploy to its original shape at a predetermined transition temperature. This feature is particularly beneficial for vascular implant applications in which the shape of the device in its compressed state eases the insertion process. The nitinol deploys as it is warmed by the surrounding tissue, expanding to take on the desired shape of a stent, filter, or other device. The transition temperature depends on the alloy's relative concentrations of nickel and titanium; a typical nickel concentration of 55–60% is used in medical devices, since this gives a transition temperature at approximately the temperature of the body (37°C).

Hazard Identification. One concern with using nitinol in implant applications is the potential release of nickel into the body. Although nickel is a dietary requirement, it is also highly toxic—known to cause dermatitis, cancer subsequent to inhalation, and acute pneumonitis from inhalation of nickel carbonyl, and to exert a toxic effect on cellular reproduction. It is a known sensitizer, with approximately 5% of the domestic population allergic to this common metal, probably through exposure from costume jewelry and clothing snaps. The biocompatibility question at hand is whether or not *in vivo* corrosion of nitinol releases unsafe levels of nickel.

Dose-Response Assessment. A search of the world medical literature revealed that the recommended safe level of exposure to nickel in intravenous fluids is a maximum of 35 µg/day (Stark, 1997). This value can be taken as an allowable limit of nickel exposure for a 70-kg (154–lb) adult.

The intravenous fluid data are based on subjects that are comparable to the patients who will be receiving nitinol implants. The data are for humans (not animals), for ill patients (not healthy workers or volunteers), and for similar routes of exposure (intravenous fluid and tissue contact). For these reasons, no safety correction factor need be applied to the allowable limit of exposure.

Exposure Assessment.   The available dose of nickel from nitinol implants can be estimated from data found in the literature. In one study, dental arch wires of nitinol were extracted in artificial saliva, and the concentration of nickel measured in the supernatant. Corrosion reached a peak at day 7, then declined steadily thereafter. The average rate of corrosion under these conditions was 12.8 $\mu g/day/cm^2$ over the first 28 days.

Risk Characterization.   A comparison of the available dose with the allowable limit for intravenous fluid levels shows that there is approximately a threefold safety margin, assuming that the implanted device is a full 1 cm^2 in surface area. (Devices with less surface area will contribute even less to the nickel concentration and have an even larger safety margin.) Considering the high quality of the data, a threefold safety margin is sufficient to justify using nitinol in vascular implants.

2.   Wound-Dressing Preparation

Today's wound dressings are highly engineered products, designed to maintain the moisture content and osmatic balance of the wound bed so as to promote optimum conditions for wound healing. Complex constructions of hydrocolloids and superabsorbers, these dressings are sometimes used in direct tissue contact over full-thickness wounds that penetrate the skin layers.

Hazard Identification.   There have been reports in the literature of patients succumbing to cardiac arrest from potassium overload, with the wound dressing as one of the important contributors of excess potassium in the bloodstream. The effects of potassium on cardiac function are well characterized. Normal serum levels for potassium are 3.8 to 4 milliequivalents per liter. As the potassium concentration rises to 5–7 mEq/L, a patient can undergo cardiac arrest and die. The biocompatibility issue to be explored is whether or not a wound-dressing formulation might release dangerous levels of potassium if used on full-thickness wounds.

Dose-Response Assessment.   An increase of approximately 1 mEq/L of potassium is unlikely to provoke mild adverse events in most patients. Assuming that the average person's blood volume is 5 liters, a one-time dose of 5 mEq of potassium may begin to cause adverse reactions. This value can be considered to be the allowable limit of potassium for most patients.

Exposure Assessment.   Let us suppose that each dressing contains 2.5 g of potassium bicarbonate. Since the molecular weight of potassium bicarbonate is 100 g/mole, each dressing contains 0.025 mole of sodium bicarbonate, or 0.025

mEq of potassium ion. If a patient were to use four dressings in a day, the available dose of potassium would be 0.1 mEq/day.

Risk Characterization. Comparing the available dose of potassium (0.1 mEq) to the allowable limit (5 mEq) shows that there is a 50-fold safety margin. Considering that patients may be small in size, may have kidney impairment, or may receive potassium from additional sources such as intravenous fluids, this safety margin is too small, and so the dressing should be reformulated.

3. Perchloroethylene Solvent

A manufacturer of metal fabricated parts uses perchloroethylene to clean the finished pieces. Perchloroethylene has many advantages as a cleaner and degreaser; it is highly volatile, does not damage the ozone layer, and is very effective as a precision cleaning solvent. The most common use of perchloroethylene is in the dry-cleaning industry, but it is also commonly used in the electronics industry to clean circuit boards.

Hazard Identification. The downside of perchloroethylene is that it is highly toxic, with a material safety data sheet several pages in length listing adverse effects ranging from dizziness to death. Biocompatibility testing on solvent-cleaned parts would be meaningless; the solvent concentration on the part is so small that any effects of the solvent would be masked by the natural biological process of the test animals. The biocompatibility question that must be answered is whether or not sufficient residual perchloroethylene remains on the cleaned metal parts to pose a health hazard.

Dose-Response Assessment. Threshold limit values (TLVs) are values that indicate the maximum level of a chemical that a healthy worker could take in on a daily basis over the course of his or her work life without experiencing any adverse effects (ACGIH, 1986; AHHA, 1980). The TLV for perchloroethylene is 50 ppm/day (50 ml of perchloroethylene per 10^3 liters of air) by inhalation. The average person inhales 12,960 liters of air per day, making this equivalent to 650 ml of perchloroethylene per day. Since the vapor density of perchloroethylene is 5.76 g/L, the TLV is equal to 3.7 g of perchloroethylene per day by inhalation.

Because TLVs for inhalation—as opposed to direct tissue exposure—are determined based on healthy individuals (not ill patients), we will divide the TLV by an uncertainty factor of 100 (i.e., 10) to account for a different route of exposure and 10 to account for healthy-to-ill persons. By this method, we obtain an allowable perchloroethylene limit of 37 mg/day.

Exposure Assessment. To calculate an available dose of perchloroethylene, we need some additional information. In this case, the manufacturer brought a number of cleaned metal pieces into equilibrium within a closed jar, then analyzed the headspace above the pieces by using a high-pressure liquid chromatography to determine the concentration of perchloroethylene released. The concentration of perchloroethylene was undetectable by high-performance liquid chromatography. Since the limits of this analytical method are 2 ppb, this value was taken as the concentration of perchloroethylene in the headspace. Taking the weight of the metal pieces, the number of pieces tested, and the volume of the headspace, it was calculated that the amount of perchloroethylene per single piece was a maximum of 1.0 ng/piece. If we suppose that a patient might be exposed to a maximum of 50 pieces over a lifetime, then the maximum available dose of perchloroethylene from the pieces would be 50 ng.

Risk Characterization. A comparison of the available dose (50 ng) to the allowable limit (37 mg/day) indicates an ample safety margin.

4. Ligature Material

A manufacturer purchases commercial black fishing line to use as a ligature in a circumcision kit. Because the ligature is not "medical grade," a cytotoxicity test is routinely conducted as an incoming inspection test. It was assumed that a negative cytotoxicity test would be associated with an acceptable incidence of skin irritation.

Hazard Identification. A newly received lot of the fishing line failed the cytotoxicity test. The extraction ratio of this material—of indeterminate surface area—was 0.2 g/ml, with a 0.1-ml aliquot of sample extract being applied to a culture dish. Thus, 0.2 g/ml $\times$ 0.1 ml = 0.02 g represents a toxic dose of fishing line.

Dose-Response Assessment. A titration curve was obtained on the sample extract. If the sample was diluted 1:2, the test was still positive; however, if the sample was diluted 1:4, the test was negative. Thus, 0.02 g/4 = 0.005 g of fishing line, the maximum dose that is not cytotoxic. This value was called the allowable limit of fishing line.

Exposure Assessment. Each circumcision kit contained about 12 in. of line, but only about 4 in. of material was ever in contact with the patient. Since an 8-yard line was determined to weigh 5 g, the available dose of fishing line was calculated to be 5 g/288 in. $\times$ 4 in. = 0.07 g.

Risk Characterization. A comparison of the available dose (0.07 g) with the allowable limit (0.005 g) convinced the manufacturer to reject the lot of fishing line.

L. Sources of Data

Data for calculating the allowable limit of exposure to a material can come from many sources, most of them promulgated by industrial and environmental hygienists and related agencies (Hayes, 1994).

Threshold limit values are time-weighed average concentrations of airborne substances. They are designed as guides to protect the health and well-being of workers repeatedly exposed to a substance during their entire working lifetimes (7–8 hr/day, 40 hr/wk). Threshold limit values are published annually by the American Conference of Governmental Industrial Hygienists (ACGIH, 1986). Biological exposure indices (BEIs) are also published annually by ACGIH. These are the maximum acceptable concentrations of a substance at which a worker's health and well-being will not be compromised.

Other published guides include workplace environmental exposure levels (WEELs), from the American Industrial Hygiene Association (AIHA, 1980); recommended exposure limits (RELs), from the U.S. National Institute for Occupational Safety and Health; and permissible exposure limits (PELs), from the U.S. Occupational Safety and Health Administration. In the United States, PELs have the force of law.

Another important limit measurement, short-term exposure limits (STELs), are defined as the maximum concentration of a substance to which workers can be exposed for a period of up to 15 min continuously, provided that no more than four excursions per day are permitted, and with at least 60 min between exposure periods. The STEL allows for short-term exposures during which workers will not suffer from irritation, chronic or irreversible tissue damage, or narcosis of sufficient degree to increase the likelihood of injury, impair self-rescue, or materially reduce work efficiency. Some substances are given a "ceiling," an airborne concentration that should not be exceeded even momentarily. Examples of substances having ceilings are certain irritants whose short-term effects are so undesirable that they override consideration of long-term hazards.

M. Uncertainty Factors

An uncertainty factor is a correction that is made to the value used to calculate an allowable limit. It is based on the uncertainty that exists in the applicability of the data to actual exposure conditions. Typically, uncertainty factors range in value from 1 to 10. For example, a correction factor of 10 might be applied for data obtained in animals rather than humans, or to allow for a different route of exposure. In other words, for every property of available data that is different from the actual application, a correction factor of between 1 and 10 is applied. If our first example had been of a small amount of data obtained in animals by a different route of exposure, an uncertainty factor of 1000 might be applied.

N. Safety Margins

A safety margin is the difference or ratio between the allowable limit (after correction by the uncertainty factor) and the available dose. How large does a safety margin need to be? Generally, a safety margin of 100× or more is desirable, but this can depend on the security of the risk under consideration, the type of product, the business risk to the company, and the potential benefits of product use.

REFERENCES

AAMI. (1997). AAMI Standards: Vol. 4, Biological Evaluation of Medical Devices, AAMI, Arlington, VA.

AAMI. (1998). AAMI Standards: Reduced Devices—Risk Management—Part 1: Applications, AAMI/ISO 14971-1, AAMI, Arlington, VA.

ACGIH. (1986). Documentation of the Threshold Limit Values for Substances in Workroom Air, 5th ed. American Conference of Governmental Industrial Hygienists, Cincinnati.

AIHA. (1980). Hygienic Guide Series, vols. I and II. American Industrial Hygiene Association, Akron, OH.

Brown, R. P. and Stratmeyer, M. (1997). Proposed Approach for the Biological Evaluation of Medical Device Materials. In: Proceedings of the Medical Design and Manufacturing East 97 Conference and Exposition, Canon Communications, Santa Monica, CA, pp. 205–209, 205–218.

Bunger, M. and Tummler, H. P (1994). Classification of active medical devices according to the medical device directive, Med. Dev. Tech., March: 33–39.

CDRH. (1992). Regulatory Requirements for Medical Devices: A Workshop Manual, Center for Device and Radiological Health, HHS publication FDA 92-4165, Washington, DC.

CDRH. (1995a). Premarket Notification (510(k)) Guidance Document for Contact Lens Care Products, Center for Device and Radiological Health, Food and Drug Administration, Washington, DC.

CDRH. (1995b). Testing Guidelines for Class III Soft (Hydrophilic) Contact Lens Solutions, Center for Device and Radiological Health, Food and Drug Administration, Washington, DC.

CDRH. (1995c). Draft Guidance for the Content of Premarket Notifications for Menstrual Tampons, Center for Device and Radiological Health, Food and Drug Administration, Washington, DC.

CFR. (1992). FDA's policy statement concerning cooperative manufacturing arrangements for licensed biologics, Fed. Reg., 57:55544.

Council directive 93/42/EEC of 14 June 1993 concerning medical devices, Off. J. Eur. Comm., 36 (July 12): 1.

Ecobichon, D. J. (1992). The Basis of Toxicology Testing, CRC Press, Boca Raton, FL.

European Committee for Standardization. (1991). CEN Annual Report 1991. Brussels.

FDLI. (1995). Compilation of Food and Drug Laws, vols. I and II; vol. III (1996), supplement (1998), Food and Drug Law Institute, Washington, DC.

European Commission. (1993). Final draft guidelines on medical device classification, MEDDEV 10/93, Brussels.

FDA. (1987). Good laboratory practice regulations: Final rule. Fed. Reg., part VI, 52(172).

FDA. (1995). EPA Bluebook Memorandum #G95: Use of International Standard ISO-

10993, Biological Evaluation of Medical Devices Part I: Evaluation and Testing, Food and Drug Administration, Washington, DC.

Fries, R. C. (1999). Medical Device Quality Assurance and Regulatory Compliance, Marcel Dekker, New York.

Gad, S. C. and Chengelis, C. P. (1998). Acute Toxicology, Academic, La Jolla, CA.

Gad, S. C. (2001). Regulatory Toxicology, 2nd ed. Taylor and Francis, London.

Gad, S. C. and Taulbee, S. (1996). Handbook of Data Recording, Maintenance and Management for the Biomedical Sciences, CRC Press, Boca Raton, FL.

Goering, P. L. and Galloway, W. D. (1989). Toxicology of medical device material, Fund. Appl. Toxicol., 13: 193–195.

The Gray Sheet. (1992). EC "medical devices" directive slated for adoption in mid-1993, EC Commission official says: CEN estimate development of 92 standards for directive, M-D-D-1 reports, Gray Sheet, Oct. 12.

The Gray Sheet. (1996a). European Union class III device approvals average 240 days or less, HIMA survey says: Study release intended to bolster support for FDA reform legislation, Gray Sheet, Feb. 26: 7–8.

The Gray Sheet (1996b). FDA 510(k) average review time for fiscal 1996 projected to be on par with FY 95 figure of 137 days: PMA average review time expected to drop to 250 days, Gray Sheet, March 25.

Haindl, H. (1997). CE marking via self-declaration, Med. Dev. Diag. Ind., Sept.: 86–90.

Hayes, A. W. (1994). Principles and Methods of Toxicology, 3rd ed. Raven Press, New York, pp. 26–58.

Heller, M. A. (1999). Guide to Medical Device Regulation, vols. 1 and 2. Thompson, Washington, DC.

ISO. (various dates). Biological Evaluation of Medical Devices. ISO 10993, parts 1–12. International Organization for Standardization, Geneva.

ISO. (1992). Biological Evaluation of Medical and Dental Materials and Devices, ISO, Brussels.

ISO. (1996). Risk and Hazard Assessment of Medical Devices, ISO 14538, ISO, Brussels.

MHW. (1995). Guidelines for basic biological tests of medical materials and devices, notification no. 99.

Japanese Pharmacopoeia XIII. (1996), Japanese Pharmacopoeia Association, Tokyo.

Kahan, J. S. (1995). Medical Devices—Obtaining FDA Market Clearance, Parexel, Waltham, MA.

Stark, N. J. (1997). Case studies: Using the world literature to reduce biocompatability testing. In: Proceedings of the Medical Design and Manufacturing East 97 Conference and Exposition, Canon Communications, Santa Monica, CA, pp. 205-1–205-7.

Stark, N. J. (1988). Conducting health-based risk assessment of medical materials, Med. Plas. Biomat., Sept./Oct.: 18–25.

USP. (2000). Biological tests-plastics. In: The United States Pharmacopoeia, XXIV § NF-19. United States Pharmacopoeial Convention, Rockville, MD, pp. 1235–38.

3

Road Map to Test Selections

Determining what testing is required for the development and approval of a new medical device can be a complex issue. This is even more the case after the issue of when to perform necessary tests is factored in. Postapproval, one must determine what ongoing testing is required to ensure continued safety of the product. Understanding the complexities requires careful consideration of some key concepts.

I. KEY CONCEPTS

There are 10 major categories to consider in evaluating and establishing the safety of a medical device, and in so doing defining what testing must be performed. These are presented in Table 3.1, and will each be considered in detail in this chapter.

II. CONDITIONS OF USE

The starting point for evaluating the safety of a near (or potential) medical device (or material for use in devices) must be to understand both how it is intended to be used (which governs the type of contact it will have with the end-use consumers—i.e., patients—and therefore the areas of potential risk and the applicable regulations) and how it is likely to be used (or misused).

Intended use starts with developing an objective statement of what purpose the device is to serve, and therefore how it is to be in contact with the patient

TABLE 3.1 Key Concepts in Medical Device Safety Assessment

 1. Condition of use
 2. Materials/components/products
 3. Chemical and physical property considerations
 4. Factors of influence
 5. Prior knowledge
 6. Types and uses of tests
 7. Reasonable man
 8. Qualification vs. process control
 9. Tiers of concern: consumer/health care provider/manufacturer
10. Sterilization

Note: These also could be thought of as areas of consideration.

[skin/body surface, only body cavity, indirectly with a fluid path (such as and most commonly the blood stream) within the body] and for how long there is to be patient contact. The categories for type of contact are drawn from the nation's regulatory guidelines presented earlier, but actual devices may fit in several categories. It is also important to know more details of the contact (e.i., what body cavity contact is with—mouth, nasal, vagina, anal, etc.).

The duration of exposure in use should also be established. This should be the cumulative duration for any patient, and not just the single time/use duration, (i.e., if a device is to be used 5 min a day each day for a week, it should be considered to have an approximately 35-minute cumulative patient exposure). For most devices, the intended use for any one patient is a single time, but if the device (say a glove) is used by a health care provider over the course of a day, cumulative exposure can be extensive.

One must also consider unintended uses or expected abuses of the device. People use devices in ways that are not planned, such as using elastic bandages to cover wounds. Such is especially (but not exclusively) the case for children and the elderly, who are more likely to be susceptible to adverse effects. It should also be kept in mind that, although many medical devices (disposable gloves and syringes, e.g.) are intended to be single-use disposables, in poorer cultures this frequently may not be the case. One cannot guard against every—or even most unusual—device usage, but should exercise some consideration of what the most likely misuses are.

III. MATERIALS, COMPONENTS, AND PRODUCTS

What is actually sold for use by or on the end-use consumer (the patient) is what is regulated by the various government agencies. This is the product, which must be evaluated for biocompatibility in conformance with applicable guidelines, in the form or forms (sterilized or unsterilized) in which it is intended to be sold.

Products are frequently composed of components, however. Simple examples are a disposable syringe (needle, barrel, plunger, lubricant, and stopper) or a surgical prep set (scrub, disinfectant, razor, etc.). Changing a component can significantly alter the biocompatibility of a product, and certain components, by the nature of both their composition and exposure to patients, are more likely to present biocompatibility problems. An example is the common disposable plastic syringe, of which billions are used each year. For the syringe, the most likely problem component is the stopper—the flexible piece at the end of the plunger. The stopper is most commonly made of natural rubber, and has direct contact with fluids entering the body (and frequently a fluid path).

Components, of course, are manufactured from or composed of materials. Materials (polymers, elastomers, steel, etc.) are the fundamental starting point for the development of a device, and are very frequently not produced by the device (or component) manufacturer, but rather are provided by an outside vendor.

Almost all biocompatability problems (the exceptions being due to sterility, sterilization, and cleanliness) for devices are due to the materials used in a device. Table 3.2 provides a concise list of material-based considerations for safety of a device.

A. Chemical and Physical Property Considerations

Engineers involved in the design and development of new medical devices are primarily concerned with the physical properties essential for the proper functioning of the device. Accordingly, the most important aspects of materials being used in device construction are its physical properties. Toxicologists and others responsible for device safety (the subject of this volume) are primarily concerned with the chemical nature and properties of materials used in devices, but must also be conversant with physical property considerations. For that reason, this section presents a primer on the chemical nature and chemical and physical properties of materials used in devices. Physical or mechanical properties can also be important for biocompatibility.

Mechanical insult is a localized, nonspecific, detrimental mechanical interaction between a device and the contacting tissue. It may be caused by rubbing, crushing, occluding, stripping, or penetrating the tissue. Rubbing may cause layers of tissues to separate from one another, resulting in the formation of blisters or bare underlying dermal layers. Crushing, or pressure damage, may result from tissue swelling beneath an inelastic device. Occlusive materials may encourage moisture and bacteria to accumulate beneath them. Tissue may be stripped when adhesive materials are removed, tearing the epidermis away from the dermis.

TABLE **3.2** Raw Material Characterization

Chemical characterization
  List materials
  List potential extractables or leachables from materials
  Physiochemical tests: USP water and isopropanol extracts
  International pharmacopoeial tests
  Infrared analysis: document polymer identification
  Chromatographic characterization
    Molecular weight distribution
    Additive and/or extract analysis
  Trace metals
  Specific gravity
  Moisture content
Physical characterization
  Hardness
  Surface characterization
  Color, opacity, or haze
  Strength properties
    Tensile/elongation
    Flexure
    Compression
  Thermal analysis
  Viscosity, melting point, refractive index
Biological characterization (nothing listed)

Tissue penetration, due to incision or puncture, will cause cells to be ruptured and physically separated from each other. Indigestible particulate matter may be shed into or left embedded in the tissue.

Microscopically, mechanical insult, like chemical insult, is characterized by inflammation. Macroscopic responses to mechanical injury are usually obvious and include dermatosis, callus, granuloma, or cyst formation. Histologically, responses to mechanical injury may include tissue infiltration by phagocytic macrophages and foreign-body giant cells, and by fribroblast, the function of which is to deposit collagen and wall off the offending material within a cyst. Whereas the tissue effects of chemical insults are generally symmetrically distributed around the sample as the offending chemical is extracted, those of mechanical insult are generally asymmetrically distributed according to the geometry of the material.

Mechanical failure includes device failure that causes injury to the organism or loss of a life support mechanism. Mechanical failure is not generally considered to be an issue of biocompatibility, although certainly it is an issue of device safety.

The majority of components of medical devices are constituted from a small number of categories of materials. The important categories of materials in device formulation and construction are the following: water, stainless steels, polymers, elastomers, silicones, and natural fibers (cotton and wood pulp, primarily). Each of these needs to be considered in turn. Additionally, biologically derived materials are seeing increased utilization in devices (Kambric et al., 1986), but are of such diverse nature that is not currently possible to adequately overview them in this volume.

These are interactions that occur between a material used in a device and the organism ("host") that it has contact with. Device materials having systemic contact with a host ("biomaterials") may be degraded by the host by a number of chemical means, which should be kept in mind when considering the use of any of the materials described in this section. These pathways of chemical degradation of biomaterials include the following:

Hydrolysis (acid, base, neutral aqueous media)
Oxidation (corrosion, chain cleavage)
Thermolysis
Photo-oxidation
Specific enzyme—catalyzed hydrolysis or oxidation
Attack by complex media (culture media, serum, blood, gastric juices, urinary fluids, phagocyte-containing fluid, etc.)
Chain cleavage due to mechanical fracture

The chemical basis of toxicity or biocompatibility problems are related to these same processes.

In theory the biocompatibility of a material could be assessed by a careful analysis of its chemical composition, but in practice the exact chemical composition is usually either proprietary or unknown and too costly to identify. It is common knowledge that virtually no plastics are pure polymers; all are modified with inadvertent contaminants and intentional additives. Fabrics purchased from the textile industry contain a variety of finish coatings. Natural materials are usually impure and vary from lot to lot. Synthetic materials contain organic residues. Metal alloys contain leachable essential trace elements.

Because of these variables, toxicologists usually adopt a different approach to establishing biocompatibility. The interaction of a material with living tissue is assessed in vivo: the material is considered biocompatible with regard to a particular mechanism of injury if there is little or no tissue response; it is considered nonbiocompatible if there is a response. Three factors are important: the rate at which an additive or contaminant leaches out of the material, the effect that the loss of additives has on the material, and the toxicity of the additive or contaminant. When a positive response occurs, the toxicologist must play chemical sleuth to identify its cause and to recommend process or formulation changes to eliminate it.

The following are some of the sources of possible toxic substances in medical device materials. Each source is then discussed separately.

Residual monomers
Residual solvents
Degradation products
By-products from irradiation
Sterilization residuals
Formulation additives
Inadvertent contaminants
Bacterial endotoxins

Residual monomers.   Polymerization results in a distribution of molecular weights. Although monomers are usually toxic, the toxicity of the polymeric unit generally decreases as the molecular weight increases. Residual monomers result from incomplete polymerization; their concentration can be controlled by carefully regulating polymerization conditions.

Residual solvents.   Solvents are often an integral part of manufacturing and may remain behind in fluid materials such as adhesives, adhesive removers, barrier pastes, gels, or lubricants. Some acrylate adhesive systems are now water-based, which eliminates the concern for residual solvents. When the solvent is an integral component of the final product, as with adhesive removers and certain barrier pastes, its presence and potential transdermal absorption must be addressed in labeling.

Degradation products.   Materials may undergo degradation during manufacture, sterilization, or storage, or after application to or implantation in the body. During manufacture, heat may thermally degrade a material; polyvinyl chloride is especially susceptible to heat and may release hydrochloric acid, resulting in an autocatalytic unzipping process. During sterilization, polytetrafluorethylene is susceptible to irradiation breakdown, resulting in the release of hydrofluoric acid. Stored materials exposed to light and oxygen may suffer ultraviolet degradation or oxidation. Implanted materials, particularly metals, may corrode or be biologically degraded (ISO, 1997).

Stabilizers added to the polymer can protect against degradation. Materials should be tested for degradation and biocompatibility only after both manufacture and a suitable aging period.

By-products from irradiation.   Gamma irradiation is becoming an increasingly common method of sterilization; 2-3 Mrad is the usual sterilization dose. It is also used to facilitate cross-linking in certain formulations. As a result, many materials undergo degradation. Polyglycolic acid, used in suture production, is virtually destroyed by irradiation. Most medical polymers decrease in molecular weight as a result of chain scission. Polypropylene and other polymers may undergo chain scission, cross-linking, and oxidation. Any material that is irradiation sterilized should be tested for biocompatibility afterward, although most medical polymers remain useful.

Sterilization residuals. Chemical sterilization with ethylene oxide has a long history of use; the main advantages are that the procedure is carried out at low temperatures and the sterilization facility need not deal with radioactive sources. Ethylene oxide, which is itself toxic, also degrades into toxic ethylene chlorohydrin and ethylene glycol. Even after extensive degassing, some materials do not release these toxic molecules. All materials that are to be ethylene oxide sterilized must be tested for toxic residuals. These are discussed in Chapter 13.

Formulation additives. Formulation additives include plasiticizers, stabilizers, antioxidants, fillers, catalysts, mold release agents, colorants, antistatic agents, preservatives, and flame retardants. Both synthetic and natural fabrics are apt to have a variety of finish coatings.

Plasticizers allow the polymeric chains of a plastic to slide past each other, providing material flexibility. Stabilizers protect the plastic against heat, oxygen, and light. Antioxidants protect it from oxidation. Fillers expand the volume of the plastic and sometimes impart mechanical properties. Catalysts are small molecules that promote polymerization. Mold release agents facilitate the release of a molded part from the mold. Colorants add color and beauty. Antistatic agents prevent electrostatic buildup. Preservatives protect against microbial degradation. Flame retardants slow the release of toxic fumes during extreme conditions of heat or flame. Coatings impart a variety of properties to fabric, such as resistance to mildew or absorbency.

Any of these additives may contribute to nonbiocompatibility. To complicate the picture, because the medical device industry uses only a small fraction of the total volume of industrial plastics, few device manufacturers are in a position to specify the exact formulation of the material they will use. (Even so-called medical-grade plastics contain additives, medical grade usually taken to mean that the material has passed certain testing regimens, usually USP grade VI, and that it is processed under clean conditions.) Manufacturers thus must frequently evaluate industrial-grade materials to obtain the mechanical and chemical properties required in the final product.

Fabric devices, like any other dermal contact product, must also be evaluated for biocompatibility. Those that will be laundered between uses present the user with less finish-coating exposure than do disposable de-

vices that bring new fabric with each use. Some finish coats are carcinogenic; others cause allergic reactions or skin irritation. Some are water-
soluble and are removed during washing. Others are organic-based and
will remain.

Inadvertent contaminants. Materials may also contain inadvertent contaminants or particulates that are introduced during manufacture. Metal
shavings from equipment wear or plastic shards from stamping processes
have been known to adulterate devices.

Bacterial endotoxins. Finally, materials may contain bacterial endotoxins,
most commonly introduced through water during manufacture. Contaminating endotoxins are of concern for devices that will be used on anything
other than intact skin on the mucous membrane. They are readily eliminated by using endotoxin-free water.

Issues around the specific primary materials used in device manufacture
should now be considered. Note that the characterization of materials is
specifically addressed in ISO 10993-14.

B. Specific Material Considerations

1. Water

In one way or another, water is involved in the production of virtually every
medical device. For many devices (particularly diagnostics), it is also incorporated into the device. Yet water tends to be invisible to many considering device
biocompatibility and safety.

Water's greatest uses are in cleaning and rinsing devices and their components. Purified water is obtained by distillation, ion-exchange treatment, reverse
osmosis, or other suitable processes. Such water is prepared from source material
complying with the regulations of the U.S. Environmental Protection Agency
(USEPA) for drinking water. Water can be a problem in device safety and biocompatibility, generally due to the presence of things in it that do not comply
with USEPA and other regulations (e.g., micro-organisms, pesticides, organics,
other pyrogens, and heavy metals), as well as contaminants from other devices
or components that may have been previously rinsed in the water (such as latex
from gloves or stoppers). Water is usually a source of problems in the production
of devices, and not in the development stage. Specific issues and standards associated with heavy metals will be addressed in Chapter 13.

2. Metals

A variety of metals sees significant use in medical devices, although with the
exception of stainless steel their use in patient contacting situations is largely
limited to implants. The uses are a reflection of the properties of the various
metals, as summarized in Table 3.3.

TABLE 3.3 Properties of Major Metals Used in Medical Devices

Material: Metals and metallic alloys	Strength	Tensile modulus	Creep modulus	Fatigue life	Lubricity	Water permeability	Water absorption	Biostability
Cobalt chrome alloys	High	High	High	High	Mod.	Low	Low	High
Nickel chrome alloys	High	High	High	High	Mod.	Low	Low	High
Nitinol alloys (shape memory alloys)	High	High	High	High	Mod.	Low	Low	High
Stainless steels	High	High	High	High	Mod.	Low	Low	Med.
Tantalum	High	High	High	High	Mod.	Low	Low	High
Titanium and titanium alloys	High	High	High	High	Mod.	Low	Low	High

Stainless steel is by far the most common metal used in devices. This ferrous alloy is widely used in surgical instruments, wire sutures, needles, screws, and implant parts, in which great strength is needed. By definition, steels are alloys of iron containing 0.002–1.5% carbon, while stainless steel contains high percentages (~10–25%) of chromium. Table 3.4 presents the American Standard Testing Materials (ASTM) specifications of the two grades of stainless steel that are commonly used for medical devices. Stainless steel is rarely a biocompatibility problem in medical devices. In some long-term implants, there can be concerns about reaction of the alloy with body fluids, but even this is unusual.

The other major metals are primarily used in surgical implants, particularly orthopedic (bone) prosthesis. These are primarily titanium and cobalt alloys, although some more exotic metals are also seeing use. Gold, palladium, and platinum, for example, are plated onto the surface of stents to provide radiopacity for placement and monitoring. Silver is used as an antimicrobial. Unlike stainless steel, not all of these metals are biologically inert. The compositions and properties of the other major metal alloys employed are summarized in Tables 3.5–3.7.

3. Polymers

Polymers are macromolecules formed by the chemical bonding of five or more identical units called monomers. In most cases the number of monomers is quite large (3500 for pure cellulose), and often is not precisely known. In synthetic polymers, this number can be controlled to a predetermined extent, for example,

TABLE 3.4 Chemical Composition of Stainless Steel

Element	Composition (%)	
	Grade 1	Grade 2
Carbon	0.08 max	0.030 max
Manganese	2.00 max	2.00 max
Phosphorus	0.030 max	0.030 max
Sulfur	0.030 max	0.030 max
Silicon	0.75 max	0.74 max
Chromium	17.00–19.00	17.00–19.00
Nickel	12.00–14.00	12.00–14.00
Molybdenum	2.00–3.00	2.00–3.00
Nitrogen	0.10 max	0.10 max
Copper	0.50 max	0.50 max
Iron	Balance	Balance

Source: ASTM F56, 1986.

TABLE **3.5** Cobalt-Based Alloys

	Wrought CoNiCrMo MoWFe	Cast wrought CoCrMo CoNiCr-	Wrought CvoCrMo	Wrought CoNiCrMo	Wrought CoNiCr- MoWFe	Wrought CoCrMo
Condition	AN	AN	AN	AN	AN	CW
Source	(1,2)	(1,3)	(4)	(5)	(1,3)	(4)
Density (g/cm³)	7.8	9.15	—	—	9.15	—
E (tensile) (GPa)	230	—	—	230	—	—
Hardness (Hv)	300	240	—	—	450	—
$\sigma_{0.2\%}$ (MPa)	455	390	240–450	275	1000	1585
σ_{UTS} (MPa)	665	880	795–1000	600	1500	1795
Elong. (min.%)	10	30	50	50	9	8

Note: AN: annealed; CW; cold worked; —unavailable. *Source*: [1]: BSI 3531 (Part 2, Sec. 4–5, Amend. 2, 1983); [2]: ASTM F90-82; [4]: ASTM F562-84; [5]: ASTM F563-83.

by shortstopping agents. (Combinations of two, three, or four monomers are called, respectively, dimers, trimers, and tetramers, and are known collectively as oligomers. Such oligomers are not polymers.) A partial list of polymers by type includes the following (Billmeyer, 1971):

I.   Inorganic: siloxane, sulfur, chains, black phosphorus, boron-nitrogen, silicones
II. Organic
   A.   Natural
      1.   Polysaccharides: starch, cellulose, pectin, seaweed gums (aga, etc.), vegetable gums (arabic, etc.)
      2.   Polypeptides (proteins): casein, albumin, globulin, keratin, insulin, DNA
      3.   Hydrocarbons: rubber and gutta percha (polyisoprene), also called elastomers
   B.   Synthetic
      1.   Thermoplastic polymers: nylon, polyvinyl chloride, polyethylene (linear), polystyrene, polypropylene, fluorocarbon resins, polyurethane, acrylate resins
      2.   Thermosetting polymers: polyethylene (cross-linked) phenolics, alkyds, polyesters
   C.   Semisynthetic cellulosics (rayon, methylcellulose acetate) and modified starches (starch acetate, etc.)

For most devices, we are concerned only with the synthetic organic polymers. The principal class of natural polymers of concern, the elastomers, will be

TABLE 3.6 Titanium and Titanium-Based Alloys

	Ti type 4	Ti6A14V	Ti5A12.5Fe	Ti6A14V	Ti6A17b	To5A12/5Fe
Condition	AN	AN	HF	HF	HF	HF
Source	[1,2]	[1,3]	[7]	[6]	[4,5]	[7]
Density (g/cm^3)	4.5	4.4	4.45	4.4	4.52	4.45
E (tensile) (GPa)	127	127	—	127	105	—
Hardness (Hv)	240–280	310–350	—	—*	400	—
$\sigma_{0.2\%}$ (MPa)	430–465	830	815	—*	800–900	900
σ_{UTS} (MPa)	550–575	900	965	—*	900–1000	985
Elong. (min.%)	15	8	16	—*	10–12	13

Note: AN: annealed; HF: hot forged; —: unavailable.

TABLE 3.7 Other Metals and Alloys

Material	Ta	Ta	Pt	Pt10Rh	Pt10Rh	W
Condition	AN	AN	CW	AN	AN	75% CWSN
Source	[1,2]	[1,2]	[1,2]	[1]	[1]	[1]
Density (g/cm^3)	16.6	16.6	21.5	20	20	19.3
E (tensile) (GPa)	186	186	147	—	—	345
Hardness (Hv)	—	—	38–40	90*	165*	225
$\sigma_{0.2\%}$ (MPa)	140	345	—	—	—	—
σ_{UTS} (MPa)	205	515	135–165	310	620	125–140
Elong. (min.%)	20–30	2	35–40	35	2	~0

Note: AN: annealed; CW: cold worked; SN: sintered bar; *: Brinell hardness; —: unavailable.

considered later in this chapter, along with the synthetic members of this class. The chief class of inorganic polymers of concern, the silicones, will likewise be considered later in this chapter.

Polymers can be categorized in a number of ways, (Haslam et al., 1972; McMurrer, 1985/1986). Homopolymers, for example, consist of only one repeating monomer unit. Table 3.8 lists the most commonly encountered homopolymers. Figure 3.1 provides the structures of some typical monomers, while Figure 3.2–3.6 provide structural illustrations of some homopolymers.

Copolymers are produced by the simultaneous polymerization of two or more dissimilar molecules. Examples include polyvinyl acetate (Figure 3.7), polyesters (Figure 3.8), and polymides (Figure 3.9). Synthetic elastomers (such

TABLE 3.8 Commonly Used Homopolymers in Medical Devices

Polyethylene
Polypropylene
Polybutylene
Polyvinylchloride
Polystyrene
Polychloroprene
Polyacrylates
Polytetrafluoroethylene
Polysiloxanes
Polysulfones
Polyamides

Source: Autian, 1980.

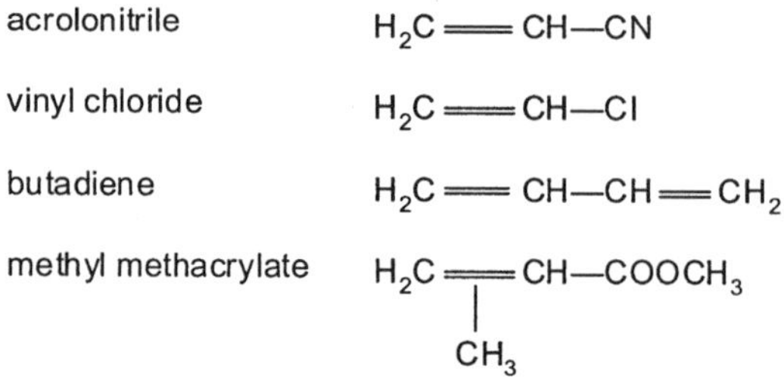

acrolonitrile $H_2C \!=\!=\! CH\!-\!CN$

vinyl chloride $H_2C \!=\!=\! CH\!-\!Cl$

butadiene $H_2C \!=\!=\! CH\!-\!CH \!=\!=\! CH_2$

methyl methacrylate $H_2C \!=\!=\! CH\!-\!COOCH_3$
                                     $|$
                                  CH_3

FIGURE 3.1   Molecular structures of four typical isomers.

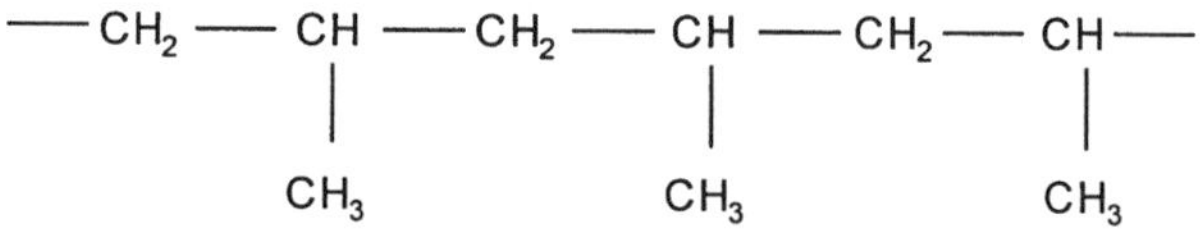

$$-CH_2 \!-\! CH \!-\! CH_2 \!-\! CH \!-\! CH_2 \!-\! CH -$$
$$\quad\quad\;\; | \quad\quad\quad\quad | \quad\quad\quad\quad |$$
$$\quad\quad CH_3 \quad\quad\;\; CH_3 \quad\quad\;\; CH_3$$

FIGURE 3.2   Structural diagram of polypropylene, a typical homopolymer, along with that of its monomeric unit (propylene).

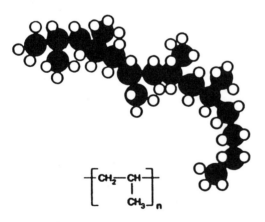

FIGURE 3.3   Structure of polypropylene, a typical homopolymer, rendered as a molecular model.

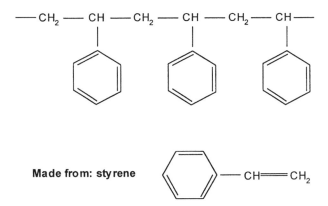

Made from: styrene

FIGURE 3.4 Structural diagram of polystyrene, a typical homopolymer, along with that of its monomeric unit (styrene).

as SBR synthetic rubber, made from styrene and butadiene) are also copolymers. This pattern continues with the terpolymers (such as ABS, shown in Figure 3.10), which consist of three different monomers.

The principle concerns with the biocompatibility of polymers are additives, residual monomers, and contaminants that are leachable in the body. As Table 3.9 shows, polymers themselves generally have very low toxicities. Partially as a reflection of their high molecular weights, true polymers themselves are not generally absorbed into the body, are not irritating, and are not sensitizers.

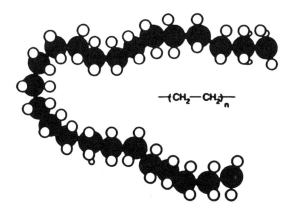

FIGURE 3.5 Structure of polyethylene, a typical homopolymer, with a structural diagram of its monomer, ethylene.

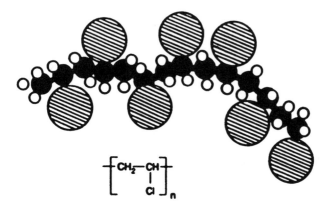

FIGURE 3.6 Structure of polyvinyl chloride (PVC), a typical homopolymer, rendered as a molecular model along with the structure of the monomeric unit (vinyl chloride).

Residual monomers, additives, and contaminants are a very different story. Each of these can be quite significant biologically.

Residual monomers are those remaining individual building block units in homopolymers, copolymers, terpolymers, and so on (as diagrammed structurally in Figures 3.1–3.10) that are not successfully incorporated into the plastic during the synthesis process. Technically, we should also include dimers, trimers, and

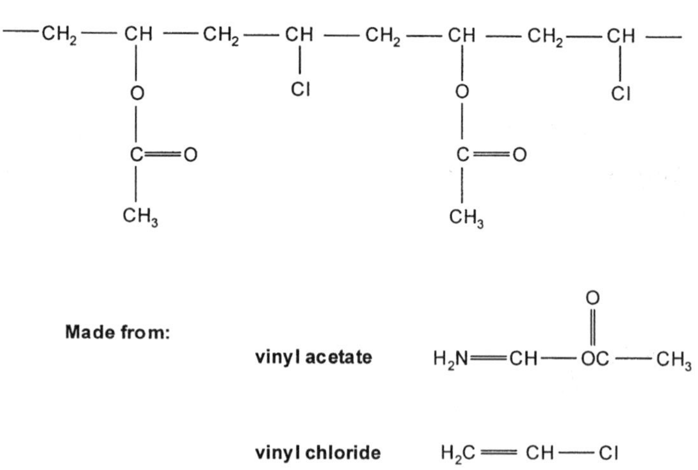

$$ \text{—CH}_2\text{—CH—CH}_2\text{—CH—CH}_2\text{—CH—CH}_2\text{—CH—} $$

Made from:

vinyl acetate $\quad H_2N = CH — OC — CH_3$

vinyl chloride $\quad H_2C = CH — Cl$

FIGURE 3.7 Structural diagram of vinyl acetate, a typical copolymer, along with the structures of its two constituent monomers (vinyl acetate and vinyl chloride).

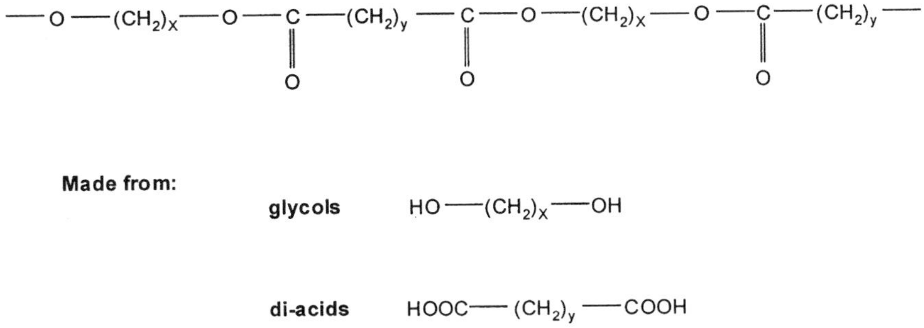

— O —(CH₂)ₓ— O — C —(CH₂)ᵧ — C — O —(CH₂)ₓ— O — C —(CH₂)ᵧ —

(with C=O groups below)

Made from:

glycols   HO —(CH₂)ₓ—OH

di-acids   HOOC— (CH₂)ᵧ —COOH

FIGURE 3.8 Structural diagram of a polyester, a typical copolymer, along with the structures of its two constituent monomers (glycols and diacids).

other small-chain fragments that are left in the polymer mass but are not chemically bound to it. Many factors help determine how much residual monomer will be left in a polymer, and how available such residuals are to a surrounding biological matrix. Some of the monomers are quite active biologically. When we test a plastic for biocompatibility, biologically available (leachable) residual monomers are a significant part of our concern. Examples of toxic monomers (and their principal toxicities) that can be found in polymers include the following:

Acrylonitrile: human carcinogen (liver, brain)
Vinyl chloride: human carcinogen (liver)
Formaldehyde: animal carcinogen (nasal)
Methylene dianline: suspect human carcinogen

A wide variety of other chemical entities are specifically incorporated into plastics to achieve desired goals of structure, performance, and processing ease.

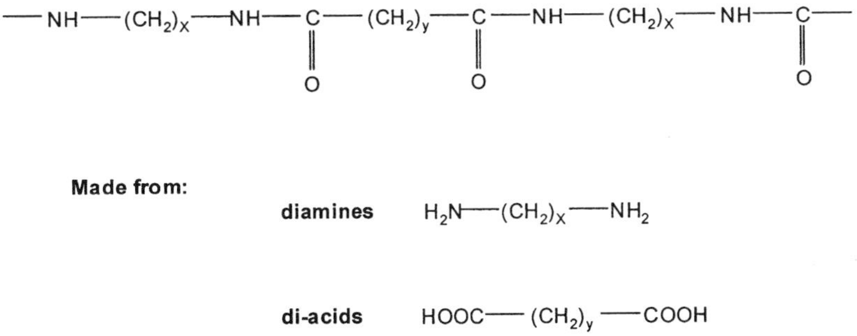

— NH —(CH₂)ₓ—NH— C — (CH₂)ᵧ— C —NH— (CH₂)ₓ— NH— C—

(with C=O groups below)

Made from:

diamines   H₂N—(CH₂)ₓ—NH₂

di-acids   HOOC— (CH₂)ᵧ —COOH

FIGURE 3.9 Structural diagram of a polymide, a typical copolymer, along with the structures of its two constituent monomers (diamines and diacids).

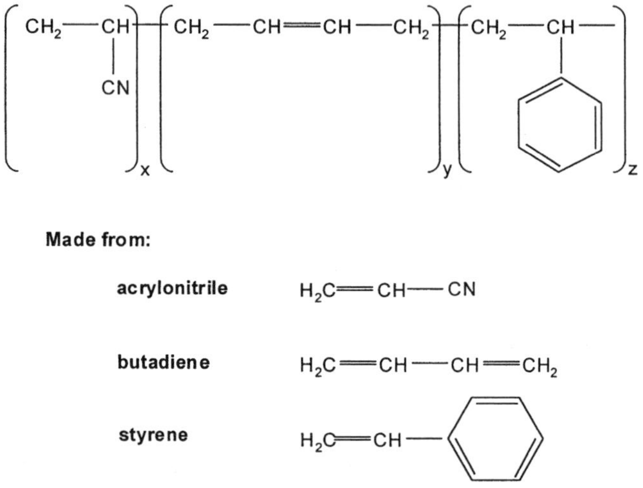

Made from:

acrylonitrile $H_2C{=}CH{-}CN$

butadiene $H_2C{=}CH{-}CH{=}CH_2$

styrene $H_2C{=}CH{-}$⬡

FIGURE 3.10   Structural diagram of ABS, a typical terpolymer, along with the structures of its three constituent monomers (acrylonitrile, butadiene, and styrene).

Table 3.10 presents a short list of the major categories of additives. Such additives can be quite significant biologically, and may be very biologically available. A historical example is diethylhexylphthalate (DEHP), a one widely used plasticizer that was found both to be an animal carcinogen and to migrate readily from plastic bags and tubing to the blood and intravenous solutions they contained (Peck et al., 1979; Sasakawa and Mitomi, 1978). Figure 3.11 presents the results of one study of DEHP migration into blood products stored in bags containing DEHP. During the processes of polymer synthesis and forming of the components

TABLE 3.9   Oral Lethalities of Common Polymers

Polymer	Rat LD_{50}(g/kg BW)
Polyethlene	>8
Polypropylene	>8
Polychloroprene latex	>40
Chlorosulfonated polyethylene	>20
Polyvinyl acetate	>25
Polyacrylonitrile	>3
Polyacrylamide	>8.2
Aromatic polyamides	>7.5

Source: Autian, 1980.

TABLE 3.10   Additives Used
in Plastics

Plasticizers
Lubricants
Antioxidants
Colorants
Emulsifiers
Stabilizers
Curing agents
UV absorbers
Blowing agents
Fillers
Release agents
Flame and fire retardants
Accelerators
Antistatic agents

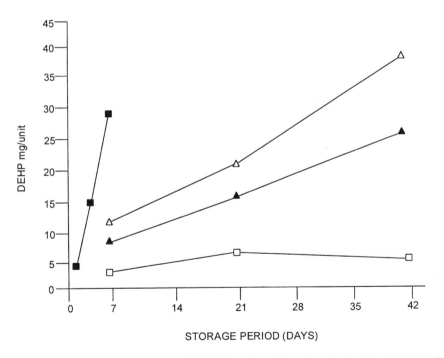

FIGURE 3.11   Average amount of DEHP in stored blood products. △ whole blood, 0–5°C; ▲ plasma fraction, 0.5°C; □ packed red cells, 0–5°C; ■ platelet concentrate, 22°C. Source: Miripol and Stern (1977).

and products, materials (e.g., solvents and mold release agents) can contaminate the polymer product (Petersen et al., 1981).

The result of the additives and contaminants being in plastic is that a range of toxic materials may be leached from many plastics. Table 3.11 presents a short list of some of the more significant of these.

For the interested reader, Kroschowitz (1990) and Dumitriu (1994) are excellent texts on polymers, particularly as they are utilized in medical devices.

4. Elastomers

The classic definition of an elastomer is a member of a class of synthetic thermosetting polymeric substances possessing rubberlike qualities (e.g., the ability to regain shape after deformation, to be stretched to at least twice its original length,

TABLE 3.11 Identified Toxic
Materials in Polymers

Aluminum
Acrylonitrile (monomer)
Arsenic
Benzene
Benzoic peroxide
Bisphenol A
Cadmium
Carbon tetrachloride
Dibutyl tin
Epoxy curing agents
Ethylene dichloride
Ethylene oxide
Formaldehyde
Ketones and hydrocarbons
Lead
Mercaptobenzothiazole
Methyl chloride
Methylene chloride
Methylene dianiline
Nickel
PAHs on carbon black
Pyrene
Tin
Tricresyl phosphate
Triphenyl phosphate

Source: Autian, 1980; Northup, 1989.

and having toughness and resistance to weathering and chemical attacks.) For our purposes, however, the natural rubbers will also be included under the term.

The chemical requirements for useful elastomers include high molecular weight, flexibility of the polymer chain, and a controlled degree of polarity and structural irregularity. These features impart cohesiveness and a lack of molecular order in the undeformed state, although natural and synthetic rubbers generally take on some aspects of crystallinity at very low temperatures or when they are highly extended.

Natural rubber is natural organic substance obtained from the sap of certain trees. Rubber is produced from a wide variety of plants, especially Hevea brasiliensis (family Euphorbiaceae), a tall softwood tree native to Brazil, but also from species of Mabea, Manihot, Sapium, Ficus, and others. The milky liquid (latex) found in the inner bark and obtained by tapping (cutting) and bark is coagulated; the oldest and simplest technique is by smoking over a fire. Plantation rubber, widely grown in Southeast Asia (particularly Malaysia), comes from trees grown from selected seeds, with trees spaced well apart; tapping similar to the method used for wild trees, but coagulation in accomplished chemically.

Most rubber used in medical devices is still of the natural variety due to economics and the better resistance of the natural product to heat. Recent concerns about latex allergies, however, have increased the move toward synthetic products.

Synthetic rubber (or the proper elastomers) comprises a family of elastic products derived chiefly from petroleum and alcohol, some of which closely resemble natural rubber some of which have quite different physical properties. Research on the chemistry of natural rubber led in the nineteenth century to the isolation of isoprene, which was reconverted into a rubberlike substance by distillation. This and other processes by which long chains of molecules were created (called polymerization) attracted continued research into the early twentieth century.

Among the most important synthetics are the butadiene-styrene copolymers; the various butadiene copolymers; the chloroprene polymer (neoprene); the polysulfide polymers (Thiokol); cis-1,4-polyisoprene, ethylene-propylene terpolymers (EPDM rubber); polyurethane rubber; the isobutylene polymers (butyl rubbers); the silicone rubbers produced by blending silicones with natural and synthetic rubbers; and plasticized vinyl chloride and vinyl acetate polymers and copolymers. These can be cross-linked with sulfur, peroxides, or similar agents. The term was later extended to include uncross-linked polyolefins that are thermoplastic; these are generally known as TPO rubbers. Their extension and retraction properties are notably different from those of thermosetting elastomers.

Many important elastomers are copolymers in which the main molecular chain is composed of carbon atoms. They are usually based on butadiene and other organic compounds obtainable from petroleum. In Buna S, the second component is styrene; in Buna N, acrylonitrile. Butyl rubber, used in pneumatic inner tubes, is a copolymer of isobutylene and isoprene. Elastomeric materials in which the main polymer chain contains atoms other than carbon include the polysulfide rubbers (Thiokols) and the silicones. We will consider the silicones as a separate class of compounds.

Like natural rubbers, synthetic rubbers can be toughened by vulcanization and improved and modified for special purposes by reinforcement with other materials.

Elastomers are used as closures in vessels, stoppers in syringes, in gloves, tubing, and condoms, and in a host of ways in other devices. The degree of curing of elastomers is particularly important in determining their biocompatibility. Natural rubbers are natural products, of course, and therefore subject to significant lot-to-lot variability in composition.

5. Silicones

Silicones (organosiloxane polymers) are a large group of siloxane polymers based on a structure of alternating silicon and oxygen atoms with any of a variety of organic radicals attached to the silicone, such as is shown in Figure 3.12 (Hardman and Torkelson, 1986; Rochow, 1951). Silicones are very widely used in devices and in the pharmaceutical industry, and in such uses the majority of the substituent organic groups are methyl (McGregor, 1953).

Silicones have an unusual array of properties. Chief among these are thermal and oxidative stability and physical properties little affected by temperature. Other important characteristics include a high degree of chemical inertness, resistance to weathering, good dielectric strength, and low surface tension. As the general formula implies, the molecular structure can vary considerably to include linear, branched, and cross-linked structures. These structural forms and the substituent (R) groups provide many combinations of useful properties that lead to a wide range of commercially important applications. Silicones include fluids, resins, and elastomers. Many derived products (e.g., emulsions, greases, adhesives, sealants, and coatings) have been developed for a large variety of uses in the device industry.

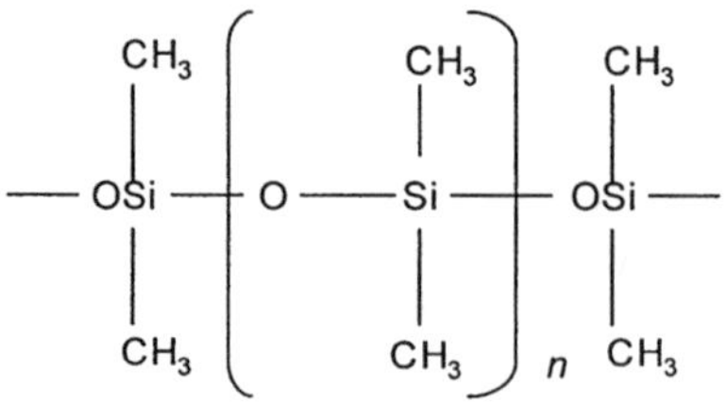

FIGURE 3.12   Example of the basic structural segment of a silicone.

Silicones can be liquids, semisolids (gels), or solids, depending on the molecular weight and degree of polymerization. Viscosity ranges from less than 1 to more than 1 million centistokes. Polymers may be straight-chain, or cross-linked with benzoyl peroxide or other free radical initiation, with or without a catalyst. They have very low surface tensions, extreme water repellency, high lubricating properties, and excellent dielectric properties, and are permeable to gases and highly resistant to attack and decomposition by biological systems (Heggers et al., 1983).

Silicones are used as adhesives, lubricants, protective coatings, wetting agents, mold release agents, surfactants, foam stabilizers, surgical membranes and implants, gaskets, and tubing in the device industry. They have been used as implantable devices since the late 1950s, and in recent years (in the form of prosthetic breast implants) have become of concern for purported health effects (Bommer et al., 1983; Laopahand et al., 1982) and have acted as potent litogens. (See the discussion of this aspect in Chapter 17.)

6. Fibers

Fibers (both natural and synthetic) are also widely used in medical devices as sutures, connectors, and binding and absorbent materials. Natural fibers that are commonly employed are silk (typically as suture material), linen, and cotton (primarily for its absorbent properties in bandages, tampons, etc.). The natural fibers do not usually cause biocompatibility problems if properly prepared, cleaned, and sterilized, although environmental contamination of the fiber is a possibility.

Synthetic fibers can be of either a durable or short-lived nature. Nylon and rayon are used for durable applications, with rayon being used as an absorbent material in the place of cotton. For suture use, absorbable materials have been developed for use as sutures, with the advantage that an additional surgical procedure is not required to remove them after wound healing is achieved (Schmitt and Polistina, 1967; Elbert et al., 1971; Frazza and Schmitt, 1971; Katz and Turner, 1970). Figure 3.13 presents structures of commonly used nonabsorbable suture materials, and Figure 3.14 those of common absorbable suture materials.

There has recently been some (seemingly unfounded) concern about the use of rayon and some other synthetic fibers due to possible contamination with diaxanes.

7. Ceramics

Ceramics are products manufactured by the action of heat on earthy raw materials (i.e., those that are neither metallic or organic), with silicon and its oxides, aluminum oxides, and complex materials known as silicates occupying a predominant position. In physical structure, ceramics may be polycrystalline, glass, combinations of multicrystals with glassy phases, or single crystals. The universal properties of ceramics that account for their enduring utility include mechanical strength

- cellulosics – cotton, linen
- polyamides (nylon)   SURGILON® (ACY)
  [NH(CH$_2$)$_6$NH-CO(CH$_2$)$_4$CO]
- polyesters (polyethyleneterephthalate)   DACRON®
  [O(CH$_2$)$_2$OCOC$_6$H$_4$CO]
- polyelefins (polypropylene)   SURGILENE® (ACY)
  [CH$_2$CH(CH$_3$)]
- protein–silk

FIGURE 3.13   The five most commonly used nonabsorbable suture materials, with the structures and trade names of the three that are synthetic.

(in spite of the brittleness); chemical durability (at both normal and elevated temperatures) against the deteriorating effects of oxygen, water (liquid or vapor), acids, bases, salts, and organic solvents; hardness contributing to resistance against erosion; and the ability to be combined with metals and other materials to make uniquely effective devices and device parts. The forming of artificial ceramics involves particle technology, including size reduction (commination), measurement, and separation; blending and packing of particles; surface chemistry and physics; rheology, or the flow of more or less plastic materials under pressure; and bonding of particles. Other sciences contribute to the understanding and control of heat treatment.

Ceramics came into being because of the useful rheological properties of the clay–water system, with its capability of being shaped, whether as a paste, a fluid suspension, or a damp, crumbly powder. Modern industrial ceramics often replace clay with organic or inorganic additives to make the raw material easier to form and to provide strength before firing (final heating). Clay-based ceramics undergo both chemical-mineralogical and physical changes during heat treatment to form new phases, including a glassy phase that often constitutes the bond between the grains in the new microstructure. Such heat treatment involves sin-

- poly(p-diozanone) – absorbed in 6 months (rats)
  [O(CH$_2$)$_2$OCH$_2$CO]   PDS® (Ethicon)
- poly(glycolic acid) – absorbed in 40-90 days (rabbits)
  [OCH$_2$CO$_2$CH$_2$CO]   DEXON® (ACY)
- poly(glycoclide-co-lactide)
  [OCH$_2$CO$_2$CH$_2$CO]$_{90}$[OCH(CH$_3$)CO$_2$CH(CH$_3$CO]$_1$ CICRYL® (Ethicon)

FIGURE 3.14   Three common absorbable suture materials, with their structures and trade names.

tering in the presence of a liquid phase. The complex series of occurrences accompanying heat treatments include gas evolution, oxidation, valence changes, chemical reactions, phase transformations, melting, shrinkage, and still other chemical and physical changes. The trend with modern ceramics technology is to simplify such changes by establishing the chemical and mineral changes before forming. Maximum density is sought in the forming batch, and compaction is achieved by applying the principles of particle packing. Then heat treatment brings about sintering in the solid state with a minimum of shrinkage, gas evolution, and attendant flaws, such as warping, cracking, or the formation of unwanted pores.

Many significant ceramic products, such as thermal insulation and filters for liquids and gases, require controlled porosity, both in terms of percentage by volume and in pore diameters and distributions. In fact, texture compromises the prime distinction between refractories, whitewares, and electronic and glass-ceramics that may otherwise be identical in chemical and mineral composition.

Ceramics see their widest use in devices as components of implants, particularly orthopedic (bone replacement) implants. The ceramics used in orthopedic applications include both the man-made (or artificial) ones and the natural ceramic of bones, dentine, and enamel—hydroxyapatite. All such ceramics may be either bioinert or bioactive, based on whether they are chemically bonded to the natural bone structure or are in direct opposition to one another.

It is also important to determine whether the ceramics are porous or not when considering their use in devices. Tables 3.12 and 3.13 summarize the significant properties of the most important ceramics used in devices.

8.   Physical Properties of Polymers, Elastomers, and Silicones

As pointed out earlier, it is important to understand the physical properties of materials used in devices. Such properties are the primary concern of engineers, but the toxicologist needs to be conversant with them to understand their importance in device performance.

Major physical properties and (if applicable) their ASTM-designated test methods are as follows (Krause et al., 1983):

> *Tensile strength*—the greatest longitudinal stress a substance can withstand without rupture (pounds per square inch; PSI); instrument: Monsanto Tensometer T-10 or Instron model # 1122 (ASTM D412).
>
> *Abrasion resistance*—1 in.^{2} sample mounted in Gardner abrasion tester (Pacific Scientific) with abrasion sponge; run 1000 passes and report weight loss as percentage (ASTM D2486).
>
> *Elongation*—at breakpoint in tensile strength measurement, determine percentage elongation (how much base is stretched before breaking; ASTM D412).

TABLE 3.12 Properties of Typical Ceramics Used in Devices

	Strength	Tensile modulus	Creep modulus	Fatigue life	Lubricity	Water permeability	Water absorption
Single-crystal alumina	High	High	High	High	Mod	Low	Low
Porous alumina	High	High	High	—	—	High	Low
Hydroxyapatite	Mod.	Mod.	High	High	—	Low	Low

TABLE 3.13 Ceramic Materials Used in Devices

Material	Al_2O_3	C	C	C	ZrO_2
Condition	HP	LTI	VT	ULTI	SHP
Source	[1,2]	[3]	[3]	[3]	[4]
Density (g/cm³)	3.93	1.7–2.2	1.4–1.6	1.5–2.2	6.1
Grain size (µm)	3–4	30–40*	10–40*	8–15*	<0.5
E (tensile) (GPa)	380	18–28	24–31	14–21	200
Hardness (Hv)	23,000	150–250	150–200	150–250	1300
σ_{UFS}(MPa)	550	280–560	70–210	350–700	1200
Σ_{UCS}(MPa)	4,500	—	—	—	—

Note: HP: high purity; LTI: low temperature isotropic; SHP: sintered, hot isostatic pressed; ULTI: ultralow temperature isotropic; VT: vitreous (glassy); *: angstroms; —:unavailable.

Modulus—during tensile strength and elongation tests, data are identified at specified percentage of elongation value (100%, 200%, 300%) and the process (PSI) measured at each elongation (ASTM D412).

Tensile set—stretch 1-in. die cut (ASTM 412c), to 300% for 3 min; relax for 3 min; measure difference; standard <10% (Monsanto T10 Tensometer ASTM F703 Sec. 7.1.2).

Tear resistance—place test bar with standard partial cut in Instron test apparatus; stretch to propagate tear to breakage (in PSI; ASTM D624).

Wear—in vivo, measure as linear reduction in thickness at the contacting surface as determined by serial X rays (Dickson, 1979; Dumbleton, 1981; McKellup et al., 1981; 1984; McKellop and Clarke, 1983; Seedhom et al., 1973; and Tillotson et al., 1971).

Hardness (compression modulus at surface) tests are as follows:

Point penetration test—degree of penetration of a given diameter point under a known force over a fixed time.

Rockwell hardness tests—nonrecoverable indentation is measured after a major load is imposed for 15 sec. followed by a 10-kg load for 15 sec. The size of major load and ball diameter is used as Rockwell hardness durometer test; Similar to Rockwell tests except that indenter is spring loaded and an equilibrium indentation load determined; indentation depth established the hardness.

Surface characterization for pre- and postimplant evaluation should include (DePalma, 1986) the following:

Porosity
Surface tension

Infrared spectroscopy
Scanning electron microscopy
Surface charge (zeta potential)
Energy dispersive X-ray analysis
Surface texture analysis (stylus)

Impact strength tests include pendulum, falling ball, and tensile impact tests. For pendulum tests (IZOD, Sharpey), a weighted pendulum is released from a fixed height and allowed to impact a fixed specimen at the bottom of the swing (notched sample). The amount of energy absorbed by the sample is then measured.

Permeability of films for polymers can be determined by permeation kinetics (Berg and von Hippel, 1985), as follows:

Use Franz diffusion cells (Crown Glass, Somerville, NJ).
40-cm-diameter disc of film (thickness important).
Measure diffusion into liquid sink with time.
Can measure analytically or by labeling techniques.

Polymeric gel testing can be done for the following:

Gel cohesivity—measure of ability of gel to resist flow; can measure with
    funnellike orifice and measure distance of gel flow in 30 min.
Gel penetration—measure of gel stiffness; a gel penetrometer measures
    this by recording the distance that a probe falls through the gel in 5 sec.

Creep resistance test characteristics include the following:

Measurements made by placing a sample under a fixed tensile load and
    measuring its elongation with time.
Magnitude of tensile load is important.
Data often presented as elongation versus time for different stress levels.

Polymers.   Surface porosity and bacterial intrusion can be a concern if pores are 0.1 mm, and can be contaminated with micro-organisms such as staphylococcus ($\sim$1 μm), streptococus ($\sim$0.8–1 μm), pseudomonas (0.5–3 μm), and TB (0.2–0.6 μm) (Freter, 1980).

Viscosity.   Viscosity is the internal resistance to flow exhibited by a fluid—the ratio of shearing stress to rate of shear. A liquid has a viscosity of 1 poise if a force of 1 dyne/cm^2 causes two parallel liquid surfaces 1 cm^2 in area and centimeter apart to move past one another at a velocity of 1 cm/sec. One poise equals 100 centipoise. Viscosity in centipoise divided by the liquid density at the same temperature gives kinematic viscosity in centistokes (CS). One hundred centistokes equal one stroke. To determine kinematic viscosity, the time is measured for an exact quantity of liquid to flow by gravity through a standard capillary. Water is the primary viscosity standard, with an accepted viscosity at 20°C of 0.01002 poise. Hydrocarbon liquids such as hexane are less viscous. Molasses may have a viscosity of several hundred centistokes, while for a very heavy lubrication oil the viscosity may be 100 centistokes. There are many empirical methods for measuring viscosity. A more thorough description of physical, mechanical, thermal, and chemical methods for polymer evaluation can be found in Shah (1998).

9. Biologically Derived Materials

There is an increasing use of biologically derived materials (typically from pigs and cattle) for tissue repair and prosthesis uses. While the normal concerns for artificially derived materials may be lessened for these, concerns of infection, particularly by such agents as prions and viruses, and of immunologically based tissue–tissue interactions are heightened.

C. Factors Influencing Test Selection

Actual decisions as to what testing is to be done are based on a complex set of reasons, some of which are pecular to the company involved and some of which are generally applicable. The author labels these reasons as "factors of influence," and believes that they can be summarized as belonging to the seven categories presented in Table 3.14. The first of these factors, regulatory requirements, was extensively covered in the first chapter. The others are discussed briefly here.

1. Perceptions

It should be kept in mind that what people believe or perceive is as important as what is real. What materials are used, how a device is designed, and what testing is done are significantly influenced by current public and health care provider beliefs. Concerns about and memories of silicones, latex, toxic shock syn-

TABLE 3.14 Factors
of Influence on Safety
Test Selection

Regulatory requirements
Perceptions
Hazard identification
Risk assessment
Animal welfare concerns
Claims
Time and economics

drome, and so on, may dictate more extensive testing than regulations. Beliefs can also influence device acceptance, such as in the case of IUDs (intrauterine devices) as contraceptive devices after the publicity around the Dalkon Shield.

2. Hazard Identification

The most fundamental requirement in testing is to quickly identify (or eliminate the possibility of) any significant hazards, their services, and how to eliminate or minimize them if they are present. Many of the tests used for medical devices are really designed to act as sensitive screens for hazards. They purposely maximize the potential to get a positive response (i.e., they are very sensitive). Such tests share a number of common characteristics (see Table 3.15) and do not establish the relevance of such findings of hazard to real-life device use.

3. Risk Assessment

The process of taking the results of toxicity and biocompatibility tests of literature findings and all other sources of information and then relating them to actual device use in the marketplace is risk assessment. The need to be able to perform a meaningful and convincing risk assessment may require the conduct of additional tests that allow for the quantification of risk (which screens usually do not). Such tests are usually focused on a single well-defined endpoint (such as mucosal irritation) as identified in a hazard identification test or screen, and have their own set of characteristics as summarized in Table 3.15. Table 3.16 speaks to those of specific toxicity tests. It should be pointed out at this point that all substances (even water and green apples) are toxic at some dose. The real-life hazard is when the dose at which harm may occur is within the realm of likely exposure. Table 3.17 address the point of relative toxicity.

4. Claims

Claims are what is said in labeling and advertising, and may be either of a positive (therapeutic or beneficial) or negative (lack of an adverse effect) nature. The

TABLE 3.15 Characteristics of Screens and Specific Toxicity Assays Screens

Assay for overt toxicity
Macroscopic, qualitative data
Dose not related to material application
Limited definition of test substance
Rapid
Usually single exposure
Small number of replicates
No internal statistical validity
Minimum false negatives and maximum false positives

TABLE 3.16 Characteristics of Specific Toxicity Assays

Assay for no adverse effect level and toxic level
Quantitative data
Systematic observations on multiple end points (health behavior, nutrition, necropsy, pathology, clinical chemistry, hematology, etc.)
Specific data on strength, identity, and purity of test material
Short or long duration
Quantitative extrapolation of safely allowed
Single well-defined end point
Formal internal statistical validity

positive or efficacy claims are not usually the direct concern of the toxicologist, although it must be kept in mind that such claims must be proved and can easily exceed the limits of the statutory definition of a device, turning the product into a drug or combination product.

Negative claims such as "nonirritating" or "hypoallergenic" also must be proved, and are generally the responsibility of the product safety professional. There are special tests for such claims.

5. Time and Economies

The final factors of influence or arbitrator of test conduct and timing are the requirements of the marketplace, the resources of the organization, and the economic worth of the product.

Plans for filings with regulatory agencies and for market launches are typically set before actual testing (or final stage development) is undertaken, as the need to be in the marketplace in a certain time frame is critical. Such timing and economic issues are beyond the scope of this volume, but must be considered.

IV. PRIOR KNOWLEDGE

The appropriate starting place for the safety assessment of any new chemical entity, particularly a potential new material for a medical device, is to first determine what is already known about the material and whether or not there are any close structural or pharmacological analogues (pharmacological analogues being agents with assumed similar pharmacological mechanisms). Such a determination requires complete access to the available literature. In using this information, one must keep in mind that there is both an initial requirement to build a data file or-base, and a need to update such a store on a regular basis. Updating a database requires not merely adding to what is already there, but also discarding out-of-date (i.e., now known to be incorrect) information and reviewing the entire structure for connections and organization.

TABLE 3.17 Classification of Chemical Hazards

		Routes of administration		
Commonly used term	Single oral dose, rats LD^{50}	Inhalation 4-hr vapor exposure mortality 1/6–4/6 rats (ppm)	Single application to skin of rabbits LD^{50}	Probable lethal dose for man
Extremely toxic	1 mg or less/kg	10	5 mg or less/kg	A taste, a drop, 1 grain
Highly toxic	1–50 mg/kg[a]	10–100	5–43 mg/kg	1 teaspoonful (4 ml)
Moderately toxic	50–500 mg/kg	100–1000	44–340 mg/kg	1 ounce (30 g)
Slightly toxic	0.5–5 g/kg	1000–10,000	0.35–2.81 g/kg	1 pint (250 g)
Practically g/kg quart or nontoxic	5–15 g/kg	10,000–100,000	22.6 or more g/kg	>1 quart or >1 liter

[a] By law, those materials with oral LD$_{50}$s of 50 mg/kg or less in rats are classified as class B poisons and must be labeled "Poison." Class A poisons are defined not by testing, but by inclusion on a regulatorily mandated list (CFR 173, section 173.326):

"S 173.326 Poison A.

(a) for the purpose of Parts 170–189 of this subchapter extremely dangerous poison. Class A. are poisonous gases or liquids of such nature that a very small amount of the gas, or vapor of the liquid, mixed air is dangerous to life. This class includes the following:

(1) Bromactone.

(2) Cyanogen.

(3) Cyanogen chloride containing less than 019 percent water.

(4) Diphosgene.

(5) Ethyldichlorarsine.

(6) Hydrocyanic acid (see Note 1 of this paragraph).

(7) [Reserved]

(8) Methyldichlorarsine.

(9) [Reserved]

(10) Nitrogen peroxide (tetroxide).

(11) [Reserved]

(12) Phosgene (diphosgene).

(13) Nitrogen tetroxide-nitric oxide mixtures containing up to 33.2 percent weight nitric oxide.

NOTE 1: Diluted solutions of hydrocyanic acid of not exceeding 5 percent strength are classed as poisonous articles. Class B (see S 173–343)."

(b) Poisonous gases or liquids, Class A. as defined in paragraph (a) of this section, except as provided in S 173.331, must not be offered for transportation by rail express.

[239 FR 18753, Dec. 29, 1964. Redesignated at 32 FR 5606, Apr. 5, 1967, and amended by

Amdt. 173-94, 41 FR 16081, Apr. 15, 1976;

Amdt. 173-94A, 41 FR 40883, Sept. 20, 1976.

Source: From Deichman and Gerard (1966) and Gad and Chengelis (1998).

The first step in any new literature review is to obtain as much of the following information as possible:

1.   Correct chemical identity, including molecular formula, Chemical Abstracts Service (CAS) registry number, common synonyms, trade names, and a structural diagram. Gosselin et al. (1984) and Ash and Ash (1994; 1995) are excellent sources of information on existing commercial products and their components and uses.
2.   Chemical composition (if a mixture) and major impurities.
3.   Production and use information.
4.   Chemical and physical properties (physical state, vapor pressure, pH, solubility, chemical reactivity, etc.).
5.   Any structurally related chemical substances that are already on the market or in production.
6.   Known or presumed biological properties.

Collecting the above information is not only important for hazard assessment (high vapor pressure would indicate high inhalation potential, just as high and low pH would indicate high irritation potential), but the prior identification of all intended use and exposure patterns may provide leads to alternative information sources. For example, drugs to be used as antineoplastics or antibiotics may already have extensive toxicology data obtainable from government or private sources. A great deal of the existing toxicity information (particularly information on acute toxicity) is not available in the published or electronic literature because of concerns about the proprietary nature of this information and the widespread opinion that it does not have enough intrinsic scholarly value to merit publication. This unavailability is unfortunate, as it leads to considerable replication of effort and expenditure of resources that could be better used elsewhere. It also means that an experienced toxicologist must use an informal search of the unpublished literature of his colleagues as a supplement to searches of the published and electronic literature.

There are now numerous published texts that should be considered for use in literature-reviewing activities. An alphabetic listing of 24 of the more commonly used hard copy sources for safety assessment data is provided in Table 3.18. Obviously, this is not a complete listing and consists of only the general multipurpose texts that have a wider range of applicability for toxicology. Texts dealing with specialized classes of agents (e.g., disinfectants) or with specific target organ toxicity (neurotoxins and teratogens) are generally beyond the scope of this text. Parker (1988) should be consulted for details on the use of these texts. Wexler (2000), Parker (1988), and Sidhu et al. (1989) should be consulted for more extensive listings of the literature and computerized databases. Such sources can be off direct (free) Internet sources (where one must beware of GIGO—garbage in, garbage out), commercial databases, and package products,

TABLE 3.18 Published Information Sources for Safety Assessment

Title	Author, date
Annual Report on Carcinogens	National Toxicology Program, 2000
Burger's Medicinal Chemistry	Wolff, 1997
Carcinogenically Active Chemicals	Lewis, 1991
Catalog of Teratogenic Agents	Shepard, 1998
Chemical Hazards of the Workplace	Proctor and Hughes, 1978
Chemically Induced Birth Defects	Schardein, 1999
Clinical Toxicology of Commercial Products	Gosselin et al., 1984
Contact Dermatitis	Cronin, 1980
Criteria Documents	NIOSH, various
Current Intelligence Bulletins	NIOSH, various
Dangerous Properties of Industrial Materials	Sax, 2000
Documentation of the Threshold Limit Values for Substances in Workroom Air	ACGIH, 1986
Encyclopedia of Toxicology	Wexler, 1998
Handbook of Toxic and Hazardous Chemicals	Sittig, 1985
Hygienic Guide Series	AIHA, 1980
Hamilton and Hardy's Industrial Toxicology	Finkel, 1983
Medical Toxicology	Ellenhorn, 1997
Merck Index	Budavari, 1989
NIOSH/OSHA Occupational Health Guidelines for Chemical Hazards	Mackison, 1981
Patty's Industrial Hygiene and Toxicology	Clayton and Clayton, 1981
Physician's Desk Reference	Barnhart, annual
Registry of Toxic Effects of Chemical Substances (RTECS)	NIOSH, 1984
Casarett and Doull's Toxicology: The Basic Science of Poisons	Klassen, 1996
Toxicology of the Eye	Grant, 1993

to mention just the major categories. Appendix C provides addresses for major free Internet sources.

A. Miscellaneous Reference Sources

There are some excellent published information sources covering some specific classes of chemicals; for example, heavy metals, plastics, resins, or petroleum hydrocarbons. The National Academy of Science series Medical and Biologic Effects of Environment Pollutants covers 10 to 15 substances considered to be environmental pollutants. CRC Critical Reviews in Toxicology is a well-known scientific journal that over the years has compiled over 20 volumes of extensive literature reviews of a wide variety of chemical substances. A photocopy of this journal's topical index will prevent one from overlooking information that may be contained in this important source. Trade organizations such as the Fragrance Industry Manufacturers Association and the Chemical Manufacturers Association have extensive toxicology databases from their research programs that are readily available to toxicologists of member companies. Texts that deal with specific target organ toxicity—neurotoxicity, hepatotoxicity, or hematotoxicity—often contain detailed information on a wide range of chemical structures. Such published information sources as the Target of Organ Toxicity series (Taylor & Francis, now halfway through revision) are examples of the types of publications that often contain important information on many industrial chemicals that may be useful either directly or by analogy. Upon discovery that the material one is evaluating may possess target organ toxicity, a cursory review of these types of texts is warranted.

For many toxicologists the online literature search has changed over the last decade, from an occasional, sporadic activity to a semicontinuous need. Usually, nontoxicology-related search capabilities are already in place in many companies, therefore all that is needed is to expand the information source to include some of the databases that cover the type of toxicology information one desires. If no capabilities exist within an organization, however, one can approach a university, consultant, or a private contract laboratory and utilize its online system at a reasonable rate. It is even possible to access most of these sources from home using a personal computer (PC). The major available online databases are as follows:

1. National Library of Medicine. The National Library of Medicine (NLM) information retrieval service contains the well-known and frequently used Medline, Toxline, and Cancerlit databases. Databases commonly used by toxicologists for acute data in the NLM service are the following:
   a. Toxline (Toxicology Information Online) is a bibliographic database covering the pharmacological, biochemical, physiological, environmental, and toxicological effects of drugs and other chemicals. It contains approximately 1.7 million citations, most of which are complete with abstract, index terms, and CAS registry numbers. Toxline citations have publication dates of 1981 to the present. Older information is on Toxline 65 (pre-1965 through 1980).
   b. Medline (Medical Information Online) is a database containing approximately 7 million references to biomedical journal articles published since 1966. These articles, usually with an English abstract, are from over 3000 journals. Coverage of previous years (back to 1966) is provided by back files, which are searchable online, that total some 3.5 million references.

    c.   Toxnet (Toxicology Data Network) is a computerized network of toxicologically oriented data banks. Toxnet offers a sophisticated search and retrieval package that accesses the following three subfiles:

        i.   Hazardous Substances Data Bank (HSDB) is a scientifically reviewed and edited data bank containing toxicological information enhanced with additional data related to the environment, emergency situations, and regulatory issues. Data are derived from a variety of sources, including government documents and special reports. This database contains records for over 4100 chemical substances.

        ii.   Toxicology Data Bank (TDB) is a peer-reviewed data bank focusing on toxicological and pharmacological data, environmental and occupational information, manufacturing and use data, and chemical and physical properties. References have been extracted from a selected list of standard source documents.

        iii.   Chemical Carcinogenesis Research Information System (CCRIS) is a National Cancer Institute-sponsored database derived from both short- and long-term bioassays on 2379 chemical substances. Studies cover carcinogenicity, mutagenicity, promotion, and cocarcinogenicity.

    d.   Registry of Toxic Effects of Chemical Substances (RTECS) is the NLM's online version of the National Institute for Occupational Safety and Health's (NIOSH) annual compilation of substances with toxic activity. The original collection of data was derived from the 1971 toxic substances lists. RTECS data contain threshold limit values, aquatic toxicity ratings, air standards, National Toxicology Program carcinogenesis bioassay information, and toxicological/carcinogenic review information. The National Institute for Occupational Safety and Health is responsible for the file content in RTECS, and for providing quarterly updates to NLM; RTECS currently covers toxicity data on more than 106,000 substances.

2.   The Merck Index.   The Merck Index is now available online for up-to-the-minute access to new chemical entities.

B. Search Procedure

As mentioned in the introduction, chemical composition and identification information should already have been obtained before the chemical is to be searched. With most information retrieval systems this is a relatively straightforward procedure. Citations on a given subject may be retrieved by entering the desired free text terms as they appear in titles, keywords, and abstracts of articles. The search is then initiated by entering the chemical CAS number and/or synonyms. If you are only interested in a specific target organ effect (e.g., carcinogenicity) or specific publication years, searches can be limited to a finite number of abstracts before requesting the printout.

Often it is unnecessary to request a full printout (author, title, abstract). You may choose to review just the author and title listing before selecting out the abstracts of interest. In the long run, this approach may save you computer time, especially if the number of citations being searched is large.

Once you have reviewed the abstracts, the last step is to request photocopies of the articles of interest. Extreme caution should be used in making any final health hazard determination based solely on an abstract or nonprimary literature source.

C. Monitoring Published Literature and Other Research in Progress

Although there are a few other publications offering similar services, the Life Sciences edition of Current Contents (Institute for Scientific Information) is the publication most widely used by toxicologists for monitoring the published literature. Current Contents monitors over 1180 major journals and provides a weekly listing by title and author. Selecting those journal you wish to monitor is one means of selectively monitoring the major toxicology journals.

Aids available to the toxicologist for monitoring research in progress are quite variable. The National Toxicology Program's (NTP) Annual Plan for Fiscal Year 1996 highlights all the accomplishments of the previous year and outlines the research plans for the coming year. The annual plan contains all projects in the president's proposed fiscal year budget that occur within the National Cancer Institute/National Institutes of Health, National Institute of Environmental Health Sciences/National Institutes of Health, National Center for Toxicological Research/Food and Drug Administration, and NIOSH/Centers for Disease Control. This report includes a list of all the chemicals selected for testing in research areas that include but are not limited to mutagenicity, immunotoxicity, teratoly/ reproduction, neurotoxicity, pharmacokinetics, subchronic toxicity, and chronic toxicity/carcinogenicity.

The annual plan also contains a bibliography of NTP publications from the previous year. A companion publication is the 1999 NTP Review of Current DHHS, DOE, and EPA Research Related to Toxicology. Similar to the annual plan, this document provides detailed summaries of both proposed and ongoing research.

Another mechanism for monitoring research in progress is by reviewing abstracts presented at the annual meetings of professional societies such as the

Society of Toxicology, Teratology Society, Environmental Mutagen Society, and American College of Toxicology. These societies usually have their abstracts prepared in printed form; for example, the current Toxicologist contains over 1700 abstracts presented at the annual meeting. Copies of the titles and authors of these abstracts are usually listed in the societies' respective journals, which, in many cases, would be reproduced and could be reviewed through Current Contents.

D. New Sources

Scientists today are more aware than ever before of the existence of what has been called the "information revolution." At no other time in recent history has so much information become available from so many different "traditional" resources, including books, reviews, journals, and meetings, as well as personal PC-based materials such as databases, alerting services, optical-disk-based information, and news media.

The good news for toxicologists interested in the safety of chemical entities of all types is that numerous new computer-based information products are available that can be extremely useful additions to current safety and toxicology libraries. These tools enable one to save considerable time, effort, and money while evaluating the safety of chemical entities.

The primary focus of this section is on the description and applications of the recent innovations of newly emerging information services based on the PC.

1. Kinds of Information

The kinds of information described here are found on three types of PC media—floppy, CD-ROM, and laser disks. The products run the gamut of allowing one to assess current developments on a weekly basis, as well as carry out more traditional reviews of historical information. The general types of information one can cover include basic pharmacology, preclinical toxicology, competitive products, and clinical safety.

The specific products discussed are as follows: two floppy disk-based products called Current Contents on Diskette and Focus On: Global Change; five CD-ROM products called Toxic Release Inventory, Material Safety Data Sheets, CCINFOdisc, Pollution/Toxicology, and Medline Ondisc; and a laser disk product entitled the Veterinary Pathology Slide Bank. We provide a brief synopsis of the major features of each as well as a description of their integration into a functional, PC-based toxicology information center (TIC).

When such a TIC is established, one will find that some unusual benefits accrue. One now has immediate and uninterrupted access to libraries of valuable and comprehensive scientific data. This access is free of "online" constraints and designed to be user friendly, with readily retrievable information available

24 h a day, 7 days a week. The retrieved information can also usually be manipulated in electronic form, so one can use it in reports and/or store it in machine-readable form as ASCII files.

The minimal hardware requirements, which are certainly adequate for all the items discussed here, are an IBM or IBM-compatible PC equipped with at least 640 K RAM, a single floppy disk drive, at least a 40-Mbyte hard disk drive, a CD-ROM drive, a VGA color monitor, and a printer. The basic point here is that hardware requirements are minimal and readily available. In the case of the laser disk products, a laser disk drive and high resolution (VGA) monitor are also required.

PC-Based Information Products: Floppy Disk-Based. We currently have ready access to a rapidly growing variety of relevant information resources. From a current awareness perspective, an excellent source of weekly information is the floppy disk-based product called Current Contents on Diskette (CCOD). Several versions are available; however, the Life Sciences version is most appropriate for this review because of its coverage on a weekly basis of over 1200 journals describing work in the biological sciences. One will note that the product has several useful features, including very quick retrieval of article citations as well as several output options (including either hard copy or electronic storage of references as well as reprint requests).

PC-Based Information Products: CD-ROM Media. The gradual emergence of this technology during the past several years has recently blossomed with the introduction of several CD-ROM products that deal with safety issues surrounding the toxicology and safety of chemicals. CD-ROM media with such information can generally be characterized by two major advantages: they are relatively easy to use and are amazingly quick in retrieving data of interest.

Toxic Release Inventory (TRI). Before embarking on a discussion of products describing health, toxicology, and safety issues, it is well to be aware of a new pilot CD-ROM version of the Environmental Protection Agency's (EPA) 1987 toxic chemical release inventory and hazardous substances fact sheets. This TRI resource, which contains information regarding the annual inventory of hundreds of named toxic chemicals from certain facilities (since 1987), as well as the toxicological and ecological effects of chemicals, is available from the National Technical Information Service (NTIS), U.S. Department of Commerce, Springfield, Virginia 22161.

The list of toxic chemicals subject to reporting was originally derived from those designed for similar purposes by the states of Maryland and New Jersey. As such, over 300 chemicals and categories are noted. (After appropriate rule making, modifications to the list can be made by the EPA.) The inventory is designed to inform the public and government officials about routine and accidental releases of toxic chemicals to the environment.

The CD-ROM version of the database can be efficiently searched with a menu-driven type of software called Search Express. It allows one to search with Boolean expressions as well as individual words and/or frequency of "hits" as a function of the number of documents retrieved on a given topic. Numerous searchable fields have been included, allowing one to retrieve information by a variety of means—for example, the compound name; the chemical registry number; the amount of material released into the air, water, or land; the location of the site of release; and the SIC code of the releasing party. One can also employ ranging methods with available numeric fields and sorting of output.

It is hoped that this shared information will help to increase the awareness, concern, and action by individuals to ensure a clean and safe environment. The TRI database is a significant contribution to that effort and the CD-ROM version is a superb medium with which to widely publicize and make accessible the findings.

Material Safety Data Sheets (MSDS). The MSDS CD-ROM is a useful resource that contains over 33,000 MSDS on chemicals submitted to the Occupational Safety and Health Administration (OSHA) by chemical manufacturers. This resource contains complete MSDS information as well as other important information such as the chemical formula, structure, physical properties, synonyms, registry number, and safety information.

Users can easily search the CD-ROM by employing the Aldrich catalog number, Chemical Abstracts Service CAS number, chemical name, or molecular formula. One can also export the chemical structures to some supported software for subsequent inclusion into work-processing programs. The product is available from Aldrich Chemical Company, Inc., 940 West St. Paul Ave., Milwaukee, WI 54233.

Canadian Centre for Occupational Health and Safety (CCINFO). This set of four CD-ROM disks contains several valuable databases of information that are updated on a quarterly basis: MSDS, CHEM Data, OHS Source, and OHS Data. The MSDS component currently contains over 60,000 MSDS supplied by chemical manufacturers and distributors. It also contains several other databases [RIPP, RIPA, and Pest Management Research Information System (PRIS)], one of which (PRIS) even includes information on pest management products, including their presence and allowable limits in food.

A second disk in the series (CHEM Data) contains comprehensive information from the CHEMINFO, RTECS, and Chemical Evaluation Search and Retrieval System (CESARS) databases, as well as recommendations on the transport of dangerous goods (TDG)/hazardous materials (49CFR).

The third and fourth disks include Occupational Health and Safety (OHS) information. These disks contain databases on resource organizations, resource people, case law, jurisprudence, fatalities, mining incidents, and ADISCAN. Furthermore, information on noise levels, NIOSH (NIOSHTEC) nonionizing radiation levels, and a document information directory system is readily retrievable. These CD-ROM materials are available from the Canadian Centre for Occupational Health and Safety, 250 Main Street East, Hamilton, Ontario L8N 1H6.

Pollution and Toxicology (POLTOX). This CD-ROM library also focuses our attention on environmental health and safety concerns. Scientists working in any industry or capacity that deals with toxic or potentially toxic chemicals will find it very useful. It allows one access to seven major databases in this field in a single search through its use of "linking" features in its software. The distributors of this product have provided us with a spectrum of information dealing with toxic substances and environmental health.

The collection of these databases include five that are available exclusively from Cambridge Scientific Abstracts (CSA)—pollution abstracts, toxicology abstracts, ecology abstracts, health and safety science abstracts, and aquatic pollution and environmental quality abstracts. The abstracts come from journals or digests published by CSA on important issues, including environmental pollution, toxicological studies of industrial chemicals and ecological impacts of biologically active chemicals, as well as health, safety, and risk management in occupational situations. The POLTOX CD-ROM contains over 200,000 records from these sources since 1981.

POLTOX also contains two other useful databases—Toxline (described earlier) and the Food Science and Technology Abstracts (FSTA) libraries. The FSTA component is a reasonably comprehensive collection of information regarding toxicological aspects of compounds found in food, including contamination, poison, and carcinogenic properties. The CD-ROM product is available from Compact Cambridge, 7200 Wisconsin Avenue, Bethesda, MD 20814.

Medline. The Medline database, which comes from the National Library of Medicine, is a superb, indispensable reference library that is particularly strong in its wide coverage of research activities in the biomedical literature. It also encompasses the areas of clinical medicine, health policy, and health care services. Each year, over 300,000 articles are reviewed and indexed into the database. The full bibliographic citations of these articles, usually including the abstract of the published work, are available from numerous vendors in CE-ROM form and are usually updated on a monthly basis.

Information can be accessed from Medline in a variety of ways: by author, title, subject, Chemical Abstracts Service registration number, keyword, publication year, and journal title. Medline Ondisc is the CD-ROM product we employ (from Dialog Information Services, Inc., 3460 Hillview Ave., Palo Alto, CA 94304). It allows access to the full Medline files back to 1984. Each year from that time until 1988 is covered on a single CD-ROM disk; starting in 1989, each disk covers only a six-month time period. The information is accessed through either an easily employed "menu-driven" system or a more standard online type of "command language."

Gower Publishing (Brookfield, VT) has published a series of "electronic handbooks'' providing approved ingredient information on materials used in cosmetics, personal care additives, food additives, and pharmaceuticals. Academic Press, through its Sci-Vision branch, has just (2000) launched an ambitious service of CD ROM-based toxicity database products that are structure-and substructure-searchable.

It is worth noting that the CD-ROM-based system has been seamlessly integrated with both record-keeping and communications (proprietary) software so that one can optionally monitor the use of the online services and easily continue searching in the Dialog online environment after using the CD-ROM-based Medline library. Another very useful feature includes the storage of one's search logic so that repetitive types of searches-over time, for example—can be done very easily.

PC-Based Information Products: Laser Disc

International Veterinary Pathology Slide Bank (IVPSB). This application represents an important complementary approach toward training and awareness using laser disc technology. The IVPSB provides a quality collection of transparencies, laser videodiscs, and interactive computer/videodisc training programs. In particular, the videodisc contains over 21,000 slides from over 60 contributors representing 37 institutions from six countries. These slides are accessible almost instantaneously because of the tremendous storage capacity and rapid random search capabilities of the videodisc through the interactive flexibility of the computer. The information available is of particular interest to toxicologists and pathologists because the visuals illustrate examples of gross lesions of infectious diseases, regional diseases, clinical signs or external microscopy, histopathology, normal histology, cytology and hematology, and parasitology.

The laser disc, a catalog of the entries, a computer database, and selected interactive programs can be obtained from Dr. Wayne Crowell, Dept. of Veterinary Pathology, University of Georgia, Athens, GA 30602.

V. TYPES AND USES OF TESTS

Safety assessment tests used for medical devices can generally be considered as either hazard identification/screens or special studies uniquely designed for specific problems or types of devices. The bulk of this book will look at how each of the significant types of such tests are performed and interpreted. Table 3.19 summarizes the common varieties of available biocompatibility tests and their objectives, as well as where in the test they are considered in detail.

A. Reasonable Man

The reasonable man is a concept in law which, though not universally applicable, still provides guidance as to what one can expect from those that use devices (and

TABLE **3.19** Common Biocompatibility Assays

Cytotoxicity—a screen for adverse short-term biological effects, specifically does it kill cultured maturation cells.

Primary dermal irritation (PDI)—evaluate potential of a single dermal exposure to cause skin irritation.

Eye irritation—evaluation potential of a single ocular exposure to cause eye irritation.

Vaginal mucosal irritation—Evaluates potential for a single exposure to irritate vaginal mucosa.

Intracutaneous reactivity—evaluates potential of a single injection of eluate to irritate or damage cutaneous tissue.

Intramuscular implant—can be from 7 to 28 days long. Does implanted device/ material damage surrounding tissue more than implanted inert "control" material?

Dermal sensitization—evaluate the potential of a material to cause delayed contact hypersensitivity.

Pyrogen/LAL—determines if detectable levels of bacterial endotoxin/fevers causing substances can be elated from material/device.

Acute systemic toxicity—determine the potential of a single dose of a material, at a predetermined level, for lethality.

Carcinogenicity—determines the potential for a material to induce and/or promote the formation of neoplasms.

Mutagenicity—determine the potential of a material to cause undesirable genetic effects.

Hemolysis—determines the potential for a product to lyse red blood cells.

what, therefore, the limits are on uses for which the manufacturer of the device should be considered responsible for ensuring safety). The standard of reasonableness is obviously open to interpretation, but does provide a conceptual basis for determining for which uses one must ensure a device is safe (and for which a precautionary label is required) and for which it is not. The "test" employed in a legal sense is one of foreseeability (i.e., would a reasonable man in the defendant's position foresee a measurable risk to the plaintiff?) (Madden, 1992).

B. Qualifications vs. Process Control

Most of this book addresses testing from the point of view of what is done to quality a product—to get it access to the marketplace. Such testing is done, at a minimum, to meet specific regulatory requirements that one can determine by consulting the appropriate guidelines. Biocompatibility testing, however, does not end once a product is approved for the marketplace; rather, some form of testing must be conducted on an ongoing basis to ensure that the lots of product that enter the marketplace over time continue to be safe. The testing to be done to ensure this is generally specified in the device master file (DMF), but what tests are done and with what frequency is left to the judgment of the manufacturer (who is, however, charged in the GMPs with conducting an adequate program of periodic testing to ensure the continued quality and safety of the product). Such testing is usually derived from the results of qualification testing and product and (manufacturing) process validation studies (Table 3.20). Careful consideration (and statistical analysis of these and the variables that are involved in the manufacturing process) generally identify which biocompatibility tests best serve to identify when the product is not as it should be, due to either the process not being in control (or there having been a series of small, incremental changes that in summation have altered the process) or when changes in vendor-supplied materials have occurred. A statistical analysis of the data will also clarify sampling strategies and the required frequency of testing. This will lead to specification of a routine testing program for lot release, most commonly utilizing the approaches shown in Table 3.21.

The Device Master File (DMF) on plant manufacturing SOPs need to specify what happens when a lot fails routine or release testing. It is sometimes wise to have a conditional two-tier test scheme, an inexpensive but somewhat sensitive screening test (such as cytotoxicity) that is performed on some specified regular basis, and a second, more specific (and expensive) test that is conducted in those cases in which a lot fails the screening test.

C. Tiers of Concern: Consumers, Health Care Providers, and Manufacturing Employees

This book focuses primarily on the tests done to meet regulatory requirements for new product approval. Such requirements are intended to ensure the safety on the end-use consumer of devices, the patients. Knowing what the intended use and claims are for a product, it is generally easy to identify what the routes, duration, and extent of ''exposure'' or ''dosing'' will be.

Patients represent only the final tier of those who will be exposed to a device, however. There are (at least) two other tiers that we must consider. The others are the health care providers and those involved in actually producing and packaging the devices. Health care providers include nurses, doctors, laboratory technicians, pharmacists, and public health workers. Though they do not use the devices on a daily basis, they will handle and apply or administer the products. As such, they will have different routes and durations of exposure that must be considered and evaluated for safety. Dermal exposure in particular is likely to be more extensive.

Likewise, those involved in manufacturing and packaging the product will have significantly different exposures. For these individuals, we must also be

TABLE 3.20   Product and Process Validation

This is a series of qualification studies to demonstrate that manufacturing pro-
    cess controls are sufficient for preproduction quality assurance requirements
    and product specifications. Testing is performed to verify the effectiveness of
    such control and to evaluate the biological effects of processing aids added
    during manufacture.
Environmental control
    Environmental monitoring program
    Microorganism identification
    Viable and nonviable particulate analysis
Manufacturing process control—initial qualification and ongoing control
    Raw material characterization (compare effects of process on characteristics
        determined in phase I)
    Infrared analysis
    Cytotoxicity
    Physiochemical tests (USP, JP, etc.)
    Other materials characterization tests
    Bioburden testing
    Process water system validation
    Purified water monograph tests, USP
    Water for injection monograph tests, USP
    Endotoxin concentrations (LAL testing)
    Quality device cleaning processes
    Package qualifications
Sterility
    Bioburden testing and organism identification
    Biological indicator studies (sport count, D-value)
    Sterilization cycle development
    Sterilization cycle validation, plan for periodic revalidation
    Dose determination studies (AAMI) plan for quarterly dose audits
    Sterility tests
    EO dissipation curve studies and assessment of use exposure levels (AAMI/
        ISO)
    Package validation
Finished product qualification—single use or reusable
    Physical testing for function and performance stability
    Chemical residues
    Testing for bacterial endotoxins
        In vitro, limulus amoebocyte lysate (LAL)
        In vivo, rabbit pyrogen tests
    Biocompatibility
        Cytotoxicity test
        Hemocompatibility test

TABLE **3.20** Continued

Special material and device tests
  Chemistry tests
  Microbiology tests
  Toxicology tests
Nonviable particulate analysis
Label claim (instructions) for reusable devices
  Decontamination
  Cleaning
  Disinfection/sterilization
Other product specific testing
Shelf-life stability qualification
  Accelerated aging studies
  Real-time aging

TABLE **3.21** Routine Testing

Release testing involves what is performed routinely to satisfy GMP and ISO requirements for finished product testing prior to the release of product for distribution. In addition, phase IV includes testing that may be incorporated into the manufacturer's quality assurance audit program by conducting periodic raw material and finished product testing in order to document that materials and product conform to specifications.
Release testing
  Endotoxin concentration limulus amebocyte lysate (LAL), USP
  Pyrogenicity rabbit test, USP
  Safety test, USP infusion/transfusion assemblies
  Sterility testing
  Microbial limit test, USP
  Cytotoxicity, USP/ISO
  Materials characterization
Periodic audit testing
  Endotoxin concentration limulus amebocyte lysate (LAL), USP
  Pyrogenicity rabbit test, USP
  Cytotoxicity raw materials finished products
  In vitro hemolysis test for blood contract products
  EO residual testing
  Materials characterization
  Physical testing
  Particulate testing
  Bioburden testing

Source: HIMA, 1985.

concerned with exposure to materials used in device construction and formulation. The potential for inhalation exposure is most likely here.

D. Sterilization and Cleanliness

It goes without saying that microbial contamination of devices must be controlled and that appropriate steps must be taken to sterilize products and materials. The subject is addressed later in this volume in some detail. It should also be remembered, however, that the means of sterilization (ethylene oxide, radiation, chemical sterilization, or steam) may both affect device quality and, in some cases, carry their own biocompatibility concerns. Here, residuals are the issue.

Finally, it must be stressed that cleanliness—in the sense of exclusion of foreign matter (even such seemingly innocuous things as lint and dust)—is essential. If such foreign materials should gain entry to the body, they can trigger dangerous immune modulated responses (Turco and Davis, 1973). FDA has specifically considered the problem of particles in medical devices from the perspective of physiological effects and provided guidance on the issue (Marlowe, 1980).

REFERENCES

American Conference of Governmental Industrial Hygienists (ACGIH). (1986). Documentation of the Threshold Limit Values for Substances in Workroom Air, 5th ed. ACGIH, Cincinnati.
American Industrial Hygiene Association (AIHA). (1980). Hygienic Guide Series, vols. I and II. AIHA, Akron, OH.
Ash, M. and Ash, I. (1994). Cosmetic and Personal Care Additives, electronic handbook. Gower, Brookfield, VT.
Ash, M. and Ash, I. (1995). Food Additives, electronic handbook, Gower, Brookfield, VT.
ASTM. (1984c). Test method for Rockwell hardness of plastics and insulating materials. In: ASTM Annual Book of Standards, American Society of Testing Materials, Philadelphia, procedure D-785-65.
ASTM. (1984d). Test method for rubber property-durometer hardness. In: ASTM Annual Book of Standards, American Society of Testing Materials, Philadelphia, procedure D-2991-71.
ASTM. (1984.). Test method for water absorption of plastics. In: ASTM Annual Book of Standards, American Society of Testing Materials, Philadelphia, procedure D-570-81.
ASTM. (1984.). Test methods for impact resistance of plastics and electrical insulating materials. In: ASTM Annual Book of Standards, American Society of Testing Materials, Philadelphia, procedure D-244-80.
ASTM. (1984.). Test methods for tensile, compressive and flexural creep and creep rupture of plastics. In: ASTM Annual Book of Standards, American Society of Testing Materials, Philadelphia, procedure D-2990-77.

ASTM-F56. (1986). Standard specification for stainless steel sheet and strip for surgical implants, Amer. Soc. Test. Mat., 13.01:7–9.

Autian, J. (1980). Plastics. In: Caserett and Doull's Toxicology: The Basic Science of Poisons, 2nd ed. (J. Doull, C. D. Klassen, and M. O. Amdur, eds.), Macmillan, New York, pp. 531–556.

Barnhart, E. R. (1999). Physician's Desk *Reference*, Medical Economics Company, Oradell, NJ.

Berg, O. G. and von Hippel, P. H. (1985). Diffusion-controlled macromolecular interactions, Ann. Rev. Biophys. Biophys. Chem., 14:131–160.

Billmeyer, F. W. (1971). Textbook of Polymer Science, Wiley, New York.

Bommer, J., Waldher, R., and Ritz, E. (1983). Silicone storage disease in long-term hemodialysis patients, Contr. Nephrol., 36:115–126.

Budavari, S. (1989). The Merck Index, 11th ed. Merck and Company, Rahway, NJ.

Clayton, D. G. and Clayton, F. E., eds. (1981). Patty's Industrial Hygiene and Toxicology, 3rd revised ed., vols. 2A, 2B, and 2C. Wiley, New York.

Cronin, E. (1980). Contact Dermatitis, Churchill Livingston, Edinburgh.

Deichmann, W. and Gerard, H. (1996). Toxicology of Drugs and Chemicals, Academic, New York.

DePalma, V. A. (1986). Apparatus for zeta potential measurement of rectangular flow cells, Rev. Sci. Instr. 51:1390–1395.

Dickson, G. (1979). Physical and chemical properties and wear, J. Dent. Res. 58:1535–1543.

Dumbleton, J. H. (1981). General considerations in friction and wear measurement. In: Tribology of Natural and Artificial Joints. Elsevier, New York, pp. 110–148.

Dumitriu, S. (1994). Polymeric Biomaterials, Marcel Dekker, New York.

Elbert, J. G., McKinney, P. W., Conn, J. Jr., Binder, P., and Beal, J. M. (1971). Polyglycolic acid synthetic absorbable sutures, Amer. J. Surg., 121(5):561–565.

Ellenhorn, M. J. (1997). Medical Toxicology, 2nd ed. Elseiver, New York.

Finkel, A. J. (1983). Hamilton and Hardy's Industrial Toxicology, 4th ed. John Wright PSG, Boston.

Frazza, E. J. and Schmitt, E. E. (1971). A new absorbable suture, J. Biomed. Mat. Res. Sym., 1:43–58.

Freter, R. (1980). Mechanism of association of bacteria with mucosal surfaces, Ciba Found. Sump., 80:36–55.

Gad, S. C. and Chengelis, C. P. (1998). Acute Toxicology, 2nd ed. Academic, San Diego, CA.

Gosselin, R. E., Smith, R. P., and Hodge, H. C. (1984). Clinical Toxicology of Commercial Products, 5th ed. Williams & Wilkins, Baltimore.

Grant, W. M. (1993). Toxicology of the Eye, 4th ed. Charles C. Thomas, Springfield, IL.

Hardman, B. and Torkelson, A. (1986). Silicones. In: Encyclopedia of Polymer Science and Engineering (H. F. Mark et al. eds.), Wiley, New York, pp. 204–308.

Haslam, J., Willis, H. A., and Squirrell, D. C. M. (1972). Identification and Analysis of Plastics, 2nd ed. Ififfe, London.

Heggers, J. P., Kassovsky, N., Parsons, R. W., Robson, M. C., Pelley, R. P., and Raine, T. J. (1983). Biocompatibility of silicone implants, Ann. Plast. Surg., 11:38–45.

HIMA Report 85-1. (1985). Guidelines for the Preclinical Safety Evaluation of Materials

Used in Medical Devices (T. J. Henry, ed.). Health Industry Manufacturers Association, Washington, DC.

Institute for Scientific Information (ISI). (1986). Current Contents—Life Sciences. ISI, Philadelphia.

ISO. (1997). ISO 10993-16 Toxicokinetic Study Design for Degradation Products and Leachables.

Kambric, H. E., Muraboyoshi, S., and Nose, Y. (1986). Biomaterials in artificial organs, Chem. Egr. News (April 14):30–48.

Katz, A. R. and Turner, R. J. (1970). Evaluation of tensile and absorption properties of polyglycolic acid sutures, Surg. Gyn. Ob. 131:701–716.

Klassen, C. D. (1996). Casarett and Doull's Toxicology, McGraw–Hill, New York.

Krause, A., Lange, A., and Ezrin, M. (1983). Plastics Analysis Guide, Hansu, New York.

Kroschowitz, J. (1990). Concise Encyclopedia of Polymer Science and Engineering, Wiley, New York.

Laopahand, T., Osman, E. M., Morley, A. R., Ward, M. K., and Kerr, D. N. S. (1982). Accumulation of silicone elastomers in regular dialysis, Proc. EDTA, 19:143–152.

Lewis, R. J. (1991). Carcinogenically Active *Chemicals*, Van Nostrand Reinhold, New York.

Mackison, F. (1981). Occupational Health Guidelines for Chemical *Hazards*, Dept. of Health and Human Services (NIOSH)/Department of Labor (OSHA) DHHS no. 81–123. U.S. Government Printing Office, Washington, DC.

Madden, M. S. (1992). Toxic Torts Handbook, Lewis Publishers, Boca Raton, FL.

Marlowe, D. E. (1980). Particles in Medical *Devices*, U.S. Food and Drug Administration, Springfield, VA; Natl. Tech. Information Service (PB81-131625).

McGregor, R. R. (1953). Silicones in pharmacy, Pharm. Internat., Jan.:24–26, 63.

McKellop, H., Clarke, I., Markolf, K., et al. (1981). Friction and wear properties of polymer, metal, and ceramic prosthetic joint materials evaluated on a multi-channel screening device, J. Biomed. Mat. Res. 15:619–653.

McKellop, H., Hosseninian, A., and Burgoyne, K. (1984). Polyethylene wear against titanium alloy compared to stainless steel and cobalt-chromium alloys, *Transactions of the Second World Congress on Biomaterials—Tenth Annual Meeting of the Society of Biomaterials*, Washington, DC, April 27–May 1.

McKellop, H. A. and Clarke, I. C. (1983). Evolution and evaluation of materials—Screening machines and joint simulators in predicting in-vivo wear phenomena. In: Functional Behavior of Orthopedic Biomaterials (P. Ducheyne, G. W. Hastings, eds.). CRC Press, Boca Raton, FL.

McMurrer, M. C., Ed. (1985/1986). *Plastics Compounding Redbook*, HBJ Publications, pp. 14–74.

Miripol, J. E. and Stern, I. J. (1977). Decreased accumulation of phthalate plasticizer during storage of blood as packed cells, Transfusion, 17:71–72.

National Institute for Occupational Safety and Health (NIOSH). NIOSH Criteria for a Recommended Standard for Occupational Exposure to XXX, Dept. of Health, Education and Welfare, Cincinnati.

National Institute for Occupational Safety and Health (NIOSH) (19XX). NIOSH Current Intelligence *Bulletins*, Dep. of Health, Education and Welfare, Cincinnati.

National Institute for Occupational Safety and Health (NIOSH) (1984). Registry of Toxic Effects of Chemical Substances, 11th ed., vols. 1–3. Dept. of Health and Human Services, DHHS no. 83-107, 1983 and RTECS supplement DHHS 84-101, Washington, DC.

National Toxicology Program. (2000). Nineteenth Annual Report on *Carcinogens*. Dept. of Health and Human Services, Washington, DC, PB 85-134633.

National Toxicology Program. (1999). Review of Current DHHS, DOE, and EPA Research Related to Toxicology, Dept. of Health and Human Services, NTP-85-056, U.S. Government Printing Office, Washington, DC.

Parker, C. M. (1988). Available Toxicology Information Sources and Their Use. In: Product Safety Evaluation Handbook (S. C. Gad, ed.). Marcel Dekker, New York, pp. 23–41.

Peck, C. C., Odom, D. G., Friedman, H. I., Albro, P. W., Hass, J. R., Brody, J. T., and Jess, D. A. (1979). Di-2-ethylehexyl phthalate (DEHP) and mono-1-ethylhexyl phthalate (MEHP) accumulation in whole blood and red cell concentrates, Transfusion, 19: 137–416.

Petersen, M. C., Vine, J., Ashley, J. J., and Nation, R. L. (1981). Leaching of 2-(2-phdroxy-ethylmercapto)benzothiazole into contents of disposable syringes, J. Pharm. Sci., 70:1139–1143.

Proctor, N. H. and Hughes, J. P. (1978). Chemical Hazards of the Workplace, Lippincott, Philadelphia.

Rochow, E. G. (1951). In Introduction to the Chemistry of the Silicones, Wiley, New York.

Sasakawa, S. and Mitomi, Y. (1978). Di-2-ethylhexylphthalate (DEHP) content of blood or blood components stored in plastic bags, Vox Sang., 34:81–86.

Sax, N. I. (2000). Dangerous Properties of Industrial Materials, 10th ed. Van Nostrand Reinhold, New York.

Schardein, J. L. (1999). Chemically Induced Birth Defects, 3rd ed. Marcel Dekker, New York.

Schmitt, E. E. and Polistina, R. A. (1967). Surgical Sutures. U.S. patent 3,297,033, American Cyanamid.

Seedhom, B., Dowson, D., and Wright, V. (1973). Wear of solid phase formed high density polyethylene in relation to the life of artificial hips and knees, *Wear*, 24:35.

Shah, V. (1998). Handbook of Plastics Testing Technology, Wiley, New York.

Shepard, T. H. (1998). Catalog of Teratogenic Agents, 9th ed. Johns Hopkins University Press, Baltimore.

Sidhu, K. S., Stewart, T. M., and Netton, E. W. (1989). Information sources and support networks in toxicology, J. Amer. Coll. Toxicol. 8:1011–1026.

Sittig, M. (1985). Handbook of Toxic and Hazardous Chemicals, 2nd. ed. Noyes, Park Ridge, NJ.

Steinemann, S. G. (1980). Corrosion of surgical implants—in vivo and in vitro tests. In: Evaluation of Biomaterials (G. D. Winter, J. L. Leroy, and K. de Groot, eds.). Wiley, New York, pp. 1–34.

Tillotson, E. W., Craig, R. G., and Peyton, F. A. (1971). Friction and wear of restorative dental materials. J. Dent. Res., 50:149–154.

Turco, S. and Davis, N. M. (1973). Clinical significance of particular matter: A review of the literature, Hosp. Pharm., 8:137–40.
Wexler, P. (2000). Information Resources in Toxicology, 3rd ed. Elsevier, New York.
Wexler, P. (1998). Encyclopedia of Toxicology, Academic, San Diego, CA.
Wolff, M. E. (1997). Burger's Medicinal Chemistry, 5th ed. Wiley, New York.

4

What to Test
Sampling and Sample Preparation

In Chapter 3 the question of what to test was explored from the aspect of state in the development process—that is, material, component, or device. In the chapters that follow this one, the issues of how to actually perform tests are explained in detail, but here the vital bridge between these is addressed—how to select individual items for testing (sampling) and how to prepare the items selected for the testing process (sample preparation). ISO 10993-12 addresses both these issues (and the selection and use of reference materials) in summary fashion.

I. SAMPLING

Sampling is simply the act of selecting the appropriate items or parts to test so that what is tested (either the product or material, or an extract of either of these) is representative of what is to actually be marketed (i.e., final product as shipped) or used in production. For an approved product, of course, the sampling will be part of an ongoing quality assurance process.

Sampling—the selection of which and how many individual data points will be collected, whether in the form of selecting which to select from an assembly line or whether or not to remove a portion of a lot of plastic for testing—is an essential step upon which all other efforts toward a good experiment or study are based. It is essential for quality control, and is a statistically driven process.

There are three assumptions about sampling that are common to most of the statistical analysis techniques that are used in safety assessment: that the sample is collected without bias, that each member of a sample is collected independently of the others, and that members of a sample are collected with replacements. Precluding bias, both intentional and unintentional, means that at the time of selection of a sample to measure, each portion of the population from which that selection is to be made has an equal chance of being selected. Ways of precluding bias are discussed elsewhere (Gad, 1998).

Independence means that the selection of any portion of the sample is not affected by and does not affect the selection or measurement of any other portion.

Finally, sampling with replacement means that in theory, after each portion is selected and measured, it is returned to the total sample pool and thus has the opportunity to be selected again. This is a corollary of the assumption of independence. Violation of this assumption (which is almost always the case in toxicology and all the life sciences) does not have serious consequences if the total pool from which samples are sufficiently large (say 20 or greater) that the chance of reselecting that portion is small anyway.

There are four major types of sampling methods—random, stratified, systematic, and cluster (Levy and Lemoshow, 1991). Random is by far the most commonly employed method in toxicology. It stresses the fulfilment of the assumption of avoiding bias. When the entire pool of possibilities is mixed or randomized, then the members of the group are selected in the order in which they are drawn from the pool.

Stratified sampling is performed by first dividing the entire pool into subsets or strata, then doing randomized sampling from each stratum. This method is employed when the total pool contains subsets that are distinctly different but in which each subset contains similar members. An example is how to determine the nature of the particle size distribution in a large batch of a powdered plastic resin. Larger pieces or particles are on the top, while progressively smaller particles have settled lower in the container, and at the very bottom, the material has been packed and compressed into aggregates. To determine a timely, representative answer, proportionately sized subsets from each layer or stratum should be selected, mixed, and randomly sampled. This method is used most commonly in material studies.

In systematic sampling, a sample is taken at set intervals (such as every fifth container of reagent or taking a sample of water from a fixed sample point in a flowing stream every hour). This is most commonly employed in quality assurance or (in the clinical chemistry lab) in quality control.

In cluster sampling, the pool is already divided into numerous separate groups (e.g., cases of product), and we select small sets of groups (e.g., several boxes of product from the selected cases), then select a few members from each set. What one gets then is a cluster of measures. Again, this is a method most commonly used in quality control or in environmental studies when the effort and expense of physically collecting a small group of units is significant.

In classic toxicology studies sampling arises in a practical sense in a limited number of situations. The most common of these are as follows:

1. Selecting a subset of animals or test systems from a study to make some measurement (which either destroys or stresses the measured system, or is expensive) at an interval during a study. This may include such cases as doing interim necropsies in a chronic study or collecting and analyzing blood samples from some animals during a subchronic study.
2. Analyzing inhalation chamber atmospheres to characterize aerosol distributions with a new generation system.
3. Analyzing a diet in which a test material has been incorporated.
4. Performing quality control on an analytical chemistry operation by having duplicate analyses performed on some materials.
5. Selecting data to audit for quality assurance and control purposes (Ryan, 1989; CDRH, 1992).

II. RANDOMIZATION

As pointed out above, randomization is an essential step in avoiding bias in sampling. Randomization is the act of assigning a number of items (plates of bacteria or test animals, e.g.) to groups in such a manner that there is an equal chance for any one item to end up in any one group. This is a control against any possible bias in assignment of subjects to test groups. A variation on this is censored randomization, which ensures that the groups are equivalent in some aspect after the assignment process is complete. The most common example of a censored randomization is one in which it is ensured that the body weights of test animals in each group are not significantly different from those in the other groups. This is done by analyzing group weights both for homogeneity of variance and by analysis of variance after animal assignment, then rerandomizing if there is a significant difference at some nominal level, such as p^{TM} 0.10. The process is repeated until there is no difference.

There are several methods for actually performing the randomization process. The three most common are use of a card assignment, use of a random number table, and use of a computerized algorithm.

For the card-based method, individual identification numbers for items (plates or animals, e.g.) are placed one at a time in succession into piles corresponding to the required test groups. The results are a random group assignment.

The random number table method requires only that one have unique numbers assigned to test subjects and access to a random number table. One simply sets up a table with a column for each group to which subjects are to be assigned. We start from the head of any one column for each group to which subjects are to be assigned. (Each time the table is used, a new starting point should be utilized.) If our test subjects number fewer than 100, we utilize only the last two digits in each random number in the table. If they number more than 99 but fewer than 1000, we use only the last three digits. To generate group assignments, we read down a column, one number at a time. As we come across digits that correspond to a subject number, we assign that subject to a group (enter its identifying number in a column), proceeding to assign subjects to groups from left to right, filling one row at a time. After a number is assigned to an animal, any duplication of its unique number is ignored. We use as many successive columns of random numbers as we may need to complete the process.

The third (and now most common) method is to use a random number generator that is built into a calculator or computer program. Procedures for generating these are generally documented in user manuals.

One is also occasionally required to evaluate whether a series of numbers (e.g., an assignment of animals to test groups) is random. This requires the use of a randomization test, of which there are a large variety. The chi-square test can be used to evaluate the goodness of fit to a random assignment. If the result is not critical, a simple sign test will work. For the sign test, we first determine the middle value in the numbers being checked for randomness. We then go through a list of numbers assigned to each group, scoring each as a + (greater than our middle number) or − (less than our middle number). The number of pulses and minuses in each group should be approximately equal.

III. SAMPLE PREPARATION

How samples are prepared for testing once selected is as critical as what samples are tested. With devices, much of sample preparation centers on the derivation of extracts for use in tests in which inclusions of an intact solid device is either inappropriate or not physically positive.

The manufacturer should choose a biologically relevant solvent system that will yield a quantity of extract sufficient to perform tests for biocompatibility. The observed biological response results from the combination of the concentration of the substances that reach the target cells and the intrinsic activity of the substances upon these cells. No single simple extraction procedure would simulate the effect of exposure to the physiological environment. For example, serum contains electrolytes, a variety of fats, and nitrogenous compounds. The extraction solution should be chemically and biologically uncomplicated, however, so that the extraction solution itself does not interfere with subsequent tests. The extraction solution should include an appropriate combination of polar and nonpolar solvents, and the extraction procedure should occur in a static condition as well as under agitation. The ratio of product to extraction solution and the time for the extraction process should reflect the quantities and dwell times occurring in the anticipated use of the device.

At least two solvents, polar and nonpolar, are used to obtain soluble extracts for those biocompatibility tests that are better performed at an elevated temperature. Polar solvent can be water, saline solution, and/or water or saline solution with alcohol. Nonpolar solvent can be cottonseed oil (CSO), sesame oil, and/or polyethylene glycol (DEG) solution. The most commonly employed solvents for extraction are characterized in Table 4.1. Culture medium may also be used for cell-based test systems, such as in cytotoxicity testing.

Extracting conditions shall attempt to exaggerate the clinical use conditions so as to define the potential toxicological hazard without causing significant changes such as fusion or melting of the material pieces or altering the chemical structure. If a device component melts or loses shape during extraction, the resulting extractant solution cannot be used in a valid test.

The results derived from tests in which the conditions of extraction were exaggerated need to be viewed in light of these exaggerations. Judgment needs to be used in interpreting the results as to their appropriateness to the actual use conditions and device potential toxicity.

The concentration of any endogenous or extraneous substances in the extract, and hence the amount exposed to the test cells, depends on the interfacial area, condition of the sample surface, the extraction volume, pH, chemical solubility, osmolarity, agitation, temperature, and other factors. These conditions should each be carefully considered. It should also be remembered that for solid polymer and elastomer components, unfinished areas (such as are exposed if an elastomeric closure or stopper piece is cut) are likely to have more leachable materials than are present in a more fully cured or finished surface.

Use of a lipophilic [such as cotton seed oil (CSO)] and a hydrophilic (generally saline) solvent system simulates likely physiologic extraction conditions in use. The addition of ethanol and PEG provides a fair representation of potential extraction conditions when the device is in extended contact with a drug or therapeutic solution (Autian, 1977).

General points or guidance for extraction include the following (AAMI, 1997):

1. The extraction shall be performed in sterile, chemically inert containers by using aseptic techniques.
2. The extraction time and temperature are dependent on the physicochemical characteristics of the material and extraction vehicle. Recommended conditions are
   a. Not less than 24 hr at 37°C.
   b. 72 hr at 50°C
   c. 24 hr at 70°C.
   d. 1 hr at 121°C

TABLE **4.1** Commonly Utilized Extractants and Vehicles

Common name: **Cottonseed oil (CSO)**
Chemical name: NA
Molecular weight: NA
Formula: Mixture of natural products; glycerides of palmitic, olive and linoleic
   acids
Density: 0.915–0.921 g/ml
Volatility: Low
Solubility/miscibility: Soluble in ether, benzene, chloroform, and DMSO. Slightly
   soluble in ethanol.
Biological considerations: Orally, serves as energy source (and therefore can al-
   ter food consumption and/or body weight). Prolonged oral administration has
   been associated with enhanced carcinogenesis.
Chemical compatibility/stability considerations: Thickens upon prolonged expo-
   sure to air. Available in USP grade.
Uses (routes): In extractions and as a vehicle for oral, dermal, vaginal, rectal,
   and subcutaneous administration.
Common name: **DMSO/dimethyl sulfoxide**
Chemical name: Sulfinylbis [methane]; CAS #67-68-5
Molecular weight: 78.13
Formula: C_2H_6OS
Density: 1.100 g/ml at 20°C
Volatility: Medium
Solubility/miscibility: Soluble in water, ethanol, acetone, ether, oils
Biological considerations: Oral LD50 (rats) = 17.9 ml/kg. Repeated dermal ex-
   posure can defat skin. Repeated oral exposure can produce corneal opacit-
   ies. Not cytotoxic to cells in primary culture at less than 0.05% (V/V). Intra-
   peritoneal LD50 (mice) = 11.6 ml/kg.
Chemical compatibility/stability considerations: Very hydroscopic liquid. Combus-
   tible.
Uses (routes): All, as a carrier at up to 5% to enhance absorption.
Common name: **Ethanol; EtOH**
Chemical name: Ethyl alcohol; CAS #64-17-5
Molecular weight: 46.07
Formula: C_2H_5OH Density: 0.789 g/ml
Volatility: High, but declines when part of mixture with water.
Solubility/miscibility: Miscible with water, acetone, and most other vehicles.
Biological considerations: Orally, will produce transient neurobehavioral intoxica-
   tion. Oral LD50(rats) = 13.0 ml/kg. Intravenous LD50 (Mice) = 5.1 ml/kg.
Chemical compatibility/stability considerations: Flammable colorless liquid avail-
   able USP grade.
Uses (routes): Extraction solvent vehicle for dermal and oral, though can be
   used in lower concentrations for most other routes. Volume of oral instillation
   should be limited to 5 ml/kg.

TABLE **4.1** Continued

Common name: **Polyethylene glycol (PEG)**
Chemical name: NA
Molecular weight: 400 (approximate average, range 380–420)
Formula: $H(OCH_2CH_2)_nOH$
Density: 1.128 g/ml
Volatility: Very low
Solubility/miscibility: Highly soluble in water. Soluble in alcohol and many organic solvents.
Biological considerations: Employed as water-soluble emulsifying/dispersing agents. Oral LD50 (mice) = 23.7 ml/kg. Oral LD50 (rats) = 30 ml/kg.
Chemical compatibility/stability considerations: Do not hydrolyze or deteriorate on storage and will not support mold growth. Clear, viscous liquid.
Uses (routes): As extraction solvent for oral administration as a vehicle full strength or mixed with water. Total dosage of PEG-400 should not exceed 5–10 ml.
Common name: **Saline**
Chemical name: Physiological saline; isotonic salt solution
Molecular weight: 18.02
Formula: 019% NaCl in water (weight to volume)
Density: As water
Volatility: Low
Solubility/miscibility: As water
Biological considerations: No limitations—preferable to water in parenteral applications.
Chemical compatibility/stability considerations: None
Uses (routes): Extraction solvent all except perocular.

Source: Gad and Chengelis, 1998; Lewis, 1993.

3. Extraction conditions should simulate as closely as possible the conditions under which the device will normally be used, therefore item a gives the preferred conditions for extraction.

The recommended conditions may be applied according to the device characteristics and specific conditions of use.

Extraction procedures using culture medium with serum can only be used under the conditions specified in item a above (i.e., not less than 24 hr at 37°C).

When agitation is considered to be appropriate, the method should be specified and reported.

When appropriate, cut the material into small pieces before extraction. For polymers, 10 mm by 50 mm pieces have been used. Molded elastomer closures should be tested intact.

The ratio between the surface area of the material and the volume of extraction vehicle shall be no more than 6 cm^2/ml. The surface area shall be calculated on the basis of the overall sample dimensions, not taking into account surface irregularity and porosity. The actual surface characteristics should be considered in the interpretation of the test results, however. If the surface area is indeterminate, then 0.1 g/ml to 0.2 g/ml shall be used.

If possible, liquid extracts shall be used immediately after preparation.

If an extract is stored, then the stability of the extract under the conditions of storage should be verified with appropriate methods.

If the extract is filtered, centrifuged, or processed by other methods prior to being applied to the cells, this must be included in the final report.

For use in direct contract tests (e.g., implantation studies), materials that have various shapes, sizes, or physical states (i.e., liquid or solid) may be tested without modification in the cytotoxicity assays.

> The preferred sample of a solid specimen should have at least one flat surface. Adjustments shall be made for other shapes and physical states.
>
> The sterility of the test specimen shall conform to the requirements in the USP.
>
> Test materials from sterilized devices that are normally supplied nonsterile but are sterilized before use shall be sterilized by the method recommended by the manufacturer and handled aseptically throughout the extraction and test procedure.
>
> The effect of sterilization methods or agents on the device should be considered in defining the preparation of the test material prior to use in the test system.
>
> Test materials from devices not required to be sterile in use shall be used as supplied and handled aseptically throughout the extraction and test procedure.
>
> Liquids shall be tested by either
>
> 1. Direct deposition.
> 2. Deposition on to a biologically inert absorbent matrix. (Filter discs have been found to be suitable.)

If appropriate, materials classed as superabsorbent shall be wetted with culture medium prior to testing.

The USP (2000) provides specific guidance for use in preparing extraction solutions for use in biological reactivity tests. These are as follows:

> Apparatus—for the tests includes the following.
> Autoclave—Use an autoclave capable of maintaining a temperature of 121 ± 2.0°, equipped with a thermometer, a pressure gauge, a vent cock, a

rack adequate to accommodate the test containers above the water level, and a water cooling system that will allow for cooling of the test containers to about (but not below) 20° immediately following the heating cycle.

Oven—Use an oven, preferably a forced-circulation model, that will maintain operating temperatures of 50° or 70° within ± 2°.

Extraction containers—Use only containers, such as ampuls or screw-cap culture test tubes, of type I glass. If used, culture test tubes are closed with screw caps having suitable elastomeric liners. The exposed surface of the elastomeric liner is completely protected with an inert solid disk 0.05 mm to 0.075 mm in thickness. A suitable disk may be fabricated from a polytetrafluoroethylene (polytef) resin.

Preparation of apparatus—Clean all glassware thoroughly with chromic acid cleansing mixture, or if necessary with hot nitric acid, followed by prolonged rinsing with water. Clean cutting utensils by an appropriate method (e.g., successive cleaning with acetone and methylene chloride) prior to use in subdividing a specimen. Clean all other equipment by thorough scrubbing with a suitable detergent and prolonged rinsing with water.

Render containers and equipment used for extraction (and in transfer and administration of test material) sterile and dry by a suitable process. (If ethylene oxide is used as the sterilizing agent, allow adequate time for completing degassing.)

A. Procedure

Preparation of sample—Both the systemic injection test and the intracutaneous test may be performed using the same extract, if desired, or separate extracts may be made for each test. Select and subdivide into portions a sample of the size indicated in Table 4.2. Note that ISO 10993 (part 12) guidance is equivalent but stated differently, as presented in Table 4.3. Remove particulate matter, such as lint and free particles, by treating each subdivided sample or negative control as follows. Place the sample into a clean, glass-stoppered, 100-ml graduated cylinder of type I glass, and add about 70 ml of water for injection. Agitate for about 30 sec, then drain off the water, repeat this step, and dry those pieces prepared for the extraction with vegetable oil in an oven at a temperature not exceeding 50°. (*Note*—Do not clean the sample with a dry or wet cloth or by rinsing or washing with an organic solvent, surfactant, etc.)

Preparation of extracts—Place a properly prepared sample to be tested in an extraction container, and add 20 ml of the appropriate extracting medium. Repeat these directions for each extracting medium required for testing. Also prepare one 20-ml blank of each medium for parallel injec-

TABLE **4.2**   Surface Area of Specimen to Be Used

Form of material	Thickness	Amount of sample for each 20 ml of extracting medium	Subdivided into
Film or sheet	<0.5 mm	Equivalent of 120 cm² total surface area. (Both sides combined.)	Strips of about 5 × 0.3 cm
	0.5 to 1 mm	Equivalent of 60 cm² total surface area. (Both sides combined.)	
Tubing	<0.5 mm (wall)	Length (in cm) = 60 cm²/ (sum of ID and OD circumferences)	Sections of about 5 × 0.3 cm
	0.5 to 1 mm (wall)	Length (in cm) = 60 cm²/ (sum of ID and OD circumferences)	
Slabs, tubing, and molded items	>1 mm	Equivalent of 60 cm² total surface area. (All exposed surfaces combined.)	Pieces up to about 5 × 0.3 cm
Elastomers	>1 mm	Equivalent of 25 cm² total surface area. (All exposed surfaces combined.)	Do not subdivide

Note: When surface area cannot be determined due to the configuration of the specimen, use 0.1 g of elastomer or 0.2 g of plastic or other polymers for every 1 ml of extracting fluid. Molded elastomeric closures are tested intact.

tions and comparisons. Extract by heating in an autoclave at 121° for 60 min, in an oven at 70° for 24 hr, or at 50° for 72 hr. Allow adequate time for the liquid within the container to reach the extraction temperature.

Note—The extraction conditions should not in any instance cause physical changes, such as fusion or melting of the sample pieces, that result in a decrease in the available surface area. A slight adherence of the pieces can be tolerated. Always add the cleaned pieces individually to the extracting medium. If culture tubes are used for autoclave extractions with vegetable oil, seal the screw caps adequately with pressure-sensitive tape.)

Cool to about room temperature (but not below 20°) shake vigorously for several minutes, and decant each extract immediately using aseptic precautions into a dry, sterile vessel. Store the extracts at a temperature between 20° and 30°, and do not use for tests after 24 hr. Of special

TABLE 4.3 Extraction Ratios

Form/material	Thickness	Surface area/volume[2a]
Nonabsorbent	Not applicable	6 cm²/ml
Absorbents and hydro-colloids[b]	Not applicable	0.1 g/(1 ml + absorption capacity)
Film, sheet, or tubing wall[c]	<0.5 mm	6 cm²/ml
	0.5 to 1 mm	3 cm²/ml
Slabs, tubing, and molded items	>1 mm	3 cm²/ml
Elastomers[d]	>1 mm	1.25 cm²/ml
Indeterminate surface area	Not applicable	0.2 g sample/ml or 0.1 g elastomer/ml

[a] Plus or minus 10%. [b] Based on a technique developed by N. J. Stark.
[c] May be subdivided into strips or sections. [d] Do not subdivide; cut edges have different extraction properties than outer surfaces.
Source: ISO, 1993.

importance are the contact of the extracting medium with the available surface area of the plastic and the time and temperature during extraction, the proper cooling, agitation, and decanting process, and the aseptic handling and storage of the extracts following extraction.

One should be aware that close reading of the requirements under MHW Notification 99 (MHW, 1999) is required; otherwise exaggerated extraction conditions may be inappropriately and erroneously employed (such as in the case of biologically derived materials such as collagen).

IV. REFERENCE MATERIALS

In nearly every biocompatibility test, reference materials are used to serve as experimental controls. Negative controls, in the form of blanks, are used in most biological evaluations in which test article extracts are prepared. The use of these blanks provides the basis for a comparison of the effects of the test material extract with a validated negative test result. Japanese (MHW) guidelines consistently refer to these as standard reference materials (SRMs).

A number of materials have been used extensively in biological testing as negative or positive controls. High-density polyethylene, obtained from the *U.S. Pharmacopoeia*, is a standard negative control. The nonreactive plastic can be implanted into living tissue and the results compared with those for a test material that has been similarly implanted. Likewise, a polyvinyl chloride formulation containing organotin additives serves well as a positive control.

V. CONCLUSION

ISO 10993-12, *Sample Preparation and Reference Materials*, clearly indicates that it is preferable to evaluate medical devices in their final product form. The reasoning is simple—the biological testing must incorporate everything involved in making the device. Obviously, the constituent materials must be safe for patient contact. Equally important to device biocompatibility are the processes and materials used during manufacturing. For most devices, the use of fluid extracts of the test materials prepared in a fashion to mimic or exaggerate the expected clinical conditions is the most appropriate technique for determining the potential effects of chemical leachables. Extraction fluid selection, extraction conditions, and material-to-extractant ratios are all outlined in the standard. The selection and use of appropriate experimental controls also is important in evaluating device materials for safety and is also covered in ISO 10993-12.

Japan (MHW) tends to specify extraction/sampling procedures independently for each test type.

REFERENCES

AAMI. (1997). Biological Evaluation of Medical Devices, AAMI, Washington, DC.

Autian, J. (1977). Toxicological evaluation of biomaterials: Primary acute toxicity screening program, Artif. Organs, 1:53–60.

CDRH. (1992). Regulatory Requirements for Medical Devices, FDA, Washington, DC.

Gad, S. C. and Chengelis, C. P. (1998). Acute Toxicology Testing, 2nd ed. Academic, San Diego, CA.

Gad, S. C. (1998). Statistics and Experimental Design for Toxicologists, 3rd ed. CRC Press, Boca Raton, FL.

ISO. (1993). 10993—Part 12: Sample Preparation and Reference Materials.

Levy, P. S. and Lemoshow, S. (1991). Sampling of Populations: Methods and Applications, J Wiley, New York.

Lewis, R. J. (1993). Hawley's Condensed Chemical Dictionary, Van Nostrand Reinhold, New York.

MHW. (1999). Guidelines for Basic Biological Tests of Medical Materials and Devices, notification 99, MHW, Japan.

Ryan, T. P. (1989). Statistical Methods for Quality Improvement, Wiley, New York.

USP. (2000). United States Pharmacopoeia XXIV § NF-19, United States Pharmacopoeia, Philadelphia.

5

Cytotoxicity Testing

The cell or tissue culture including cytotoxicity methods is a fair predictor of biocompatibility when used together with other appropriate tests (Wilsnack, 1976; Gad, 2000). Several highly specialized cell culture methods are available to monitor the biocompatibility of the raw materials used in manufacturing the device or auditing the manufacturing process. Cell or tissue culture testing offers several advantages, including the following:

It is simple, rather inexpensive, and easy to perform.
It allows testing of a biomaterial on human tissue.
It is sensitive to toxic material.
It is easy to manipulate and allow more than one end-point investigation.
It can be used to construct a dose-response curve.
It can give quick and quantitative results and allows direct access or direct observation or measurement.

Although cell or tissue culture offer many advantages, its use is currently limited to screening the biomaterials, therefore cytotoxicity results should be used for biocompatibility in conjunction with other tests.

The objective of cell cytotoxicity testing is to screen the biocompatibility of the polymer and elastomer portions of medical devices or medical device components using mammalian cell cultures. Cytotoxicity is a useful method for screening material. It can also serve as a quality control mechanism for audit or batch testing programs, and is a basic part of all device biocompatibility evaluation (AAMI, 1997; CDRH, 1992; ISO, 1993). It is one of the oldest assays de-

117

signed specifically to screen plastics for toxicity (Rosenbluth et al., 1965). Given the extreme sensitivity of this test, materials found to be cytotoxic must be assessed along with the results of in vivo and other studies to evaluate the risk to human health. Unlike the other studies utilized in biocompatibility testing, cytotoxicity is not a pass or fail test. Failure in cytotoxicity is generally grounds for performing a confirmatory test such as an implantation or intracutaneous reactivity (Barile, 1994).

I. BACKGROUND

The great majority of toxic compounds are chemically stable and produce their characteristic effects by interference with biochemical or physiological homeostatic mechanisms. This means that a full understanding of the pharmacology of leachable toxics is essential. In the case of drugs, it has been estimated that some 80% of adverse reactions are the result of exaggerated pharmacological responses. Many adverse events are the consequence of disturbance of normal physiology and do not result in cell death. This is one reason that cytotoxicity assays on their own cannot provide a full assurance of safety.

Cytotoxicity, the causing of cell death, is often the consequence of exposure to a harmful chemical, but the number of cells that must be killed before the function of a tissue or organism is noticeably impaired is highly variable. Some cell types, notably the epithelia, including the liver, have the ability to regenerate in response to insult while others, most notably neurons, cannot. Some organs, such as the liver, lung, and kidney, have a substantial reserve capacity in excess of normal requirements, and normal body function can be maintained in the presence of marked impairment.

Cytotoxicity assays measure loss of some cellular or intercellular structure and/or functions, including cell death. They are generally simple to perform, are reproducible, and have a clearly defined endpoint. Predictability based on comparison with in vivo standard (e.g., lethality, irritation and implantation) tests may be variable for a variety of reasons, however, including the fact that the assay systems are continually exposed, whereas in vivo there are biological protective measures in operation. Some assays may not be universally capable of detecting all chemical classes of irritants because of the endpoint used.

There are several factors to consider when selecting a cell line for these tests. These include the following:

Precise nature of the study
Availability of the cell or tissue
Relevance to intended use
Need or acceptability of the use of primary culture, early passage cultures, or established cell line

Need to use differentiated cell or cell line

Requirement for metabolic activation and the compatibility with S9 or other metabolizing systems

Easily identifiable markers or endpoints

Ease of handling and storage

Absence of special growth requirements

Published information on the use

Experience

A variety of cell lines have been used, including corneal epithelial cells, lung fibroblasts, Chinese hamster ovary (CHO) cells, canine renal cells, HeLa (human tumor cell line) cells, and microorganisms. Some cell lines used with success by FRAME (the Fund for the Replacement of Animals in Medical Experiments) are BCL-D1 (a human embryo lung finite-lived fibroblastlike cell), CHO, RL4 (rat liver), L929 (fibrobalstic mouse subcutaneous), HeLa, and BHK (fibroblastic baby hamster kidney cell). The popular human cell line W138 has been replaced with many new cell lines or explant cultures of human origin because W138 is no longer available in a quantity to meet the demand. The Japanese recommend the V79 cell line.

Differentiated cells are used to evaluate the effects materials may have on specific tissues. Differentiated cells are generally nonfibrobalstic cells that are different from transformed and fibroblastic cells, such as L cells, which are used in ASTM cytotoxicity test methods. Differentiated cells have organ-specific or tissue-specific functions and have specific biological end points or measurable characteristics. Liver cells, which are differentiated cells, have all or some liver functions.

Most cells in culture are fibroblasts. Primary cells that are taken directly from an animal often are difficult to establish in culture and become fibroblasts, losing the normal functions of growing differentiated cells. Numerous conditions have to be optimized for obtaining good growth of differentiated cells. Most cultured cells have a fibroblastic appearance, although they may not be true fibroblasts. For example, cells grown under nonoptimum conditions can temporarily take an appearance of fibroblasts. The fibroblasts in culture can take over cultures because they grow readily on plastic surfaces. The recent success in growing differentiated cells was partially due to techniques that have been developed to remove and limit the growth of fibroblasts to allow other cells to grow. The properties of the cell cultures usually depend on the cultivation conditions, and normal cells can grow in culture only for a limited number of generations.

The test in differentiated cells is important for at least two reasons. First, the tissue-type specific features of differentiated cells may modulate the effects of chemicals on the fundamental properties of cells. Second, it is important to determine the effects of chemicals on specific cell functions or responses. Culture systems for growing epithelial, liver, or embryonic cells have been developed only recently. The number of available differentiated cells for biocompatibility testing is currently small, but there is significant development in this area.

A very large number of end points for cytotoxicity assays have been described, some of which are given in Table 5.1. The possible cytotoxicity end points are (Caldwell, 1993; Northup, 1986; 1987; 1992) as follows:

Microscopic examination of cell morphology, membrane integrity, and fragility
Cell population and density
Cell adhesiveness
Cytopathic effect
Total protein content
Rate of growth
Rate of protein synthesis
Total DNA content
Rate of DNA synthesis
Colony-forming efficiency
Tryphan blue uptake and other dye uptake
Biochemical assays of enzymes

Much of the initial work on the range of cytotoxicity assays that have been developed (and their end point measurement methods) was done with the goal

TABLE 5.1 Examples of End Point Measurements Used in Cytotoxicity Assays

Method	Basis/end point	Reference
Microphysiometry	Metabolic rate measurement	Bruner et al. (1991)
Uridine uptake inhibition	Membrane damage	Shopsis and Sathe (1984)
Neutral red uptake	General cytotoxicity	Borenfreund and Puemer (1984; 1985; 1987)
Neutral red release	Cell membrane injury	Rohde (1992)
Leucine incorporation	General cytotoxicity	Sina et al. (1992)
Total protein	General cytotoxicity	Riddell et al. (1986)
Fluorescein leakage	Cell membrane injury	Rohde (1992)
Colony-forming efficiency	Lethal cytotoxicity	North-Root et al. (1982)
MTT dye reduction	Mitochondrial damage	Sina et al. (1992)
Crystal violet staining	Lethal cytotoxicity	Itagaki et al. (1991)
Alkaline phosphatase release	Membrane injury	Scaife (1985)
Intracellular ATP	General metabolic toxicity	Kemp et al. (1985)

of developing an in vitro alternative to the rabbit eye irritation test. A few of the more commonly used methods are briefly described below.

A. Crystal Violet Staining

Itagaki et al. (1991) employed a simple technique using cultured HeLa S3 cells or SIRC cells (an established line of rabbit corneal cells) in the presence of serial dilutions of the test material. After the incubation period, crystal violet was used to stain residual viable cells. The IC_{50} was calculated; that is, the concentration of test material inhibiting growth of cells by 50%. Using various surfactants they found good correlations between the IC_{50} and the maximum in vivo eye irritation scores for the materials tested.

B. Silicone Microphysiometer

This is a light-addressable potential sensor device that can be used to indirectly measure the rate of production of acidic metabolite from cells placed in a biosensor flow chamber. The end point calculated is the MRD_{50}; that is, the concentration of test material required to reduce the metabolic rate by 50% (Bruner et al., 1991). Mouse fibroblasts have been used as the test cell. Bagley et al. (1991) found that the MRD_{50} for a variety of materials correlated well with the maximum average score for in vivo eye irritation.

C. Microtox Test

This test utilizes changes in luminescence from Photobacterium phosphoreum, which is generated through a process linked to respiration by NAADH and flavin mononucleotide (Bulich, 1990). Light output is measured photometrically before and after the addition of the test substance and an EC_{50} value calculated; that is, 50% reduction in light emission. Bagley et al. (1992) found that in general test substances with the highest in vivo irritation gave the lowest EC_{50} values.

D. Neutral Red Uptake Assay

In this procedure, cells—usually mouse fibroblasts or CHO cells—are exposed to the test material and then to neutral red. Retention of neutral red indicates cell viability. Bagley et al (1991) found that in general the concentration of test material required to reduce neutral red uptake decreased as the in vivo irritant potential of the test material increased. Attention needs to be paid to the technical aspects of incubation, as emphasized by Blein et al. (1991), who found that correlation with materials with an extreme pH were underestimated because of the buffering effect of the culture medium, and that volatile materials were also underestimated, probably because of loss of material.

Several intertest comparisons have been undertaken. Sina et al. (1992) compared leucine incorporation, MTT (tetrazolium(3-(4,5-dimethylthiazol-2-yl)2 diphenyl tetrazolium bromide) dye reduction, and neutral red uptake in corneal epithelial cells and Chinese hamster lung fibroblasts. None of the end point target cell combinations accurately predicted in vivo eye irritation in this series, but the MTT dye reduction method gave the best overall correlation.

II. CYTOTOXICITY ASSAYS

Cytotoxicity assays assess the effect of test material on a particular aspect of cell or intercellular function, or of lethal cytotoxicity. They therefore give a measure of potential to cause cell and tissue injury and as such may be used as a screen for predicting local tissue injury, including eye injury. The appropriate choice of the test cell and end point indicator for certain chemical classes may give a reasonable prediction of the potential for eye irritation. The choice of the screening cytotoxicity assay, or assays, should in part be determined by past experience, the likely mechanism for an irritant response, and the chemistry of the material tested.

In vitro assays such as cytotoxicity serve to assess acute toxic effects, and in far larger organisms are most effective in predicting local tissue irritation effects. Such experiments using cultured cells utilize a variety of methods based on either a fresh isolate from fragments of tissue or cell suspension (primary cell culture), which grow to confluence and then age and die, or single cell clones (continuous cell culture), which have an indefinite capacity to grow and replicate. The continuous cell lines have the advantage of being consistent, reliable, and reproducible. They act as a standard with a documented history, they have fewer biological variables, and they may be tuned to particular toxicity concerns by using a variety of tissues and species with a range of doses and exposure periods. As a result these methods can be very efficient in screening, and are often more sensitive than acute toxicity tests in animals. Early cell culture methods merely estimated the numbers of living or dead cells, but now morphological analysis by electron microscopy reveals a spectrum of microcellular changes, and cell function tests measure biochemical parameters, indicating the nature of cell stress.

Although many modifications have been made, cell culture tests are of four main types: gel diffusion, direct contact, extract dilution, and cell function tests.

Gel diffusion uses agar or agarose to cover a cell monolayer. A sample of the material or extract is placed on top of the gel, providing a concentration gradient of diffusibles. Agarose allows a faster diffusion of uncharged molecules and is as sensitive as the rabbit intramuscular implantation test.

Direct contact of the test material onto a culture layer is more sensitive than the rabbit intramuscular implantation test, but care must be taken to avoid physical damage to the cells by pressure or movement of the sample.

Extracts may be serially diluted in the nutrient media and provide a quantitative comparison with reference extracts. Inevitably the correlation with animal tests will depend on the nature of the eluants.

Cell function tests are a very precise way of registering cellular response to any insult. In particular, inhibition of cell growth can be measured with considerable sensitivity.

With increasing complexity of test methodology, the results may be less reproducible, and increasing sensitivity may not assist the prediction of risk to humans, as the impact of a material on the body systems may be much less intense than in the culture plate.

As discussed above, several tissue culture methods are available for testing biomaterials. These are divided into two major groups: one tests the toxicity of a soluble extract of the material, and the other tests the toxicity by the direct contact of cells with the material or components of the device.

Examples of cytotoxicity test methods using extracts include the following:

Fluid medium tissue culture assay
Inhibition of cell growth assay
Cloning efficiency assay

Fluid medium tissue culture evaluates the cellular damage caused by the test extract on a confluent monolayer culture. The text extract is incorporated into the culture medium, which is usually double strength ($2\times$) minimum essential medium supplemented with serum and other essential nutrients at the maintenance level. The toxic effect on the monolayer, such as cell lysis and microscopic observation of cell morphology changes, is usually checked after 24 and 48 hr. Cell lysis can be scored by direct microscopic observation or with the use of radiolabels or tryphan blue dye uptake.

The inhibition of cell growth is a more informative test requiring more time and skill. Distilled water extract is incorporated into the tissue culture medium and inoculated with the cells in the tissue culture tubes. After 72 hr, the extent of cell growth is determined by total protein assay, such as the Lowery photometric method, on the removed cells from the individual tubes.

The cloning efficiency assay is more informative, sensitive, and quantitative, and required even more skill. The cloning efficiency assay's procedure and end point are similar, but are more accurate, sensitive, and direct than cell growth inhibition or fluid medium methods. The cloning efficiency assay normally uses a CHO cell line and a single-cell cloning technique to estimate the tox insult induced in cloning efficiency. The number of cells in the initial inoculum is considerably less than those plated to get confluent cultures (approximately 1×10^5 or less cells in a 100×15 mm petri dish, compared to 1×10^6 or more cells). The initial inocula are incubated for approximately 24 hr before these growing cells are treated with the tissue culture medium containing the test extract. The cytotoxic effect of the extract is determined by measuring the ability of the treated cells to form colonies during seven subsequent days of incubation. The cloning efficiency of the treated cultures is compared to that of the control. The agar overlay method can be used to evaluate the toxicity of the extracts, but it is primarily used for the direct contact cytotoxicity tests of the solid test sample.

Several tests are available to test cytotoxicity by direct contact. These include the following:

ASTM F813, practice for direct contact cell culture evaluation of materials for medical devices

ASTM F895 test method for agar diffusion cell culture screening for cytotoxicity

ASTM F1027, standard practice for assessment of tissue and cell compatibility of orificial prosthetic materials and devices

NIH publication no. 85–2185, "Guidelines for Blood-Material Interactions"

HIMA report: "Guidelines for the Preclinical Safety Evaluation of Materials Used in Medical Devices"

Others tests, including many device-specific toxicity guidance documents on toxicity testing

In addition, the agar overlay tissue culture method and fluid medium tissue culture method can be used for direct contact cytotoxicity testing. In the fluid medium method, the test material or device is placed directly on the growing monolayer cell surface. In the agar overlay method, the solid test sample is placed on or in the agar layer containing the vital stain, such as neutral red over the growing monolayer of cells. The response is evaluated grossly and microscopically and graded according to the zone index, the size of the cytopathic area, the lysis index, and percentage of cell lysis.

Proper cytotoxicity testing should include at least one test with extract and one direct contact test, if feasible.

In addition, differentiated cells are used to evaluate the effects materials may have on specific tissues. Differentiated cells are generally nonfibroblastic cells, which are different from transformed and fibroblastic cell lines, such as L cells used in ASTM cytotoxicity test methods. Differentiated cells have organ-specific or tissue-specific functions and have specific biological end points or measurable characteristics. Liver cells, which are differentiated cells, have all or some liver functions.

Most cells in culture are fibroblasts. Primary cells that are taken directly from an animal often are difficult to establish in culture and become fibroblasts, losing the normal functions of growing differentiated cells. Numerous conditions have to be optimized for obtaining good growth of differentiated cells. Most cultured cells have a fibroblastic appearance, although they may not be true fibroblasts. For example, cells grown under nonoptimum conditions can temporarily take on an appearance of fibroblasts. The fibroblasts in culture can take over cultures because they grow readily on plastic surfaces. The recent success in growing differentiated cells was partially due to techniques that have been developed to remove and limit the growth of fibroblasts to allow other cells to grow. The properties of the cell cultures usually depend on the cultivation conditions, and normal cells can grow in culture only for a limited number of generations.

The test in differentiated cells is important for at least two reasons. First, the tissue-type specific features of differentiated cells may modulate the effects of chemicals on the fundamental properties of cells. Second, it is important to determine the effects of chemicals on specific cell functions or responses. Culture systems for growing epithelial, liver, or embryonic cells have been developed only recently. The number of available differentiated cells for biocompatibility testing is currently small, but significant developments in this area are coming. Information in this area can be found in Gad (2000).

The three specific tests prescribed by ISO (and USP, 2000) are presented below.

A. Agar Diffusion Test

This test is designed for elastomeric closures in a variety of shapes. The agar layer acts as a cushion to protect the cells from mechanical damage while allowing the diffusion of leachable chemicals from the polymeric specimens. Extracts of materials that are to be tested are applied to a piece of filter paper.

Sample preparation—Use extracts prepared as directed, or use portions of the test specimens having flat surfaces not less than 100 mm² in surface area.

Procedure—Prepare the monolayers in 60-mm-diameter plates using 7 ml of cell culture preparation. Aspirate the culture medium from the monolayers, and replace it with serum-supplemented culture medium containing not more than 2% of agar. Place the flat surfaces of sample preparation, USP negative control plastic RS (to provide a negative control), and either USP positive bioreaction extract RS or USP positive bioreaction solid RS (to provide a positive control) in duplicate cultures in contact with the solidified agar surface. Incubate all cultures for not less than 24 hr at 37 ± 1°, preferably in a humidified incubator containing 5 ± 1% of carbon dioxide. Examine each culture around each sample, negative control, and positive control under a microscope using cytochemical stains if desired.

Interpretation of results—The biological reactivity (cellular degeneration and malformation) is described and rated on a scale of 0 to 4 (Table

TABLE 5.2 Reactivity Grades for Agar Diffusion Test

Grade	Reactivity	Description of reactivity zone
0	None	No detectable zone around or under specimen
1	Slight	Zone limited to area under specimen
2	Mild	Zone extends less than 0.5 cm beyond specimen
3	Moderate	Zone extends 0.5 to 1.0 cm beyond the specimen
4	Severe	Zone extends greater than 1.0 cm beyond specimen but does not involve entire dish

5.2). Measure the response obtained from the negative control and the positive control. The test system is suitable if the observed response corresponds to the labeled biological reactivity grad of the relevant reference standard. Measure the response obtained from the sample preparation. The sample meets the requirements of the test if none of the cell culture exposed in the sample shows greater than a mild reactivity (grade 2). Repeat the test if the suitability of the system is not confirmed.

B. Direct Contact Test

This test is designed for materials in a variety of shapes. The procedure allows for simultaneous extraction and testing of leachable chemicals from the specimen with a serum-supplemented medium. The procedure is not appropriate for very low- or high-density materials that could cause mechanical damage to the cells.

Sample preparation—Use portions of the test specimen having flat surfaces not less than 100 mm^2 in surface area.

Procedure—Prepare the monolayers in 35-mm-diameter plates using 2 ml of cell suspension. Aspirate the culture medium from the cultures, and replace it with 0.8 ml of fresh culture medium. Place a single sample preparation, USP negative control plastic RS (to provide a negative control), and USP positive bioreaction solid RS (to provide a positive control) in each of duplicate cultures. Incubate all cultures for not less than 24 hr at 37 ± 1° in a humidified incubator, preferably containing 5 ± 1% of carbon dioxide. Examine each culture around each sample, negative control, and positive control under a microscope, using cytochemical stains if desired.

Interpretation of results—Proceed as directed for interpretation of results under the agar diffusion test using Table 5.3. The sample meets the requirements of the test if none of the cultures treated with the sample shows greater than a mild reactivity (grade 2). Repeat the test if the suitability of the system is not confirmed.

TABLE **5.3** Reactivity Grades for Direct Contact Test and for Elution Test

Grade	Reactivity	Conditions of all cultures
0	None	Discrete intracytoplasmic granules; no cell lysis
1	Slight	More than 20% of the cells are round, loosely attached, and without intracytoplasmic granules; occasional lysed cells are present
2	Mild	More than 50% of the cells are round and devoid of intra-cytoplasmic granules; extensive cell lysis and empty areas between cells
3	Moderate	Greater than 70% of the cell layers contain rounded cells and/or are lysed
4	Severe	Nearly complete destruction of the cell layers

C. Elution Test

This test is designed for the evaluation of extracts of polymeric materials. The procedure allows for extraction of the specimens at physiological or nonphysiological temperatures for varying time intervals. It is appropriate for high-density materials and for dose-response evaluations.

Sample preparation—Prepare as directed in preparation of extracts, using ether sodium chloride injection (0.9% NcCl) or serum-free mammalian cell culture media as extraction solvents. If the size of the sample cannot be readily measured, a mass of not less than 0.1 g of elastomeric material or 0.2 g of plastic or polymeric material per ml of extraction medium may be used. Alternatively, use serum-supplemented mammalian cell culture media as the extracting medium to more closely simulate physiological conditions. Prepare the extracts by heating for 24 hr in an incubator, preferably containing $5 \pm 1\%$ of carbon dioxide. Maintain the extraction temperature at $37 \pm 1°$, because higher temperatures may cause denaturation of serum proteins.

Procedure—Prepare the monolayers in 35-mm-diameter plates using 2 ml of cell culture preparation. Aspirate the culture medium from the monolayers, and replace it with either extracts of the sample, USP negative control plastic RS (to provide a negative control), or USP positive bioreaction extract RS (to provide a positive control). The serum-supplemented and serum-free cell culture media extracts are tested in duplicate without dilution (100%). The sodium chloride injection extract is diluted with serum-supplemented cell culture medium and tested in duplicate at 25% extract concentration. Incubate all cultures for 48 hr at $37 \pm 1°$ in an incubator, preferably containing $5 \pm 1\%$ of carbon dioxide. Examine

each culture at 48 hr under a microscope, using cytochemical stains if
desired.

Interpretation of results—Proceed as directed for interpretation of results
under agar diffusion test, but using Table 5.3. Repeat the test if the suitability of the system is not confirmed. The sample meets the requirements of the test if the cultures treated with the samples show no greater
than a mild reactivity (grade 2). If the cultures treated with the sample
show a significantly greater reaction than the cultures treated with the
negative control, repeat the test with several quantitative dilutions of the
extracts.

For each of these three procedures, it should be kept in mind that while
USP requires that tests be performed in duplicate, ISO requires that they be done
in triplicate.

D. Correlation with In Vivo Results

Cytotoxicity testing for medical devices is a very useful screening tool, but it
must be kept firmly in mind that the correlation of results from these assays with
intact animal tests (and with observed effects in humans) is very limited. This
issue was researched more than 20 years ago (Wilsnack et al., 1973; Wilsnack,
1976) with side-by-side comparisons of cytotoxicity results with those of animal
tests conducted on the same samples. The results demonstrated limited correlation
and "the ellipsoid effect," the best correlation being between extreme results in
the different tests.

The author has also tried to correlate the results of cytotoxicity and concurrent animal tests (particularly subcutaneous injection and implantation tests, in
which one would expect the best case), only to find that there were high levels
of false negatives and positives, though predominantly the latter. Investigators
are thus cautioned to not place too much faith and weight on the results of these
assays.

III. CONCLUSION

Cytotoxicity tests, as an initial screen for toxicities of both plastics and elastomers
and of leachates from them, have been in use since the 1960s (Rosenbluth et al.,
1965), but have also been recognized for a long time to be limited to effectively
serving only as screens that in effect say "look at this and evaluate/consider
further." This limitation to use as screens as opposed to as definitive tests is due
to at best the moderate correlation of their results with in vivo findings (Wilsnack,
1976). Regulatory agencies recognize the limitations of these test systems, and

users should bear in mind the categorical (as opposed to truly quantitative) nature of results.

REFERENCES

AAMI. (1997). Biological Evaluation of Medical Devices, Association for the Advancement of Medical Instrumentation, Arlington, VA, pp. 69–82.

Bagley, D. M., Rizvi, P. Y., Kong, B. M., and DeSalva, S. J. (1991). Factors affecting the use of the hens' egg chorioallantoic membrane assay as a model for eye irritation potential, Toxicol. Cut. Ocul. Toxicol., 10:95–104.

Barile, F. A. (1994). Introduction to in Vitro Cytotoxicity, Mechanisms and Methods, CBC Press, Boca Raton, FL.

Blein, O., Adolphe, M., Lakhdar, B., et al. (1991). Correlation and validation of alternative methods to the Draize eye irritation test (OPAL project), Toxicol. in Vitro, 5:555–557.

Borenfreund, E. and Puerner, J. (1985). Toxicity determined in vitro by morphological alterations and neutral red absorption, Toxicol. Lett., 24:119–124.

Borenfreund, E. and Puerner, J. A. (1987). Short-term quantitative in vitro cytotoxic assay involving an S-9 activating system, Cancer Lett., 34:243–248.

Borenfreund, E. L. and Puerner, J. (1984). A simple quantitative procedure using monolayer cultures for cytotoxicity assays (HTD/NR-90), J. Tis. Cul. Meth., 9(1):7–9.

Bruner, L. H., Kain, D., Roberts, D. A., and Parker, R. D. (1991). Evaluation of seven in vitro alternatives for ocular safety testing, Fund. Appl. Toxicol., 17:136–149.

Bulich, A. A., Tung, K. K., and Scheibner, G. (1990). The luminescent bacteria toxicity test: Its potential as an in vitro alternative, J. Biolumin. Chemilumen., 5:71–77.

Caldwell, J. (1993). Biochemical basis of toxicity. In: General and Applied Toxicology (B. Ballantyne, T. Marrs, and P. Turner, eds.). Stockton, New York, pp. 169–183.

CDRH. (1992). Regulatory Requirements for Medical Devices, Food and Drug Administration, Rockville, MD.

Gad, S. C. (2000). In Vitro Toxicology, 2nd ed., Taylor and Francis, Philadelphia.

ISO. (1993). ISO/DIS 10993-5, Biological Testing of Medical and Dental Materials and Devices—Part 5: Tests for Cytotoxicity: In Vitro Methods.''

Itagaki, H., Hagino, C., Kato, S., Kobayashi, T., and Umeda, M. (1991). An in vitro alternative to the Draize eye irritation test: Evaluation of the crystal violet staining method, Toxicol. in Vitro, 5:139–143.

Kemp, R. B., Meredith, R. W. J., and Gamble, S. H. (1985). Toxicity of commercial products on cells in culture: A possible screen for the Draize eye irritation test, Food Chem. Toxicol., 23:267–270.

North-Root, H., Yackvien, F. Demetrulias, J., Gacula, M. Jr., and Heinze, J. E. (1982). Evaluation of an in vitro cell toxicity test using rabbit corneal cells to predict the eye irritation potential of a surfactant. Toxicol. Lett., 14:207–212.

Northup, S. J. (1986). Mammalian cell culture models. In: Handbook of Biomaterials Evaluation (A. F. Von Recum, ed.) Macmillan, New York, pp. 209–225.

Northup, S. J. (1987). Cytotoxicity tests of plastics and elastomers, Pharmacopoeial Forum, 13:2939–2942.

Northup, S. (1992) Cytotoxicity and mutagenicity. In: Guidelines for Blood Material Interactions (P. Didisheim, L. Harker, and B. Ratner, eds.), ASTM, Philadelphia.
Riddell, R. J., Clothier, R. H., and Balls, M. (1986). An evaluation of three in vitro cytotoxicity assays, Food Chem. Toxicol., 24:469–477.
Rohde, B. H. (1992). In vitro methods in ophthalmic toxicology. In: Ophthalmic Toxicol-
   ogy (G. C. Y. Chiou, ed.). Raven, New York, pp. 109–165.
Rosenbluth, S. A., Weddington, G. R., Guess, W. L., and Autian, J. (1965). Tissue culture
   method for screening toxicity of plastic materials to be used in medical practice,
   J. Pharm Sci., 54:156–159.
Scaife, M. C. (1985). An in vitro cytotoxicity test to predict the oculara irritancy potential
   of detergent products, Food Chem. Toxicol., 23:253–258.
Shopsis, C. and Sathe, J. (1984). Uridine uptake inhibition as a cytotoxic test: Correlation
   with the Draize test, Toxicology, 29:195–296.
Sina, J. F., Ward, G. J., Laszeh, M. A., and Gautheron, P. D. (1992). Assessment of
   cytotoxic assays as predicators of ocular irritation of pharmaceuticals, Fund. Appl.
   Toxicol., 18:515–521.
USP. (2000). The United States Pharmacopoeia XXIV § NF-19, United States Pharmacopeial Convention, Rockville, MD.
Wilsnack, R. E. (1976). Quantitative cell culture biocompatibility testing of medical devices and correlation to animal tests, Biomat. Med. Dev. Art. Org., 4:235–261.
Wilsnack, R. E., Meyer, F. J., and Smith, J. G. (1973). Human cell culture toxicity testing
   of medical devices and correlation to animal tests, Biomat. Med. Dev. Art. Org.,
   1:543–562.

6

Blood Compatibility

I. INTRODUCTION

Hemocompatibility—a lack of significant adverse interactions of a device with the found elements of the blood—is one of the most complex of the standard safety concerns for devices to be evaluated. Properly done as an independent entity, it would also be the most expensive of the standard, short-term responses end point to endnote. ISO 10993 part 4 (*Selection of Tests for Interactions with Blood*) presents 25 different categories of assays for these evaluations.

Few materials have consistently shown good hemocompatibility in both arterial and venous blood flow environments. Results obtained from laboratory animals may not apply to man, and results from one test system cannot be correlated to those obtained from a different test system. In vitro results may not be good predictors of what happens in vivo (Didisheim et al., 1984; Lindon et al., 1978). Any hemocompatibility statement should be linked to the intended use and conditions for which the statement is valid.

Blood-material interaction can range from minimal protein adsorption to activation of coagulation, complement, and destruction of cells. Complicated mechanisms that interact with medical devices exist in the cardiovascular system. Devices vary enormously in type, function, and duration of blood contact (Cooper et al., 1987; Dewangee, 1987), therefore a multidisciplinary approach to hemocompatibility testing is important. This includes in vitro static and dynamic tests, acute extracorporeal tests, tests of cardiovascular devices in animals, and clinical studies. Most commonly only the in vitro static tests are performed. Complex interactions are operative between the surfaces of devices/materials and the blood, based on both chemical and physical parameters (Zaslavsky et al., 1978).

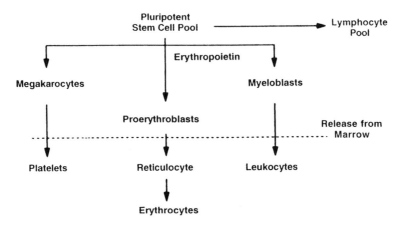

FIGURE 6.1   Representation of the genesis of formed blood elements arising from the bone marrow.

A thorough review of the normal function and structure of the hematopoietic system is a discipline in itself and far beyond the range of this chapter. Irons (1985), Brown (1984), and Williams et al. (1995) should be consulted by those interested in background information. Figures 6.1 and 6.2 provide a rudimentary overview of the pathways involved in the generation and differentiation of the formed elements of the blood.

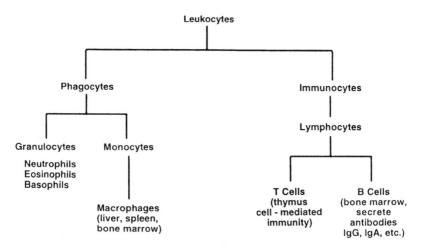

FIGURE 6.2   Representation of the differentiation of leukocytes into white blood cells.

The FDA and the Tripartite Subcommittee (1986) requirements for hemato-compatibility evaluation for most devices that were not implants in the vascular system were frequently met in part by performing a simple hemolysis test. The ASTM guidelines (ASTM, 1987) and NIH (1985) called for a more stringent approach. Under ISO-10993-4, either externally communicating devices with indirect or circulating contact with the blood stream, or implant devices in the vascular system must be evaluated. It is recommended that this evaluation look at five different end points (test categories: thrombosis, coagulation, platelets, hematology, and immunology). Table 6.1 summarizes the representation tests available to evaluate each of these end points.

Each of these categories, of course, is a potential type of interaction between the blood and the materials used in the devices.

Devices contacting and therefore potentially having an interaction with the blood are categorized by ISO as follows:

A. Noncontact Devices

An example is in vitro diagnostic devices, and these have no testing requirements.

B. External Communicating Devices

These are devices that contact the circulating blood and serve as a conduit into the vascular system. Examples include but are not limited to those below.

External communicating devices that serve as an indirect blood path include but are not limited to:

Cannulae
Extension sets
Devices for the collection of blood
Devices for the storage and administration of blood and blood products
(e.g., tubing, needles, and bags)

Indirect blood path devices are assigned the simplest testing strategy by ISO. A profile of six relatively inexpensive in vitro tests is recommended: one test for thrombosis, one for coagulation, one for platelet count, two hematology tests, and a complement activation panel for immunology. Additional optional tests may also be required.

External communicating devices in contact with circulating blood include but are not limited to:

Cardiopulmonary bypass
Extracorporeal membrane oxygenators
Hemodialysis equipment
Donor and therapeutic apheresis equipment

TABLE 6.1 ISO 10993-4: Selection of Tests for Interaction with Blood (Representative Tests)

Test categories	Level I methods	Level II methods	Comments
Thrombosis	Light microscopy (adhered platelets, leukocytes, aggregates, erythrocytes, fibrin, etc.)	SEM	Light microscopy can be replaced by scanning electron microscopy if the nature of the material presents technical problems for light microscopy.
Coagulation	Partial thromboplastin time (nonactivated)	FPA, D-Dimer, etc.	
Platelets	Platelet count	PF-4, thromboxane B2	
Hematology	Leukocyte count and differential; hemolysis (plasma hemoglobin)	Reticulocyte count	Hemolysis is regarded as an especially significant screening test to perform in this category because of its measurement of red blood cell membrane fragility in contact with materials and devices. The method used should be one of the normative standard test methods for hemolysis.
Immunology	C3a, C5a, RCC Bb, iC3b, C4d, SC5b-9	Cytokines and mRNAs	A panel including the last four tests encompasses the various complement activation pathways.

Devices for absorption of specific substances from the blood
Interventional cardiology and vascular devices
Percutaneous circulatory support systems
Temporary pacemaker electrodes

Circulating blood devices are assigned a somewhat more complex testing strategy, reflecting the fact that circulating blood must flow through the device; hence device patency becomes an issue. Again, tests from the five basic categories are recommended by ISO. Additional optional tests are also listed.

TABLE 6.2 Abbreviations

Abbreviation	Meaning
Bb	Product of alternate pathway complement activation
β-TG	Beta-thromboglobulin
C-4d	Product of classic pathway complement activation
C-3a, C5a	(Active) complement split products from C3 and C5
D-Dimer	Specific fibrin degradation products (F XIII cross-linked fibrin)
ECMO	Extracorporeal membrane oxygenator
E.M.	Electron microscopy
FDP	Fibrin/fibrinogen degradation products
FPA	Fibrinopeptide A
F_{1+2}	Prothrombin activation fragment 1 + 2
iC3b	Product of central C complement activation
IL-1	Interleukin-1
IVC	Inferior vena cava
MRI	Magnetic resonance imaging
PAC-1	Monoclonal antibody that recognizes the activated form of platelet surface glycoprotein IIb/IIIa
PET	Positron emission topography
PF-4	Platelet factor 4
PT	Prothrombin time
PTT	Partial thromboplastin time
RIA	Radioimmunoassay
S-12	Monoclonal antibody that recognizes the alpha granule membrane component GMP140 exposed during the platelet release reaction
SC5b-9	Product of terminal pathway complement activation
TAT	Thrombin-antithrombin complex
TCC	Terminal complement complex
TT	Thrombin time
VWF	von Willebrand factor

C. Implant Devices

These are devices that are placed largely or entirely within the vascular system. Examples include but are not limited to:

Mechanical or tissue heart valves
Prosthetic or tissue vascular grafts
Circulatory support devices (ventricular-assist devices, artificial hearts, intra-aortic balloon pumps)
Inferior vena cava filters

TABLE 6.3 External Communicating Devices

Test category	Method	Comments
Level 1: Blood path, indirect		
Thrombosis	Light microscopy (adhered platelets, leukocytes, aggregates, erythrocytes, fibrin, etc.)	Light microscopy can be replaced by scanning EM if the nature of the material presents technical problems for light microscopy
Coagulation	PTT (nonactivated)	
Platelets	Platelet count	
Hematology	Leukocyte count and differential: hemolysis (plasma hemoglobin)	Hemolysis is regarded as an especially significant screening test to perform in this category because of its measurement of red blood cell membrane fragility in contact with materials and devices. The method used should be one of the normative standard test methods for hemolysis.
Immunology	C3a, C5a, TCC, Bb, iC3b, C4d, SC5b-9	A panel including the last four tests encompasses the various complement activation pathways.
Level 2 (optional)		
Thrombosis	Scanning EM	
Coagulation	Coagulation factor assays, including: FPA, D-dimer, F_{1+2}, PAC-1, s-12, TAT	
Platelets	PF-4, β-TG, thromboxane B2, ^{111}In-labeled platelet survival	

Stents

Arteriovenous shunts

Blood monitors

Internal drug delivery catheters

Pacemaker electrodes

Intravascular membrane oxygenators (artificial lungs)

The ISO guidelines also provide detailed guidance as to tests to be performed for each of these types of devices. This guidance is summarized in Tables 6.3 through 6.7. Table 6.2 provides a codex for the significant aberrations utilized in Tables 6.2 through 6.7. Not covered in these tables are the specialized cases associated with cardiovascular devices.

TABLE 6.4 External Communicating Devices (Level 1: Circulating Blood)

Test category	Method	Comments
Thrombosis	Percentage occlusion; flow reduction; gravimetric analysis (thrombus mass); light microscopy (adhered platelets, leukocytes, aggregates, erythrocytes, fibrin, etc.); pressure drop across device	Light microscopy can be replaced by scanning EM if the nature of the material presents technical problems for light microscopy. Pressure drop not recommended for devices intended for PR.
Coagulation	PTT (nonactivated)	
Platelets	Platelet count; platelet aggregation; template bleeding time	
Hematology	Leukocyte count and differential: hemolysis (plasma hemoglobin)	Hemolysis is regarded as an especially significant screening test to perform in this category because of its measurement of red blood cell membrane fragility in contact with materials and devices. The method used should be one of the normative standard test methods for hemolysis.
Immunology	C3a, C5a, TCC, Bb, iC3b, C4d, SC5b-9	A panel including the last four tests encompasses the various complement activation pathways.

TABLE 6.5   External Communicating Devices (Level 2: Optional)

Test category	Method	Comments
Thrombosis	Scanning EM (platelet adhesion and aggregation; platelet and leukocyte morphology; fibrin)	
Coagulation	Specific coagulation factor assays; FPA, D-dimer, F_{1+2}, PAC-1, S-12, TAT	
Platelets	PF-4, β-TG; thomboxane B2; gamma imaging of radiolabeled platelets; ^{111}In-labeled platelet survival	^{111}In-labeling is recommended for PR only.
Hematology	Reticulocyte count; activation specific release products of peripheral blood cells (i.e., granulocytes)	
Immunology	C3a, C5a, TCC, Bb, iC3b, C4d, SC5b-9	A panel including the last four tests encompasses the various complement activation pathways.

II. STANDARD TESTS

Among the wide range of tests described in Tables 6.3 through 6.7, are a number that are most commonly performed. Theses are available at most contract research laboratories and hospitals, and include (besides the simple tests presented here) determination of the numbers and types of formed elements of the blood (Lewis et al., 1990) and other end points such as the absorption of specific formed elements of the blood (such as lymphocytes) on the surfaces of polymers and ceramics (Yokoyama et al., 1986). These may require more specialized equipment and approaches than are generally available.

A. Hemolysis Tests

The simplest and most commonly conducted menocompatibility test is the homolysis test. In the direct contact hemolysis test the intact test article is placed in a solution of saline and a small amount of whole red blood is added. After a period of incubation (1 hr at 37°C) the supernate is decanted and assayed for hemoglobin. The concentration of hemoglobin is proportional to the number of red cells that lysed.

TABLE **6.6** Implant Devices (Level 1)

Test category	Method	Comments
Thrombosis	Percentage occlusion; flow reduction; autopsy of device (gross and microscopic); autopsy of distal organs (gross and microscopic)	
Coagulation	PTT (nonactivated), PT, TT; plasma fibrinogen, FDP	
Platelets	Platelet count; platelet aggregation	
Hematology	Leukocyte count and differential; hemolysis (plasma hemoglobin)	Hemolysis is regarded as an especially significant screening test to perform in this category because of its measurement of red blood cell membrane fragility in contact with materials and devices. The method used should be one of the normative standard test methods for hemolysis.
Immunology	C3a, C5a, TCC, Bb, iC3b, C4d, SC5b-9	A panel including the last four tests encompasses the various complement activation pathways.

The percentage of hemolysis is calculated by the following equation:

$$Percentage\ hemolysis = \frac{A - B}{C} \times 100$$

where A is the absorbance of the test sample, B is the absorbance of a negative control, and C is the absorbance of a positive control.

Hemolysis tests evaluate the acute in vitro hemolytic properties of materials, especially those intended for use in contact with blood. The concentration of substances that produce hemolysis is generally higher than that needed to produce a cytotoxic effect. The result of hemolysis testing can be correlated with acute in vivo toxicity tests. A hemolysis test is rapid, requires simple equipment, gives easily interpretable quantitative results, and can be performed in the presence of the material or on the extract. The results are compared to the controls and expressed as the percentage of hemolysis.

TABLE 6.7   Implant Devices (Level 2: Optional)

Test category	Method	Comments
Thrombosis	Scanning EM; angiography	
Coagulation	Specific coagulation factor assays; FPA, D-dimer, F_{1+2}, PAC-1, S-12, TAT	
Platelets	^{111}In-labeled platelet survival PF-4, β-TG; thomboxane B2; gamma imaging of radiolabeled platelets	
Hematology	Reticulocyte count; activation specific release products of peripheral blood cells (i.e., granulocytes)	
Immunology	IL-1 and other cytokines; detection of messenger-RNA specific for cytokines	

The average life span of red cells is 120 days. When the life span is shortened, whatever the cause, there is said to be a hemolytic process, and when the marrow fails to replace the lost cells quickly enough a hemolytic anemia develops.

The term hemolytic is rather misleading, as it implies actual lysis or bursting of the red cells in the circulation. Sometimes this does occur, and then it is known as intravascular hemolysis. More often, however, the cells are damaged or in some way inadequate, and are then removed from the circulating blood by macrophages in the spleen in the usual way. This process is known as extravascular hemolysis. One of the most common tests for hemolysis is the osmotic fragility test.

The membranes surrounding most cells in animal tissues are semipermeable, which means that they allow the passage of water but prevent the passage of dissolved substances. When two solutions of different concentration are separated by such a membrane, water passes from the more dilute solution to the more concentrated one, until the concentration on both sides is equal. This tendency for water to flow in one direction is called osmosis, and the pressure exerted as it does so is known as the osmotic pressure.

Two solutions of equal concentration are known as "isotonic." When their concentrations are unequal the more dilute solution is "hypotonic" (hypo = low) and the more concentrated solution is "hypertonic" (hyper = over, above).

If red cells are to retain their shape and function properly, the hemoglobin solution inside the cell and the plasma outside the cell must be isotonic. Similarly, when dealing with red cells in the laboratory, solutions must be isotonic with the contents of the cell.

B. The Osmotic Fragility Test

The degree of hemolysis of cells in hypotonic solutions depends largely on their shape. Cells that are already spherocytic are easily lysed; that is, they are more fragile. Target cells, on the other hand, are more resistant to lysis than normal cells.

A series of solutions are prepared containing salt concentrations from 0.3 grams to 0.6 grams per 100 ml. A volume of blood is then added to each of these, and after half an hour the degree of hemolysis is found by spinning down the intact red cells and measuring the color intensity of the supernatant. A normal control blood must always be treated in the same way for the purpose of comparison and to check the quality of the reagents (Kirk et al., 1975). The process proceeds as follows:

1. Method
   a. Place two rows of seven 10-ml tubes in a rack, and label one row Ti-T7 (test) and the other row C1-C7 (control).
   b. Label another four tubes T. Std., T. Blank, C. Std., and C. Blank. Place these in the appropriate places in the rack.
   c. Using one row only, set up tubes as follows:

Tube	1	2	3	4	5	6	7	Std.	Blank
1% NaCl (ml)	3.0	3.5	4	4.5	5.0	5.5	6.0	—	10
Distilled water (ml)	7	6.5	6.0	5.5	5.0	4.5	4.0	10	—
Final NaCl concentration (g %)	0.3	0.35	0.4	0.45	0.5	0.55	0.6		

   d. Mix the solutions carefully, then transfer 5 ml from each tube to the corresponding tube of the second row. This ensures that each concentration is the same for test and control.
   e. To the test row add 0.05 ml of control blood in the same way.
   g. Mix all the tubes and allow them to stand at room temperature for 30 min.
   h. Mix them again, then centrifuge all the tubes at 3000 rev/min for 5 min.
   i. Using the appropriate blank, read the color intensities of the test row in a colorimeter, using an Ilford 625 green filter. Take care not to disturb

the red cell layer when transferring the clear supernatants to the cuvettes for reading.

  j. Repeat the procedure with the control row, taking care to change the blank.

2. Calculation and results: You now have two sets of eight readings, including the standards. The standards, which are cells in water, represent 100% hemolysis. They are different from each other, because the hemoglobin levels of the two bloods are different.

Using one set of readings, calculate the percentage hemolysis in each tube.

$$\text{Percentage hemolysis} = \frac{\text{Test reading}}{\text{Standard reading}} \times 100$$

Calculate the second set of results in the same way. The results are best expressed in the form of a graph showing the percentage hemolysis against the NaCl concentrations.

3. Factors influencing the results.

  a. The blood must be as fresh as possible, preferably less than 4 hr old. Cells deteriorate on standing and begin to lyse spontaneously.

  b. Defibrinated or heparinized blood is most suitable for this test, as such blood would not contain any extra salts. Blood anticoagulated with ethyl-enediamine-tetra-acetic acid (EDTA) is used also.

  c. The ratio of blood to saline affects the results; a ratio of $1:100$ is usually used.

  d. The pH of the saline also affects the results. In order to standardize this, a stock solution of buffered saline that is osmotically equivalent to 10% NaCl may be prepared, as follows:

Sodium chloride (NaCl):   10.80 grams
Disodium hydrogen phosphate ($Na_2PO_4.2H_2O$):   27.21 grams
Sodium dihydrogen phosphate ($NaH_2PO_4.2H_2$:   4.86 grams
Distilled water to 2 liters.

This solution is diluted 1 in 10 just before use.

4. Normal range

  a. Slight hemolysis: 0.45–0.4 g% NaCl.

  b. Complete hemolysis: 0.35–0.3 g% NaCl

C. Erythrocyte Stability

The erythrocyte stability test provides a sensitive measure of the interaction of leachable substances with the plasma membrane of erythrocytes and is reflected as changes in the osmotic fragility of the erythrocytes. This test can detect leachables at concentrations slightly below the sensitive levels of many cytotoxicity systems.

Hypotonic saline or distilled water (as described above under hemolysis) can be adjusted to the required tonicity. Extractors are adjusted to give osmolarity appropriate to hemolyze about 50% of the erythrocytes. Usually rabbit blood is used, diluted with isotonic saline to about 1% hematocrit. One-tenth ml of this stock erythrocyte solution is added to 5 ml of hypotonic extract, and the surviving cells are counted. The relative hemolysis, the number of cells lysed in the extract versus the number of cells lysed in the control, is reported. By performing the tests with a series of dilutions of the extract, the concentration of extract at which no detectable change occurs can be established and compared with data from other materials or from extracts prepared under different conditions. Cell size distribution profiles can also be obtained in this test, giving an indication of the degree of swelling or morphologic changes.

D. Whole Blood Clotting Time

Whole blood clotting time may be measured by modifying the Lee–White method or other relevant tests. Thrombin time, prothrombin time, and/or platelet counts should be included.

Partial thromboplastin time (PTI)
Shortened time = activation of intrinsic pathway
Sensitive to all known clotting factors except VII and XII
Prothrombin time (PT)
Measures activation of extrinsic pathway
Measures time required for recalcified plasma to clot in presence of thromboplastin
Thrombin time (TT)
Useful in detecting inhibitors of the thrombin–fibrinogen reaction
Measure the availability of functional fibrinogen

E. Thrombogenicity

Testing for thrombogenicity is normally done by examining platelet and fibrinogen turnover and observing thrombus formation and resulting emboli. Because thrombogenicity tests are usually difficult, controversial, and expensive, manufacturers should contact FDA to choose the proper model and test protocol (as briefly described below).

Thrombosis is the formation or existence of a blood clot within the vascular system. When associated with a device, it can be a life-threatening event because the clot, called a thrombus, can occlude a vessel and stop the blood supply to an organ or body part. If detached, the thrombus becomes an embolus and may occlude a vessel at a distance from the original site. When measuring thrombosis,

the test end point is the size of clot formation or the adherence of platelets, leukocytes, erythrocytes, or other aggregates on the test device.

In the *light microscopy* method, an intact sample may be exposed to whole
blood ex vivo. Ex vivo means away from or outside of the body, and in ex vivo
experiments, some of an animal's blood is caused to bypass the normal circulatory system and pass through or across a device, then flow back into the animal's
body. Light microscopy is used to scan the material for evidence of thrombus
formation. Alternatively, the material or device may be excised after a suitable
period of exposure in vivo, then scanned for thrombus formation using a light
microscope. Thrombosis "tests" give a yes or no answer; there is either thrombus
formation or there is not.

Percentage occlusion, flow reduction, and gravimetric analysis are all attempts to quantify the amount of thrombus formation. Percentage occlusion is
visually assessed after a device has been in use and has been removed. Percentage
occlusion is a measure of the severity of the thrombotic process in a conduit.
Flow reduction is a measure of the drop in rate or volume of blood flow through
a device after a period of implantation. Gravimetric analysis is a weight measure
of thrombus mass after removal of the mass from a device after a period of use.

Scanning electron microscopy is a method of visually assessing a device
on a micron scale. When used on explanted materials or devices it may give a
closer visual assessment of thrombus formation, capsular formation, or device
performance.

Angiography (an X ray of blood vessels that have been made radio-opaque
by the injection of a dye) is a method of taking an X ray of the vasculature
following injection of a radiopague substance to obtain a description of the blood
vessels or the arterial pulse.

F. Complement Activation

Inappropriate or excess complement activation may lead to unwanted tissue damage or cause cardiopulmonary distress in patients (Henderson, 1989). Complement activation is usually measured by the conversion of C_3 to C_{3a} and/or C_5 to
C_{5a}. The hemolytic complement expressed in CH_{50} is generally not sensitive
enough to detect complement activation caused by biomaterials and is not acceptable as a complement activation assay.

The classic complement system consists of nine separate protein components (C_1 through C_9) acting in sequence. When activated, complement components interact sequentially with one another in a cascade. Activation of some
complement components results in the cleavage of a component into two fragments. In some cases, the larger fragments join other activated fragments and
the smaller fragments, such as C_{3a} and C_{5a}, have inflammatory properties. The
C_{3a} and C_{5a} cause vasodilation and increase capillary permeability.

G. Protein Adsorption

The adsorption of plasma protein is generally the first event that occurs when blood contacts a foreign surface (Lemm and Unger, 1980). This protein layer has a great influence on the thrombogenicity of a material. One of the more commonly used techniques is the radiolabeling of protein with ^{125}I. The measurements consist of the following three steps:

> Exposing a solid surface to a solution containing the radiolabeled proteins
> Rinsing to remove all but the adsorbed protein
> Measuring the radioactivity retained by the surface

This technique provides a direct measurement of the amount of protein adsorbed on a surface. Protein adsorption can also be studied from flowing solutions in specially designed flow chambers. Recently, real-time spectrophotometric measurements of dynamic protein adsorption have been done by Fourier and transformed into infrared-attenuated total reflectance.

H. Coagulation

Coagulation refers to the process of blood clotting, which results from the initiation of a cascading enzymatic pathway in which the product of one reaction is an enzyme that catalyzes another subsequent reaction. The outcome of coagulation is the formation of a clot or thrombus. When measuring coagulation, the test end point is enzyme activation or suppression (not thrombus formation).

Clotting time, as designed by Lee and White, is probably the earliest coagulation test developed. It is not discussed in ISO 10993 part 4, although it is still frequently used to screen materials for blood compatibility. A sample of blood is removed from an animal exposed to a material or device. The time at which the blood is withdrawn is noted as accurately as possible. The syringe is emptied into a small glass tube, which is rotated endwise every 30 sec. The point at which the blood no longer flows from its position but maintains its surface contour when inverted is taken as the end point. Normal clotting time in humans is about 6.5 min.

Thromboplastin is the third blood coagulation factor (factor III). Partial thromboplastin time is the clotting time of recalcified citrated plasma upon the addition of partial thromboplastin obtained from mammalian brain or lung. Shortening of the PTT following contact with a material indicates activation of coagulation factors, and a prolonged PTT suggests a deficiency. A blood sample, as citrated plasma, is obtained from an animal that has been exposed to the intact material. An excess of calcium ions and thromboplastin are added and the time to clotting measured.

Prothrombin is a circulating protein that forms thrombin when acted upon by thrombokinase. Prothrombin time is related to prothrombin concentration and the accessory factors, factor V, factor VII, and factor X. In the presence of thromboplastin, clotting time depends on the concentrations of these four factors. A blood sample is obtained from an animal that has been exposed to the intact material. An excess of calcium ions and thromboplastin is added and the time to clotting measured. A prolonged PT indicates a deficiency of prothrombin, factors V, VII, X, or fibrinogen, indicating that the implant has inactivated, absorbed, or otherwise interfered with the concentration of these proteins.

Thrombin is a protein found in shed blood. Formed from prothrombin, it reacts with soluble fibrinogen, converting it to fibrin, which forms the basis of blood clots. Thrombin time is the time required for plasma to clot when a solution of thrombin is added. A blood sample as plasma is obtained from an animal that has been exposed to the intact material. A solution of thrombin is added to the plasma and the time to clotting measured. A prolonged TT indicates a deficiency in fibrinogen.

Plasma fibrinogen is a protein in the blood that forms fibrin when acted upon by thrombin and calcium. A sample of plasma is obtained from an animal that has been exposed to the intact material. Active fibrinogen is measured indirectly by using a commercially available TT assay. Thrombin time is dependent on fibrinogen and can be an accurate measure of its active concentration.

Fibrin/fibrinogen degradation products are by-products of degraded fibrin and/or fibrinogen. A sample of plasma is obtained from an animal that has been exposed to the intact material. An immunoassay is performed by exposing the plasma to fibrin/fibrinogen antibodies per the instructions in commercially available tests.

Specific coagulation factor assays for fibrinopeptide A, D dimer (a fibrin degradation product), F_{1+2} (prothrombin activation fragment 1+2), PAC-1 (a monoclonal antibody that recognizes the activated form of platelet surface glycoprotein IIb/IIIa), S-12 (a monoclonal antibody that recognizes the alpha granule membrane component 9GMP140 exposed during the platelet release reaction), or TAT (thrombin-antithrombin complex) may be performed on blood samples taken from animals exposed to intact implanted material.

I. Platelets

1. Platelet Count

Platelets are flat, round cells found in the circulating blood. They play an important role in blood coagulation, hemostasis, and thrombus formation. When a small vessel is injured, platelets adhere to each other and the edges of the injury and form a plug. The plug or blood clot soon retracts and stops the loss of blood. A blood sample is obtained from an animal that has been exposed to the intact material and the number of platelets per mm^3 is determined. Normal human values are 200,000 to 300,000.

2. Platelet Aggregation

Platelet aggregation is induced when cells at the site of injury secrete epinephrine, or when collagen, thrombin, or other agents are produced at the site. Platelet aggregation can by induced in vitro by the addition of these agents exogenously. To evaluate the ability of platelets to aggregate, plasma is placed in a beaker and the exogenous agents added with constant stirring. As the platelets aggregate the plasma becomes progressively clearer. An optical system (aggregometer) is used to detect the change in light transmission. Delayed or reduced platelet aggregation, or spontaneous aggregation, is a sign of platelet activation.

Assays for PF-4 (platelet factor 4), β-TG (beta-thromboglobulin), or thromboxane B2 may be performed on blood samples taken from animals exposed to intact implanted material.

Gamma imaging of radiolabeled platelets may be performed using [111]Indium-labeled platelets. Platelet survival times may be determined in situ in animals exposed to intact implanted material.

III. CONCLUSION

Though hematocompatibility has long been identified as a concern for medical devices and biomaterials (Mason, 1972; Autian, 1977; Wilsnack and Bernadyn, 1979), it is only recently that the standards for evaluation of the relevant end points have come to utilize available technology (ISO-10993-4).

Currently, for materials and for devices with limited (in either extent of duration) exposure to the circulated blood, a limited battery of in vitro evaluations as described in Table 6.1 should be adequate to ensure hematocompatibility. For devices with extended contact with circulating blood (systemic circulation), however, a much more extensive evaluation, including at least an in vivo study in a suitable model species, should be considered.

REFERENCES

ASTM F 756-87. (1987). Standard Practice for Assessment of Hemolytic Properties of Materials, Washington, DC.

Autian, J. (1977). Toxicological evaluation of biomaterials: primary acute toxicity screening program, Art. Organs, 1:53–60.

Brown, B. A. (1984). Hematology: Principles and Procedures, Lea and Febiger, Philadelphia.

Cooper, S. L., Fabrizius, D. J., and Grasel, T. G. (1987). Methods of assessment of thrombosis ex vivo. In: Blood in Contact with Natural and Artificial Surfaces, vol. 516 (E. F. Leonard, V. T. Turitto, and L. Vroman, Eds.). Ann. NY Acad. Sci., pp. 572–585.

Dewangee, M. K. (1987). Methods of assessment of thrombosis in vivo. In: Blood in

Contact with Natural and Artificial Surfaces, vol. 516 (E. F. Leonard, V. T. Turitto, and L. Vroman, Eds.). Ann. NY Acad. Sci., pp. 541–571.

Didisheim, P., Dewanjee, M. K., Kaye, M. P., Frisk, C. S., Fass, D. N., Tirrell, M. V., and Xillman, P. E. (1984). Nonpredictability of long-term in vivo response from short-term in vitro or ex vivo blood/material interactions. Trans. Am. J. Soc. Art. Int. Organs, 30:370–376.

Henderson, L. W. (1989). Immunotoxicology of blood-synthetic membrane interactions, Fund. Appl. Toxicol., 13:228–234.

Irons, R. D., ed. (1985). Toxicology of the Blood and Bone Marrow, Raven, New York.

ISO. (1993). ISO-10993-part 4, Selection of Tests for Interactions with Blood.

Kirk, C. J. C., Peel, R. N., James, K. R., and Kershaw, Y. (1975). Basic Medical Laboratory Technology, Wiley, New York.

Lemm, N. and Unger, V. (1980). Adsorption of blood proteins on different polymer surfaces in vitro. In: Evaluation of Biomaterials (G. D. Winter, J. L. Leary, and K. deGroot, Eds.). Wiley, New York.

Lewis, S. M., Rowan, R. M., and Kubota, F. (1990). Recommended methods for the visual determination of white cell and platelet count, J. Clin. Pathol., 43:932–936.

Lindon, N. N., Rodvien, R., Brier, D., et al. (1978). In vitro assessment of interaction of blood with model surfaces, J. Lab. Clin. Med., 92:904–914.

Mason, R. G. (1972). Some methods of in vitro estimation of the blood compatibility of biomaterials, Bull. NY Acad. Med., 48(2):407–424.

NIH. (1985). Guidelines for Blood–Materials Interactions, Report of the National Heart, Lung, and Blood Institute-Working Group, NIH publication no. 85-2185, Sept. 1985.

Tripartite Biocompatibility Guidance for Medical Devices. (1986). Prepared by toxicology subgroup of the Tripartite subcommittee on medical devices, Sept. 1986.

Williams, W. J., Bentley, R., Erslev, A. J., and Rundles, R. W. (1995). Hematology, 3rd ed. McGraw–Hill, New York.

Wilsnack, R. E. and Bernadyn, S. A. (1979). Blood compatibility of medical device materials as measured by lymphocyte function, Biomat. Med. Dev. Art. Organs, 7(4): 527–546.

Yokoyama, M., Nakahashi, T., Nishimura, T., Maeda, M., Inoue, S., Kataoka, K, and Sakurai, Y. (1986). Adhesion behavior of rat lymphocytes to poly (ether)-poly (amino acid) block and graft copolymers, J. Biomed. Mat. Res., 20:867–878.

Zaslavsky, B. Y., Ossipov, N. N., and Rogozhin, S. V. (1978). Action of surface-active substances on biological membranes. III. Comparison of hemolytic activity of ionic and nonionic surfactants, Bhiochim. Biophys. Acta, 510:15–159.

7

Irritation and Pyrogenicity

Irritation studies assess the short-term and generally localized hazards of medical devices in the immediate region of their applications. Topical local (tissue) tolerance effects are almost entirely limited to irritation. Though this usually means dermal irritation, it can also be vaginal, rectal, nasal, or ocular. All but ocular irritation use some version of a common subjective rating scale (see Table 7.1) to evaluate responses.

Most commonly recognized is the use of this scale in the primary dermal irritation (PDI) test, which is performed for those agents that are to be administered to patients by application to the skin. As with all local tolerance tests, it is essential that the material be evaluated in "condition of use"; that is, in the final product, and applied to test animals in the same manner that the device is to be used clinically. If appropriate (under applicable regulations) or necessary due to the nature or mode of use of the device, an extract can be evaluated. Such extracts are generally evaluated in the intracutaneous reactivity test.

Additionally, there is a requirement for devices to evaluate the potential pyrogenicity of the final product (and generally, on a quality control basis of subsequent appropriately selected samples of production lots) if

The label claims that the device is pyrogen-free
The device comes in contact with blood or spinal fluid
The device is an intraocular lens

TABLE 7.1 Evaluation of Local Tissue Reactions in Tissue Irritation Studies

Method basis/end point	Reference
Erythema and eschar formation	
No erythema	0
Very slight erythema (barley perceptible)	1
Well-defined erythema	2
Moderate to severe erythema	3
Severe erythema (beet redness) to slight eschar formation (injuries in depth)	4
Necrosis (death of tissue)	+N
Eschar (sloughing and scar formation)	+E
Edema formation	
No edema	0
Very slight edema (barely perceptible)	1
Slight edema (edges of area well-defined by definite raising)	2
Moderate edema (raised approximately 1 mm)	3
Severe edema (raised more than 1 mm and extending beyond the area of exposure)	4
Total possible score for primary irritation	8

Source: Draize et al., 1944.

I. DERMAL IRRITATION

Skin irritation testing is performed to demonstrate the potential toxicity of the device; that is, for initiating or aggravating damage through its contact with the skin (Draize, 1955; 1959). Primary skin irritation is usually done according to the regulations of the Consumer Product Safety Commission, Title 16, Chapter II, Part 1500, or some variation thereof (e.g., ISO 10993) (ASTM, 1981). The purpose of the study is to determine the dermal irritation potential of the test article to the intact and abraded skin of the rabbit.

Skin absorption occurs through a process of binding, partitioning, and diffusion of test materials on and into the skin. Penetration has been assessed in vivo by measuring the amount of test substances at different times at different layers of the skin. Blood levels of the test sample have been measured in this test.

A complicated series of chemical and physiological responses result in primary skin irritation. When skin is exposed to toxic substances, the Draize rabbit skin test, first outlined by John Draize in 1944, remains an important source of safety information for government and industry. In this test, the dermal irritation caused by a substance is investigated by observing changes ranging from erythema and edema to ulceration produced in rabbit skin when irritants are applied.

These skin reactions are produced by diverse physiologic mechanisms, although they are easily observed visually and by palpitation.

Evaluation of materials for their potential to cause dermal irritation and corrosion due to acute contact has been common for industrial chemicals, cosmetics, agricultural chemicals, and consumer products since at least the 1930s (Generally, pharmaceuticals are only evaluated for dermal effects if they are to be administered topically—and then by repeat exposure tests, which will not be addressed here.) As with acute eye irritation tests, one of the earliest formal publications of a test method (although others were used) was that of Draize et al. in 1944 (Geller et al., 1985; SOT, 1989). The methods currently used are still basically those proposed by Draize et al., and have changed very little since 1944. Although these methods (unlike their near relatives, the eye irritation tests) have not particularly caught the interest and spotlight of concern of the animal welfare movement, there are efforts underway to develop alternatives that either don't use animals or are performed in a more humane and relevant (to human exposure) manner.

Among the most fundamental assessments of the safety of a product, or indeed of any material that has the potential to be in contact with a significant number of people in our society, are tests in animals that seek to predict potential skin irritation or corrosion. Like all the other tests in what is classically called range finding, tier I, or acute battery, the tests used here are among the oldest designs and are currently undergoing the greatest degree of scrutiny or change. Currently all the established test methods for these end points use the same animal model—the rabbit (almost exclusively the New Zealand White)—though some other animal models have been proposed.

Virtually all have the potential to contact the skin of people. In fact, many (cosmetics and shampoos, e.g.) are intended to have skin contact. The greatest number of medical device problems are skin conditions, indicating the large extent of dermal exposure where none is intended.

Testing is performed to evaluate the potential occurrence of two different yet related end points. The broadest application of these is an evaluation of the potential to cause skin irritation, characterized by erythema (redness) and edema (swelling). Severity of irritation is measured in terms of both the degree of these two parameters and how long they persist. There are two types of irritation tests, each designed to address a different concern.

1. Primary (or acute) irritation, a localized reversible dermal exposure response resulting from a single application of, or exposure to, a chemical without the involvement of the immune system.
2. Cumulative irritation, a reversible dermal response resulting from repeated exposure to a substance. (Each individual exposure is not capable of causing acute primary irritation.)

Although most regulations and common practice characterize an irritation that persists for 14 days past the end of exposure as other than reversible, the second end point of concern with dermal exposure—corrosion per se—is assessed in separate test designs. These tests start with a shorter exposure period (4 hr or less) to the material of concern, and then evaluate simply whether tissue has been killed or not (or, in other words, if necrosis is present or not).

It should be clear that if a material is found to have less than severe dermal irritation potential, it will not be corrosive, and therefore need not be tested separately for the corrosion endpoint.

The adult human has 1.8 m^2 of skin, varying in thickness from 0.02 in. on the eyelids to 0.12 to 0.16 in. on the back, palms, and soles of the feet (Hipp, 1978). The epidermis, the outer portion of the skin, is several layers thick, covers the entire surface of the body, and is referred to as the horny layer or *stratum corneum*. It is the first line of defense against physical, chemical, and thermal exposure. The skin is host to normal bacterial flora consisting of *Micrococci* and *Corynebacterium*, which play an important role in the protection against infection. The melanocyte system, responsible for skin colonization, is located at the interface of the epidermis and the dermis. New cells are constantly being formed from the basal layer and slowly migrate to the surface, replenishing themselves approximately every two weeks (Monash and Blank, 1958).

Irritation is generally a localized reaction resulting from either a single or multiple exposure to a physical or chemical entity at the same site. It is characterized by the presence of erythema (redness), edema, and may or may not result in cell death. The observed signs are heat (caused by vessel dilation and the presence of large amounts of warm blood in the affected area), redness (due to capillary dilation), and pain (due to pressure on the sensory nerves). The edema often observed is largely due to plasma, which coagulates in the injured area, precipitating a fibrous network to screen off the area, thereby permitting leukocytes to destroy exogenous materials by phagocytosis. If the severity of injury is sufficient, cell death may occur, thereby negating the possibility of cellular regeneration. Necrosis is a term often used in conjunction with cell death, and is the degeneration of the dead cell into component molecules that approach equilibrium with surrounding tissue (Montagna, 1961).

A. Primary Dermal Irritation Test

I. Rabbit testing procedure
  A. A group of at least 8 to 12 New Zealand White rabbits are screened for the study.
  B. All rabbits selected for the study must be in good health; any rabbit exhibiting sniffles, hair loss, loose stools, or apparent weight loss is rejected and replaced.

C. One day (at least 18 hr) prior to application of the test substance, each rabbit is prepared by clipping the hair from its back and sides using a small animal clipper. A no. 10 blade is used to remove long hair and a no. 40 blade is used to remove the remaining hair.

D. Six animals with skin sites that are free from hyperemia or abrasion (due to shaving) are selected. Skin sites that are in the telogen phase (resting stage of hair growth) are used. Those skin sites that are in the anagen phase (stage of active growth, indicated by the presence of a thick undercoat of hair) or not used.

II. Study procedure

A. As many as four areas of skin, two on each side of the rabbit's back, can be utilized for sites of administration.

B. Separate animals are not required for an untreated control group. Each animal serves as its own control.

C. Besides the test substance, a positive control substance (a known skin irritant—1% sodium lauryl sulfate in distilled water) and a negative control (an untreated patch) are applied to the skin. When a vehicle is used for diluting, suspending, or moistening the test substance, a vehicle control patch is required, especially if the vehicle is known to cause any toxic dermal reactions of if there is insufficient information about the dermal effects of the vehicle.

D. The intact (free of abrasion) sites of administration are assigned a code number. Up to four sites can be used, as follows:
1. Test substance
2. Negative control
3. Positive control
4. Vehicle control (if required)

E. Application sites should be rotated from one animal to the next to ensure that the test substance and controls are applied to each position at least once.

F. Each test or control substance is held in place with a 1-in. × 1-in. 12-ply surgical gauze patch. The gauze patch is applied to the appropriate skin site and secured with 1-in.-wide strips of surgical tape at the four edges, leaving the center of the gauze patch nonoccluded.

G. If the test substance is a solid or semisolid, a 0.5-gram portion is weighed and placed on the gauze patch. The test substance patch is placed on the appropriate skin site and secured. The patch is subsequently moistened with 0.5 ml of physiological saline.

H. When the test substance is in flake, granule, powder, or other particulate form, the weight of the test substance that has a volume of 0.5 ml (after compacting as much as possible without crushing or altering the individual particles, such as by tapping the measuring container) is used whenever this volume weight is less than 0.5 grams. When applying powders, granules, and the like, the gauze patch designated for the test sample is secured to the appropriate skin site with one of four strips of tape at the most ventral position of the animal. With one hand, the appropriate amount of sample measuring 0.5 ml is carefully poured from a glycine weighing paper onto the gauze patch that is held in a horizontal (level) position with the other hand. The patch containing the test sample is then carefully placed into position on the skin and the remaining three edges are secured with tape. The patch is subsequently moistened with 0.5 ml of physiological saline.

   I.   If the test substance is a liquid, a patch is applied and secured to the appropriate skin site. A 1-ml tuberculin syringe is used to measure and apply 0.5 ml of test substance to the patch.

   J.   The negative control site is covered with an untreated 12-ply surgical gauze patch (1 in. $\times$ 1 in.).

   K.   The positive control substance and vehicle control substance are applied to the gauze patch in the same manner as a liquid test substance.

   L.   The entire trunk of the animal is covered with an impervious material (e.g., Saran Wrap) for a 24-hr period of exposure. The Saran Wrap is secured by wrapping several long strips of athletic adhesive tape around the trunk of the animal. The impervious material aids in maintaining the position of the patches and retards the evaporation of volatile test substances.

   M.   An Elizabethan collar is fitted and fastened around the neck of each test animal. The collar remains in place for the 24-hr exposure period. The collars are utilized to prevent removal of wrappings and patches by the animals, while allowing the animals food and water *ad libitum*.

   N.   The wrapping is removed at the end of the 24-hr exposure period. The test substance skin site is wiped to remove any test substance still remaining. When colored test substances (e.g., dyes) are used, it may be necessary to wash the test substance from the test site with an appropriate solvent or vehicle (one that is suitable for the substance being tested). This is done to facilitate accurate evaluation for skin irritation.

   O.   Immediately after the removal of the patches, each 1 in. $\times$ 1 in. test or control site is outlined with an indelible marker by dotting each of the four corners. This procedure delineates the site for identification.

III.   Observations

   A.   Observations are made of the test and control skin sites 1 hr after removal of the patches (25 hr postinitiation of application). Erythremia and edema are evaluated and scored on the basis of the designated values presented earlier in Table 7.1.

    B.   Observations are again performed 46 and 72 hr after application and the scores are recorded.

    C.   If necrosis is present or the dermal reaction is unusual, the reaction should be described. Severe erythema should receive the maximum score (4), and +N should be used to designate the presence of necrosis and +E the presence of eschar.

    D.   When the test substance produces dermal irritation that persists 72 hr postapplication, daily observations of test and control sites are continued on all animals until all irritation caused by the test substance resolves until day 14 postapplication.

IV. Evaluation of results

    A.   A *subtotal irritation value* for erythema and eschar formation is determined for each rabbit by adding the values observed at 25, 48 and 72 hr postapplication.

    B.   A *subtotal irritation value* for edema formation is determined for each rabbit by adding the values observed at 25, 48, and 72 hr postapplication.

    C.   A *total irritation score* is calculated for each rabbit by adding the subtotal value for erythema or eschar formation to the subtotal irritation value for edema formation.

    D.   The *primary dermal irritation index* (PDII) is calculated for the test substance or control substance by dividing the sum of the total irritation scores by the number of observations (three days × six animals = 18 observations).

    E.   The categories of the PDII are as follows. (This categorization of dermal irritation is a modification of the original classification described by Draize et al., 1944.)

          PDII = 0.0   Nonirritant
          >0.0–0.5   Negligible irritant
          >0.5–2.0   Mild irritant
          >2.0–5.0   Moderate irritant
          >5.0–8.0   Severe irritant

    Other abnormalities, such as atonia or desquamation, should be noted and recorded.

B. In Vitro Alternatives

Extensive progress has been made in devising alternative in vitro systems for evaluating the dermal irritation potential of chemicals since this author last reviewed the field (Gad and Chengelis, 1998). Table 7.2 overviews 20 proposed

TABLE 7.2 In Vitro Dermal Irritation Test Systems

System	End point	Validation data?[a]	References
Test I			
Excised patch of perfused skin	Swelling	No	Dannenberg et al. (1987)
Mouse skin organ culture	Inhibition of incorporation of [³H]-thymidine and [¹⁴C]-leucine labels	No	Kato et al. (1992)
Mouse skin organ culture	Leakage of LDH and GOT	Yes	Bartnik et al. (1989)
Test II			
TESTSKIN—cultured surrogate skin patch	Morphological evaluation (?)	No	Bell et al. (1989)
Cultured surrogate skin patch	Cytotoxicity	No	Naughton (1989)
Test III			
Human epidermal keratinocytes (HEKs)	Release of labeled arachidonic acid	Yes	DeLeo et al. (1988)
Fibroblasts	Acids	Yes	Lamont et al. (1989)
HEKs	Cytotoxicity	Yes	Gales et al. (1989)
HEKs	Cytotoxicity (MIT)	Yes	Swisher et al. (1988)
HEKs, dermal fibroblasts	Cytotoxicity	Yes	Babich et al. (1989)
HEKs	Inflammation mediator release	No	Boyce et al. (1988)

Cultured Chinese hamster ovary	Increase in β-hexosaminidase levels in the media	No	Lei et al. (1986)
Cultured $C_3H10T_{1/2}$ and HEK cells	Lipid metabolism inhibition	No	DeLeo et al. (1987, 1988)
Cultured cells			
BHK21/C13	Cell detachment	Yes	Reinhardt et al. (1987)
BHK21/C13	Growth inhibition		
primary rat thymocytes	Increased membrane permeability		
Rat periodontal mast cells	Inflammation mediator release	Yes (surfactants)	Prottey and Ferguson (1976)
Test IV			
Hen's egg	Morphological examination		Reinhardt et al. (1987)
SKINTEX—protein mixture	Protein coagulation	Yes	Gordon et al. (1990); Bason et al. (1991)
Test V			
Structure-activity relationship (SAR) model	NA	Yes	Enslein et al. (1987)
SAR model	NA	No	Firestone and Guy (1986)

[a] Evaluated by comparison of predictive accuracy for a range of compounds compared with animal test results. Not validated in the sense used in this chapter. *Note:* NA = not applicable.

systems that now constitute five very different approaches. This is an effort that extends back to the early 1960s (Choman, 1963).

The first approaches (I) uses patches of excised human or animal skin maintained in some modification of a glass diffusion cell that maintains the moisture, temperature, oxygenation, and electrolyte balance of the skin section. In this approach, after the skin section has been allowed to equilibrate for some time, the material of concern is placed on the exterior surface and wetted (if not liquid). Irritation is evaluated either by swelling of the skin (a crude and relatively insensitive method for mild and moderate irritants), by an evaluation of the inhibition of uptake of radiolabeled nutrients, or by measurement of leakage of enzymes through damaged membranes.

The second set of approaches (II) utilizes a form of surrogate skin culture comprising a mix of skin cells that closely mirror key aspects of the architecture and function of the intact organ. These systems seemingly offer a real potential advantage, but to date the "damage markers" employed (or proposed) as predictors of dermal irritation have been limited to cytotoxicity.

The third set of approaches (III) is to use some form of cultured cell (either primary or transformed), with primary human epidermal keratinocytes (HEKs) preferred. The cell cultures are exposed to the material of interest, then ectotoxicity, release of inflammation markers, or decrease of some indicator of functionality (lipid metabolism, membrane permeability, or cell detachment) is measured.

The fourth group (IV) contains two miscellaneous approaches—the use of the membrane from a hen's egg with morphological evaluation of damage being the predictor of the end point (Reinhardt et al., 1987), and the SKINTEX system, which utilizes the coagulation of a mixture of soluble proteins to predict dermal response.

Finally, in group V there are two structure–activity relationship models that use mathematical extensions of past animal results correlated with structure to predict the effects of new structures.

Many of these test systems are in the process of evaluating their performance against various small groups of compounds for which the dermal irritation potential is known. Evaluation by multiple laboratories of a wider range of structures will be essential before any of these systems can be generally utilized.

II. OCULAR IRRITATION TESTING

Ocular irritation is significantly different from the other local tissue irritation tests for a number of reasons (Grant, 1993). For the medical device industry, eye irritation testing is performed when the device is intended to be put into the eye as a means or route of application for ocular therapy. There are a number of special tests applicable to medical devices that are beyond the scope of this chapter, since they are intended to assess potential effects or irritation of a specific device. These are addressed later in the chapter on special cases (Chapter 15). In general, however, it is desired that an eye irritation test that is utilized by this group be both sensitive and accurate in predicting the potential to cause irritation in humans. Failing to identify human ocular irritants (lack of sensitivity) is to be avoided, but of equal concern is the occurrence of false positives.

A. Primary Eye Irritation Test

The primary eye irritation test was originally intended to predict the potential for a single splash of chemical into the eye of a human being to cause reversible and/or permanent damage. Since the introduction of the original Draize test over 50 years ago (Draize et al., 1944), ocular irritation testing in rabbits has both developed and diverged. Indeed, there is clearly no longer a single test design that is used, and different objectives are pursued by different groups using the same test. This lack of standardization has been recognized for some time and attempts have been made to address standardization of at least the methodological aspects of the test, if not the design aspects.

One widely used study design, which begins with a screening procedure as an attempt to avoid testing severe irritants or corrosives in animals goes as follows:

I. Test article screening procedure
   A. Each test substance will be screened in order to eliminate potentially corrosive or severely irritating materials from being studied for eye irritation in the rabbit.
   B. If possible, the pH of the test substance will be measured.
   C. A primary dermal irritation test will be performed prior to the study.
   D. The test substance will not be studied for eye irritation if it is a strong acid (pH of 2.0 or less) or strong alkali (pH of 11.0 or greater), and/or if the test substance is a severe dermal irritant (with a PDII of 5 to 8) or causes corrosion of the skin.
   E. If it is predicted that the test substance does not have the potential to be severely irritating or corrosive to the eye, continue to the rabbit screen procedure.

II. Rabbit screening procedure
   A. A group of at least 12 New Zealand White rabbits of either sex are screened for the study. The animals are removed from their cages and placed in rabbit restraints. Care should be taken to prevent mechanical damage to the eye during this procedure.
   B. All rabbits selected for the study must be in good health. Any rabbit exhibiting sniffles, hair loss, loose stools, or apparent weight loss is rejected and replaced.
   C. One hour prior to instillation of the test substance, both eyes of each

rabbit are examined for signs of irritation and corneal defects with a handheld slit lamp. All eyes are stained with 2.0% sodium fluorescein and examined to confirm the absence of corneal lesions. *Fluorescein staining*: Cup the lower lid of the eye to be tested and instill one drop of a 2% (in water) sodium fluorescein solution onto the surface of the cornea. After 15 sec, thoroughly rinse the eye with physiological saline. Examine the eye, employing a handheld long-wave ultraviolent illuminator in a darkened room. Corneal lesions, if present, appear as bright yellowish-green fluorescent areas.

D. Only nine of the 12 animals are selected for the study. The nine rabbits must not show any signs of eye irritation and must show either a negative or minimum fluorescein reaction (due to normal epithelial desquamation).

III. Study procedure

A. At least 1 hr after fluorescein staining, the test substance is placed in one eye of each animal by gently pulling the lower lid away from the eyeball to form a cup (conjunctival cul-de-sac) into which the test material is dropped. The upper and lower lids are then gently held together for 1 sec to prevent immediate loss of material.

B. The other eye remains untreated and serves as a control.

C. For testing liquids, 0.01 ml of the test substance is used.

D. For solids or pastes, 100 mg of the test substance is used.

E. When the test substance is in flake, granular, powder, or other particulate form, the amount that has a volume of 0.01 ml (after gently compacting the particles by tapping the measuring container in a way that will not alter their individual form) is used whenever this volume weighs less than 10 mg.

F. For aerosol products, the eye should be held open and the substance administered in a single 1-sec burst at a distance of about 4 in. directly in front of the eye. The velocity of the ejected material should not traumatize the eye. The dose should be approximated by weighing the aerosol can before and after such treatment. For other liquids propelled under pressure, such as substances delivered by pump sprays, an aliquot of 0.01 ml should be collected and instilled in the eye as for liquids.

G. The treated eyes of six of the rabbits are not washed following instillation of the test substance.

H. The treated eyes of the remaining three rabbits are irrigated for 1 min with room temperature tap water, starting 20 sec after instillation.

I. To prevent self-inflicted trauma by the animals immediately after instillation of the test substance, the animals are not immediately returned to their cages. After the test and control eyes are examined and graded at 1 hr postexposure, the animals are returned carefully to their respective cages.

IV. Observations

  A. The eyes are observed for any immediate signs of discomfort after instilling the test substance. Blepharospasm and/or excessive tearing are indicative of irritating sensations caused by the test substance, and their duration should be noted. Blepharospasm does not necessarily indicate that the eye will show signs of ocular irritation.

  B. Grading and scoring of ocular irritation are performed in accordance with Table 7.3. The eyes are examined and grades of ocular reactions are recorded.

  C. If signs of irritation persist at day 7, readings are continued on days 10 and 14 after exposure or until all signs of reversible toxicity are resolved.

  D. In addition to the required observation of the cornea, iris, and conjunctiva, serious effects (e.g., pannus, rupture of the globe, or blistering of the conjunctivae) indicative of a corrosive action are reported.

  E. Whether or not toxic effects are reversible depends on the nature, extent, and intensity of damage. Most lesions, if reversible, will heal or clear within 21 days, therefore if ocular irritation is present at the 14-day reading, a 21-day reading is required to determine whether the ocular damage is reversible or nonreversible.

B. Alternatives

Testing for a potential to cause irritation or damage to the eyes remains the most active area for the development (and validation) of alternatives and the most sensitive area of animal testing in biomedical research. This has been true since the beginning of the 1980s. Table 7.4 presents an overview of the reasons for pursuing such alternatives. The major reason, of course, has been the pressure from public opinion.

Indeed, many of the in vitro tests now being evaluated for other end points (e.g., skin irritation and lethality) are adaptations of test systems first developed for eye irritation uses. A detailed review of the underlying theory of each test system is beyond the scope of this chapter. Frazier et al. (1987) performed such a review, and Table 7.5 presents an updated version of the list of test systems overviewed in that volume.

There are six major categories of approachs to in vitro systems. Replacing the rabbit would require some form of battery of such test systems. Many individual systems, however, might constitute effective screens in defined situations. The first five of these aim at assessing portions of the irritation response, including alterations in tissue morphology, toxicity to individual complete cells or tissue

TABLE 7.3 Scale of Weighted Scores for Grading the Severity of
Ocular Lesions

Reaction criteria	Score
I. Cornea	
A. Opacity degree of density (area that is most dense is taken for reading)	
1. Scattered or diffuse area, details of iris clearly visible	1
2. Easily discernible translucent area, details of iris slightly obscured	2
3. Opalescent areas, no details of iris visible, size of pupil barely discernible	3
B. Area of cornea involved	
1. One-quarter (or less) but not zero	1
2. Greater than one-quarter, less than one-half	2
3. Greater than one-half, less than whole area	3
4. Greater than three-quarters, up to whole area	4
Scoring equals A × B × 5; total maximum = 80[a]	
II. Iris	
A. Values	
1. Folds above normal, congestion, swelling, circumcorneal ingestion (any one or all of these or combination of any thereof), iris still reacting to light (sluggish reaction is possible)	1
2. No reaction to light, hemorrhage, gross destruction (any one or all of these)	2
Scoring equals A × B (where B is the area of the iris involved, graded as "under cornea"); total maximum = 10	
III. Conjunctivae	
A. Redness (refers to palpebral conjunctivae only)	
1. Vessels definitely injected above normal	1
2. More diffuse, deeper crimson red, individual vessels not easily discernible	2
3. Diffuse beefy red	3
B. Chemosis	
1. Any swelling above normal (include initiating membrane)	1
2. Obvious swelling with partial eversion of the lids	2
3. Swelling with lids about half closed	3
4. Swelling with lids about half closed to completely closed	4
C. Discharge	
1. Any amount different from normal (does not include small amount observed in inner canthus of normal animals)	1
2. Discharge with moistening of the lids and hair just adjacent to the lids	2
3. Discharge with moistening of the lids and considerable area around the eye	3
Scoring (A + B + C) × 2; total maximum = 20	

Note: The maximum total score is the sum of all scores obtained from the cornea, iris, and conjunctivae.
[a] All A × B = Σ (1–3) × Σ (1–4) for six animals.

TABLE 7.4 Rationales for Seeking in Vitro Alternatives for Eye Irritancy Tests

1. Avoid whole animal and organ in vivo evaluation.
2. Strict Draize scale testing in the rabbit assesses only three eye structures (conjunctiva, cornea, iris), and traditional rabbit eye irritancy tests do not assess cataracts, pain, discomfort, or clouding of the lens.
3. In vivo tests assess only inflammation and immediate structural alternations produced by irritants (not sensitizers, photoirritants or photoallergens). Note, however, that the test was (and generally is) intended to evaluate any pain or discomfort.
4. Technical training and monitoring are critical (particularly in view of the subjective nature of evaluation).
5. Rabbit eye tests do not perfectly predict results in humans, if the objective is either the total exclusion of irritants or the identification of truly severe irritants on an absolute basis (i.e., without false positives or negatives). Some (i.e., Reinhardt et al., 1985) have claimed that these tests are too sensitive for such uses.
6. There are structural and biochemical differences between rabbit and human eyes that make extrapolation from one to the other difficult. For example, Bowman's membrane is present and well developed in man (8–12 μm thick) but not in the rabbit, possibly giving the cornea greater protection.
7. Lack of standardization.
8. Variable correlation with human results.
9. Large biological variability between experimental units.
10. Large, diverse and fragmented databases which are not readily comparable.

physiology, inflammation or immune modulation, and alterations in repair and/ or recovery processes. These methods have the limitation that they assume that one of the component parts can or will predict effects in the complete organ system. While each component may serve well to predict the effects of a set of chemical structures that determine part of the ocular irritation response, a valid assessment across a broad range of structures will require the use of a collection or battery of such tests.

The sixth category contains tests that have little or no empirical basis, such as computer-assisted structure–activity relationship models. These approaches can only be assessed in terms of how well or poorly they perform. Table 7.5 presents an overview of all six categories and some of the component tests within them, updated from the assessment by Frazier et al. (1987), along with references for each test.

Given that there are now some 70 or more potential in vitro alternatives, the key points along the route to the eventual objective of replacing the in vivo

TABLE 7.5   In Vitro Alternatives for Eye Irritation Tests

I.   Morphology
  A.   Enucleated superfused rabbit eye system (Burton et al., 1981)
  B.   Balb/c 3T3 cells/morphological assays (HTD) (Borenfreund and Puerner, 1984)
II. Cell toxicity
  A.   Adhesion/cell proliferation
    1.   BHK cells/growth inhibition (Reinhardt et al., 1985)
    2.   BHK cells/colony formation efficiency (Reinhardt et al., 1985)
    3.   BHK cells/cell detachment (Reinhardt et al., 1985)
    4.   SIRC cells/colony forming assay (North-Root et al., 1982)
    5.   Balbe/c 3T3 cells/total protein (Shopsis and Eng, 1985)
    6.   BCL/D1 cells/total protein (Balls and Horner, 1985)
    7.   Primary rabbit corneal cells/colony forming assay (Watanabe et al., 1988)
  B.   Membrane integrity
    1.   LS cells/dual dye staining (Scaife, 1982)
    2.   Thymocytes/dual fluorescent dye staining (Aeschbacher et al., 1986)
    3.   LS cells/dual dye staining (Kemp et al., 1983)
    4.   RCE-SIRC-P815-YAC-1/Cr release (Shadduck et al., 1985)
    5.   L929 cells/cell variability (Simons, 1981)
    6.   Bovine red blood cell/hemolysis (Shadduck et al., 1987)
    7.   Mouse L929 fibroblasts-erythrocin C staining (Frazier, 1988)
    8.   Rabbit corneal epithelial and endothelial cells/membrane leakage (Meyer
         and McCulley, 1988)
    9.   Agarose diffusion (Barnard, 1989)
  C.   Cell metabolism
    1.   Rabbit corneal cell cultures/plasminogen activator (Chan, 1985)
    2.   LS cells/ATP assay (Kemp et al., 1985)
    3.   Balb/c 3T3 cells/neutral red uptake (Borenfreund and Puerner, 1985)
    4.   Balb/c 3T3 uridine uptake inhibition assay (Shopsis and Sathe, 1984)
    5.   HeLa cells/metabolic inhibition test (MIT-24) (Selling and Ekwall, 1985)
    6.   MDCK cells/dye diffusion (Tchao, 1988)
III. Cell and tissue physiology
  A.   Epidermal slice/electrical conductivity (Oliver and Pemberton, 1985)
  B.   Rabbit ileum/contraction inhibition (Muir et al., 1983)
  C.   Bovine cornea/corneal opacity (Muir et al., 1984)
  D.   Proposed mouse eye/permeability test (Maurice and Singh, 1986)
IV. Inflammation/immunity
  A.   Chorioallantoic membrane (CAM)
    1.   CAM (Leighton et al., 1983)
    2.   HET-CAM (Luepke, 1985)
  B.   Bovine corneal cup model/leukocyte chemotactic factors (Elgebaly et al., 1985)
  C.   Rat peritoneal mast cells/histamine release (Jacaruose et al., 1985)
  D.   Rat peritoneal mast cells/serotonin release (Chasin et al., 1979)
  E.   Rat vaginal explant/prostaglandin release (Dubin et al., 1984)
  F.   Bovine eye cup/histamine (Hm) and leukotriene C4 (LtC4) release (Benassi et
       al., 1986)
V.   Recovery/repair
  A.   Rabbit corneal epithelial cells-wound healing (Jumblatt and Neufeld, 1985)
VI. Other
  A.   EYTEX assay (Gordon and Bergman, 1986; Soto et al., 1988)
  B.   Computer-based structure-activity (SAR) (Enslein, 1984, Enslein et al., 1988)

---

test systems are thus: (1) How do we select the best candidates from this pool? (2) How do we want to use the resulting system (as a screen or test)? (3) How do we select, develop, and validate the system or systems that will actually be used?

There have been limited-scale validations of many of these tests. Most of the individual investigators have performed such "validations" as part of their development of the test system, and in a number of cases trade association have sponsored comparative and/or multilaboratory validations. At least for screening, several systems should be appropriate for use, and in fact are used now by several commercial organizations. In terms of use within defined chemical structural classes, use of in vitro systems for testing of chemicals for nonhuman exposure should supplant traditional in vivo systems once validated on a broad scale by multiple laboratories. Broad use of single tests based on single end points (such as cytotoxicity) is not likely to be successful, as demonstrated by such efforts as those of Kennah et al. (1989).

III. OTHER NONPARENTERAL ROUTE IRRITATION TESTS

Mucosal irritation may be evaluated by a number of tests, although each of them has serious limitations. In the cheek pouch mucosal test, intact samples or sample extracts are inserted into the cheek pouches of Chinese hamsters. In the vaginal mucosal tests, sample extracts are injected into the vagina of albino rabbits. Rabbits in estrous may give false positive results. In the penile mucosal tests, sample extracts are dripped onto the expressed penises of albino rabbits. Most of the sample is removed when the penis is withdrawn into the body. The oral mucosa and rectal mucosa may also be evaluated. Methods for these tests are set forth in ISO 10993, part 10.

The design of vaginal, rectal, penile, and nasal irritation studies is less formalized, but follows the same basic pattern as the primary dermal irritation test. The rabbit is the preferred species for vaginal and rectal irritation studies, but the monkey and dog have also been used for these (Chvapil et al. 1979; Eckstein et al., 1969; Lilly et al., 1972; Lindhe et al., 1970; Muller et al., 1988; Nixon et al., 1972; Bernstein and Carlish, 1979; Kaminsky and Willigan, 1982; Davidson et al., 1982; Haugen, 1980). Both the rabbit and rat have commonly seen use for nasal irritation evaluations. Defined quantities (typically 1.0 ml) of test solutions or suspensions are instilled into the orifice in question. For the vagina or rectum inert bungs are usually installed immediately thereafter to continue exposure for a defined period of time (usually the same number of hours as future human exposure). The orifice is then flushed clean, and 24 hr after exposure it is examined and evaluated (graded) for irritation using the scale in Table 7.1.

IV. PARENTERAL IRRITATION/TOLERANCE

There are a number of special concerns about the safety of materials that are routinely injected (parenterally administered) into the body. By definition, these concerns are all associated with materials that are the products of the pharmaceutical and (in some minor cases) medical device industries. Such parenteral routes include three major ones—IV (intravenous), IM (intramuscular), and SC (subcutaneous)—and a number of minor routes (such as intra-arterial) that are not considered here.

These unusual concerns include irritation (vascular, muscular, or subcutaneous), pyrogenicity, blood compatibility, and sterility (Avis, 1985). The background of each of these, along with the underlying mechanisms and factors that influence the level of occurrence of such an effect, are briefly discussed below.

A. Irritation

Tissue irritation upon injection and the accompanying damage and pain, is a concern that must be addressed for the final formulation, which is to be either tested in humans or marketed, rather than for the active ingredient. This is because most irritation factors are either due to or influenced by aspects of formulation design. (See Avis, 1985, for more information on parenteral preparations.) These factors are not independent of the route (IV, IM, or SC) that will be used, and in fact (as discussed later) are part of the basis for selecting between the various routes.

The lack of irritation and tissue damage at the injection site is sometimes called *tolerance*. Some of the factors that affect tolerance are not fully under the control of an investigation and are also unrelated to the material being injected. These include body movement, temperature, and animal age. Factors that can be controlled, but are not inherent to the active ingredient, include solubility, tonicity, and pH. Finally, the active ingredient and vehicle can have inherent irritative effects and factors, such as solubility (in the physiological milieu into which they are being injected), concentration, volume, molecular size, and particle size. Gray (1978) and Ballard (1968) discuss these factors and the morphological consequences that may occur if they are not addressed.

B. Pyrogenicity

Pyrogenicity is the induction of a febrile (fever) response induced by the parenteral (usually IV or IM) administration of exogenous material. Pyrogenicity is usually associated with microbiological contamination of a final formulation, but it is now of increasing concern because of the growing interest in biosynthetically produced materials. Generally, ensuring sterility of product and process will guard against pyrogenicity for traditional pharmaceuticals. For biologically produced products, the FDA has promulgated the general guideline that no more than 5.0 units of endotoxin may be present per mg of drug substance.

V. PARENTERAL ROUTES

There are at least 13 different routes by which to inject material into the body, including the following:

1. Intravenous
2. Subcutaneous
3. Intramuscular
4. Intra-arterial
5. Intradermal
6. Intralesional
7. Epidural
8. Intrathecal
9. Intracisternal
10. Intracardiac
11. Intraventricular
12. Intraocular
13. Intraperitoneal

Each of these routes has devices involved in the administration of the injected or infused agent. Only the first three are discussed in any detail here. Most of these routes of administration place a drug directly or indirectly into systemic circulation. There are a number of these routes, however, by which the drug exerts a local effect, in which case most of the drug does not enter systemic circulation (e.g., intrathecal, intraventricular, intraocular, intracisternal). Certain routes of administration may exert both local and systemic effects, depending on the characteristics of the drug and excipients (e.g., subcutaneous).

The choice of a particular parenteral route will depend on the required time of onset of action, the required site of action, and the characteristics of the fluid to be injected, among other factors.

Muscle irritation is the local inflammation, pain, and damage that results from the parenteral injection of pharmaceuticals into a muscle mass. It is due to a range of physicochemical factors as well as chemical/biological interactions, and is particularly of concern with antibiotics.

A. Test Systems for Parenteral Irritation

There are no regulatory guidelines or suggested test methods for evaluating agents for muscular or vascular irritation. Since such guidelines are lacking but the evaluation is necessary, those responsible for these evaluations have tried to develop and employ the most scientifically valid procedures.

Hagan (1959) first suggested a method for assessing IM irritation, although the need was first identified 10 years before (Nelson et al., 1949). His approach, however, did not include a grading system for evaluation of the irritation, and the method used the sacrospinalis muscles, which are somewhat difficult to dissect or repeatedly inject.

Shintani et al. (1967) developed and proposed the methodology that currently seems to be more utilized (USP, 2000). It uses the lateral vastus muscle and includes a methodology for evaluation, scoring, and grading of the irritation. Additionally, Shintani et al. investigated the effects of several factors, such as the pH of the solution, drug concentration, volume of injection, effect of repeated injections, and time to maximum tissue response.

B. Acute Intramuscular Irritation in the Male Rabbit

1. Overview of study design
   Each rabbit is injected as follows.

Site (m. vastus lateralis)	Treatment (1.0 ml/site)
Left	(Test article)
Right	(vehicle)

Day 1:   Injection of all treatment groups (9 rabbits)

Day 2:   Sacrifice and evaluation: 24-hr posttreatment group (3 rabbits)

Day 3:   Sacrifice and evaluation: 48-hr posttreatment group (3 rabbits)

Day 4:   Sacrifice and evaluation: 72-hr posttreatment group (3 rabbits)

2. Administration
   2.1   Route: The test article is injected into the vastus lateralis of each rabbit.
   2.2   Dose: The dose selected is chosen to evaluate the severity of irritation, and represents a concentration that might be used clinically. This volume has been widely used in irritation testing.
   2.3   Frequency: Once only.
   2.4   Duration: 1 day.
   2.5   Volume: 1.0 ml per site.
3. Test system
   3.1   Species, age, and weight range: Male New Zealand White rabbits weighing 2 to 5 kg are used. The New Zealand White rabbit has been widely used in muscle irritation research for many years,

and is a reasonably sized, even-tempered animal that is well adapted to the laboratory environment.

3.2 Selection: Animals to be used in the study are selected on the basis of acceptable findings from physical examinations and body weights.

3.3 Randomization: Animals are ranked by body weight and assigned a number between 1 and 3. The order of number assigned (e.g., 1-3-2) is chosen from a table of random numbers. Animals assigned number 1 are in the 24-hr posttreatment group, and those assigned number 3 are in the 72-hr posttreatment group.

4. In-life observations

4.1 Daily observations: Once daily following dosing.

4.2 Physical examinations: Once within the 2 weeks before the first dosing day.

4.3 Body weight: Should be determined once before the start of the study.

4.4 Additional examinations may be done by the study director to elucidate any observed clinical signs.

5. Postmortem procedures

5.1 Irritation is evaluated as follows: Three rabbits are sacrificed by a lethal dose of barbiturate at approximately 24, 48, or 72 hr after dosing. The left and right lateral vastus muscles of each rabbit are excised. The lesions resulting from injections are scored for muscle irritation on a numerical scale of 0 to 5, as shown in Table 7.6 (Shintani et al., 1967).

The average score for the nine rabbits is then calculated, and a category of irritancy is then assigned based on Table 7.7.

TABLE 7.6 Muscle Irritation Evaluation

Reaction criteria	Score
No discernible gross reaction	0
Slight hyperemia and discoloration	1
Moderate hyperemia and discoloration	2
Distinct discoloration in comparison with the color of the surrounding area	3
Brown degeneration with small necrosis	4
Widespread necrosis with an appearance of cooked meat, and occasionally an abscess involving the major portions of the muscle	5

TABLE 7.7 Muscle Irritation
Categorization

Average score	Grade
0.0 to 0.4	None
0.5 to 1.4	Slight
1.5 to 2.4	Mild
2.5 to 3.4	Moderate
3.5 to 4.4	Marked
4.5 or greater	Severe

C. Acute Intravenous Irritation in the Male Rabbit

The design here is similar to the IM assay, except that injections are made into the veins in specific muscles masses.

1. Overview of study design
   Rabbits will be injected as follows:

Group	Number of animals	Treatment site	Evaluation
1	2	m. vastus lateralis (left) and cervi-codorsal subcutis (left) m. vastus lateralis (right) and cervi-codorsal subcutis (right)	24 hr
2	2	m. vastus lateralis (left) and cervi-codorsal subcutis (left) m. vastus lateralis (right) and cervi-codorsal subcutis (right)	72 hr
3	2	auricular vein (left) auricular vein (right)	24- and72-hr evaluations

Day 1: Injection of all groups (6 rabbits)
Day 2: Evaluation of group 3 (2 rabbits); sacrifice and evaluation of group 1 (2 rabbits)
Day 4: Evaluation of group 3 (2 rabbits); sacrifice and evaluation of group 2 (2 rabbits)

2. Administration
   2.1. Intramuscular: M. vastus lateralis
   2.2. Subcutaneous: Cervicodorsal subcutis
   2.3. Intravenous: Auricular vein
   2.4. Dose: The doses and concentration selected are chosen to evaluate the severity of irritation. The dose volumes have been widely used in irritation testing.
   2.5. Frequency: Once only.
   2.6. Duration: 1 day.
   2.7. Volume: M vastus lateralis and cervicodorsal subcutis: 1.0 ml per site; auricular vein: 0.5 ml per site.
3. Test system
   3.1. Species, age, and weight range: Male New Zealand White rabbits weighing 2 to 5 kg are used.
   3.2. Selection: Animals to be used in the study are selected on the basis of acceptable findings from physical examinations.
   3.3. Randomization: Animals are ranked by body weight and assigned a number between 1 and 3. The order or numbers assigned (e.g., 1-3-2) are chosen from a table of random numbers. Animals assigned number 1 are in group 1, those assigned number 2 are in group 2, and those assigned number 3 are in group 3.
4. In-life observations
   4.1. Daily observations: Once daily following dosing.
   4.2. Physical examinations: Once within the 2 weeks before the first dosing day.
   4.3. Body weight: Determined once before the start of the study.
   4.4. Additional examinations may be done by the study director to elucidate any observed clinical signs.
5. Postmortem procedures
   5.1. Intramuscular irritation is evaluated as follows: Rabbits are sacrificed by a lethal dose of barbiturate approximately 24 and 72 hr after dosing. The left and right lateral vastus muscles of each rabbit are excised. The reaction resulting from injection is scored for muscle irritation using the scale shown in section 5.3.
   5.2. Subcutaneous irritation is evaluated as follows: Rabbits are sacrificed by a lethal dose of barbiturate approximately 24 and 72 hr after dosing. The subcutaneous injection sites are exposed by dissection, and the reaction is scored for irritation on a scale of 0 to 5, as in Table 7.6.
   5.3. Intravenous irritation is evaluated as follows: Rabbits are sacrificed by a lethal dose of barbiturate following the 72-hr irritation evaluation. The injection site and surrounding tissue are grossly

evaluated at approximately 24 and 72 hr after dosing on a scale of 0 to 3, as follows:

Reaction criteria	Score
No discernible gross reaction	0
Slight erythema at injection site	1
Moderate erythema and swelling with some discoloration of the vein and surrounding tissue	2
Severe discoloration and swelling of the vein and surrounding tissue with partial or total occlusion of the vein	3
Average score per site	Irritancy grade
0.0 to 0.4	None
0.5 to 1.4	Slight
1.5 to 2.4	Moderate
2.5 or greater	Severe

5.4. Additional examinations may be done by the study director to elucidate the nature of any observed tissue change.

D. Alternatives

Intramuscular and IV injection of parenteral formulations of pharmaceuticals can produce a range of discomfort, including pain, irritation, and/or damage to muscular or vascular tissue. These are normally evaluated for prospective formulations before use in humans by histopathologic evaluation of damage in intact animal models, usually the rabbit. Attempts have been made to make this in vivo methodology both more objective and quantitative based on measuring the creatinine phosphokinase released in the tissue surrounding the injection site (Meltzer et al., 1970; Sidell et al., 1974). Currently a protocol utilizing a cultured skeletal muscle cell line (L6) from the rat as a model has been evaluated in an interlaboratory validation program among 11 pharmaceutical laboratories. This methodology (Young et al., 1986) measures creatine kinase levels in media after exposure of the cells to the formulation of interest, and predicts in vivo results for antibiotics and a fair correlation for a broader range of parenteral drug products. Likewise, Williams et al. (1987), Laska et al. (1991), and Kato et al. (1992) have proposed a model that uses cultured primary skeletal muscle fibers from the rat. Damage is evaluated by the release of creatinine phosphokinase. An evaluation using six parenterally administered antibiotics (ranking their EC_{50} values) showed good relative correlation with in vivo results.

Another proposed in vitro assay for muscle irritancy for injectable formulations is the red blood cell hemolysis assay (Brown et al., 1989). Water-soluble formulations in a 1:2 ratio with freshly collected human blood are gently mixed for 5 min. The percentage of red blood cell survival is then determined by measuring differential absorbance at 540 mm. This value is then compared to values for known irritants and nonirritants. This assay reportedly accurately predicts muscle irritation against a very small group of compounds (four).

VI. INTRACUTANEOUS IRRITATION

The intracutaneous irritation test is a sensitive acute toxicity screening test and is generally accepted for detecting potential local irritation by extracts from a biomaterial. Extracts of material obtained with nonirritation polar and nonpolar extraction media are suitable, and sterile extracts are desirable.

A. Intracutaneous Test

This test is designed to evaluate local responses to the extracts of materials under test following intracutaneous injection into rabbits.

Test Animal.   Select healthy, thin-skinned albino rabbits whose fur can be clipped closely and whose skin is free from mechanical irritation or trauma. In handling the animals, avoid touching the injection sites during observation periods, except to discriminate between edema and an oil residue. Rabbits that have been previously used in unrelated tests, such as the *pyrogen test*, and that have received the prescribed rest period, may be used for this test, provided that they have clean, unblemished skin.

Procedure.   Agitate each extract vigorously prior to withdrawal of injection doses to ensure even distribution of the extracted matter. On the day of the test, closely clip the fur on the animal's back on both sides of the spinal column over a sufficiently large test area. Avoid mechanical irritation and trauma. Remove loose hair by means of a vacuum. If necessary, swab the skin lightly with diluted alcohol, and dry the skin prior to injection. More than one extract from a given material can be used per rabbit if you have determined that the test results will not be affected. For each *sample* use two animals and inject each intracutaneously, using one side of the animal for the sample and the other side for the *blank*, as outlined in Table 7.8. (*Note*: Dilute each gram of the extract of the sample prepared with *polyethylene glycol 400* (and the corresponding *blank*) with 7.5 volumes of *sodium chloride injection* to obtain a solution having a concentration of about 120 mg of polyethylene glycol per ml.)

Examine injection sites for evidence of any tissue reaction, such as erythema, edema, and necrosis. Swab the skin lightly, if necessary, with diluted

TABLE 7.8 Intracutaneous Test

Extract or blank	Number of sites (per animal)	Dose (µl per site)
Sample	5	200
Blank	5	200

alcohol to facilitate reading of injection sites. Observe all animals at 24, 48, and 72 hr after injection. Rate the observations on a numerical scale for the extract of the sample and for the blank, using Table 7.1. Reclip the fur as necessary during the observation period.

If each animal at any observation period shows an average reaction to the *sample* that is not significantly greater than to the *blank*, the *sample* meets the requirements of this test. If at any observation period the average reaction to the sample is questionably greater than the average reaction to the blank, repeat the test using three additional rabbits. On the repeat test, the average reaction to the sample in any of the three animals is not significantly greater than the blank.

B. Pyrogenicity

Pyrogenicity is the induction of a febrile (fever) response by the parenteral (usually IV or IM) administration of exogenous material, usually (but not always) bacterial endotoxins. Pyrogenicity is usually associated with microbiological contamination of a final formulation or product but is now increasingly of concern because of the increase in interest in biosynthetically produced materials. In general, ensuring the sterility of product and process will guard against pyrogenicity. Pyrogenicity testing is performed extensively in the medical device industry. If a device is to be introduced directly or indirectly into the fluid path, it is required that it be evaluated for pyrogenic potential (USP, 2000a, European Pharmacopoeia, 1990).

The USP pyrogen test using rabbit or the limulus amebocyte lysate (LAL) test can be used to support pyrogen-free claims. If the LAL test is used, the LAL test method must either meet the FDA's document titled *Guideline on Validation of the Limulus Amebocyte Lysate Test as an End-Product Endotoxin Test for Human and Animal Parental Drugs, Biological Products, and Medical Devices,* or a 510(k) or PMA application must be submitted for the LAL test.

The bacterial endotoxin limit for medical devices is 0.5 EU/ml. Manufacturers may retest LAL test failures with another LAL test or the USP rabbit pyrogen test. Medical devices that contact cerebrospinal fluid should have less than 0.06 EU/ml of endotoxin.

In vitro pyrogenicity testing (or bacterial endotoxin testing) is one of the great success stories for in vitro testing. Some 15 years ago, the LAL test was developed, validated, and accepted as an in vitro test for estimating the concentration of bacterial endotoxins that may be present in or on a sample of the article(s) to which the test is applied. The test uses LAL that has been obtained from aqueous extracts of the circulating amebocytes of the horseshoe crab, *Limulus polyphemus* and that has been prepared and characterized for use as an LAL reagent for gel-clot formation (Cooper, 1975; Weary and Baker, 1977). The test's limitation is that it detects only the pyrogens of gram-negative bacteria. This is generally not significant (at least for use in lot release assays), since most environmental contaminants that gain entrance to sterile products are gram-negative (Bulich et al., 1981; Devleeschouwer et al., 1985).

Where the test is conducted as a limit test, the specimen is determined to be positive or negative to the test judged against the endotoxin concentration specified in the individual monograph (USP, 2000c). Where the test is conducted as an assay of the concentration of endotoxin with calculation of confidence limits of the result obtained, the specimen is judged to comply with the requirements if the result does not exceed (1) the concentration limit specified in the individual monograph and (2) the specified confidence limits for the assay. In either case the determination of the reaction end point is made with parallel dilutions of redefined endotoxin units.

Since LAL reagents have also been formulated to be used for turbidimetric (including kinetic) assays or colorimetric readings, such tests may be used if shown to comply with the requirements for alternative methods. These tests require the establishment of a standard regression curve, and the endotoxin content of the test material is determined by interpolation from the curve. The procedures include incubation for a preselected time of reacting endotoxin and control solutions with LAL reagent and reading the spectrophotometric light absorbance at suitable wavelengths. In the case of the turbidimetric procedure the reading is made immediately at the end of the incubation period. In the kinetic assays, the absorbance is measured throughout the reaction period and rate values are determined from those readings. In the colorimetric procedure the reaction is arrested at the end of the preselected time by the addition of an appropriate amount of acetic acid solution prior to the readings. A possible advantage in the mathematical treatment of results if the test is otherwise validated and the assay suitably designed, could be the confidence interval and limits of potency from the internal evidence of each assay itself.

C. Reference Standard and Control Standard Endotoxins

The reference standard endotoxin (RSE) is the USP endotoxin reference standard, which has a defined potency of 10,000 USP EU per vial. Constitute the entire contents of one vial of the RSE with 5 ml of LAL reagent water, vortex for not less than 20 min, and use this concentrate for making appropriate serial dilutions. Preserve the concentrate in a refrigerator for making subsequent dilutions for not more than 14 days. Allow it to reach room temperature, if applicable, and vortex it vigorously for not less than 5 min before use. Vortex each dilution for not less than 1 min before proceeding to make the next dilution. Do not use stored dilutions. A control standard endotoxin (CSE) is an endotoxin preparation other than the RSE that has been standardized against the RSE. If a CSE is a preparation not already adequately characterized, its evaluation should include characterizing parameters both for endotoxin quality and performance (e.g., reaction in the rabbit) and for suitability of the material to serve as a reference (e.g., uniformity and stability). To ensure consistency in performance, detailed procedures for its weighing and/or constitution and use should also be included. Standardization of CSE against the RSE using an LAL reagent for the gel-clot procedure may be effected by assaying a minimum of four vials of the CSE or four corresponding aliquots, where applicable, of the bulk CSE and one vial of the RSE as directed under test procedure, but using four replicate reaction tubes at each level of the dilution series for the RSE and four replicate reaction tubes similarly for each vial or aliquot of the CSE. If the dilutions for the four vials or aliquots of the CSE cannot all be accommodated with the dilutions for the one vial of the RSE on the same rack for incubation, additional racks may be used for accommodating some of the replicate dilutions for the CSE, but all of the racks containing the dilutions of the RSE and CSE are incubated as a block. In such cases, however, the replicate dilution series from the one vial of the RSE are accommodated together on a single rack and the replicate dilution series from any one of the four vials or aliquots of the CSE are not divided between racks. The antilog of the difference between the mean log 10 end point of the RSE and the mean log 10 end point of the CSE is the standardized potency of the CSE, which is then converted to and expressed in units/ng under stated drying conditions for the CSE or units per container, whichever is appropriate. Standardize each new lot of CSE prior to use in the test. Calibration of a CSE in terms of the RSE must be with the specific lot of LAL reagent and the test procedure with which it is to be used. Subsequent lots of LAL reagent from the same source and with similar characteristics need only to be checked for the potency ratio. The inclusion of one or more dilution series made from the RSE when the CSE is used for testing will enable observation of whether or not the relative potency shown by the latter remains within the determined confidence limits. A large lot of a CSE may, however, be characterized by a collaborative assay of a suitable design to provide a representative relative potency and the within-laboratory and between-laboratory variance.

A suitable CSE has a potency of not less than 2 EU/ng and not more than 50 EU/ng, where in bulk form under adopted uniform drying conditions (e.g., to a particular low moisture content and other specified conditions of use) and a potency within a corresponding range where filled in vials of a homogeneous lot.

D. Preparatory Testing

Use an LAL agent of confirmed label or determined sensitivity. In addition, where there is to be a change in a lot of CSE, LAL reagent, or another reagent, conduct tests of a prior satisfactory lot of CSE, LAL, and/or other reagent in parallel on changeover. Treat any containers or utensils employed so as to destroy extraneous surface endotoxins that may be present, such as by heating in an oven at 250°F or above for sufficient time.

The validity of test results for bacterial endotoxins requires an adequate demonstration that specimens of the article (or of solutions, washings, or extracts thereof to which the test is to be applied) do not of themselves inhibit or enhance the reaction or otherwise interfere with the test. Validation is accomplished by testing untreated specimens or appropriate dilutions thereof, concomitantly with and without known and demonstrable added amounts of RSE or a CSE, and comparing the results obtained. Appropriate negative controls are included. Validation must be repeated if the LAL reagent source or the method of manufacture or formulations of the article is changed.

Test for confirmation of labeled LAL regent sensitivity. Confirm the labeled sensitivity of the particular LAL reagent with the RSE (or CSE) using not less than four replicate vials, under conditions shown to achieve an acceptable variability of the test; namely, the antilog of the geometric mean log 10 lystate gel-clot sensitivity is within 0.5 to 2.0, where the labeled sensitivity is in EU/ml. The RSE (or CSE) concentrations selected to confirm to LAL reagent label potency should bracket the stated sensitivity of the LAL reagent. Confirm the labeled sensitivity of each new lot of LAL reagent prior to use in the test.

1. Inhibitions or Enhancement Test

Conducts assays, with standard endotoxin, or untreated specimens in which there is no endogenous endotoxin detectable, and of the same specimens to which endotoxin has been added as directed under test procedures, but use no fewer than four replicate reaction tubes at each level of the dilution series for each untreated specimen and for each specimen to which endotoxin has been added. Record the end points (E, in units/ml) observed in the replicates. Take the logarithms (e) of the end points, and compute the geometric means of the log end points for the RSE (or CSE) for the untreated specimens and for specimens containing endotoxin by the formula antilog, e/f, where e is the sum of the log end points of the dilution series used and f is the number of replicate end points in each case. Compute the amount of endotoxin in the specimen to which endotoxin has been added. The test is valid for the article if this result is within twofold of the known added amount of endotoxin. Alternatively, if the test has been appropriately set up, the test is valid for the article if the geometric mean end point dilution for the specimen to which endotoxin has been added is within one twofold dilution of the corresponding geometric mean end point dilution of the standard endotoxin.

Repeat the test for inhibition or enhancement using specimens diluted by a factor not exceeding that given by the formula, x/y. (See Maximum Valid Dilution, below.) Use the least dilution sufficient to overcome the inhibition or enhancement of the known endotoxin for subsequent assays of endotoxin in test specimens.

If endogenous endotoxin is detectable in the untreated specimens under the conditions of the test, the article is unsuitable for the inhibition or enhancement test, or it may be rendered suitable by removing the endotoxin present by ultrafiltration or by appropriate dilution. Dilute the untreated specimen (as constituted, where applicable, for administration or use) to a level not exceeding the maximum valid dilution, at which no endotoxin is detectable. Repeat the test for inhibition or enhancement using the specimens at those dilutions.

E. Test Procedure

In preparing for and applying the test, observe precautions in handling the specimens in order to avoid gross microbial contamination. Washings or rinsings of devices must be with LAL reagent water in volumes appropriate to their use, and where applicable, of the surface area that comes into contact with body tissues or fluids. Use such washings or rinsings if the extracting fluid has been in contact with the relevant pathway or surface for not less than 1 hr at a controlled room temperature (15–30°C). Such extracts may be combined, where appropriate.

For validating the test for an article, for endotoxin limit tests or assays, or for special purposes where so specified, testing of specimens is conducted quantitatively to determine response end points for gel-clot readings. Usually graded strengths of the specimen and standard endotoxin are made by multifold dilutions. Select dilutions so that they correspond to a geometric series in which each step is greater than the next lower step by a constant ratio. Do not store diluted endotoxin, because of its loss of activity by absorption. In the absence of supporting data to the contrary, negative and positive controls are incorporated into the test.

Use no fewer than two replicate reactions tubes at each level of the dilution series for each specimen under test. Whether the test is employed as a limit test or as a quantitative assay, a standard endotoxin dilution series involving no fewer than two replicate reaction tubes is conducted in parallel. A set of standard endotoxin dilution series is included for each block of tubes, which may consist of a number of racks for incubation together, provided the environmental conditions within blocks are uniform.

F. Preparation

Since the form and amount per container of standard endotoxin and of LAL reagent may vary, constitution and/or dilution of contents should be as directed in the labeling. The pH of the test mixture of the specimen and the LAL reagent is in the range of 6.0–7.5 unless specifically directed otherwise in the individual monograph. The pH may be adjusted by the addition of sterile, endotoxin-free sodium hydroxide or hydrochloric acid or suitable buffers to the specimen prior to testing.

1. Maximum Valid Dilution

The maximum valid dilution (MVD) is appropriate to injections or to solutions for parenteral administration in the form constituted or diluted for administration, or where applicable, to the amount of drug by weight if the volume of the dosage form for administration could be varied. Where the endotoxin limit concentration is specified in the individual monograph in terms of volume (in EU/ml), divide the limit by γ, which is the labeled sensitivity (in EU/ml) of the lysate employed in the assay, to obtain the MVD factor. Where the endotoxin limit concentration is specified in the individual monograph in terms of weight or of units of active drug (in EU/mg or in EU/unit), multiply the limit by the concentration (in mg/ml or in units/ml of the drug in the solution tested or of the drug constituted according to the label instructions, whichever is applicable), and divide the product of the multiplication by γ to obtain the MVD factor. The MVD factor so obtained is the limit dilution factor for the preparation for the test to be valid.

G. Procedure

To 10 × 75-mm test tubes add aliquots of the appropriately constituted LAL reagent and the specified volumes of specimens, endotoxin standard, negative controls, and a positive product control consisting of the article, or of solutions, washings, or extracts thereof, to which the RSE (or a standardized CSE) has been added at a concentration of endotoxin of 2 for LAL reagent (see under test for confirmation of labeled LAL reagent sensitivity). Swirl each gently to mix and place in an incubating device such as a water bath or heating block, accurately recording the time at which the tubes are so placed. Incubate each tube, undisturbed, for 60 ± 2 min at 37 ± 1°C, and carefully remove it for observation. A positive reaction is characterized by the formation of a firm gel that remains when inverted through 180°. Record such a result as a positive (+). A negative result is characterized by the absence of such a gel or by the formation of a fiscous gel that does not maintain its integrity. Record such a result as a negative (−). Handle the tubes with care, and avoid subjecting them to unwanted vibrations, or false-negative observations may result. The test is invalid if the positive product control or the endotoxin standard does not show the end point concentration to be within ±twofold dilutions from the label claim sensitivity of the LAL reagent or if any negative control shows a gel-clot end point.

H. Calculation

Calculate the concentration of endotoxin (in units/ml or in units/gram or mg) in or on the article under test by the formula: pS/U, where S is the antilog of the geometric mean log 10 of the end points, expressed in EU/ml for the standard endotoxin; U is the antilog of elf, where e is the log 10 of the end point dilution factors expressed in decimal fractions, and f is the number of replicate reaction tubes read at the end point level for the specimen under test; and p is the correction factor for those cases in which a specimen of the article cannot be taken directly into test but is processed as an extract, solution, or washing.

Where the test is conducted as an assay with sufficient replication to provide a suitable number of independent results, calculate for each replicate assay the concentration of endotoxin in or on the article under test from the antilog of the geometric mean log end point ratios. Calculate the mean and the confidence limits from the replicate logarithmic values of all the obtained assay results by a suitable statistical method.

I. Interpretation

The article meets the requirements of the test if the concentration of endotoxin does not exceed that specified in the individual monograph, and the confidence limits of the assay do not exceed those specified.

1. Rabbit Pyrogen Test

The U.S. *Pharmacopeia* describes a pyrogen test using rabbits as a model. This test, which is the standard for limiting risks of a febrile reaction to an acceptable level, involves measuring the rise in body temperature in a group of three rabbits for 3 hr after injection of 10 ml of test solution.

Apparatus and Diluents. Render the syringes, needles, and glassware free of pyrogens by heating at 250°F for not less than 30 min or by any other suitable method. Treat all diluents and solutions by washing and rinsing the devices or parenteral injection assemblies in a manner that will ensure that they are sterile and pyrogen-free. Periodically perform control pyrogen tests on representative portions of the diluents and solutions that are used for washing and rinsing the apparatus.

Temperature Recording. Use an accurate temperature-sensing device, such as a clinical thermometer or thermistor or similar probe, that has been calibrated to ensure an accuracy of $\pm 0.1°$ and has been tested to determine that a maximum reading is reached in less than 5 min. Insert the temperature-sensing probe into the rectum of the test rabbit to a depth of not less than 7.5 cm, and after a period of time not less than that previously determined as sufficient, record the rabbit's temperature.

Test Animals. Use healthy, mature rabbits. House the rabbits individually in an area of uniform temperature (between 20°C and 23°C) free from disturbances likely to excite them. The temperature should vary no more than $\pm 3°C$ from the selected temperature. Before using a rabbit for the first time in a pyrogen test, condition it for not more than 7 days before use by a sham test that includes all of the steps as directed under procedure, except injection. Do not use a rabbit for pyrogen testing more frequently than once every 48 hr nor prior to 2 weeks following a maximum rise in its temperature of 0.6° or more while being subjected to the pyrogen test, or following its having been given a test specimen that was adjusted to be pyrogenic.

Procedure. Perform the test in a separate area designated solely for pyrogen testing and under environmental conditions similar to those under which the animals are housed. Withhold all food from the test rabbits during the period of the test. Access to water is allowed at all times, but may be restricted during the test. Its probes measuring rectal temperature remain inserted throughout the testing period. Restrain the rabbits with loose-fitting Elizabethan collars that allow the rabbits to assume a natural resting posture. Not more than 30 min prior to the injection of the test dose, determine the "control temperature" of each rabbit. This is the base for the determination of any temperature increase resulting from the injection of a test solution. In any one group of test rabbits, use only those whose control temperatures do not vary by more than 1°C from each other, and do not use any rabbit having a temperature exceeding 39.8°C.

Unless otherwise specified in the individual protocol, inject 10 ml of the test solution per kg of body weight into an ear vein of each of three rabbits, completing each injection within 10 min after the start of administration. The test solution is either the product, constituted if necessary as directed in the labeling, or the material under test. For pyrogen testing of devices or injection assemblies, use washings or rinsings of the surfaces that come in contact with the parenterally administered material or with the injection site or internal tissues of the patient. Ensure that all test solutions are protected from contamination. Perform the injection after warming the test solution to a temperature of 37°C $\pm$ 2°. Record the temperature at 1, 2, and 3 hr subsequent to the injection.

Test Interpretation and Continuation. Consider any temperature decreases as zero rise. If no rabbit shows an individual rise in temperature of 0.6° or more above its respective control temperature and if the sum of the three individual maximum temperature rises does not exceed 1.4°, the product meets the requirements for the absence of pryogens. If any rabbits shows an individual temperature rise of 0.6° or more or if the sum of the three individual maximum temperature rises exceeds 1.4°, continue the test using five other rabbits. If not more than three of the eight rabbits show individual rises in temperature of 0.6° or more, and if the sum of the eight individual maximum temperature rises does not exceed 3.7°, the material under examination meets the requirements for the absence of pyrogens.

J. Factors Affecting Irritation Responses and Test Outcome

The results of local tissue irritation tests are subject to considerable variability because of relatively small differences in test design or technique. Weil and Scala (1971) arranged and reported on the best known of several intralaboratory studies to clearly establish this fact. Though the methods presented above have proven to give reproducible results in the hands of the same technicians over a period of years (Gad et al., 1986) and contain some internal controls (the positive and vehicle controls in the PDI) against large variabilities in results or the occurrence of either false positives or negatives, it is still essential to be aware of those factors that may systematically alter test results. These factors are summarized below.

1. In general, any factor that increases absorption through the stratum corneum or mucous membrane will also increase the severity of an intrinsic response. Unless this factor mirrors potential exposure conditions, it may in turn adversely affect the relevance of test results.
2. The physical nature of solids must be carefully considered both before testing and in interpreting results. Shape (sharp edges), size (small particles may abrade the skin due to being rubbed back and forth under the occlusive wrap), and rigidity (stiff fibers or very hard particles will be physically irritating) of solids may all enhance an irritation response.
3. Solids frequently give different results when they are tested dry than if wetted for the test. As a general rule, solids are more irritating if moistened. (Going back to item 1, wetting is a factor that tends to enhance absorption.) Care should also be taken as to moistening agent; some (few) batches of U.S. *Pharmacopeia* physiological saline (used to simulate sweat) have proven to be mildly irritating to the skin and

mucous membrane on their own. Liquids other than water or saline should not be used.

4. If the treated region on potential human patients will be a compromised skin surface barrier (e.g., if it is cut or burned) some test animals should likewise have their application sites compromised. This procedure is based on the assumption that abraded skin is uniformly more sensitive to irritation. Experiments, however, have shown that this is not necessarily true; some materials produce more irritation on abraded skin, while others produce less (Guillot et al., 1982; Gad et al., 1986).

5. The degree of occlusion (in fact, the tightness of the wrap over the test site) also alters percutaneous absorption and therefore irritation. One important quality control issue in the laboratory is achieving a reproducible degree of occlusion in dermal wrappings.

6. Both the age of the test animal and the application site (saddle of the back vs. flank) can markedly alter test outcome. Both of these factors are also operative in humans, of course (Mathias, 1983), but in dermal irritation tests, the objective is to remove all such sources of variability. In general, as an animal ages, sensitivity to irritation decreases. For the dermal test, the skin on the middle of the back (other than directly over the spine) tends to be thicker (and therefore less sensitive to irritations) than that on the flanks.

7. The sex of the test animals can also alter study results, because both regional skin thickness and surface blood flow vary between males and females.

8. Finally, the single most important (yet also most frequently overlooked) factor that influences the results and outcome of these (and, in fact, most) acute studies is the training of the staff. In determining how test materials are prepared and applied and in how results are ''read'' against a subjective scale, both accuracy and precision are extremely dependent on the technicians involved. To achieve the desired results, initial training must be careful and inclusive. Just as important, some form of regular refresher training must be exercised—particularly in the area of scoring of results. Using a set of color photographic standards as a training and reference tool is strongly recommended. Such standards should clearly demonstrate each of the grades in the Draize dermal scale.

9. It should be recognized that local tissue tolerance (or ''irritancy'') tests are designed with a bias to preclude false negatives, and therefore tend to exaggerate results in relation to what would happen in humans. Findings of negligible irritancy (or even in the very low mild irritant range) should therefore be of no concern unless the product under test is to have large-scale and prolonged dermal contact.

VII. PROBLEMS IN TESTING (AND THEIR RESOLUTIONS)

Some materials, by either their physicochemical or toxicological natures, generate difficulties in the performance and evaluation of dermal irritation tests. The most commonly encountered of these problems are presented below.

1. Compound volatility. One is sometimes required or requested to evaluate the potential irritancy of a liquid that has a boiling point between room temperature and the body temperature of the test animal. As a result, the liquid portion of the material will evaporate off before the end of the testing period. There is no real way around the problem; one can only make clear in the report on the test that the traditional test requirements were not met, although an evaluation of potential irritant hazard was probably achieved (for the liquid phase would also have evaporated from a human that it was spilled on).

2. Pigmented material. Some materials are strongly colored or discolor the skin at the application site. This makes the traditional scoring process difficult or impossible. One can try to remove the pigmentation with a solvent. If successful, the erythema can then be evaluated. If use of a solvent fails or is unacceptable, one can (wearing thin latex gloves) feel the skin to determine if there is warmth, swelling, and/or rigidity—all secondary indicators of the irritation response.

3. Systemic toxicity. On rare occasions, the dermal irritation study is begun only to have the animals die very rapidly after test device is applied.

REFERENCES

Aeschbacher, M., Reinhardt, C. A., and Zbinden, G. (1986). A rapid cell membrane permeability test using fluorescent dyes and flow cytometry, Cell. Bio. Toxicol., 2: 247.

ASTM. (1981). Standard Practice for Testing Biomaterials in Rabbits for Primary Skin Irritation, F719–81, Washington, DC.

Avis, K. E. (1985). Parenteral preparations. In: Remington's Pharmaceutical Sciences (A. R. Gennaro, Ed. Mack, Easton, PA, pp. 1518–1541.

Babich, H., Martin-Alguacil, N., and Borenfreund, E. (1989). Comparisons of the cytotoxicities of dermatotoxicants to human keratinocytes and fibroblasts in vitro. In: In Vitro Toxicology: New Directions (A. M. Goldberg, Ed.). Mary Ann Liebert, New York, pp. 153–167.

Ballard, B. E. (1968). Biopharmaceutical considerations in subcutaneous and intramuscular drug administration, J. Pharm. Sci., 57:357–378.

Balls, M., and Horner, S. A. (1985). The FRAME interlaboratory program on in vitro cytotoxicology, Food Chem. Toxicol., 23:205–213.

Barnard, N. D. (1989). A Draize alternative, Animals Agenda, 6:45.

Bartnik, F. G., Pittermann, W. F., Mendoft, N., Tillmann, U., and Kunstler, K. (1989). Skin organ culture for the study of skin irritancy, Third International Congress of Toxicology, Brighton, U.K.

Bason, M., Harvell, J., Gordon, V., Maibach, H. (1991). Evaluation of the SKINTEX system, presented at the Irritant Contact Dermititis Symposium, Groningen, Netherlands, Internat. J. Derm., 30:623–626.

Bell, E., Gay, R., and Swiderek, M., (1989). Use of fabricated living tissue and organ equivalents as defined in higher order systems for the study of pharmacologic responses to test substances, presented at the NATO Advanced Research Workshop, Pharmaceutical Application of Cell and Tissue Culture to Drug Transport, Bandol, France, Sept. 4–9, 1989.

Benassi, C. A., Angi, M. R., Salvalaoi, L., and Bettero, A. (1986). Histamine and leukotriene C4 release from isolated bovine sclerachoroid complex: A new in vitro ocular irritation test, Chim. Agg., 16:631–634.

Bernstein, M. L., and Carlish, K. (1979). The induction of hyperkeratotic white lesions in hamster cheek pouches with mouthwash, Oral Surg., 48:517.

Borenfreund, E., and Puerner, J. A. (1984). A simple quantitative procedure using monolayer cultures for cytotoxicity assays, J. Tis. Cult. Meth., 9:7–9.

Borenfreund, E., and Peurner, J. A. (1985). Toxicity determined in vitro by morphological alterations and Neutral Red absorption, Toxicol. Lett., 24:119–124.

Boyce, S. T., Hansbrough, J. F., and Norris, D. A. (1988). Cellular responses of cultured human epidermal keratinocytes as models of toxicity to human skin. In: Progress in in Vitro Toxicology (A. M. Goldberg, Ed.). Mary Ann Liebert, New York, pp. 23–37.

Brown, S., Templeton, D., Prater, A., and Potter, C. J. (1989). Use of an in vitro hemolysis test to predict tissue irritancy in an intramuscular formulation, J. Parenter. Sci. Tech., 43:117–120.

Bulich, A. A., Greene, M. W., Isenberg, D. L. (1981). Reliability of bacterial compounds and complex effluents. In: Aquatic Toxicology and Hazard Assessment (D. R. Branson and K. L. Dickson, Eds.). American Society for Testing and Materials (ASTM), Washington, DC, pp. 338–347.

Burton, A. B. G., York, M., and Lawrence, R. S. (1981). The in vitro assessment of severe eye irritation, Food Cosmet. Toxicol., 19:471–480.

Chan, K. Y. (1985). An in vitro alternative to the Draize test. In: In Vitro Toxicology: Alternative Methods in Toxicology, vol. 3 (A. M. Goldberg, Ed.). Mary Ann Liebert, New York, pp. 405–422.

Chasin, M., Scott, C., Shaw, C., and Persico, F. (1979). A new assay for the measurement of mediator release from rat peritoneal mast cells, Int. Arch. Allergy Appl. Immunol., 58:1–10.

Choman, B. R. (1963). Determination of the resopnse of skin to chemical agents by an in vitro procedure, J. Invest. Derm., 44:177–182.

Chvapil, M., Chvapil, T. A., Owen, J. A., Kantor, M., Ulreich, J. B., and Eskelson, C. (1979). Reaction of vaginal tissue of rabbits to inserted sponges made of various materials, J. Biomed. Mat. Res., 13:1.

Cooper, J. F. (1975). Principles and applications of the limulus test for pyrogen in parenteral drugs, Bull. Parenter. Drug Assoc., 3:122–130.

Dannenberg, A. M., Moore, K. G., Schofield, B. H., et al. (1987). Two new in vitro methods for evaluating toxicity in skin (employing short-term organ culture). In: Alternative Methods in Toxicology, Vol. 5 (A. M. Goldberg, Ed.). Mary Ann Liebert, New York, pp. 115–128.

Davidson, W. M., Sheinis, E. M., and Shepherd, S. R. (1982). Tissue reaction to orthodontic adhesives, Amer. J. Orthod., 82:502.

DeLeo, V., Hong, J., Scheide, S., Kong, B., DeSalva, S., and Bagley, D. (1988). Surfactant-induced cutaneous primary irritancy: An in vitro model-assay system development. In: Progress in in Vitro Technology (A. M. Goldberg, Ed.). Mary Ann Liebert, New York, pp. 39–43.

DeLeo, V., Midlarsky, L., Harber, L. C., Kong, B. M., and DeSalva, S. (1987). Surfactant-induced cutaneous primary irritancy: An in vitro model. In: Alternative Methods in Toxicology, vol. 5 (A. M. Goldberg, Ed.). Mary Ann Liebert, New York, pp. 129–138.

Devleeschouwer, M. J., Cornil, M. F., and Dony, J. (1985). Studies on the sensitivity and specificity of the limulus amebocyte lysate test and rabbit pyrogen assays, Appl. Environ. Microbio., 50:1509–1511.

Draize, J. H. (1955). Dermal Toxicity, Association of Food and Drug Officials of the U.S., FDA, Washington, DC, pp. 46–59.

Draize, J. H. (1959). Dermal Toxicity. Appraisal of the Safety of Chemicals in Foods, Drugs, and Cosmetics, Austin, TX, Association of Food and Drug Officials of the United States, Texas State Dept. of Health.

Draize, J. H., Woodard, G., and Clavery, H. O. (1944). Method for the study of irritation and toxicity of substances applied topically to the skin and mucous membranes, J. Pharm. Exp. Ther., 82:237–390.

Dubin, N. H., De Blasi, M. C., et al. (1984). Development of an in vitro test for cytotoxicity in vaginal tissue: Effect of ethanol on prostanoind release. In: Acute Toxicity Testing: Alternative Approaches. Alternative Methods in Toxicology, vol. 2 (A. M. Goldberg, Ed.). Mary Ann Liebert, New York, pp. 127–138.

Eckstein, P., Jackson, M. C. N., Millman, N., and Sobrero, A. J. (1969). Comparison of vaginal tolerance tests of spermicidal preparations in rabbits and monkeys, J. Repro. Fert. 20:85–93.

Elgebaly, S. S., Nabawi, K., Herkbert, N., O'Rourke, J., and Kruetzer, D. L. (1985). Characterization of neutrophil and monocyte specific chemotactic factors derived from the cornea in response to injury, Invest. Ophthal. Vis. Sci., 26:320.

Enslein, K. (1984). Estimation of toxicology end points by structure-activity relationships, Pharm. Rev., 36:131–134.

Enslein, K., Blake, V. W., Tuzzeo, T. M., Borgstedt, H. H., Hart, J. B., and Salem, H. (1988). Estimation of rabbit eye irritation scores by structure-activity relationships, In Vitro Toxicol., 2:1–14.

Enslein, K., Borgstedt, H. H., Blake, B. W., and Hart, J. B. (1987). Prediction of rabbit skin irritation severity by structure–activity relationships, In Vitro Toxicol., 1:129–147.

European Pharmacopoeia. (1990). Part V.2.1.9. Pyrogens.

Firestone, B. A., and Guy, R. H. (1986). Approaches to the prediction of dermal absorption and potential cutaneous toxicity. In: In Vitro Toxicology, vol. 3 Alternative Methods in Toxicology (A. M. Goldberg, Ed.). Mary Ann Liebert, New York, pp. 516–536.

Frazier, J. M. (1988). Update: A critical evaluation of alternatives to acute ocular irritancy testing. In: Progress in in Vitro Toxiciology (A. M. Goldberg, Ed.). Mary Ann Liebert, New York, pp. 67–75.

Frazier, J. M., Gad, S. C., Goldberg, A. M., and McCulley, J. P. (1987). A Critical Evaluation of Alternatives to Acute Ocular Irritancy Testing, Mary Ann Liebert, New York.

Gad S. C., and Chengelis, C. P. (1998). Acute Toxicity: Principles and Methods, 2nd ed., Academic, San Diego, CA.

Gad, S. C., Walsh, R. D., and Dunn B. J. (1986). Correlation of ocular and dermal irritancy of industrial chemicals, Ocular Derm. Toxicol. 5(3):195–213.

Gales, Y. A., Gross, C. L., Karebs, R. C., and Smith, W. J. (1989). Flow cytometric analysis of toxicity by alkylating agents in human epidermal keratinocytes. In: In Vitro Toxicology: New Directions (A. M. Goldberg, Ed.). Mary Ann Liebert, New York, pp. 169–174.

Geller, W., Kobel, W., Seifert, G. (1985). Overview of animal test methods for skin irritation, Fund. Chem. Toxicol., 23(2): 165–168.

Gordon, V. C., and Bergman, H. C. (1986). Eyetex, an in Vitro Method for Evaluation of Optical Irritancy, report 26, National Testing Corporation, Washington, DC.

Gordon, V. C., Kelly, C. P., Bergman, H. C. (1990). Evaluation of SKINTEX, an in vitro method for determining dermal irritation, Toxicologist, 10(1):78.

Grant, M. W. (1993). Toxicology of the Eye, 4th ed. Thomas, Springfield, IL.

Gray, J. E. (1978). Pathological evaluation of infection injury. In: Sustained and Controlled Release Drug Delivery Systems (J. Robinson, Ed.). Marcel Dekker, New York, pp. 351–405.

Guillot, J. P., Gonnet, J. F., Clement, C., Caillard, L., and Trahaut, R. (1982). Evaluation of the cutaneous-irritation potential of 56 compounds, Fund. Chem. Toxicol., 201: 563–572.

Hagan, E. C. (1959). Appraisal of the Safety of Chemicals in Foods, Drugs and Cosmetics, Association of Food and Drug Officials of the United States, Austin, TX, p. 19.

Haugen, E. (1980). The effect of periodontal dressings on intact mucous membrane and on wound healing: A methodological study, Acta Odontol. Scand., 8:363.

Hipp, L. I. (1978). The skin and industrial dermatosis, Nati. Safety News, April.

Jacaruso, R. B., Barlett, M. A., Carson, S., and Trombetta, L. D. (1985). Release of histamine from rat peritoneal cells in vitro as an index or irritational potential, J. Toxicol. Cut. Ocular Toxicol., 4:39–48.

Jumblatt, M. M., and Neufeld, A. H. (1985). A tissue culture model of human corneal epithelium. In: In Vitro Toxicology. Alternative Methods in Toxicology, vol. 3 (A. M. Goldberg, Ed.). Mary Ann Liebert, New York, pp. 391–404.

Kaminsky, M. and Willigan, D. A. (1982). PH and the potential irritancy of douche formulations to the vaginal mucosa of the albino rabbit and rat, Fund. Chem. Toxicol., 20:193.

Kato, I., Harihara, A., and Mizushima, Y. (1992). An in vitro method for assessing muscle irritation of antibiotics using rat primary cultured skeletal muscle fibers, Toxicol. Appl. Pharmacol., 117:194–199.

Kemp, R. V., Meredith, R. W. J., Gamble, S., and Frost, M. (1983). A rapid cell culture technique for assaying the toxicity of detergent based products in vitro as a possible screen for high irritants in vivo, Cytobio., 36:153–159.

Kemp, R. V., Meredith, R. W. J., and Gamble, S. (1985). Toxicity of commercial products on cells in suspension: A possible screen for the Draize eye irritation test, Food Chem. Toxicol., 23:267–270.

Kennah, H. E., Albulescu, D., Hignet, S., and Barrow, C. S. (1989). A critical evaluation of predicting ocular irritancy potential from an in vitro cytotoxicity assay, Fund. Appl. Toxicol., 12:281–290.

Lamont, G. S., Bagley, D. M., Kong, B. M., and DeSalva, S. J. (1989). Developing an alternative to the Draize skin test: Comparison of human skin cell responses to irritants in vitro. In: In Vitro Toxicology: New Directions (A. M. Goldberg, Ed.). Mary Ann Liebert, New York, pp. 183–184.

Laska, D. A., Williams, P. D., Reboulet, J. T., Morris, R. M. (1991). The L6 muscle cell line as a tool to evaluate parental products for irritation, J. Parenter. Sci. Tech., 45(2):77–82.

Lei, H., Carroll, K., Au, L., and Krag, S. S. (1986). An in vitro screen for potential inflammatory agents using cultured fibroblasts. In: In Vitro Toxicology: Alternative Methods in Toxicology, vol. 3 (A. M. Goldberg, Ed.). Mary Ann Liebert, New York, pp. 74–85.

Leighton, J., Nassauer, J., Tchao, R., and Verdone, J. (1983). Development of a procedure using the chick egg as an alternative to the Draize test. In: Product Safety Evaluation: Alternative Methods in Toxicology, vol. 1 (A. M. Goldberg, Ed.). Mary Ann Liebert, New York, pp. 165–177.

Lilly, G. E., Cutcher, J. L., and Henderson, M. D. (1972). Reaction of oral and mucous membranes to selected dental materials, J. Biomed. Mat. Res., 6:545.

Lindhe, J., Heyden, G., Svanberg, G., Loe, H., and Schiott, C. R. (1970). Effect of local applications of chlorhexidine on the oral mucosa of the hamster, J. Periodont. Res., 5:177.

Luepke, N. P. (1985). Hen's egg chorioallantoic membrane test for irritation potential, Food Chem. Toxicol., 23:287–291.

Mathias, C. G. T. (1983). Clinical and experimental aspects of cutaneous irritation. In: Dermatoxicology (F. M. Margulli and H. T. Maibach, Eds.). Hemisphere, New York, pp. 167–183.

Maurice, D. and Singh, T. (1986). A permeability test for acute corneal toxicity, Toxicol. Lett., 31:125–130.

Meltzer, H. Y., Morozak, S., and Bozer, M. (1970). Effect of intramuscular injections on serum creatinine phosphokinase activity, Amer. J. Med. Sci., 259:42–48.

Meyer, D. R. and McCulley, J. P. (1988). Acute and protracted injury to cornea epithelium as an indication of the biocompatability of various pharmaceutical vehicles. In: Progress in in Vitro Toxicology (A. M. Goldberg, Ed.). Mary Ann Liebert, New York, pp. 215–235.

Monash, S. and Blank, H. (1958). Location and reformation of epithelial barrier to water vapor, Arch. Derm., 78:710–714.

Montagna, W. (1961). The Structure and Function of the Skin, 2nd ed., Academic, New York.

Muir, C. K., Flower, C., and Van Abbe, N. J. (1983). A novel approach to the search for in vitro alternatives to in vivo eye irritancy testing, Toxicol. Lett., 18:1–5.

Muller, P., Raabe, G., Horold, J., and Juretzek, U. (1988). Action of chronic peracetic acid (wofasteril) administration on the rabbit oral mucosa, vaginal mucosa and skin, Exp. Path., 34:223.

Naughton, G. K. (1989). A physiological skin model for in vitro toxicity studies. In: Alternative Methods in Toxicology, vol. 7 (A. M. Goldberg, Ed.). Mary Ann Liebert, New York.

Nelson, A. A., Price, C. W., Welch, H. (1949). Muscle irritation following the injection of various penicillin preparations in rabbits, J. Amer. Pharm. Assoc., 38:237–239.

Nixon, G. A., Buehler, E. V., and Newman, E. A. (1972). Preliminary safety assessment of disodium etidronate as an additive to experimental oral hygiene products, Toxicol. Appl. Pharm., 22:661.

North-Root, H., Yackovich, J., Demetrulias, F. J., Gucula, N., and Heinze, J. E. (1982). Evaluation of an in vitro cell toxicity test using rabbit corneal cells to predict the eye irritation potential of surfactants, Toxicol. Lett., 14:207–212.

Oliver, G. J. A. and Pemberton, M. A. (1985). An in vitro epidermal slice technique for identifying chemicals with potential for severe cutaneous effects, Food Chem. Toxicol., 23:229–232.

Prottey, C. and Ferguson, T. F. M. (1976). The effect of surfactants upon rat peritoneal mast cells in vitro, Food Chem. Toxicol., 14:425.

Reinhardt, C. A., Aeschbacher, M., Bracker, M., and Spengler, J. (1987). Validation of three cell toxicity tests and the hen's egg test with guinea pig eye and human skin irritation data. In: In Vitro Toxicology—Approaches to Validation. Alternative Methods in Toxicology, vol. 5 (A. M. Goldberg, Ed.). Mary Ann Liebert, New York, pp. 463–470.

Reinhardt, C. A., Pelli, D. A., and Zbinden, G. (1985). Interpretation of cell toxicity data for the estimation of potential irriation, Food Chem. Toxicol., 23:247–252.

Scaife, M. C. (1982). An investigation of detergent action on in vitro and possible correlations with in vivo data, Internat. J. Cosmet. Sci., 4:179–193.

Selling, J. and Ekwall, B. (1985). Screening for eye irritancy using cultured Hela cells, Xenobiotica, 15:713–717.

Shadduck, J. A., Everitt, J., and Bay, P. (1985). Use of in vitro cytotoxicity to rank ocular irritation of six surfactants. In: In Vitro Toxicology. Alternative Methods in Toxicology, vol. 3 (A. M. Goldberg, Ed.). Mary Ann Liebert, New York, pp. 641–649.

Shadduck, J. A., Render, J., Everitt, J., Meccoli, R. A., and Essexsorlie, D. (1987). An approach to validation: Comparison of six materials in three tests. In: In Vitro Toxicology—Approaches to Validation. Alternative Methods in Toxicology, vol. 5 (A. M. Goldberg, Ed.). Mary Ann Liebert, New York, pp. 75–78.

Shintani, S., Yamazaki., M., Nakamura, M., and Nakayama, I. (1967). A new method to determine the irritation of drugs after intramuscular injections in rabbits, Toxicol. Appl. Pharm., 11:293–301.

Shopsis, C. and Eng, B. (1985). Uridine uptake and cell growth cytotoxicity tests: comparison, applications, and mechanistic studies. J. Cell Biol. 101:87a.

Shopsis, C. and Sathe, S. (1984). Uridine uptake inhibition as a cytotoxicity test: Correlation with the Draize test, Toxicology, 29:195–206.

Sidell, F. R., Claver, D. L., and Kaminskis, A. (1974). Serum creatine phosphokinase activity after intramuscular injection, JAMA, 228:1884–1887.

Simons, P. J. (1981). An alternative to the Draize test. In: The Use of Alternatives in Drug Research (A. N. Rowan and C. J. Startmann, Eds.). MacMillan, London.

SOT. (1989). Position paper: Comments on the LD 50 and acute eye and skin irritation tests, Fund. Appl. Toxicol., 13:621–623.

Soto, R. J., Servi, M. J., and Gordon, V. C. (1988). Evaluation of an alternative method of ocular irritation. In: Progress in in Vitro Toxicology (A. M. Goldberg, Ed.). Mary Ann Liebert, New York, pp. 289–296.

Swisher, D. A., Prevo, M. E., and Ledger, P. W. (1988). The MTT in vitro cytotoxicity test: Correlation with cutaneous irritancy in two animal models. In: Progress in in Vitro Toxicology (A. M. Goldberg, Ed.). Mary Ann Liebert, New York, pp. 265–269.

Tchao, R. (1988). Trans-epithelial permeability of fluorescein in vitro as an assay to determine eye irritants. In: vol. 6 Alternative Methods in Toxicology, (A. M. Goldberg, ed.) Mary Ann Liebert New York, 1988, pp. 271–283.

USP. (2000a). Pyrogen test. In: United States Pharmacopeia, XXIV § NF-19, USP Convention, Rockville, MD, p. 1515.

USP. (2000b). Intramuscular irritation test. In: United States Pharmacopeia, XXIV § NF-19, USP Convention, Rockville, MD, pp. 1180–1183.

USP. (2000c). Bacterial endotoxins test. In: United States Pharmacopeia, XXIV § NF-19, USP Convention, Rockville, MD, pp. 1493–1495.

Watanabe, M., Watanabe, K., Suzuki, K., et al. (1988). In vitro cytotoxicity test using primary cells derived from rabbit eye is useful as an alternative for Draize testing. In: Progress in in Vitro Toxicology (A. M. Goldberg, Ed.). Mary Ann Liebert, New York, pp. 285–290.

Weary, M. and Baker, B. (1977). Utilization of the limulus amebocyte lysate test for pyrogen testing of large volume parenterals, administration sets and medical devices, Bull. Parenter. Drug Assoc., 31:1127–133.

Weil, C. S. and Scala, R. A. (1971). Study of intra- and interlaboratory variability in the results of rabbit eye and skin irritation tests, Toxicol. Appl. Pharmacol., 19:276–360.

Williams, P. D., Masters, B. G., Evans, L. D., Laska, D. A., and Hattendorf, G. H. (1987). An in vitro model for assessing muscle irritation due to parenteral antibiotics, Fund. Appl. Toxicol., 9:10–17.

Young, M. F., Trobetta, L. D., and Sophia, J. V. (1986). Correlative in vitro and in vivo study of skeletal muscle irritancy, Toxicologist, 6(1):1225.

8

Immunotoxicology

The evaluation of the immunotoxicity of medical devices as part of their biocompatibility assessment is currently an area of great controversy and concern in both the industry and regulating bodies. Traditionally, and in terms of current regulatory requirements, simple dermal sensitization has been adequate for evaluating this end point, in spite of the fact that the association between implanted or indwelling devices and granuloma formation has been known for some time (Adams, 1983; Anderson, 1988; Black, 1981; Burkitt et al., 1986; Woodward and Salthouse, 1986; Unanue, 1994; Salthouse, 1982; Marchant et al., 1985). Recent history (with latex and silicones) has brought the adequacy of this approach into question, however.

The immune system is a highly complex system of cells involved in a multitude of functions, including antigen presentation and recognition, amplification, and cell proliferation with subsequent differentiation and secretion of lymphokines and antibodies (Bick, 1985). The end result is an integrated system responsible for defense against foreign pathogens and spontaneously occurring neoplasms that if left unchecked may result in infection and malignancy. To be effective, the immune system must be able to both recognize and destroy foreign antigens. To accomplish this, cellular and soluble components of diverse function and specificity circulate through blood and lymphatic vessels, thus allowing them to act at remote sites and tissues. For this system to function in balance and harmony requires regulation through cell-to-cell communications and precise recognition of self versus nonself. Immunotoxicants can upset this balance if they are lethal to one or more of the cell types or alter membrane morphology and receptors. There are several undesired immune system responses that may poten-

tially occur upon repeated exposure to a medical device material that may ultimately present barriers to its development, including the following:

> Down-modulation of the immune response (immunosuppression), which
> may result in an impaired ability to deal with neoplasia and infections.
> This is of particular concern if the devise is intended or likely to be used
> in patients with pre-existing conditions, such as cancer, severe infection,
> or immunodeficiency diseases.
> Up-modulation of the immune system (i.e., autoimmunity).
> Direct adverse immune responses to the agent itself in the form of hypersen-
> sitivity responses (anaphylaxis and delayed contact hypersensitivity).
> Direct immune responses to the device that limit or nullify its utility (i.e.,
> the development of neutralizing antibodies to be a delivered agent).

Immunotoxicology has evolved over the last 20 years as a specialty within
toxicology that brings together knowledge from basic immunology, molecular biology, microbiology, pharmacology, and physiology. As a discipline, immunotoxicology involves the study of the adverse effects that xenobiotics have on the immune system. As listed above, several different types of adverse immunological
effects may occur, including immunosuppression, autoimmunity, and hypersensitivity. Although these effects are clearly distinct, they are not mutually exclusive.
For example, immunosuppressive drugs that suppress suppressor-cell activity can
also induce autoimmunity (Hutchings et al., 1985), and agents that are immunoen-
hancing at low doses may be immunotoxic at high doses. Chemical xenobiotics
may be in the form of natural or man-made environmental chemicals—pharmaceuticals and biologicals that are pharmacologically, endocrinologically, or toxicologically active. Although in general xenobiotics are not endogenously produced, immunologically active biological response modifiers that naturally occur in the body
should also be included, since many are now known to compromise immune function when present in pharmacologically effective doses (Koller, 1987).

Although the types of immunological responses to various xenobiotics may
be similar, the approach taken for screening potential immunological activity
will vary, depending on the application of the compound. In contrast to potential
environmental exposures, medical devices and biomaterials are developed with
intentional but restricted human exposure, and their biological effects are extensively studied in surveillance.

Currently, immunotoxicology in medical device safety assessment is addressed both by regulatory requirements and guidelines and by existing practice.
Notable exceptions are the testing requirements for delayed contact hypersensitivity for surface-contacting devices and antigenicity/anaphylaxis testing for devices
to be registered in Japan.

Over the last few years, however, the FDA has more frequently requested
that specific tests be performed to address potential immunotoxic concerns. In

1993, the FDA issued draft guidelines for immunotoxicity testing in the revision of the "Redbook" (FDA, 1993). Although these guidelines have been established through the Center for Food Safety and Applied Nutrition, it has become apparent that other centers within the FDA may extend the usage of these guidelines to cover testing for human and veterinary pharmaceuticals. There is also the realization, however, that the draft guidelines may require some revision to make them applicable to device testing. Immunotoxicology assessment of devices has not yet been addressed by the International Conference on Harmonization (ICH), a multinational effort that is aimed at harmonizing the toxicology testing requirements and protocols for worldwide pharmaceutical and device registrations (Koeter, 1995). This topic may come up for discussion at future conferences. CDRH (1997) has, however, promulgated guidelines for devices.

Unanticipated immunotoxicity is infrequently observed with drugs that have been approved for marketing. With the exception of drugs that are intended to be immunomodulatory or immunosuppressive as part of their therapeutic mode of action, there is little evidence that drugs or devices cause unintended functional immunosuppression in man (Gleichman et al., 1989). Hypersensitivity (allergy) and autoimmunity are frequently observed, however, and are serious consequences of some therapies (DeSwarte, 1986). An adverse immune response in the form of hypersensitivity is one of the most frequent safety causes for withdrawal of drugs that have already made it to market (see Table 8.1) and accounts for approximately 15% of adverse reactions to xenobiotics (de Weck, 1983). In addition, adverse immune responses such as this (usually urticaria and frank rashes) are the chief "unexpected" finding in clinical studies. These findings are unexpected in that they are not predicted by preclinical studies because there is a lack of good preclinical models for predicting systemic hypersensitivity responses, especially to orally administered agents. As a consequence, the unexpected occurrence of hypersensitivity in the clinic may delay or even preclude further development and commercialization. A primary purpose for preclinical immunotoxicology testing is thus to help us detect these adverse effects earlier in development before they are found in clinical trials.

I. OVERVIEW OF THE IMMUNE SYSTEM

A thorough review of the immune system is not the intent of this chapter, but a brief description of the important components of the system and their interactions is necessary for an understanding of how xenobiotics can affect immune function. A breakdown at any point in this intricate and dynamic system can lead to immunopathology.

The immune system is divided into two defense mechanisms: nonspecific or innate, and specific or adaptive mechanisms that recognize and respond to foreign substances. Some of the important cellular components of nonspecific

TABLE 8.1   Drugs Withdrawn from the Market Due to Dose- and Time-Unrelated Toxicity Not Identified in Animal Experiments

Compound	Adverse reaction	Year of introduction	Years on the market
Aminopyrine	Agranulocytosis	Approx. 1900	75
Phenacetin	Interstitial nephritis	Approx. 1900	83
Dipyrone	Agranulocytosis	Approx. 1930	47
Clioquinol	Subacute myelo-optic neuro-pathy	Approx. 1930	51
Oxyphenisatin	Chronic active hepatitis	Approx. 1955	23
Nialamide	Liver damage	1959	19
Phenoxyorioazine	Liver damage	1961	5
Mebanazine	Liver damage	1963	3
Ibufenac	Hepatotoxicity	1966	2
Practolol	Oculomucocutaneous syndrome	1970	6
Alclofenace	Hypersensitivity	1972	7
Azaribine	Thrombosis	1975	1
Ticynafen	Nephropathy	1979	1
Benoxaprofen	Photosensitivity, hematoxicity	1980	2
Zomepirac	Urticaria, anaphylactic shock	1980	3
Zimelidine	Hepatotoxicity	1982	2

Source: Adapted from Bakke et al., 1984.

and specific immunity are described in Table 8.2. The nonspecific immune components are the phagocytic cells, such as the monocytes, macrophages, and polymorphic neutrophils (PMNs).

The specific or adaptive immune system is characterized by memory, specificity, and the ability to distinguish self from nonself (Battisto et al., 1983), although recently this basic self–nonself paradigm has been challenged by the alternative hypothesis that the immune system actually responds to some form of "danger" manager (Pennisi, 1996). The important cells of the adaptive immune system are the lymphocytes and antigen-presenting cells that are part of nonspecific immunity. The lymphocytes, which originate from pluripotent stem cells located in the hematopoietic tissues of the liver (fetal) and bone marrow, are composed of two general cell types: T and B cells. The T cells differentiate in the thymus and are made up of three subsets: helper, suppressor, and cytotoxic. The B cells, which have the capacity to produce antibodies, differentiate in the bone marrow or fetal liver. The various functions of the T cells include presenting antigen to B cells, helping B cells to make antibody, killing infected cells, regulat-

TABLE 8.2 Cellular Components of the Immune System and Their Functions

Cell subpopulations	Markers[a]	Functions
Nonspecific immunity		
Granulocytes		Degranulate to release mediators
Neutrophils (blood)		
Basophils (blood)		
Eosinophils (blood)		
Mast cells (connective tissue)		
Natural killer (NK) cells		Nonsensitized lymphocytes; directly kill target cells
Retucykiendothelial	CD14; HLA-DR	Antigen processing, presentation, and phagocytosis (humoral and some cell-mediated responses)
Macrophage (peritoneal, pleural, alveolar spaces)		
Histiocytes (tissues)		
Monocytes (blood)		
Specific immunity		
Humoral immunity		
Activated B cells	CD19; CD23	Proliferate; form plasma cells
Plasma cells		Secrete antibody; terminally differentiated
Resting		Secrete I_gM antibodies (primary response)
Memory		Secrete I_gG antibodies (secondary response)
Cell-mediated immunity		
T-Cell types		
Helper (T_k)	CD4; CD25	Assists in humoral immunity; required for antibody production
Cytotoxic (T_k)	CD8; CD25	Targets lysis
Suppressor (T_s)	CD8; CD25	Suppresses/regulates humoral and cell-mediated responses

[a] Activation surface markers detected by specific monoclonal antibodies; can be assayed with flow cytometry.

ing the level of the immune response, and stimulating cytotoxic activity of other cells, such as macrophages (Male et al., 1987).

Activation of the immune system is thought to occur when antigen-presenting cells (APCs) such as macrophages and dendritic cells take up antigen via F_c or complement receptors, process the antigen, and present it to T cells. (See Figure 8.1.) Macrophages release soluble mediators such as interleukin 1 (IL-1), which stimulate T cells to proliferate. Antigen-presenting cells must present antigen to T cells in conjunction with the class II major histocompatibility complex

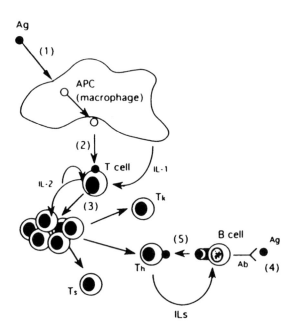

FIGURE 8.1   A simplified schematic of the immunoregulatory circuit that regulates the activation of T cells and B cells involved in humoral (T-cell dependent) and cell-mediated immunity. (1) Antigen (Ag) is processed by the APCs expressing class II MHC molecules. (2) Antigen plus class II MHC is then presented to antigen-specific T-helper cells (CD4+) which stimulate secretion of IL02. (3) IL-2 in turn stimulates proliferation (clonal expansion) of T cells and differentiation into T-suppressor (T_s), T killer (T_k), and T-helper (T_h) effector cells. The expanded clone has a higher likelihood of finding the appropriate B cell that has the same antigen and class II molecules on its surface. (4) Next, the antigen binds to an antibody (Ab) on the surface of a specific B cell. (5) The B cell, in turn, processes the antigen and presents it (plus class II MHC) to the specific T_h cell. The T_h cell is then stimulated to secrete additional interleukins (ILs) that stimulate clonal expansion and differentiation of the antigen-specific B cell.

(MHC) proteins that are located on the surface of the T cells. The receptor proteins and the T3 cell are a complex of the Ti molecule that binds antigen, the MHC proteins, and the T3 molecular complex, which is often referred to as the CD3 complex. Upon stimulation, T cells proliferate, differentiate, and express interleukin-2 (IL-2) receptors. T cells also produce and secrete IL-2, which in turn acts on antigen-specific B cells, causing them to proliferate and differentiate into antibody-forming (plasma) cells.

Antibodies (Table 8.3) circulate freely in the blood or lymph and are important in neutralizing foreign antigens. The various types of antibodies involved in humor-genes (polymorphisms) that encode diversity to the variable region of the antibody. B cells are capable of generating further diversity to antibody specificity by a sequence of molecular events involving somatic mutations, chromosomal rearrangements during mitosis, and recombinations of gene segments (Roitt et al., 1985).

The immune system is regulated in part by feedback inhibition involving complex interactions between the various growth and differentiation factors listed in Table 8.4. Since antigen initiates the signal for the immune response, elimination of antigen will decrease further stimulation (Male et al., 1987). T suppressor cells (T_s) also regulate the immune response and are thought to be important in

TABLE **8.3** Antibodies Involved in the Humoral Immune Response

Antibodies	Serum conc. mg ml^{-1} (%)	Characteristics/functions
IgG	10–12 (80%)	Monomeric structure (γ-globulin); secreted from B cells during secondary response; binds complement; can cross placenta
IgM	1–2 (5–10%)	Pentameric structure; secreted from B cells during primary response; potent binder of complement; high levels indicative of systemic lupus erythematosus or rheumatoid arthritis; cannot across placenta.
IgA	3–4 (10–15%)	Dimeric or monomeric structures; found in seromucous secretions (breast milk); secreted by B cells associated with epithelial cells in GI tract, lung, etc.
IgD	0.03 (<1%)	Monomer; extremely labile; functions not well known.
IgE	<0.0001	Reaginic antibody involved in immediate hypersensitivity; anthelminthic; does not bind complement.

Source: Extracted and modified from Clark, 1983.

TABLE 8.4   Cells and Mechanisms Involved in Cell-Mediated Cytotoxicity

Cell type	Mechanism of cytotoxicity
T_k cells	T_k cells that are specifically sensitized to antigens on target cells interact directly with target cells to lyse them.
T_D cells	Cells involved in delayed hypersensitivity that act indirectly to kill target cells; T_D cells react with antigen and release cytokines that can kill target cells.
NK cells	Nonspecific T cells that react directly with target cells (tumor cells) without prior sensitization.
Null cells	Antibody-dependent cell-mediated cytotoxicity (ADCC) involving non-T/non-B cells (null cells) with F_c receptors specific for antibody-coated target cells.
Macrophages	Nonspecific, direct killing of target by phagocytosis; also involved in presenting antigen to specific T_k cells that can then mediate cytotoxicity as described above.

the development of tolerance to self antigens. In addition to the humoral immune system or the branch that is modulated by antibody, cell-mediated immunity and cytotoxic cell types play a major role in the defense against virally infected cells, tumor cells, and cells of foreign tissue transplants. Cytotoxic T_k cells (T killer cells) recognize antigen in association with Class I molecules of MHC, while natural killer cells (NK cells) are not MHC effector cell, but rather cause lysosomal degranulation, and calcium influx into the targeted cell. The various types of cells involved in cell-mediated cytotoxicity and their mechanisms of action are outlined in Table 8.5.

A. Immunotoxic Effects

The immune system is a highly integrated and regulated network of cell types that require continual renewal to achieve balance and immunocompetence. The delicacy of this balance makes the immune system a natural target for cytotoxic drugs or their metabolites. Since renewal is dependent on the ability of cells to proliferate and differentiate, exposure to agents that arrest cell division can subsequently lead to reduced immune function or immonosuppression. This concept has been exploited in the development of therapeutic drugs intended to treat leukemias, autoimmune disease, and chronic inflammatory diseases and to prevent transplant rejection. Some drugs may adversely modulate the immune system secondarily to their therapeutic effects, however.

Two broad categories of immunotoxicity have been defined on the basis of suppression or stimulation of normal immune function. Immunosuppression is a down-modulation of the immune system characterized by cell depletion, dysfunction, or dysregulation that may subsequently result in increased susceptibility to infection and tumors. By contrast, immunostimulation is an increased or exaggerated immune responsiveness that may be apparent in the form of a tissue-damaging allergic hypersensitivity response or pathological autoimmunity. As knowledge of the mechanisms involved in each of these conditions has expanded, however, the distinction between them has become less clear. Some agents can cause immunosuppression at one dose or duration of exposure and immunostimulation at others. For instance, the chemotherapeutic drug cyclophosphamide is in most cases immunosuppressive; however, it can also induce autoimmunity (Hutchings et al., 1985). Likewise, dimethylnitrosamine, a nitrosamine detected in some foods, has been shown to have both suppressing and enhancing effects on the immune system (Yoshida et al., 1989).

1. Immunosuppression

The various cells of the immune system may differ in their sensitivity to a given xenobiotic, thus immunosuppression may be expressed as varying degrees of reduced activity of a single cell type or multiple populations of immunocytes. Several lymphoid organs such as the bone marrow, spleen, thymus, and lymph nodes may be affected simultaneously, or the immunodeficiency may be isolated to a single tissue, such as the Peyer's patches of the intestines. The resulting deficiency may in turn lead to an array of clinical outcomes of varying ranges of severity. These outcomes include increased susceptibility to infections, increased severity or persistence of infections, or infections with unusual organisms (e.g., system fungal infections). Immunosuppression can be induced in a dose-related manner by a variety of therapeutic agents at dose levels lower than those required to produce overt clinical signs of general toxicity. In addition, immunosuppression can occur without regard to genetic predisposition, given that a sufficient dose level and duration of exposure has been achieved.

Humoral immunity is characterized by the production of antigen-specific antibodies that enhance phagocytosis and destruction of micro-organisms through opsonization, thus deficiencies of humoral immunity (B lymphocytes) may lead to reduced antibody titers and are typically associated with acute gram-positive bacterial infections (i.e., Streptococcus). Although chronic infection is usually associated with dysfunction of some aspect of cellular immunity, chronic infections can also occur when facultative intracellular organisms such as *Listeria or Mycobacterium* evade antibodies and multiply within phagocytic cells.

Since cellular immunity results in the release of chemotactic lymphocytes that in turn enhance phagocytosis, a deficiency in cellular immunity may also result in chronic infections. Cellular immunity is mediated by T cells, macrophages, and NK cells involved in complex compensatory networks and secondary changes. Immunosuppressive agents may act directly by lethality to T cells or indirectly by blocking mitosis, lymphokine synthesis, lymphokine release, or

TABLE 8.5 Growth and Differentiation Factors of the Immune System

Factors	Cell of origin	Primary immune functions
Interleukins[a]		
IL-1	Macrophage, B and T cells	Lymphocyte-activating factor; enhances activation of T and B cells, NK cells, and macrophages
IL-2	T cells (T_h)	T-cell growth factor; stimulates T-cell growth and effector differentiation; stimulates B-cell proliferation/differentiation
IL-3	T cells (T_h)	Mast-cell growth factor; stimulates proliferation/differentiation of mast cells, neutrophils, and macrophages
IL-4	T cells (T_h), mast cells, B cells	B-cell growth factor; induces proliferation/differentiation of B cells and secretion of IgA, IgG_1, and IgE; promotes T-cell growth; activates macrophages
IL-6	T cells, fibroblasts, monocytes	Stimulates growth/differentiation of B cells and secretion of IgG; promotes IL-2-induced growth of T cells
IL-7	Bone marrow stromal cells	Stimulates pre-B- and pre-T-cell growth/differentiation; enhances thymocyte proliferation
IL-8	Monocytes, fibroblasts	Neutrophils chemotaxis
IL-9	T cells	Stimulates T cells and mast cells
IL-10	T cells	Stimulates mast cells and thymocytes; induction of class II MHC

Factor	Source	Function
Interferons (INF)		
α-INF	Leukocytes and mast cells	Antiviral; increases NK-cell function, B-cell differentiation, potentiates macrophage production of IL-1
β-INF	Fibroblasts, epithelial cells	Antiviral; potentiates macrophage production of IL-1; increases NK-cell function
γ-INF	T cells (T_h), cytotoxic T cells	Antiviral; activates macrophages; induces MHC class II expression on macrophages, epithelial, and endothelial cells
Tumor necrosis factors (TNF)		
TNFα	Macrophage, B and T cells	Catectin; promotes tumor cytotoxicity; activates macrophages and neutrophils; enhances IL-2 receptor expression on T cells; inhibits antibody secretion
TNFβ	T cells (T_h), NK cells	Lymphotoxin; promotes T-cell-mediated cytotoxicity, B-cell activation
Colony-stimulating factors (CSF)	Stem cells	Promotes growth and differentiation of
Granulocyte CSF	Myeloid	Granulocytes and macrophages
Macrophage CSF	Myeloid	Macrophages and granulocytes
Granulocytes-macrophage CSF	Myeloid	Granulocytes, macrophages, eosinophils, mast cells, and pluripotent progenitor cells

[a] Includes lymphokines, monokines, and cytokines produced by T cells, macrophages, and other cells, respectively. Source: Extracted and modified from Golub and Green, 1991.

membrane receptors to lymphokines. In addition, cellular immunity is involved in the production and release of interferon, a lymphokine that ultimately results in blockage of viral replication (Table 8.5). Viruses are particularly susceptible to cytolysis by T cells since they often attach to the surface of infected cells. Immunosuppression of any of the components of cellular immunity may thus result in an increase in protozoan, fungal, and viral infections as well as opportunistic bacterial infections.

Immune depression may result unintentionally as a side effect of cancer chemotherapy or intentionally from therapeutics administered to prevent graft rejection. In fact, both transplant patients administered immunosuppressive drugs and cancer patients treated with chemotherapeutic agents have been shown to be at a high risk of developing secondary cancers, particularly of lymphoreticular etiology (Penn, 1977). Most of these drugs are alkylating or cross-linking agents that by their chemical nature are electrophilic and highly reactive with nucleophilic macromolecules (protein and nucleic acids). Nucleophilic sites are ubiquitous, and include amino, hydroxyl, mercapto, and histidine functional groups. Immunotoxic agents used in chemotherapy may thus induce secondary tumors through direct genotoxic mechanisms (i.e., DNA alkylation).

Reduced cellular immunity may also result in increased malignancy and decreased viral resistance through indirect mechanisms by modulating immune surveillance of aberrant cells. T lymphocytes, macrophage cells, and NK cells are all involved in immunosurveillance through cytolysis of virally inflected cells or tumor cells, each by a different mechanism (Table 8.2) (Burnet, 1970). In addition to the common cell types described in Table 8.2, at least two other types of cytotoxic effector cells of T cell origin have been identified, each of which has a unique lytic specificity phenotype and activity profile (Merluzzi, 1985). Of these, both LAK and TIL cells have been shown to lyse a variety of different tumor cells; TIL cells, however, have 50 to 100 times more lytic activity than LAK cells. Most tumor cells express unique surface antigens that render them different from normal cells. Once detected as foreign, they are presented to the T helper cells in association with MHC molecules to form an antigen–MHC complex. This association elicits a genetic component to the immunospecificity reaction. T helper cells subsequently direct the antigen complex toward the cytotoxic T lymphocytes, which possess receptors for antigen–MHC complexes. These cells can then proliferate, respond to specific viral antigens or antigens on the membranes of tumor cells, and destroy them (Yoshida et al., 1989).

In contrast, the macrophages and NK cells are involved in nonspecific immunosurveillance in that they do not require prior sensitization with a foreign antigen as a prerequisite for lysis and are not involved with MHC molecules. The enhancement of either NK cell function or macrophage function has been shown to reduce metastasis of some types of tumors. Macrophage cells accumulate at the tumor site and have been shown to lyse a variety of transformed tumor cells (Volkman, 1984). Natural killer cells are involved in the lysis of primary autochthonous tumor cells. Migration of NK cells to tumor sites has been well documented. Although not clearly defined, it appears that they can recognize certain proteinaceous structures on tumor cells and lyse them with cytolysin.

2. Immunostimulation

A variety of drugs as well as environmental chemicals have been shown to have immunostimulatory or sensitizing effects on the immune system, and these effects are well documented in humans exposed to drugs (DeSwarte, 1986). The drug or metabolite can act as a hapten and covalently bind to a protein or other cellular constituent of the host to appear foreign and become antigenic. Haptens are low-molecular-weight substances that are not in themselves immunogenic but will induce an immune response if conjugated with nuclophilic groups on proteins or other macromolecular carriers. In both allergy and autoimmunity, the immune system is stimulated or sensitized by the drug conjugate to produce specific pathological responses. An allergic hypersensitivity reaction may vary from one that results in an immediate anaphylactic response to one that produces a delayed hypersensitivity reaction or immune complex reaction. Allergic hypersensitivity reactions result in a heightened sensitivity to nonself antigens, whereas autoimmunity results in an altered response to self antigens. Unlike immunosuppression, which nonspecifically affects all individuals in a dose-related manner, both allergy and autoimmunity have a genetic component that creates susceptibility in those individuals with a genetic predisposition. Once sensitized, susceptible individuals can respond to genetic predisposition and to even minute quantities of the antigen.

3. Hypersensitivity

The four types of hypersensitivity reactions (''sensitization'') as classified by Coombs and Gell (1975) are outlined in Table 8.6. The first three types are immediate antibody-mediated reactions, whereas the fourth type is a cellular-mediated delayed-type response that may require 1 to 2 days to occur after a secondary exposure. Type I reactions are characterized by an anaphylaxis response to a variety of compounds, including proteinaceous materials and pharmaceuticals, such as penicillin. Various target organs may be involved, depending on the route of exposure. For example, the gastrointestinal tract is usually involved with food allergies, the respiratory system with inhaled allergens, the skin with dermal exposure, and smooth muscle vasculature with systemic exposure. The type of response elicited often depends on the site of exposure and includes dermatitis and urticaria (dermal), rhinitis and asthma (inhalation), increased gastrointestinal emptying (ingestion), and systemic anaphylactic shock (parenteral).

TABLE 8.6 Types of Hypersensitivity Responses

Type and designation[a]	Components	Effects	Mechanism
I. Immediate	Mast cells; IgE	Anaphylaxis, asthma, uriticaria, rhinitis, dermatitis	IgE binds to mast cells to stimulate release of humoral factors
II. Cytoxic	Antibodies	Hemolytic anemia, Goodpasture's disease	IgG and IgM bind to cells (e.g., RBCs), fix complement (opsinization), then lyse cells
III. Immune complex (arthus)	Antigen-antibody complexes (Ag-Ab)	SLE rheumatoid arthritis, glomerular nephritis, serum sickness, vasculitis	Ag-Ab complexes deposit in tissues, and may fix complement
IV. Delayed hypersensitivity	T$_D$ cells; macrophages	Contact dermatitis, tuberculosis	Sensitized T cells induce a delayed hypersensitivity response upon challenge

Source: Based on classification system of Coombs and Gell, 1975.

Type I Hypersensitivity. During an initial exposure, IgE antibodies are produced and bind to the cell surface of mast cells and basophils. Upon subsequent exposures to the antigen, reaginic IgE antibodies bound to the surface of target cells at the F_c region (mast cells and basophils) and become cross-linked (at the F_{ab} regions) by the antigen. Cross-linking causes distortion of the cell surface and IgE molecule, which in turn activates a series of enzymatic reactions, ultimately leading to degranulation of the mast cells and basophils. These granules contain a variety of pharmacological substances (Table 8.7), such as histamines, serotonins, prostaglandins, bradykinins, and leukotrienes (SRS-A and ECR-A) Upon subsequent challenge exposures, these factors are responsible for eliciting an allergic reaction through vasodilation and increased vascular permeability. The nasal passages contain both mast cells and plasma cells that secrete IgE antibodies. Allergic responses localized in the nasal mucosa result in dilation of the local blood vessels, tissue swelling, mucus secretion, and sneezing. Reactions localized in the respiratory tract, also rich in mast cells and IgE, result in allergic asthma response. This condition is triggered by the release of histamine and SRS-A, which induce constriction of the bronchi and alveoli, pulmonary edema, and mucous secretions that block the bronchi and alveoli, together resulting in severe difficulty in breathing. In the case of a challenge dose of a drug administered systemically, the reactive patient may have difficulty breathing within minutes of exposure and may experience convulsions, vomiting, and low blood pressure. The effects of anaphylactic shock and respiratory distress, if severe, may ultimately result in death.

Antibiotics containing β-lactam structures, such as penicillin and cephalosporins, are the most commonly occurring inducers of anaphylactic shock and

TABLE 8.7 Proteins and Soluble Mediators Involved in Hypersensitivity

Factor	Origin	Characteristics/functions
Histamine	Mast cells, basophils	Contraction of smooth muscle; increases vascular permeability
Serotonin	Mast cells, basophils	Contraction of smooth muscle; leukotriene
SRS-A	Lung tissue	(Slow-reacting substance of anaphylaxis); Contraction of smooth muscle; acidic polypeptide
ECF-A	Mast cells	(Eosinophilic chemotactic factor of anaphylaxis); attracts eosinophils; small peptide
Prostaglandins	Various tissues	Modifies release of histamine and serotonin from mast cells and basophils

Source: Extracted and modified from Clark, 1983.

drug hypersensitivity in general. Other hypersensitivity reactions may include urticarial rash, fever, bronchospasm, serum sickness, and vasculitis, with reported incidences of all types varying from 0.7–10% (Idsøe et al., 1968) and the incidence of anaphylactoid reactions varying from 0.04–0.2%. When the β-lactam ring is opened during metabolism, the pencilloyl moiety can form covalent conjugates with nucleophilic sites on proteins. The penicilloyl conjugates can then act as haptens to form the determinants for antibody induction. Although most patients who have received penicillin produce antibodies against the metabolite benzylpeniclloyl, only a fraction experience allergic reaction (Garratlz and Petz, 1975), which suggests a genetic component to susceptibility.

Type II Hypersensitivity. Type II cytolytic reactions are mediated by IgG and IgM antibodies that can fix complement, opsonize particles, or induce antibody-dependent cellular cytolysis reactions. Erythrocytes, lymphocytes, and platelets of the circulatory system are the major target cells that interact with the cytolytic antibodies, causing depletion of these cells. Hemolytic anemia (penicillin, methyldopa), leukopenia, thrombocytopenia (quinidine), and/or granulocytopenia (sulfonamide) may result. Type II reactions involving the lungs and kidneys occur through the development of antibodies (autoantibodies) to the basement membranes in the alveoli or glomeruli, respectively. Prolonged damage may result in Goodpasture's disease, an autoimmune disease characterized by pulmonary hemorrhage and glomerulonephritis. Several other autoimmune-type diseases have been associated with extended treatments with D-penicillamine and other pharmaceuticals. Various types of autoimmune responses and examples of drug-induced autoimmunity are discussed in further detail later in this section.

Type III Hypersensitivity. Type III reactions (arthus) are characterized as an immediate hypersensitivity reaction initiated by antigen–antibody complexes that form freely in the plasma instead of at the cell surface. Regardless of whether the antigens are self or foreign, complexes mediated by IgG can form and settle into the tissue compartments of the host. These complexes can then fix complement and release C3a and C5a fragments that are chemotactic for phagocytic cells. Polmorphonuclear leukocytes are then attracted to the site, where they phagocytize the complexes and release hydrolytic enzymes into the tissues. Additional damage can be caused by binding to and activating platelets and basophils, which in the end results in localized necrosis, hemorrhage, and increased permeability of local blood vessels. These reactions commonly target the kidney, resulting in glomerulonephritis through the deposition of the complexes in the glomeruli.

Some devices and antibiotics (β-lactam) have been reported to produce glomerular nephritis in humans that has been attributed to circulating immune complexes. These complexes have also been observed in preclinical toxicology studies with baboons treated with a β-lactam antibiotic prior to the appearance of any biochemical or clinical changes (Descotes and Mazue, 1987). In addition, immunoglobulin complexes have been observed in rats treated with gold, and autologous immune complex nephritis has been observed in guinea pigs (Ueda et al., 1980). Similar evidence of immunomediated nephrotoxicity has been reported in rheumatoid arthritis patients administered long-term treatments with gold compounds; proteinuria has been observed in approximately 10% of these patients.

Other target organs such as the skin with lupus, the joints with rheumatoid arthritis, and the lungs with pneumonitis, may be affected. The deposition of antigen–antibody complexes through the circulatory system results in a syndrome referred to as serum sickness, which was quite prevalent prior to 1940 (Clark, 1983), when serum for diphtheria was commonly used. Serum sickness occurs when the serum itself becomes antigenic as a side effect from passive immunization with heterologous antiserum produced from various sources of farm animals. The antitoxin for diphtheria was produced in a horse and administered to humans as multiple injections of passive antibody. As a consequence, these people often became sensitized to the horse serum and developed a severe form of arthritis and glomerulonephritis caused by deposition of antigen–antibody complexes. Clinical symptoms of serum sickness present as urticarial skin eruptions, arthralgia or arthritis, lymphadenopathy, and fever. Drugs such as sulfonamides, penicillin, and iodides can induce a similar type of reaction. Although uncommon today, transplant patients receiving immunosuppressive therapy with heterologous anti-lymphocyte serum or globulins may also exhibit serum sickness (Ueda et al., 1980).

Type IV Delayed-Type Hypersensitivity (DTH). Delayed-type hypersensitivity reactions are T-cell mediated with no involvement of antibodies. These reactions, however, are controlled through accessory cells, suppressor T cells, and monokine-secreting macrophages, which regulate the proliferation and differentiation of T cells. The most frequent form of DTH manifests itself as contact dermatitis. The drug or metabolite binds to a protein in the skin or the Langerhans cell membrane (class II MHC molecules), where it is recognized as an antigen and triggers cell proliferation. After a sufficient period of time for migration of the antigen and clonal expansion (latency period), a subsequent exposure will elicit a dermatitis reaction. A 24- to 48-hr delay often occurs between the time of exposure and the onset of symptoms to allow time for infiltration of lymphocytes to the site of exposure. The T cells (CD4$^+$) that react with the antigen are activated and release lymphokines that are chemotactic for monocytes and macrophages. Although these cells infiltrate to the site via the circulatory vessels, an intact lymphatic drainage system from the site is necessary since the reaction is initiated in drainage lymph nodes proximal to the site (Clark, 1983). The release (degranulation) of enzymes and histamines from the macrophages may then result in tissue damage. Clinical symptoms of local dermal reactions may include a rash (not limited to the sites of exposure) itching, and/or burning sensations. Erythema is generally observed in the area around the site, which may become thickened and hard to the touch. In severe cases, necrosis may appear in the center of the site, followed by desquamation during the healing process. The immune-enhancing drugs isoprinosine and avridine have been shown to induce a delayed-type hypersensitivity reaction in rats (Exon et al., 1986).

A second form of delayed-type hypersensitivity response is similar to that of contact dermatitis in that macrophages are the primary effector cells responsible for stimulating CD4+ T cells. This response is not necessarily localized to the epidermis, however. A classical example of this type of response is demonstrated by the tuberculin diagnostic tests. To determine if an individual has been exposed to tuberculosis, a small amount of fluid from tubercle bacilli cultures is injected subcutaneously. The development of induration after 48 hr at the site of injection is diagnostic of prior exposure.

Shock similar to that of anaphylaxis may occur as a third form of a delayed systemic hypersensitivity response. Unlike anaphylaxis, however, IgE antibodies are not involved. This type of response may occur 5 to 8 hr after systemic exposure and can result in fatality within 24 hr following intravenous or intraperitoneal injection.

A fourth form of delayed hypersensitivity results in the formation of granulomas. If the antigen is allowed to persist unchecked, macrophages and fibroblasts are recruited to the site to proliferate, produce collagen, and effectively "wall off" the antigen. A granuloma requires a minimum of one to two weeks to form.

4. Autoimmunity

As with hypersensitivity, in autoimmunity the immune system is stimulated by specific responses that are pathogenic, and both tend to have a genetic component that predisposes some individuals more than others. As is the case with hypersensitivity, however, the adverse immune response of drug-induced autoimmunity is not restricted to the drug itself, but also involves a response to self antigens.

Autoimmune responses directed against normal components of the body may consist of antibody-driven humoral responses and/or cell-mediated, delayed-type hypersensitivity responses. T cells can react directly against specific target organs, or B cells can secrete autoantibodies that target self. Autoimmunity may occur spontaneously as the result of a loss of regulatory controls that initiate or suppress normal immunity, causing the immune system to produce lymphocytes reactive against its own cells and macromolecules, such as DNA, RNA, or erythrocytes.

Although autoantibodies are often associated with autoimmune reactions, they are not necessarily indicative of autoimmunity (Russel, 1981). Antinuclear antibodies can occur normally with aging in some healthy women without autoimmune disease, and all individuals have B cells with the potential of reacting with self antigens through Ig receptors (Dighiero et al., 1983). The presence of an antibody titer to a particular immunogen indicates that haptenization of serum albumin has occurred as part of a normal immune response. If cells are stimulated to proliferate and secrete autoantibodies directed against a specific cell or cellular component, however, a pathological response may result. The tissue damage associated with autoimmune disease is usually a consequence of type II or III hypersensitivity reactions that result in the deposition of antibody–antigen complexes.

Several diseases have been associated with the production of autoantibodies against various tissues. For example, an autoimmune form of hemolytic anemia can occur if the antibodies are directed against erythrocytes, Similarly, antibodies that react with acetylcholine receptors may cause myasthenia gravis, those directed against glomerular basement membranes may cause Goodpasture's syndrome, and those that target the liver may cause hepatitis. Other forms of organ-specific autoimmunity include autoimmune thyroiditis (as seen with amiodarone) and juvenile diabetes mellitus, which result from autoantibodies directed against the tissue-specific antigens thyroglobulin and cytoplasmic components of pancreatic islet cells, respectively. In contrast, systemic autoimmune diseases may occur if the autoantibodies are directed against an antigen that is ubiquitous throughout the body, such as DNA or RNA. For example, systemic lupus erythematosus (SLE) occurs as the result of autoimmunity to nuclear antigens that form immune complexes in the walls of blood vessels and basement membranes of tissues throughout the body.

The etiology of renal autoimmunity is not well established and is confounded by factors such as age, sex, and nutritional state, as well as genetic influences on pharmacological and immune susceptibility. Unlike idiopathic autoimmunity, which is progressive or characterized by an alternating series of relapses and remissions, drug-induced autoimmunity is thought to subside after the drug is discontinued. This is not certain, however, since a major determining factor for diagnosis of a drug-related disorder is dependent on the observation of remission upon withdrawal of the drug (Bigazzi, 1988).

One possible mechanism for xenobiotic-induced autoimmunity involves xenobiotic binding to autologous molecules, which then appear foreign to the immunosurveillance system. If a self antigen is chemically altered, a specific T helper (T_h) cell may see it as foreign and react to the altered antigenic determinant portion, allowing an autoreactive B cell to react to the unaltered hapten. This interaction results in a carrier–hapten bridge between the specific T_h and autoreactive B cell, bringing them together for subsequent production of autoantibodies specific to the self antigen that was chemically altered (Weigle, 1980). Conversely, a xenobiotic may alter B cells directly, including those that are autoreactive. The altered B cells may thus react to self antigens independent from T_h-cell recognition and in a nontissue-specific manner.

Another possible mechanism is that the xenobiotic may stimulate nonspecific mitogenicity of B cells. This could result in a polyclonal activation of B cells with subsequent production of autoantibodies. Alternatively, the xenobiotic may stimulate mitogenicity of T cells that recognize self, which in turn activates B cell production of antibodies in response to self molecules. There is also evidence to suggest that anti-DNA autoantibodies may originate from somatic mutations in lymphocyte precursors with antibacterial or antiviral specificity. For example, a single amino acid substitution resulting from a mutation in a monoclonal antibody to polyphorlcholine was shown to result in a loss of the original specificity and an acquisition of DNA reactivity similar to that observed for anti-DNA antibodies in SLE (Talal, 1987).

The mechanism of autoimmunity may also entail interaction with MHC structures determined by the HLA alleles. Individuals carrying certain HLA alleles have been shown to be predisposed to certain autoimmune diseases, which may account in part for the genetic variability of autoimmunity. In addition, metabolites of a particular drug may vary between individuals to confound the development of drug-induced autoimmunity. Dendritic cells, such as the Langerhans cells of the skin and B lymphocytes that function to present antigens to T_h cells, express Class-II MHC structures. Although the exact involvement of these MHC structures is unknown, Gleichmann et al. (1989) have theorized that self antigens rendered foreign by drugs such as D-penicillamine may be presented to T_h cells by MHC Class-II structures. An alternate hypothesis is that the drug or a metabolite may alter MHC Class-II structures on B cells, making them appear foreign to T_h cells.

A number of different drugs have been shown to induce autoimmunity in susceptible individuals. A syndrome similar to that of SLE was described in a patient administered sulfadizine in 1945 by Hoffman. (See Bigazzi, 1985.) Sulfonamides were one of the first classes of drugs identified to induce an autoimmune response, while to date over 40 other drugs have been associated with a similar syndrome.

Autoantibodies to red blood cells and autoimmune hemolytic anemia have been observed in patients treated with numerous drugs, including procainamide, chlorpropamide, captopril, cefalexin, penicillin, and methyldopa (Logue et al., 1970; Kleinman et al., 1984). Hydralazine- and procainamide-induced autoantibodies may also result in SLE. Approximately 20% of patients administered methyldopa for several weeks for the treatment of essential hypertension developed a dose-related titer and incidence of autoantibodies to erythrocytes, 1% of which presented with hemolytic anemia. Methyldopa does not appear to act as a hapten but appears to act by modifying erythrocyte surface antigens. IgG autoantibodies then develop against the modified erythrocytes.

Some metals that are used therapeutically have also been shown to induce autoimmune responses. Gold salts used to treat arthritis may induce formation of antiglomerular basement membrane antibodies, which may lead to glomerulo-nephritis similar to that seen in Goodpasture's disease. (See type II hypersensitiv-ity.) Since gold is not observed at the site of the lesions (Druet et al., 1982), it has been hypothesized that the metal elicits an antiself response. Lithium, used to treat manic depression, is thought to induce autoantibodies against thyroglobulin, which in some patients results in hypothyroidism. In studies with rats, levels of antibodies to thyroglobulin were shown to increase significantly in lithium-treated rats compared to controls immediately after immunization with thyroglob-ulin. Rats that were not immunized with throglobulin did not produce circulation antithroglobulin antibodies upon receiving lithium, however, and there was no effect of lithium on lymphocytic infiltration of the thyroid in either group (Hass-man et al., 1985).

In addition, silicone-containing medical devices, particularly breast pros-theses, have been reported to cause serum sickness-like reactions, scleroder-malike lesions, and an SLE-like disease termed human adjuvant disease (Kuma-gai et al., 1984; Guillaume et al., 1984). Some patients may also present with granulomas and autoantibodies. Human adjuvant disease is a connective tissue or autoimmune disease similar to that of adjuvant arthritis in rats and rheumatoid arthritis in humans. Autoimmune disease-like symptoms usually develop 2 to 5 years after implantation in a small percentage of people who receive implants, which may indicate that there is a genetic predisposition similar to that for SLE. An early hypothesis is that the prosthesis or injected silicone plays an adjuvant role by enhancing the immune response through increased macrophage and T cell helper function. There is currently controversy as to whether silicone as a foreign body induces a nonspecific inflammation reaction, a specific cell-medi-ated immunological reaction, or no reaction at all. There is strong support to indicate that silicone microparticles can act as haptens to produce a delayed hy-persensitivity reaction in a genetically susceptible population of people, however.

II. EVALUATION OF THE IMMUNE SYSTEM

A. Regulatory Positions

The pharmaceutical and medical device industries are increasingly concerned with whether preclinical testing of their products should include routine immuno-toxicologic screening or be done on an "as needed basis," triggered by the toxi-cological profile of the xenobiotic established in routine preclinical safety testing (Bloom et al., 1987). Although the FDA has not yet officially released guidelines for immunotoxicity testing of pharmaceuticals, recent drug development efforts in the areas of biotechnology, prostaglandins, interleukins, and recombinant bio-logical modifiers have elicited the expectation that the development of antibodies (neutralizing and otherwise) should be evaluated in at least one of the animal models used to assess general systemic toxicity. More to the point, draft guidelines have been released for devices (CDRH, 1997).

Federal attention and efforts to identify and control substances that may harm the immune system are discussed in a background paper by the Congressional Office of Technology Assessment (U.S. Congress, 1991). The National Academy of Science has convened a panel of immunotoxicologists to discuss the importance of immunotoxicology testing. The chemical industry has been a proponent of using a battery of assays to assess chemical-induced immunotoxicity, hence guidelines for a two-tiered screen approach have been proposed by the National Toxicology Program (NTP) (Luster et al., 1988). This strategy, which was developed for nontherapeutic chemicals and environmental contaminants that have different safety standards, does not address some of the safety issues and test strategy issues that are unique to pharmaceuticals. The FDA has drafted a similar two-leveled approach (Hinton, 1992) for assessing immunotoxicity of food colors and additives; however, these guidelines are likewise not necessarily relevant for testing pharmaceuticals. Since direct food additives are meant for human consumption and are tested thoroughly in animal toxicology tests, however, this strategy may be more applicable to pharmaceuticals than the strategy of the NTP. In all of these testing schemes, the initial tier generally includes a fundamental histopathologic assessment of the major components of the immune system. Additional tiers are then added to more precisely evaluate the functionality of the components that appeared to be adversely affected in the first tier of tests. These test strategies are primarily geared toward the detection of chemical-induced immunosuppression, thus the effectiveness of these test schemes for detecting immunostimulation has not yet been determined (Spreafico, 1988).

The NTP defines the first tier of assays (Table 8.8) to include an assessment of immunopathology: humoral, cell-mediated, and nonspecific immunity such as NK cell activity. The second tier (Table 8.9) includes a more comprehensive battery that should be used once functional changes are observed in the tier I assays. The tier II assays focus on mechanisms of immunotoxicity such as depletion of specific cell subsets by flow cytometry analysis or evaluation of secondary immune responses by examining IgG response. Cell-mediated immunity is assessed through a functional assay that looks at the ability of cytotoxic T cells to kill target cells, and nonspecific immunity is evaluated by examining various functions of macrophages: (1) the ability to phagocytize inert fluorescent beads or radiolabeled chicken erythrocytes and (2) the ability to produce cytokines such as IL-1 or macrophage activation factor. The ultimate immune test would be to examine the effects of xenobiotics on the intact animal's response to challenge by viral, bacterial, or parasitic pathogens or by neoplastic cells. The ability of the immune system to compensate, or conversely, its inability to compensate for loss or inhibition of its components is fully examined through host resistance mechanisms. This tiered test approach has been validated with 50 selected com-

TABLE 8.8 Tier I Screen

Parameter	Procedures
Immunopathology	Routine hematology-complete and differential count; routine toxicology information-weights of body, immune organs (spleen and thymus), liver, and kidney; histopathology of immune organs.
Humoral-mediated immunity	LPS (lipopolysaccharide) mitogen response or $F(ab)_2$ mitogenic response; enumeration of plaques by IgM antibody-forming cells to a T-dependent antigen (SRBCs; serum IgM concentration).
Cell-mediated immunity	Lymphocyte mitogenic response to concanavalin A and mixed lymphocyte response to allogeneic lymphocytes; local lymph node assay.
Nonspecific immunity	Natural killer cell activity.

Source: Adapted from Luster et al., 1988; Vos et al., 1989.

pounds, and results from these studies have shown that the use of only two or three immune tests are sufficient to predict known immunotoxic compounds in rodents with a >90% concordance (Luster et al., 1992a, b). Specifically, the use of either a humoral response assay for plaque-forming colonies (PFC response) or determination of surface marker expression in combination with almost any other parameter significantly increased the ability to predict immunotoxicity when compared to the predictivity of any assay alone.

The FDA guidelines for immunotoxicity testing of food additives start with a type 1 battery of tests. Type 1 tests can be derived from the routine measurements and examinations performed in short-term and subchronic rodent toxicity studies, since they do not require any perturbation of the test animals (immunization or challenge with infectious agents). These measurements include hematology and serum chemistry profiles, routine histopathologic examinations of immune-associated organs and tissues, and organ and body weight measurements, including thymus and spleen. If a compound produces any primary indicators of immunotoxicity from these measurements, more definitive immunotoxicity tests, such as those indicated in the preceding paragraph, may be recommended on a case-by-case basis.

The following is a brief explanation of some of the indicators that may be used to trigger additional definitive testing and a description of some of the most commonly used assays to assess humoral, cell-mediated, or nonspecific immune dysfunction, which are common to most immunotoxicology test strategies.

TABLE 8.9   Tier II Screen

Parameter	Procedures
Immunopathology	Enumeration of T and B cells and subsets; immunocytochemistry of lymphoid tissues; inumeration of cell types and numbers in the bone marrow.
Humoral-mediated immunity	Enumeration of secondary antibody (IgG) response to SRBCs.
Cell-mediated immunity	Cytotoxic T lymphocyte killing; delayed type hypersensitivity response; mouse ear swelling test (MEST; Gad et al., 1986a,b); guinea pig maximization test (Magnusson and Kligman, 1969).
Nonspecific immunity	Macrophage function—in vitro phagocytosis of fluorescent covaspheres, killing of *Listeria monocytogenes* or of tumor cells [basal and activated by macrophage activating factor (MAF)].
Host resistance	Bacterial models—*Listeria monocytogenes* (mortality or spleen clearance); *Streptococcus* species (mortality); viral models—influenza (mortality); parasitic models—*Plasmodium yoelii* (parasitemia) or *Trichinella spiralis* (muscle larvae counts and worm expulsion); syngeneic tumor models—PYB6 sarcoma (tumor incidence); B16F10 melanoma (lung burden).

Source: Adapted from Luster et al., 1988, and Vos et al., 1989, unless otherwise indicated.

B.   CDRH Testing Framework

The CDRH draft document (1997) actually sets forth a concise and step-wise approach to evaluating the potential immunotoxicity risks of devices (Figure 8.2; Table 8.10.) If the process in Figure 8.2 identifies a potential for hazard, then the tests specified in Table 8.10 are employed to evaluate those risks.

C.   Immunopathologic Assessments

Various general toxicological and histopathologic evaluations of the immune system can be made as part of routine preclinical safety testing to obtain a preliminary assessment of potential drug-related effects on the immune system. At necropsy, various immunological organs of the immune system such as thymus, spleen, and lymph nodes are typically observed for gross abnormalities and weighed in order to detect decreased or increased cellularity. Bone marrow and

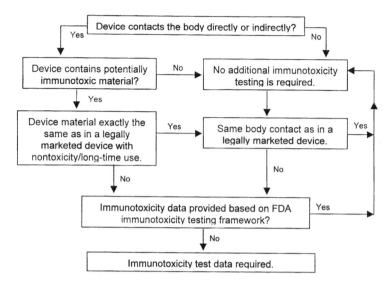

FIGURE 8.2   CDRH risk assessment immunotoxicity flow chart.

peripheral blood samples are also taken to evaluate abnormal types and/or frequencies of the various cellular components.

Organ and Body Weights.   Changes in absolute weight, organ-to-body weight ratios, and organ-to-brain weight ratios of tissues such as thymus and spleen are useful general indicators of potential immunotoxicity. These measures are nonspecific for immunotoxicity, however, since they may also reflect general toxicity and effects on endocrine function that can indirectly affect the immune system.

Hematology.   Hemacytometers or electronic cell counters can be used to assess the numbers of lymphocytes, neutrophils, monocytes, basophils, and eosinophils in the peripheral blood, while changes in relative ratios of the various cell types can be assessed by microscopic differential evaluation. Similar evaluations can be performed with bone marrow aspirates, where changes may reflect immunotoxicity to the pluripotent stem cells and newly developing lymphoid precursor cells. Potential hematological indicators of immunotoxicity include altered white blood cell counts or differential ratios, lymphocytosis, lymphopenia, or eosinophilia. Changes in any of these parameters can be followed up with more sophisticated flow cytometric analyses or immunostaining techniques that are useful for phenotyping the various types of lymphocytes (B cell, T cell) and the T-cell subsets (CD4+ and CD8+) on the basis of unique surface markers. Decreases or increases in the percentages of any of the cell populations relative to controls,

TABLE 8.10 CDRH Immunotoxicity Testing Matrix

Body contact	Contact duration	Immunological effects				
		1	2	3	4	5
Surface device skin	<24 hr (A)	pmb				
	24–30 days (B)	pmb				
	>30 days (C)	pmb				
Mucosal membrane	A	pmb	pmb			
	B	pmb	pmb	mb		
	C	pmb	pmb	mb	mb	mb
Breached/compromised surface	A	pmb	pmb			
	B	pmb	pmb	mb	mb	mb
	C	pmb	pmb	mb	mb	mb
External comm. device blood path, direct and indirect	A	pmb	pmb			
	B	pmb	pmb	mb	pmb	pmb
	C	pmb	pmb	mb	pmb	mb
Tissue/bone/dentin communicating	A	pmb	pmb			
	B	pmb	all	mb	pmb	mb
	C	pmb	all	mb	pmb	mb
Implant devices	A	pmb	pmb	mb		
	B	pmb	all	mb	pmb	mb
	C	pmb	all	mb	pmb	mb

Note: P: plastics/polymers; B: biological material; M: metals; 1: hypersensitivity; 2: inflammation; 3: immunosuppression; 4: immunostimulation; 5: autoimmunity.

or in the ratios of B cells/T cells or CD4+/CD8+ cells may be indicators of immunotoxicity.

Clinical Chemistry. Nonspecific clinical chemistry indicators of potential immune dysfunction include changes in serum protein levels in conjunction with changes in the albumin-to-globulin (A/G) ratio. Immunoelectrophoretic analysis of serum proteins can then be performed to quantify the relative percentages of albumin and the α-, β-, and γ-globulin fractions. To perform these assays, a drop of serum (antigen) is placed into a well cut in a gel, then the gel is subjected to electrophoresis so that each molecule in the serum moves in the electric field according to its charge. This separation is then exposed to specific antiserum, which is placed in a trough cut parallel to the direction in which the components have moved. By passive diffusion, the antibody reaches the electrophoretically separated antigen and reacts to form Ag-Ab complexes. The γ-globulin fractions can be separated and further quantified for the relative proportions of IgG, IgM, IgA, and IgE using similar techniques.

Serum concentrations of immunoglobulin classes and subclasses can also be measured using various techniques such as radioimmunoassays (RIAs) or enzyme-linked immunosorbent assays (ELISAs). In the ELISA, antigens specific for each class of immunoglobulin can be adsorbed onto the surfaces for microtiter plates. To determine the quantity of each antibody in a test sample, an aliquot of antiserum is allowed to react with the adsorbed antigens. Unreacted molecules are rinsed off and an enzyme-linked anti-Ig is then added to each well. Next, substrate is added and the amount of color that develops is quantified using a spectrophotometric device. The amount of antibody can then be extrapolated from standard curves since the amount of color is proportional to the amount of enzyme-linked antibody that reacts. Variations in levels of a given antibody may indicate the decreased ability of B cells or decreased numbers of B cells producing that antibody. In addition, serum autoantibodies to DNA, mitochondria, and parietal cells can be used to assess autoimmunity. Serum cytokines (IL-1, IL-2, and γ-interferon) can also be evaluated using immunochemical assays to evaluate macrophage, lymphocyte, and lymphokine activity; prostaglandin E_2 can also be measured to evaluate macrophage function.

CH50 determinations can be used to analyze the total serum complement and are useful for monitoring immune complex diseases (Sullivan, 1989). Activation of complement (Table 8.11) in the presence of autoantibodies is indicative of immune complex diseases and autoimmunity. The various components of the complement system (C3, C4) can also be measured to assess the integrity of the system. For instance, low serum concentrations of C3 and C4 with a concomitant decrease in CH50 may indicate activation of complement, while a low C4 alone is a sensitive indicator of reduced activation of the complement system. Since C3 is used as an alternate complement pathway, it usually measures high,

TABLE 8.11   The Complement System

Response factors	Origin	Characteristics/functions
Complement fixation	Serum	Critical component of humoral immune response leading to lysis of cell membranes, chemotaxis, and phagocytosis.
C1		Binds with IgG or IgM on membrane of the target cell to initiate activation of complement cascade
C4 and C2		Activated by C1; act together as a complex to activate C3; exposes a membrane site recognizable to granulocytes and macrophages, resulting in opsonization.
C3 and C5	Liver, macrophage	C3 binds to C42 complex to form C423; C5 binds to C423 to form C4235; provides sites for C6 and C7.
C6 and C7		C6 and C7 bind to C5 site to result in C567.
C8		One molecule of C567 binds with C8 to result in C5678.
C9		Up to six C9 molecules can bind with C5678 to trigger lysis by disrupting the lipid layer of the cell membrane.

therefore a low C3 with a normal C4 may indicate an alternate pathway of activation.

Histopathology.   Histopathologic abnormalities can be found in lymphoid tissues during gross and routine microscopic evaluations of the spleen, lymph nodes, thymus, bone marrow, and gut-associated lymphoid tissues such as Peyer's patches and mesenteric lymph nodes. Microscopic evaluations should include descriptive qualitative changes, such as types of cells, densities of cell populations, proliferation in known T and B cells areas (e.g., germinal centers), relative numbers of follicles and germinal centers (immune activation), and the appearance of atrophy or necrosis. In addition, unusual findings such as granulomas and scattered, focal mononuclear cell infiltrates in nonlymphoid tissues may be observed as indicators of chronic hypersensitivity or autoimmunity. A complete histopathologic evaluation should also include a quantitative assessment of cellularity through direct counts of each cell type in the various lymphoid tissues. In addition, changes in cellularity of the spleen can be more precisely quantitated from routine H & E (hematoxylin and eosin) sections using morphometric analysis of the germinal centers (B cells) and periarteriolar lymphocyte sheath (T cells).

Similar morphometric measurements can be made of the relative areas of the cortex and medulla of the thymus. If changes in cellularity are apparent from routinely stained histopathology sections, special immunostaining (immunoperoxidase or immunofluorescence) of B cells in the spleen and lymph nodes using polyclonal antibodies to IgG, or immunostaining of the T cells and their subsets in the spleen using mono-polyclonal antibodies to their specific surface markers, can be used to further characterize changes in cellularity.

Numerous physiological and environmental factors such as age, stress, nutritional deficiency, and infections may affect the immune system (Sullivan, 1989), thus adverse findings in animal studies may reflect these indirect immunotoxic effects rather than the direct immunotoxic potential of a chemical or drug. Indirect immunotoxic effects may be assessed through histopathologic evaluations of endocrine organs, such as the adrenals and pituitary.

It is also well known that the functional reserves of the immune system can allow biologically significant, immunotoxic insults to occur without the appearance of morphological changes. In addition, there is some built-in redundancy in the system in that several mechanisms may produce the same outcome. For instance, cytotoxic T cells may alone be sufficient to protect the organism against a bacterial infection; however, the body will also produce antibodies for future protection. If one mechanism is insufficient to fight off infection, the second mechanism can thus serve as a backup. Because of this functional reserve, adverse effects may remain subclinical until the organism is subjected to undue stress or subsequent challenge (Bloom et al., 1987), therefore routine immunopathologic assessments as part of standard preclinical toxicity tests may not be sufficient to detect all immunotoxins. Although changes detected in routine toxicological and pathological evaluations are nonspecific and of undetermined biological significance to the test animal, they can be invaluable as flags for triggering additional testing.

D. Humoral Immunity

As described previously, the humoral immune response results in the proliferation, activation, and subsequent production of antibodies by B cells following antigenic exposure and stimulation. The functionality and interplay between the three primary types of immune cells (macrophage, B cells, and T cells) required to elicit a humoral response can be assessed through various in vitro assays using cells from the peripheral blood or lymphoid tissues.

Antibody PFC Assay. The number of B cells producing antibody (PFC) to a T-dependent antigen such as sheep red blood cells (SRBCs) can be assessed in vitro following in vivo exposure to the test article and antigen (ex vivo tests). The PFC response to a T-dependent antigen is included as a tier I test by the NTP since it appears to be the most commonly affected functional parameter of exposure to immunosuppressants. This test is designated as a type 2 test in the FDA Redbook, however, since it requires an in vivo immunization of the animals with antigen and thus cannot be evaluated as part of an initial toxicity screen.

Although this assay requires that B cells be fully competent in secreting antibodies, T cells and macrophage cells are also essential for the proper functioning of humoral immunity. This assay is nonspecific, however, in that it cannot determine which cell type(s) is (are) responsible for dysfunction. Macrophage cells are needed to process antigen and produce IL-1. T cells are needed for several functions, including antigen recognition of surface membrane proteins and B-cell maturation through the production of various lymphokines that stimulate growth and differentiation. Sheep red blood cells (SRBCs) are most commonly used as the T-dependent antigen, although T cell independent antigens may also be useful to rule out T helper dysfunction as a cause of immunodysfunction.

The PFC assay has evolved from methodology originally developed as a hemolytic plaque assay (or Jerne plaque assay) by Nils Jerne to quantitate the number of antibody-forming cells in a cell suspension plated with red blood cells (RBCs) onto agar plates (Jerne and Nordin, 1963). In its present form, animals are treated in vivo with the test compound, immunized with approximately 5×10^8 SRBCs administered intravenously within 2 to 3 days posttreatment, and then sacrificed 4 days (IgM) or 6 days (IgG) later. Antibody-producing spleen cell suspensions are then mixed in vitro with SRBCs, placed onto covered slides, and incubated for a few hours in the presence of complement. During incubation, antibody diffuses from the anti-SRBC-producing cells and forms Ag-Ab complexes on the surfaces of nearby SRBCs, resulting in the formation of small clear plaques on the slide. Plaques are then counted and expressed as PFCs/10^6 spleen cells. A dose-related reduction in PFCs is indicative of immunosuppression.

B-Cell Lymphoproliferation Response. The NTP has classified this assay as a tier I test since mitogenesis can be performed easily in tandem with other tests to provide an assessment of the proliferative capacity of the cells (Luster et al., 1988). Since this assay is performed ex vivo with peripheral blood (or spleen) and is well characterized for use in various animal species, it has also been included as an expanded type 1 test in the revised Redbook.

The proliferation of peripheral blood or splenic B cells following stimulation with lipopolysaccharide (LPS) or other mitogens (pokeweed mitogen extract) is another measurement of humoral immunity. LPS (a bacterial lipopolysaccharide) is a B-cell-specific mitogen that stimulates polyclonal proliferation (mitosis) as part of the natural sequence of antigen recognition, activation, and clonal expansion. The mitogen does not interact with just one particular antigen-specific clone, but with all cells bearing the carbohydrate surface marker for which it is specific. Since mitogens are both polyclonal and polyfunctional, they can stimulate a wider spectrum of antigenic determinants than antigens, which can only stimulate a low number (10^{-6}) of specific cells.

In this assay, lymphocytes from animals treated in vivo are cultured in vitro in microtiter plates in the presence of tritiated [^{3}H]thymidine (or uridine) using a range of at least three concentrations of mitogen to optimize the response. Lymphocytes can be obtained aseptically from peripheral blood or from single cell suspensions of spleen cells that are prepared by pushing the tissue through sterile gauze or 60-mesh wire screens. A decrease in DNA synthesis (incorporation of ^{3}H) as compared to the unexposed cells of control animals may indicate that the B cells were unable to respond to antigenic stimulation. Alternative methodology employs an 18 to 20 hr incubation with ^{125}I-labeled iododeoxyuridine ([^{125}I]IUdR) and fluorodeoxyuridine (FudR) (White et al., 1985). After incubation, the cells are collected onto filter disks and then counted with a gamma counter.

Assays such as this that use polyclonal mitogens for activation may not be as sensitive as specific antigen-driven systems (Luster et al., 1988). In addition, suppression of the mitogen response does not always correlate with the PFC response. Since mitogenesis represents only a small aspect of B-cell function and maturation, this end point is not sensitive to early events that may affect activation, or later events that may affect differentiation of B cells into antibody-secreting cells (Klaus and Hawrylowicz, 1984).

E. Cell-Mediated Immunity

T Cell Lymphoproliferation Response. This assay is analogous to the B cell lymphoproliferative response assay described above, thus this assay is also classified as a tier I test by the NTP and as an expanded type 1 test in the revised draft of the Redbook.

T cells from the peripheral blood or spleen undergo blastogenesis and proliferation in response to specific antigens that evoke a cell-mediated immune response. T cell proliferation is assessed using T-cell-specific mitogens such as the plant lectins, concanavalin A (Con A), and phytohemagglutinin (PHA) or T-cell-specific antigens (e.g., tuberin, *Listeria*). Uptake of ^{3}H as an indicator of DNA synthesis is used as described above for evaluating B cell proliferation. T cell mitogens do not just stimulate synthesis of DNA, but in fact they also stimulate the expression of cell-specific function. For instance, Con A can trigger the expression of T helper, suppressor, and cytotoxic effector cells, and either mitogen may induce the expression (or re-expression of memory cells) of the differentiated function (Clark, 1983). Since cell populations responsive to Con A are thought to be relatively immature compared to those that are stimulated with PHA, the parallel usage of both mitogens may be useful for distinguishing the affected subset (Tabo and Paul, 1973). A secondary response to T cell antigens such as purified protein derivative of tuberculin (PPD) or tetanus toxoid can also be assessed.

Mixed Lymphocyte Response (MLR) Assay. This assay has been shown to be sensitive for the detection of chemical-induced immunosuppression and is a recommended tier I assay by the NTP (Luster et al., 1988). In addition, it has been shown to be predictive of host response to transplantation and of general immunocompetence (Harmon et al., 1982).

The mixed lymphocyte response assay assesses the ability of T cells to recognize foreign antigens on allogenic lymphocytes, and thus is an indirect measure of the cell-mediated ability to recognize graft or tumor cells as foreign. Responder lymphocytes from animals treated in vivo with the test compound are mixed with allogeneic stimulator lymphocytes that have been treated in vitro with mitomycin C or irradiated to render them unable to respond (Bach and Voynow, 1966). Both cell types are cultured in vitro for 3 to 5 days, then incubated with ^{3}H for an additional 6 hr. Once the radiolabel is incorporated into the DNA of the responding cells, the DNA is extracted and the amount of radioactive label is measured to quantitate proliferation of the responder cells of drug-treated animals compared to those of the controls.

Cytotoxic T Lymphoctye (CTL) Mediated Assay. This assay is similar to the MLR assay and can be performed in parallel or as a tier II follow-up to the MLR assay.

The CTL assay ascertains the ability of cytotoxic T cells to lyse an allogeneic target cell or the specific target cell type with which they were immunized. In general, the cytolytic response of activated effector cells is assessed by measuring the amount of radioactivity (^{51}Cr) that is released from the target cell. When performed in conjunction with the MLR assay, lymphoid cells of the two strains are cultured together in vitro as described above; however, ^{51}Cr is added to the culture after 4 to 5 days (instead of ^{3}H). Both responder and target cells are labeled with the ^{51}Cr, which is taken up rapidly by the cells through passive diffusion but is released slowly as long as the cell membrane is intact. Furthermore, since chromium is reduced from Cr^{6+} to Cr^{3+}, which enters the cells at a much slower rate than Cr^{6+}, the ^{51}Cr released from the damaged target cells is not significantly reincorporated into undamaged cells (Clark, 1983), which would reduce the sensitivity of the assay. The amount of chromium released into the medium and recovered in the supernatant of the mixture of the cells is thus directly proportionate to the extent of lysis of the target cells by the sensitized responder cells.

In a capillary tube assay developed in 1962 by George and Vaughan, the inhibition of migration of macrophage cells can be used to access normal T-cell function. (See Clark, 1983.) T cells are obtained from the peripheral blood of animals treated in vivo with a test article and injected with an antigen (e.g., tuberculin). If these T cells are functioning normally, they should release migration inhibition factor (MIF). As a consequence, the macrophages, which generally show a propensity for migration upon stimulation with the antigen, should show an MIF-induced reduction in migratory behavior.

Delayed-Type Hypersensitivity (DTH) Response. The DTH response assay is considered to be a comprehensive tier II assay for cell-mediated immunity by the NTP.

To express a DTH inflammatory response, the immune system must be capable of recognizing and processing antigen, blastogenesis and proliferation of T cells, migration of memory T cells to the challenge site of exposure to antigen, and subsequent production of inflammatory mediators and lymphokines that elicit the inflammatory response. By measuring a DTH response to an antigen, these assays thus assess the functional status of both the afferent (antigen recognition and processing) and efferent (lymphokine production) arms of cellular immunity. Various antigens have been used for assessing DTH, including keyhole limpet hemocyanin (KLH), oxazolone, dinitrochlorobenzene, and SRBCs (Vos, 1977; Godfrey and Gell, 1978; Luster et al., 1988).

In one such assay described by White et al. (1985), mice previously treated with the test article are sensitized to SRBCs by inoculation of SRBCs into the hind footpad and 4 days later challenged in the same footpad. Seventeen hr following the challenge, they are injected intravenously with ^{25}I-labeled human serum albumin (HSA), then sacrificed 2 hr later. Both hind feet are then radioassayed in a gamma counter (the second foot serves as a control for background infiltration of the label). With a normal functioning cell-mediated response, ^{125}I-labeled HSA will extravasate into the edematous area produced by the DTH response (Paranjpe and Boone, 1972). In general, a decrease in the extravasation of ^{125}I-labeled HSA is indicative of immunosuppression of the efferent arm of the cell-mediated immune system.

To assess specifically the afferent arm of the DTH response, the proliferation of the popliteal lymph node cells to SRBCs can also be measured (White et al., 1985). As described above, mice treated with the test article are sensitized to SRBCs by inoculation of SRBCs into the hind footpad. However, 1.5 hr later they are challenged intraperitoneally with FUdR, and 2 hr later they are administered [^{125}I]IUdR intravenously (instead of ^{125}I-labeled HSA). Mice are sacrificed 24 hr after challenge and both popliteal lymph nodes are removed and counted in a gamma counter.

Similar assays for DTH have been traditionally performed with the antigen *Mycobacterium tuberculosis*, which preferentially elicits a cell-mediated response. In this assay a small amount of antigen contained in the supernatant fluid from the medium in which the pathogen was grown is injected into the footpad.

Upon challenge, a visible and palpable lump should appear by 48 hr. The amount of swelling is then measured and compared with the footpad that did not receive the challenge. Alternatively, methods used by NTP employ a modified ^{125}I-labeled uridine (UdR) technique to measure the monocyte influx at the challenge site (ear) injected with KLH antigen. This assay has been shown to correlate well with decreased resistance to infectious disease (Luster et al., 1988). One should note, however, that regardless of which technique is used, anti-inflammatory drugs may produce false-positive results in this type of assay.

F. Nonspecific Immunity

Natural Killer Cell Assays. This assay is a tier I test for nonspecific immunity in the NTP testing scheme (Luster et al., 1988) and is proposed as an additional type 1 test in the draft Redbook.

Like cytotoxic T cells, NK cells have the ability to attack and destroy tumor cells or virus-infected cells. Unlike T cells, however, they are not antigen-specific, do not have unique, clonally distributed receptors, and do not undergo clonal selection. In in vitro or ex vivo tests, target cells (e.g., YAC-1 tumor cells) are radiolabeled in vitro or in vivo with ^{51}Cr and incubated in vitro with effector NK cells from the spleens of animals that had been treated with a xenobiotic. This assay can be run in microtiter plates over the range of various ratios of effector/target cells. Cytotoxic activity is then measured by the amount of radioactivity released from the damaged tumor cells, as was previously described for cytotoxic T cells. This assay can also be performed in vivo, where YAC-1 cells labeled with [^{125}I]IUdR are injected directly into mice and NK cell activity is correlated with its level of radioactivity (Riccardi et al., 1979). Immunotoxicity observed as reduced NK cell activity is correlated with increased tumorigenesis and infectivity.

Macrophage Function. Several assays are available to measure various aspects of macrophage function, including quantitation of resident peritoneal cells, antigen presentation, cytokine production, phagocytosis, intracellular production of oxygen-free radicals (used to kill foreign bodies), and direct tumor-killing potential. Techniques for quantitation of peritoneal cells and functional assays for phagocytic ability are classified as comprehensive tier II test by the NTP and as additional type 1 tests in the draft Redbook.

Macrophage cells and other PMNs contribute to the first-line defense of nonspecific immunity through their ability to phagocytize foreign materials, including pathogens, tumor cells, and fibers (e.g., silica, asbestos). Xenobiotics can affect macrophage function by direct toxicity to macrophages or by modulating their ability to become activated. Differential counts of resident peritoneal cells can be made as rapid, preliminary assessment of macrophage function for xenobiotics that are not administered parenterally.

Numerous in vitro assays can be employed to assess common function of macrophages and PMNs, including adherence to glass, migration inhibition, phagocytosis, respiratory activity (chemiluminescent assays or nitroblue tetrazolium), and target cell killing. In one such assay, the chemotactic response to soluble attractants is evaluated using a Boyden chamber with two compartments that are separated by a filter. Macrophage cells or PMNs from treated animals are placed in one side and a chemotactic agent in the other. Chemotaxis is then quantified by counting the number of cells that pass through the filter. In another assay, the ability of the macrophages to phagocytize foreign materials can be evaluated by adding fluorescent latex beads to cultures containing macrophage cells, then determining the proportion of cells that have phagocytized the beads using either a fluorescent microscope or flow cytometry (Duke et al., 1985). Similar functions can be evaluated by incubating the cells with known amounts of bacteria. The cells are then removed by filtration or centrifugation, the remaining fluid is plated onto bacterial nutrient agar, and after a few days of incubation, the bacterial colonies are counted. Furthermore, the efficiency of the cells to kill the bacteria once phagocytized can be assayed by lysing the cells and plating the lysate onto bacterial agar.

Various in vivo assessments of macrophage function have also been used. For example, peritoneal exudate cell (PEC) recruitment can be assessed using eliciting agents such as *Corynebacterium parvum*, MVE-2, or thioglycolate (Dean et al., 1984). In one such assay (White et al., 1985), mice are injected intraperitoneally with thioglycolate and sacrificed 5 days later. The peritoneal cavity is then flushed with culture medium. The cell suspension is then counted, the cell concentration is adjusted to a known density (2×10^5 ml^{-1}), and the cells are cultured for 1 hr in 24-well culture dishes. Adherent cells are then washed with medium, and aliquots of ^{51}Cr-labeled SRBCs that were opsonized with mouse IgG are added to each well and incubated for various times. This same system can be used to assess adherence to and chemotaxis of the PECs (Laskin et al., 1981). Phagocytosis can also be evaluated in vivo by measuring the clearance of injected particles from the circulation and the accumulation of the particles in lymphatic tissues such as the spleen.

Mast Cell/Basophil Function. The function of mast cells and basophils to degranulate can be evaluated using a passive cutaneous anaphylaxis test (Cromwell et al., 1986). Serum containing specific anaphylactic (IgE) antibodies from donor animals previously exposed to a known antigen is first administered by intradermal (or subcutaneous) injection into unexposed host animals. After a sufficient latency period to allow binding of the donor IgE to the host tissue mast cells, the animals are administered a second intravenous injection of the antigen. The anaphylactic antibodies present in the serum will stimulate normally functioning mast cells to degranulate (release histamines) and produce a marked inflammatory response. Using similar in vitro assays with mast cells and basophils, the quantities of histamines that are released from the cells can be measured directly in the culture medium.

G. Host-Resistance Assays

Host-resistance assays can be used to assess the overall immunocompetence of the humoral or cell-mediated immune systems of the test animals (host) to fend off infection with pathogenic microbes or to resist tumorigenesis and metastasis. These assays are performed entirely in vivo and are dependent on all of the various components of the immune system to be functioning properly. These assays thus may be considered to be more biologically relevant than in vitro tests that only assess the function of cells from one source and of one type. Since these assays require that the animal be inoculated with a pathogen or exogenous tumor cell, they cannot be performed as part of a general preclinical toxicity assessment, and are thus classified as type 2 tests in the revised Redbook. These assays are also included a tier II tests by the NTP.

Similar host-resistance assays are used to evaluate the immunosurveillance of spontaneous tumors, which is assessed as the capacity of the organism to reject grafted syngeneic tumors. Various animal-bearing tumor models (Pastan et al., 1986) and host-resistance models have been used to assess immunotoxicity. Several of the host-resistance assays utilize cultured tumor cell lines such as PYB6 sarcoma and B16F10 melanoma cells that are used with Fischer 344 rats. For example, the PYB6 sarcoma model uses death as an end point. In this assay, syngeneic mice are injected with the PYB6 sarcoma cells and death due to tumor is recorded daily. In another routinely used assay, animals that have been treated with a xenobiotic are injected with either B16F10 melanoma cells or Lewis lung carcinoma cells, then approximately 20 days later they are sacrificed and pulmonary tumors are measured and counted.

H. Hypersensitivity

Type I Hypersensitivity.   Although there are acceptable systems for evaluating type I (immediate) reactions following systemic exposure, there are no reliable animal models for predicting type I reactions following dermal applications or oral administration of drug. Repeated exposure of a xenobiotic is required to produce a type I response. A drug in the form of a hapten must covalently bind to macromolecules (proteins, nucleic acids) before it can initiate a primary antibody response. Once sensitized, even the smallest exposure to the xenobiotic can elicit a rapid, intensive IgE antibody-mediated inflammatory response. With the exception of antivirals and chemotherapeutic drugs, most drugs should not be reactive with biological nucleophiles since these drugs are usually screened out as mutagens or carcinogens in preclinical safety studies. Type I hypersensitivity, however, is a particular problem with biotechnology products themselves (e.g., insulin, growth hormones, interleukins), trace impurities from the producing organisms (e.g., *E. coli* proteins, mycelium), or the vehicles used to form emulsions (Matory et al., 1985).

The production of neutralizing antibodies to recombinant DNA protein products or their contaminants may be assayed using ELISAs or IRAs. A suitable animal model used to evaluate the potential for a type I response to protein hydrolysates is detailed in the U.S. *Pharmacopoeia*. This test is very sensitive for testing proteins administered by the parenteral route, but is of little value for low-molecular-weight drugs and those that are administered orally (Descotes and Mazue, 1987). Active systemic anaphylaxis can be assessed in guinea pigs following systemic exposure to the test compound. For dermal exposures, however, rabbits or guinea pigs must be exposed to the test article by intradermal injections and then evaluated for their ability to mount a systemic anaphylactic response. The passive cutaneous anaphylaxis test (as described above for mast cells) can also be used to assess a potential anaphylactic response to a test compound. The serum containing potential anaphylactic (IgE) antibodies from donor animals previously exposed to the test compound is first administered by intradermal (or subcutaneous) injection into unexposed host animals. After a latency period, the animals are administered an intravenous injection of the test compound together with a dye. If anaphylactic antibodies are present in the serum, the subsequent exposure to the test compound will cause a release of vasoactive amines (degranulation of mast cells), ultimately resulting in the migration of the dye to the sites of the intradermal serum injection.

Types II and III Hypersensitivity. No simple animal modes are currently available to assess type II (antibody-mediated cytotoxicity) hypersensitivity reactions. IgE antibodies and immune complexes in the sera of exposed animals can be assayed using ELISA or RIA techniques that require the use of specific antibodies to the drug.

Type III (immune complex-related disease) reactions have been demonstrated by the presence of proteinuria and immune complex deposits in the kidneys of the Brown–Norway, Lewis, and PVG/C rat strains. Susceptibility to the deposition and the subsequent lesions (glomerulonephritis), however, are often variable and dependent on the strain (Bigazzi, 1985). For example, despite the appearance of clinical signs and proteinuria, after 2 months administration of mercuric chloride, detectable levels of circulating antinuclear autoantibodies can no longer be observed in the Brown–Norway strain (Bellon et al., 1982). By contrast, in PVG/C rats administered mercuric chloride, immune complex deposition and antinuclear autoantibodies are present for longer periods of time. Proteinurea is not observed, however (Weening et al., 1978).

Type IV Hypersensitivity. There are several well-established preclinical models for assessing type IV (delayed-type) hypersensitivity reactions following dermal exposure, but not for predicting this response after systemic exposure.

The dermal exposure mode is the only currently required and widely performed immunotoxicity assay on devices.

Type IV hypersensitivity responses are elicited by T lymphocytes and are controlled by accessory cells and suppressor T cells. Macrophages are also involved in that they secrete several monokines, which results in proliferation and differentiation of T cells. There are thus numerous points along this intricate pathway in which drugs may modulate the final response. To achieve a type IV response, an initial high-dose exposure to repeated lower-dose exposures are applied to the skin. The antigen is carried from the skin by Langerhans cells and presented to cells in the thymus to initiate T cell proliferation and sensitization. Once sensitized, a second "challenge" dose will elicit an inflammatory response. Before sensitivity can be assessed, each of the models used to evaluate dermal hypersensitivity thus requires as a minimum

An initial induction exposure
A latency period for expression
A challenge exposure

A preliminary test for acute irritancy is also required to ensure that the initial dose is sufficient to stimulate sensitization and that the challenge dose is sufficient to ensure expression of the response without producing irritation, which would confound the response. To confirm suspected sensitization or to determine a threshold dose, each assay may also include a second challenge dose one to two weeks after the first challenge, at the same or lower concentrations. To increase penetration of the test article, various methods of abrasion (e.g., tape stripping) and occlusive coverings may also be used. Assessing materials to determine if they can act as delayed contact dermal sensitizers in humans is different on a number of grounds from the other tests we have looked at so far, and indeed from most of the other test systems presented later in this book. These differences all stem from how the immune system, which is the mechanistic basis for this set of adverse responses, functions.

Bringing about this Coombs type IV hypersensitivity response (which we will call sensitization) requires more than a single exposure to the causative material, both in humans and in test animals. Unlike irritation responses, sensitization occurs in individuals in an extremely variable manner. A portion of the human population is considerably more liable to be sensitized, while others are infrequently affected, and the response, once sensitization is achieved, becomes progressively more severe with each additional exposure. All three of these characteristics are due to the underlying mechanism for the response, and influence the manner in which we conduct tests. These factors mean that in vivo test systems require multiple exposures of animals and tend to underpredict the potential for an adverse response in those individuals who are most susceptible to sensitization, but because the response to repeated exposures of even minimal amounts of material in these susceptible individuals can lead to such striking adverse responses, we must be concerned about them.

A number of factors influence the potential for a chemical to be a sensitizer in humans, and in turn also influence the performance of test systems. These are summarized in Table 8.12. Various test systems manipulate these in different ways.

There are a number of references that explore and discuss the underlying immune system mechanisms and operation in greater detail. Particularly recommended is Gibson et al., (1983).

1. Objectives and General Features

Given the considerations of mechanism, degree of concern about protecting people, and practicality, the desired characteristics of a sensitization test include the following:

1. Be reproducible
2. Involve fairly low technical skill so that it may be performed as a general laboratory test
3. Not involve the use of exotic animals or equipment
4. Use relatively small amounts of test material
5. Be capable of evaluating almost any material of interest
6. Be sensitive enough to detect weak sensitizers (i.e., those that would require extensive exposure to sensitize other than the most sensitive individuals)
7. Predict the relative potency of sensitizing agents accurately

Several of these desired characteristics are mutually contradictory; as with most other test systems, each method for detecting dermal sensitization incorporates a set of compromises.

TABLE 8.12 Factors Influencing Delayed-Type Sensitization Responses

1. Percutaneous absorption of agent.
2. Genetic status of host.
3. Immunological status of host.
4. Host nutrition.
5. Chemical and physical nature of potential sensitizing agent.
6. Number, frequency, and degree of exposures of immune system to potential antigen.
7. Concurrent immunological stimuli (e.g., adjuvants, inoculations, and infections). System can be "up-modulated" by mild stimuli or overburdened by excessive stimulation.
8. Age, sex, and pregnancy (by influencing factors 1, 3, and 4 above).

All the in vivo tests have some common features, however. The most striking is that they involve at least three (and frequently four) different phases—they are multiphasic. These phases are, in order, the irritation/toxicity screen, the induction phase, the challenge phase, and (often) the rechallenge phase.

Irritation/Toxicity Screen. All assays require knowledge of the dermal irritancy and systemic toxicity of the test material(s) to be used in the induction, challenge, and rechallenge. These properties are defined in this pretest phase. Most tests desire (or will allow) mild irritation in the induction phase. Most tests desire (or will allow) mild irritation in the induction phase, but no systemic toxicity. Generally, a nonirritating concentration is required for the challenge and for any rechallenge, as having irritation present either confounds the results or precludes having a valid test. As will be discussed in the sections on the individual tests, even a carefully designed screen does not necessarily provide the desired guidance in selecting usable concentrations. During this phase, solvent systems are also selected.

Induction Phase. This requires exposing the test animals to the test material several times over a period of days or weeks. A number of events must be accomplished during this phase if a sensitization response is to be elicited. The test material must penetrate through the epidermis and into the dermis, where it must interact with dermis protein. The protein-test material complex must be perceived by the immune system as an allergen. Finally, the production of sensitized T cells must be accomplished. Some assays enhance the sensitivity of the induction phase by compromising the natural ability of the epidermis to act as a barrier. These enhancement techniques include irritation of the induction site, intradermal injection, tape stripping, and occlusive dressings. In contrast, events such as the development of a scab over the induction site may reduce percutaneous absorption. The attention of the immune system can be drawn to the induction site by the intradermal injection of oil-coated bacteria (Freund's complete adjuvant, which serves as a mild immunological stimulant).

Challenge Phase. This consists of exposing the animals to a concentration of the test material, which would normally not be expected to cause a response (usually an erythema-type response). The responses in the test animals and the control animals are then scored or measured.

Rechallenge Phase. This is a repeat of the challenge phase and can be a very valuable tool if used properly. Sensitized animals can be rechallenged with the same test material at the same concentration used in the challenge in order to assist in confirming sensitization. Sensitized animals can be rechallenged with different concentrations of the allergen to evaluate dose response relationships. Animals sensitized to an ingredient to evaluate can be challenged to a formulation containing the ingredient to evaluate the potential of the formulated product to elicit a sensitization under adverse conditions. Conversely, animals that responded (sometimes unexpectedly) to a final formulation can be challenged with the formulation without the suspected sensitizer or to the ingredient that is suspected to be the allergen. Cross-reactivity can be evaluated; that is, the ability of one test material to elicit a sensitization response following exposure in the induction phase to a different test material. A well-designed rechallenge is important and should be considered at the same time that the sensitization evaluation is being designed since the rechallenge must be run within 1 to 2 weeks after the primary challenge. Unless plans have been made for a possible rechallenge, one may have to reformulate a test material or obtain additional pure ingredient and perhaps run additional irritation/toxicity screens before the rechallenge can be run. The ability of the sensitized animals to respond at a rechallenge being run shortly after the challenge is limited. In addition, some assays use sham-treated controls, and these must be procured while the induction phase is in progress. One additional piece of information must be kept in mind when evaluating a rechallenge. The animal does not differentiate between an induction exposure and a challenge exposure. If one is using an assay that involves three induction exposure and a challenge exposure, then at the rechallenge, the animal has received four induction exposures. This "extra" induction may serve to strengthen a sensitization response.

After the study is done, one must evaluate the data and decide how to translate then to the human condition. We will look at this problem toward the end of this chapter.

2. History

Koch's initial observation of tuberculin reactivity was made in humans and guinea pigs. Although the rabbit and guinea pig have both been considered the animals of choice for evaluating adverse skin reactions of chemicals, from the beginning guinea pigs have been the animals of choice for predictive tests. Though it is widely believed that this is due to a relatively higher degree of susceptibility to dermal sensitization, the preference was actually based on availability, ease of handling, and the fact that the albino animal has a clear, pale skin that is easily denuded of hair and on which an erythema response is easy to distinguish.

Landsteiner and Jacobs (1935) first proposed a formalized predictive test in guinea pigs. Later, Landsteiner and Chase (1942) used low-molecular-weight chemicals to sensitize guinea pigs and developed the theory of complete antigen formations being due to hapten–protein interactions.

The basis of modern predictive tests is the Draize test, as established by Landsteiner and Draize et al. (1944). It consists of 10 intradermal injections of the test compound into the skin of albino guinea pigs during the 3-week induction period and a single intracutaneous challenge application 14 days after the last induction injection. A standardized 0.1% test concentration is used for induction and challenge. This method was widely used and recommended until the end of the 1960s. Its disadvantage is that only strong allergens are detected, while well-known moderate allergens fail to sensitize the animals at all.

Starting in 1964, however, a wide variety of new test designs started to be proposed. Buehler (1964; 1965) proposed what is now considered the first modern test (described in detail in this chapter), which used an occlusive patch to increase test sensitivity. The Buehler test is the primary example of the so-called epidermal methods, which have been criticized for giving false-negative results for moderate to weak sensitizers such as nickel.

A new generation of tests was established by using Freund complete adjuvant (FCA) during the induction process to stimulate the immune system, independent of both the type of hapten and the method of application; that is, whether or not the substance is incorporated in the adjuvant mixture. It is claimed that this family of tests displays the same level of susceptibility to sensitization in guinea pigs as is normally observed in humans (Cronin and Agrup, 1970). The adjuvant tests include the guinea pig maximization test (Maurer et al., 1975; 1980), split adjuvant test (Maguire and Chase, 1967), and the epicutaneous maximization test (EMP) (Guillot and Gonnet, 1985).

Finally, during the last few years, a test system that uses albino mice instead of guinea pigs—the mouse ear swelling test (MEST) (Gad et al., 1985a, b) and local lymph node assay (LLNA) (Kimber et al., 1986)—have been proposed as alternatives.

This chain of development should be expected to continue, and the overall quality and utility of tests should improve. Four tests will be presented and compared in this volume, as each has features and operating characteristics that make it alliterative in particular circumstances and cause it to be representative of other available tests. These are the Buehler, guinea pig maximization, split adjuvant, and MEST.

Modified Buehler Procedure.   This is a closed patch procedure for evaluating test substances for potential delayed contact dermal sensitization in guinea pigs. The procedure, based on that described by Buehler (1965), is practical for test substances that cannot be evaluated by the traditional intradermal injection procedure of Landsteiner and Jacobs or by the guinea pig maximization test (GPMT) for skin sensitization testing. The closed patch procedure is performed when a test substance either is highly irritating to the skin by the intradermal injection route of exposure or cannot be dissolved or suspended in a form allowing injection. It is also the method of choice for some companies. This procedure, which is one version of the Buehler test, complies with the test standards set forth in the Toxic Substances Control Act (TSCA, 1979) and other regulatory test rules, and is presented diagramatically in Figure 8.3. There are other versions that also comply.

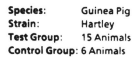

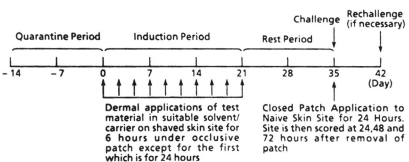

FIGURE 8.3 Study design for modified Buehler test for delayed contact dermal sensitization in the guinea pig.

Animals

1. Young albino female guinea pigs, weighing between 300 and 400 grams are used.

2. Although several proposed test rules suggest the use of male guinea pigs, the female sex is preferred because the aggressive social behavior of males may result in considerable skin damage that might interfere with the interpretation of challenge reactions. This concern occurs because animals are group housed (Marzulli and Maibach, 1996).

3. Animals that show poor growth or are ill in any way are not used, since illness markedly decreases the response. Animals with skin marked or scarred from fighting are avoided. The guinea pigs are observed for at least 2 weeks to detect any illness before starting a study.

4. The guinea pigs are identified by a cage card and marking pen or any other suitable method. There are no regulatory requirements, however, for the identification of individual animals.

5. The guinea pigs are randomly assigned to the test and negative control groups, consisting of at least 15 and at least six animals each, respectively. If a pretest group is necessary, as many animals as are needed for that group are also randomized.

Pretest Screen

1. If practical, the dermal irritation threshold concentration should be established for the test substance prior to the first induction applica-

tion. A concentration of the test substance that produces minimal or no irritation (erythema and/or edema formation) is determined. The highest concentration that produces no irritation is preferred for the dermal sensitization study challenge dose.

2. Those animals randomly assigned to the pretest group are used.
3. Each animal is prepared by clipping a 1-in.-square area of hair from the left upper flank using a small animal clipper with a no. 40 blade.
4. The test substance is diluted, emulsified, or suspended in a suitable vehicle. Vehicles are selected on the basis of their solubilizing capacity for the test substance and on their ability to penetrate the skin.
5. Different concentrations of the test substance are tested on the pretest group of guinea pigs; a few animals are used for each concentration tested.
6. A volume of 0.15 ml is applied to a patch consisting of a cotton pad (2.5 × 2.5 cm) occluded with impermeable surgical tape, or placed in a Hilltop-style occlusive ''chamber.''
7. The patch is applied to the shaved left flank of a guinea pig. The patch is held firmly in place for 24 hr by wrapping the trunk of the animal with a 3-in.-wide elastic bandage. A 2-in.-wide strip of tape is used to line the center adhesive side of the bandage in order to prevent skin damage from the adhesive.
8. After 24 hr of exposure, the wrappings and patches are removed.
9. Observations of skin reactions (erythema and/or edema formation) are recorded 48 hr after application.
10. A judgment is made as to which concentration will be used for the dermal sensitization study based on the dermal irritation data that have been collected. The highest concentration that produces minimal or no dermal irritation is selected.

Induction Phase

1. Test group and control group guinea pigs are weighed at the beginning of the study and weekly thereafter.
2. Test control group guinea pigs are clipped as described earlier in this procedure.
3. If the test substance is a liquid (solution, suspension, or emulsion), a volume of 0.15 ml of the highest concentration found to be nonirritating in a suitable vehicle (as determined in the pretest portion of this procedure) is applied to a patch consisting of a cotton pad (1 in. × 1 in.) occluded with impermeable surgical tape. If the test substance is

TABLE 8.13 Evaluation of Skin Reactions

Skin reaction	Value
Erythema and eschar formation	
No erythema	0
Very slight erythema (barely perceptible)	1
Well-defined erythema	2
Moderate to severe erythema	3
Severe erythema (beef redness) to slight eschar formation (injuries in-depth)	4
Necrosis (death of tissue)	+N
Eschar (sloughing)	+E
Edema formation	
No edema	0
Very slight edema (barely perceptible)	1
Slight edema (edges of area well-defined by definite raising)	2
Moderate edema (raised approximately 1 mm)	3
Severe edema (raised more than 1 mm and extending beyond the area of exposure)	4

Source: Draize, 1959.

a solid or semisolid 0.5 g* is applied. If the test substance is a fabric, a 1-in. square is moistened with 0.5 ml of physiological saline before application.

4. The first induction patch is applied to the clipped left flank of each test group guinea pig. The patch is held firmly in place for 24 hr by wrapping the trunk of each animal with a 3-in.-wide elastic bandage. A 2-in.-wide strip of tape is used to line the center adhesive side of the bandage in order to prevent skin damage from the adhesive. A 2-in. length of athletic adhesive tape is placed over the bandage wrap as a precautionary measure to prevent unraveling.
5. After 24 hr of exposure, the wrappings and patches are removed and disposed of in a plastic bag.
6. Each dermal reaction, if any, is scored on the basis of the designated values for erythema and edema formation presented in Table 8.13. Ob-

* When the test substance is in flake, granule, powder, or other particulate form, the weight of the test substance that has a volume of 0.5 ml (after compacting as much as possible without crushing or altering the individual particles, such as by tapping the measuring container) is used whenever this volume weighs less than 0.5 grams.

servations are made 48 hr after initiation of the first induction application. Resulting dermal irritation scores are recorded.

7. After the initial induction application, subsequent induction applications (2–10) are made on alternate days (three times weekly) until a total of 10 treatments is administered. Each of these patches is removed after 6 hr of exposure. It should be noted that some use a modification that calls for one application per week for 3 weeks.

8. Observations are made 24 and 48 hr after initiation of each subsequent induction application. Dermal scores of the remaining nine induction applications are recorded.

9. Clipping the hair from the left flank induction sites of test group animals and corresponding sites on negative control group animals is performed just prior to each subsequent induction application. Only the test group guinea pigs receive the induction applications.

Challenge Phase

1. Fourteen days after the tenth induction application, all 10 test group (and three of five control group) guinea pigs are prepared for challenge application by clipping a 1-in. square of hair from the right side, the side opposite that which was clipped during the induction phase.

2. A challenge dose, using freshly prepared test substance (solution, suspension, emulsion, semisolid, solid, or fabric), is applied topically to the right side (which has remained untreated during the induction application) of test group animals. The left side, which has previously received induction applications, is not challenge-dosed.

3. The concentration of the challenge dose is the same as that used for the first induction application. (It must be a concentration that does not produce dermal irritation after one 24-hr application.)

4. Each of three negative control group guinea pigs is challenge-dosed on the right flank at approximately the same time that the test group guinea pigs are challenge-dosed.

5. All patches are held in contact with the skin for 24 hr before removal.

6. The skin sites are evaluated using the scoring system for erythema and edema formation presented in Table 8.13. Observations are made 48, 72, and 96 hr after initiation of the challenge application. Skin reactions are recorded.

Rechallenge Phase

1. If the test substance is judged a nonsensitizing agent after the first challenge application, causes dermal sensitization in only a few ani-

mals, or causes dermal reactions that are weak or questionable, then a second and final challenge application will be performed on each test animal 7 days after the initiation of the first challenge dose.

2. Controls from the first challenge application are not rechallenged because they have been exposed to the test substances and are no longer true negative controls. The three remaining naive control group animals (not used for the first challenge) are challenged for comparison to the test group animals.

3. The procedure used for the first challenge application will be used for the second challenge application (including reclipping, patching method, and duration of exposure). Either the same concentration or a new concentration (higher or lower) of test substances may be used, depending on the results of the first challenge. Observations are made 48, 72, and 96 hr after initiation of the rechallenge application and the skin reactions are recorded.

4. When a rechallenge application is performed, the data from both challenges are compared. If neither challenge produces a positive dermal reaction, the classification of the test substance is based on both challenge applications. If one challenge application (whether it is the first or second) produces a greater number of positive dermal reactions than the other, the classification of the test substance is based on the challenge with the most positive responses.

5. Two or more unequivocally positive responses in a group of 15 animals should be considered significant. A negative, equivocal, or single response probably assures that a substance is not a strong sensitizer, although this is best confirmed by further testing with human subjects (NAS, 1977).

Interpretation of Results

1. Judgment concerning the presence or absence of sensitization is made for each animal. The judgment is made by comparing the test animal's challenge responses to its first induction treatment response, as well as to those challenge responses of negative control animals.

2. Challenge reactions to the test substance that are stronger than challenge reactions to negative controls or to those seen after the initial induction application should be suspected as results of sensitization (NAS, 1977). A reaction that occurs at 48 hr but resolves by 72 hr or 96 hr, should be considered a positive response as long as it is stronger than that displayed by controls at the same time interval.

Strengths and Weaknesses   There are a number of both advantages and disadvantages to the Buehler methodology, which has been in use for 20 years.

The relative importance and merits of each depend on the intended use of the material. The three advantages are as follows:

1. Virtually no false positives (in fact, in the experience of the author when the pretest is properly conducted, there are no false positives), compared to human experience, are generated by this test.
2. The techniques involved are easy to learn and very reproducible.
3. The Buehler-style test does not overpredict the potency of sensitizers; that is, materials that are identified as sensitizers are truly classified as very strong, weak, or in between—not all (or nearly all) as very strong.
4. There is a large database in existence for the Buehler-style test. Unfortunately, the vast majority is not in the published literature.

Likewise, there are three disadvantages associated with the Buehler-style test.

1. The test gives a high rate of false negatives for weak sensitizers and a detectable rate of false negatives for moderate sensitizers; that is, the method is somewhat insensitive, particularly if techniques for occlusive wrapping are inadequate.
2. The test takes a long time to complete. If animals are on hand when started, the test is 5 to 6 weeks long. As few laboratories keep a pool of guinea pigs on hand (especially as they are the most expensive of the common lab species), the usual case is that 8 to 10 weeks is the minimum time required to get an answer from this test.
3. The test uses a relatively large amount of test material. In the normal acute ''battery,'' the guinea pig test systems use more material than any other test systems, unless an acute inhalation study is included. With 10 induction applications, this is particularly true for the Buehler-style test.

Guinea Pig Maximization Test. The GPMT was developed by Magnusson and Kligman (1969; 1970; Magnusson, 1975) and is considered a highly sensitive procedure for evaluating test substances for potential dermal sensitization. The procedure presented here is illustrated in Figures 8.4 and 8.5, and is one common version of the test.

Animals

1. Young adult female guinea pigs, weighing between 250 and 350 grams at the initiation of the study, are used.
2. Although several proposed test rules suggest the use of male guinea pigs, the female sex is preferred because the aggressive social behavior of males may result in considerable skin damage that might interfere with the interpretation of challenge reactions.

Stage	INDUCTION		CHALLENGE	RECHALLENGE
Day	0	7	21	28
TEST GROUP (15)	A. 0.1 ml Substance ID B. 0.1 ml FCA ID C. 0.1 ml Substance + FCA ID	Closed Patch-48 H Application of Substance	Closed Patch-24 H Substance Vehicle	Closed Patch-24 H Vehicle
TEST GROUP (15)	A. 0.1 ml Vehicle ID B. 0.1 ml FCA ID C. 0.1 ml Vehicle + FCA ID	Closed Patch-48 H Application of Vehicle	Closed Patch-24 H Substance Vehicle	Closed Patch-24 H Substance

FIGURE 8.4   Study design for guinea pig maximization test for predicting delayed dermal sensitization.

3. Animals that show poor growth or are ill in any way are not used, since illness markedly decreases the response. Animals with skin marked or scarred from fighting are avoided. The guinea pigs are observed for at least 2 weeks to detect any illness before starting the study.
4. The guinea pigs are randomly assigned to two groups: (1) a test group

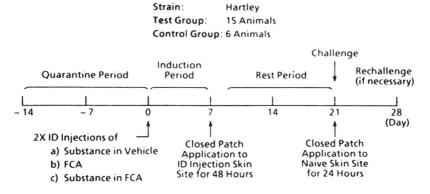

Species: Guinea Pig
Strain: Hartley
Test Group: 15 Animals
Control Group: 6 Animals

FIGURE 8.5   Injection and patching of animals in GPMT.

consisting of 15 animals; and (2) a control group consisting of six animals. If a pretest group is necessary, as many animals as are needed for that group are also randomized.

5. Test and control group guinea pigs are weighed one week prior to dosing (day 7), on the day of dosing (day 0), and weekly thereafter.

Pretest

1. Several animals are used to pretest the test substance and vehicles to determine the topical dermal irritation threshold concentration.
2. These animals are shaved on the left flank, to which is applied a 2 × 2 cm filter paper patch that contains 0.1 ml of test concentration.
3. The trunks of the animals are wrapped for 24 hr with a 3-in.-wide elastic bandage to hold the patch in contact with the skin.
4. Wrappings are removed after the 24-hr exposure, and based on skin reactions at 48 hr, a concentration of the test substance to be used is determined. Dermal irritation values are recorded for future reference.
5. In addition, several guinea pigs are utilized to determine a concentration (generally between 1–5%) of test substance in vehicle and in Freund's complete adjuvant (FCA) emulsion that can be injected id without eliciting a strong local or systemic toxic reaction.
6. The hair is clipped in an area of approximately 4 × 6 cm from the upper shoulder region of these animals.
7. Several concentrations of test substances (1–5%) can be injected in the same animal to compare local dermal reactions produced by the different concentrations.
8. If systemic toxicity is suspected, however, each concentration should be tested in separate animals to determine local and systemic effects.
9. The dermal reactions (erythema, edema, and diameter) are recorded 24 hr after the id injections.

Induction Stage 1 (Day 0)

1. The hair in an area of 4 × 6 cm is clipped from the shoulder region of each test and control group guinea pig on day 0.
2. Three pairs of id injections are made with a glass 1-ml tuberculin syringe with a 26-gauge needle, each pair flanking the dorsal midline.
3. The three pairs of id injections for *test group* animals are as follows:
   a. 0.1-ml test substance in appropriate vehicle.
   b. 0.1-ml FCA emulsion alone.
   c. 0.1-ml test substance in FCA emulsion.
4. The three pairs of id injection for *control group* animals are as follows:
   a. 0.1-ml vehicle alone.

    b.   0.1 FCA emulsion alone.

    c.   0.1-ml vehicle in FCA emulsion

5.   The injections in steps 1 and 2 above are given close to each other and nearest the head; injection 3 is given most posteriorly.

6.   The date, time, and initials of those individuals performing the id injections are recorded. Immediately before injection, an emulsion is prepared by blending commercial FCA with an equal volume of house distilled water or other solvent as appropriate.

    a.   Water-soluble test materials are dissolved in the water phase prior to emulsification.

    b.   Oil-soluble or water-insoluble materials are dissolved or suspended in FCA prior to adding water.

    c.   Paraffin oil, peanut oil, or propylene glycol can be used for dissolving or suspending water-insoluble materials.

    d.   A homogenizer is used to emulsify the FCA alone and the test substance in either FCA or vehicle prior to the id injections.

    e.   The concentration of the test substance for id injections is adjusted to the highest level that can be well tolerated locally and generally.

7.   The adjuvant injection infiltration sometimes causes ulceration, especially when it is superficial, which lasts several weeks. These lesions are undesirable, but do not invalidate the test results, except for lowering the threshold level for skin irritation.

Induction Stage 2 (Day 7)

1.   Test substance preparation

    a.   The concentration of the test substance is adjusted to the highest level that can be well tolerated.

    b.   If the test substance is an irritant, a concentration is chosen that causes a weak to moderate inflammation (as determined by the pretest).

    c.   Solids are micronized or reduced to a fine powder and then suspended in a vehicle, such as petrolatum or propylene glycol.

    d.   Water-and-oil-soluble test substances are dissolved in an appropriate vehicle.

    e.   The concentration of the test substance for id injections is adjusted to the highest level that can be well tolerated locally and generally.

2.   The same area over the shoulder region that received id injections on day 0 is again shaved on both test and control guinea pigs.

3.   A volume of 0.3 ml of a mildly irritating concentration (if possible) of the test substance (determined by the pretest) is spread over a 1 × 2 in. filter of each test group animal.

4. The control group animals are exposed to 0.3 ml of 100% vehicle using the same procedure.
5. The date, time, and initials of those individuals performing the second induction are recorded.
6. The dressings of both groups are left in place for 48 hr before removal.

Challenge Stage (Day 21)

1. An area of hair (1.5 × 1.5 in.) on both flanks of the guinea pigs (15 test and three controls) is shaved.
2. A 1 × 1 in. patch with a nonirritating concentration of test substance in vehicle (as determined by the pretest) is applied to the left flank and a 1 × 1 inch patch with 100% vehicle is applied to the right flank.
3. The torso of each guinea pig is wrapped in an elastic bandage to secure the patches for 24 hr.
4. The date, time, and initials of those individuals performing the challenge dose are recorded.
5. The patches are removed 24 hr after application.

Rechallenge (Day 28)

1. If the first challenge application of test substance does not cause dermal sensitization, causes dermal sensitization in only a few animals, or causes dermal reactions that are weak or questionable, then a second challenge application of test substance to the 15 test group guinea pigs will be conducted on day 28 (one week after the first challenge). The three remaining naive control group animals (not used for the first challenge) are challenged for comparison to the test group animals.
2. The three negative control group animals used on day 21 will not be rechallenged. These animals will be terminated because they were exposed to the test substance during the first challenge and are no longer negative controls.
3. A 1 × 1 in. patch with a nonirritating concentration of test substance in vehicle is applied to the right flank of test and control group animals. The left flanks are not dosed.
4. The date, time, and initials of those individuals performing the rechallenge dose are recorded.
5. Steps 3 and 5 are followed as for challenge state (day 21).

Observations: Challenge and/or Rechallenge Readings

1. Twenty-one hr after removing the patch, the challenge area on each flank is cleaned and clipped, if necessary.
2. Twenty-four hr after removing the patch, the first reading of dermal reactions is taken.

3. The dermal reactions are scored on a four-point scale.
    0—no reaction
    1—scattered mild redness
    2—moderate and diffuse redness.
    3—intense redness and swelling
4. Forty-eight hr after removing the patch, the second reading is taken and the scores are recorded.

Interpretation of Results

1. Both the intensity and duration of the test responses to the test substance and the vehicle are evaluated.
2. The important statistic in the GPMT is the frequency of sensitization and not the intensity of challenge responses. A value of 1 is considered just as positive as a value of 3 (as long as the values for controls are zero).
3. The test agent is a sensitizer if the challenge reactions in the test group clearly outweigh those in the control group. A reaction that occurs at 24 hr but resolves by 48 hr after removal of patches should be considered a positive response, as long as it is stronger than that displayed by the controls. The sensitization rate (percentage of positive responders) is based on the greatest number of animals showing a positive response, whether it is from the 24-hr data or the 48-hr data after removal of patches.
4. When a second challenge application is performed, the data from both challenges are compared. If neither challenge produces a positive dermal reaction, the classification of the test substance is based on both challenge applications. If one challenge application (whether it is the first or second) produces a greater number of positive dermal reactions than the other, the classification of the test substance is based on the challenge with the most positive responses.
5. Under the classification scheme of Kligman (1966; shown in Table 8.14), the test substance is assigned to 1 of 5 classes, according to the percentage of animals sensitized, ranging from a weak grade I to an extreme grade V.

The advantages and disadvantages of the GPMT can be summarized as follows, starting with the advantages:

1. The test system is sensitive and effectively detects weak sensitizers. It has a low false negative rate.
2. If properly conducted, there are no false positives; that is, materials identified as potential sensitizers will act as such at some incidence level in humans.

TABLE 8.14 Sensitization Severity
Grading Based on Incidence of
Positive Responses

Sensitization rate (%)	Grade	Classification
0–8	I	Weak
9–28	II	Mild
29–64	III	Moderate
65–80	IV	Strong
81–100	V	Extreme

Source: Kligman, 1966.

3. There is a large database available on the evaluation of compounds in this test system, and many people are familiar with the test system.

The disadvantages, meanwhile, are as follows:

1. The test system is sensitive; it overpredicts potency for many sensitizers. There is no real differentiation among weak, moderate, and strong sensitizers; virtually all positive test results identify a material as strong.
2. The techniques involved (particularly the id injections) are not easy. Some regulatory officials have estimated that as many as 35% of the laboratories that try cannot master the system to get it to work reproducibly.
3. Although not as long as the Buehler, the test still takes a minimum of 4 weeks to produce an answer.
4. The test uses a significant amount of test material.
5. One cannot evaluate fibers or other materials that cannot be injected (e.g., solids that cannot be finely ground and/or suspended or that are highly irritating or toxic by the IV route).
6. The irritation pretest is critical. Failure to detect irritation in this small group of animals does not guarantee against irritation in test animals at challenge.

Mouse Ear Swelling Test (MEST). Several of the disadvantages associated with the previous three test systems, both stated and unstated, are reflections of limitations of the guinea pig as a model and the methodology of evaluating response in terms of observing and subjectively "grading" skin erythema.

Since Crowle (1959a, b) formally proved that passive transfer of delayed-type contact hypersensitivity exists in the mouse, research immunologists have generated a wealth of information in attempts to understand the DTH response in this species (Asherson and Ptak, 1968).

In particular, they have demonstrated that thymus-derived cells are necessary for inducing a DTH response (DeSousa and Parrott, 1969). Also, the mouse has been used to investigate immunosuppressive properties of certain drugs, such as fluorinated steroids and corticosteroids. All of these have led to the development of a formalized test procedure, the MEST.

The MEST is a procedure based on that described by Gad et al. (1985 a, b; 1986; 1987) for evaluating test substances for their potential to cause dermal sensitization in mice. This procedure evaluates contact sensitization by quantitatively measuring mouse ear thickness. This method is shown diagrammatically in Figures 8.6–8.8.

Animals

1. CF-1 or Balb/C female mice, 6 to 8 weeks old, are used. The mice are observed for at least 1 week to detect any signs of illness before starting a study. Mice that show poor growth or signs of illness are excluded from use on a test.
2. Any mouse displaying redness on either ear prior to the start of a test should be replaced.
3. Mice, which have been randomly placed in cages upon arrival, are assigned to groups (a maximum of five per cage) by labeling cage

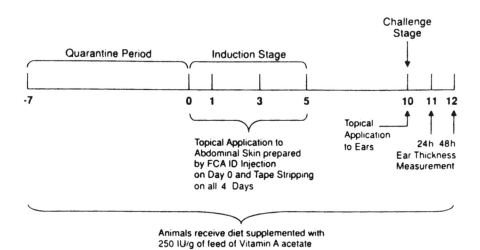

FIGURE 8.6   Study design for optimized mouse ear swelling test.

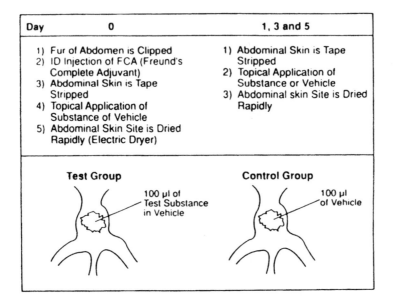

FIGURE 8.7   MEST induction stage procedures.

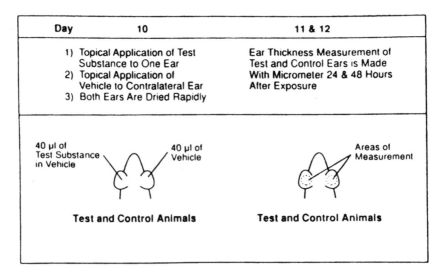

FIGURE 8.8   MEST challenge stage procedures.

cards. For each test substance investigated a pretest group of at least eight mice, a test group of at least 15 mice, and a control group of at least 10 mice are utilized. For 2 weeks prior to initiation of testing (starting on arrival), animals are given a diet supplemented with vitamin A (Thorne, et al., 1991).

4. Because animals are not individually marked, they will always be handled one at a time when each phase of this procedure is performed. The following procedure is conducted to prevent mixing animals during each phase (e.g., shaving, id injections, tape stripping, and dosing). All mice are removed from their original cage and placed in an empty cage for holding. One mouse is removed from the holding cage at a time, the phase activity is performed, and then the mouse is returned to its original cage. This step will be repeated for each of the remaining mice in the holding cage.

Pretest

1. A dermal (abdomen and ear) irritation and toxicity probe study is conducted 1 week prior to the actual MEST in order to establish the maximum concentration of test substance that produces minimal irritation to the abdomen (belly) region after a single topical application on each of 4 days (if the substance does have the potential to irritate skin) and to establish a concentration of test substance that is nonirritating to the ear after a single topical application. Also, dose levels of the test substance that produce systemic toxicity can be established during the pretest.

2. The test substance is diluted, emulsified, or suspended in a suitable vehicle. A vehicle (e.g., acetone, 70% ethanol, 25% ethanol, or methyl ethyl ketone) that should be able to solubilize the test substance and be volatile is selected.

3. Two mice from the pretest group are used to test each concentration of test substance. As many as four concentrations can be evaluated. The same mice used for belly irritation are also used for ear irritation testing.

4. On day 0, the first day of the pretest, each animal is prepared by clipping the hair from the belly region using a small animal clipper with a no. 40 blade.

5. After clipping the belly, the outer layers of epidermis (stratum corneum) of each mouse are removed from the shaved belly region with a tacky transparent tape (1-in. wide). This procedure is referred to as tape stripping. On day 0, the belly skin of each mouse is tape stripped until the application region appears shiny. While an assistant supports the dorsal portion of the mouse, the tape is pressed firmly over the

clipped belly region and quickly removed. This procedure is repeated as many times as needed.

6. After tape stripping the belly, a volume of 100 µl of test substance is applied to the belly region using a microliter pipette. At the same time, the test substance is applied to the ventral surface (10 µl) and dorsal surface (10 µl) of the left ear of the mouse using a microliter pipette.

7. On day 1, 24 hr after dosing the ears, the thickness of all probe animal ears is measured using an Oditest model D, 1000 thickness gauge.

    a. Ether is used to anesthetize the mice in a fume hood while the ears are measured.

    b. When a mouse reaches the "surgical anesthesia" stage, it is removed from the jar and gently placed on the countertop of the fume hood, which is prepared with a protective lining.

    c. While supporting the mouse with one hand, the other hand is used to press the finger lever on the Oditest gauge in order to open the flat measurement contacts. One ear of the mouse is then inserted between the contacts until it is positioned with approximately 1 to 2 mm of the outer edge of the ear showing. After positioning the ear, the finger lever is released to allow the contacts to clamp onto the ear. The measurement is read from the gauge after the indicator needle is stabilized. If desired, one or two more measurements can be rapidly made to be certain of a reproducible reading.

    d. Once a reading is obtained, the other (contralateral) ear is measured in the same manner. The animal's body is turned over in order to position the other ear for measurement.

    e. Measurements are recorded.

8. On subsequent days 1, 2, and 3, the belly region is first tape stripped five times and then a volume of 100 µl of test substance is applied topically to the belly region using a microliter pipette.

9. On day 4, 24 hr after the last topical application, the belly skin of all animals is observed for dermal irritation. A description of the results is recorded.

10. If any signs of systemic toxicity are observed on any of the pretest days, they should be noted.

11. Based on the results of the pretest data, a judgment is made as to which concentration will be used for topical induction applications to the belly and for topical challenge application to the ear. A minimal or mildly irritating concentration is preferable for induction, and the highest nonirritating concentration possible is used for challenge application.

Induction Stage

1. Day 0
   a. The belly of each test and control group mouse is clipped free of hair.
   b. Immediately after clipping, two id injections of FCA emulsion are made at separate sites in the skin of the shaved belly (each site flanks the ventral midline). Approximately 20µl of FCA emulsion is injected with a glass tuberculin syringe with a 30-gauge needle attached. Injections are performed in test and control mice.
   c. Following the id injections, the belly skin of test and control group animals is tape stripped until the site gives a shiny appearance.
   d. After tape stripping the belly, a volume of 100 µl of test substance (at a concentration determined by the pretest) is topically applied to the belly skin of test group animals with a microliter pipette. Control animals receive a dose of 100 µl of vehicle.
2. Days 1, 2, and 3
   a. The skin of the bellies of test and control group animals is tape stripped five times.
   b. After tape stripping, a volume of 100 µl of test substance is topically applied to the belly skin of test group animals and a volume of 100 µl of vehicle/solvent is topically applied to control group animals.

Challenge Stage

1. Day 10: Each test group mouse and each of five control group mice is dosed with 10 µl of a concentration of test substance (determined by the pretest data) on the ventral side of the left ear and 10 µl on the dorsal side of the left ear. The contralateral right ear is dosed with 10 µl of 100% vehicle on the ventral side and 10 µl on the dorsal side.
2. Day 11: Ear thickness measurements are made 24 hr after challenge dosing. The procedure described in Section 7, parts a, b, c, d under "Pretest" is used.
3. Day 12: Each thickness measurement is made again 48 hr after challenge dosing.

Rechallenge

1. If the test substance is judged a nonsensitizing agent after the first challenge application, causes dermal sensitization in only a few animals, or causes ear swelling that is weak or questionable, then a second and final challenge application will be performed on each test animal on day 17.

2. The five control group mice from the first challenge are not rechallenged because they have been exposed to the test substance and are no longer true negative controls. The five remaining naive control group animals (not used for the first challenge) are challenged for comparison to the test group animals.

3. The procedure used for the first challenge application will be used for the rechallenge application. Either the same concentration or a new concentration (higher or lower) of test substance may be used, depending on the results of the first challenge.

4. Measurement of both ears is performed on days 18 and 19 (24 and 48 hr after rechallenging, respectively). Each thickness measurement is recorded.

Interpretation of Results

1. Judgment concerning the presence or absence of sensitization is made for each animal. The judgment is based on the percentage difference ($\%\nabla$) between test and control ears. A "positive" sensitization response is considered to have occurred if the test ear of an animal is at least 20% thicker than the control ear.

2. The percentage of animals in a test group that is considered "positive" is then calculated and recorded as percentage of responders.

3. The negative control group ear thickness measurements are used to identify any possible dermal irritation reactions, which would be interpreted as false positive dermal sensitization responses.

4. In addition, the percentage of ear swelling is calculated for the test group. The left (A) and right (B) ear thickness measurements are added. The percentage of ear swelling equals the sum of A (test ear thicknesses) divided by the sum of B (control ear thicknesses), multiplied by 100.

    Ear swelling (%) = A/B $\times$ 100

5. When a second challenge application is performed, the data from both challenges are compared. If neither challenge procedure produces a positive sensitization reaction, the classification of the test substance is based on both challenge applications. If one challenge application (whether it is the first or second) produces a greater number of positive dermal reactions than the other, the classification of the test substance is based on the challenge with the most positive responses.

6. Two or more unequivocally positive responses in a group of 15 animals should be considered significant. A negative, equivocal, or single response probably assures that a substance is not a strong sensitizer, al-

though this is best confirmed by further testing with human subjects (NAS, 1977).

Strengths and Weaknesses   The MEST offers distinct advantages compared to the guinea pig dermal sensitization procedures:

1. The mouse is markedly less expensive.
2. Less vivarium space is required.
3. The duration of the test is shorter.
4. Less test substance is utilized.
5. The overall cost of the test is significantly less.
6. The test is objective, rather than subjective.
7. Materials that stain the skin may be easily evaluated. Several of the materials evaluated were colored and very difficult to evaluate by existing methods.
8. The test has a low false negative rate and no false positive rate, if properly performed.
9. The test seems to do a more accurate job of predicting relative hazard to humans.

Disadvantages include the following:

1. The database, though now not small, is not as extensive as that for GPMT or Buehler tests.
2. Fewer people have experience with the test system.
3. The regulatory status of data from the test system is unclear at present.

III. LOCAL LYMPH NODE ASSAY

This method has developed out of the work of Ian Kimber and associates (Kimber et al., 1986; Kimber and Dearman, 1994; Kimber and Weisenberger, 1989). It has the advantage over the other methods discussed in this chapter in that it provides an objective and quantifiable end point. The method is based on the fact that dermal sensitization requires the elicitation of an immune response. This immune response requires proliferation of a lymphocyte subpopulation. The LLNA relies on the detection of increased DNA synthesis via titriated thymidine incorporation. Sensitization is measured as a function of lymph node cell proliferative responses induced in a draining lymph node following repeated topical exposure of the test animal to the test article. Unlike the other tests discussed in this chapter, this assay looks only at induction because there is no challenge phase.

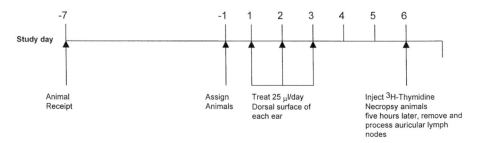

FIGURE 8.9   The mouse local lymph node assay.

The typical test (illustrated in Figure 8.9) is performed using mice—normally female CBA mice 6 to 10 weeks of age. Female BALB/c and ICR mice have also been used. After animal receipt, they are typically acclimated to standard laboratory husbandry conditions for 7 to 10 days. The usual protocol will consist of at least two groups (vehicle control and test article treated) of five mice each. They are treated on the dorsal surface of both ears with 25 µl (on each ear) of test article solution for three consecutive days. Twenty-four to 48 hr after the last test article exposure, the animals are given a bolus (0.25 ml) dose of [^{3}H]thymidine (20 µCi with a specific activity of 5.0–7.0 Ci/mmol) in phosphate buffered saline via a tail vein. Five hr after the injection, the animals are euthanized by CO_2 asphyxiation and the auricular lymph nodes are removed.

After removal, the lymph nodes can either be pooled by group or processed individually. Single cell suspensions are prepared by gentle mechanical disaggregation through a nylon (100 µm) mesh. Cells are washed twice by centrifugation in an excess of PBS. After the final supernatant wash is removed, the cells are precipitated with cold 5% trichloroacetic acid (TCA) and kept at 4°C for 12 to 18 hr. The precipitate is then pelleted by centrifugation and resuspended in 1 ml 5% TCA, and the amount of radioactivity is determined by liquid scintillation counting, using established techniques for tritium.

The data are reduced to the stimulation index (SI).

$$SI = \frac{H(\text{dpm}) \text{ treated group}}{H(\text{dpm}) \text{ control group}}$$

An SI of 3 or greater is considered a positive response; that is, the data support the hypothesis that the test material is a sensitizer.

The test article concentration is normally the highest nonirritating concentration. Several concentrations could be tested at the same time should one wish to establish a dose-response curve for induction. The test is easiest to perform if the vehicle is a standard nonirritating organic, such as acetone, ethanol, or dimethylformamide, or a solvent-olive oil blend. Until a laboratory develops its own historical control base, it is also preferable to include a positive control group. Either 0.25% dinitricholorobenzene or 0.05% oxazalone are recommended for positive controls. If the vehicle for the positive control is different from the vehicle for the test material, two vehicle control groups may be necessary.

This method has been extensively validated in two international laboratory exercises (Basketter et al., 1991; Loveless et al., 1996). In the earlier work (Basketter et al., 1991), there was good correlation between the results obtained with guinea pig tests and those obtained with the LLNA. In the more recent report, for example, five laboratories correctly identified dinitrochlorobenzene and oxazalone as sensitizers and the fact that p-aminobenzoic acid was not (Loveless et al., 1996). Arts and colleagues (1996) demonstrated that rats could be used as well as mice. Interestingly, they validated their assay (for both rats and mice) using BrDU uptake and immunohistochemical staining (rather than [^{3}H] thymidine) to quantitated lymph node cell proliferation.

This method is relatively quick and inexpensive because it uses relatively few mice (which are much less expensive than guinea pigs) and takes considerably less time than traditional guinea pig assays. It has an advantage over other methods in that it does not depend on a somewhat subjective scoring system and produces an objective and quantifiable end point. It does require a radiochemistry laboratory. Unless one already has an appropriately equipped laboratory used for other purposes (most likely metabolism studies), setting one up for the sole purpose of running the LLNA does not make economic sense. The standard version of the test has been adopted by OECD and ICVAM (see Figure 8.10), but also has been shown to have a modest false positive rate (misidentifying strong irritants as sensitizers).

A. Test System Manipulation (for All In Vivo Test Systems)

Increasing percutaneous absorption will increase test sensitivity. Factors that will increase absorption (and techniques for achieving them) include the following:

1. Increase surface area of solids.
2. Hydrate region of skin exposed to chemical. This can be done by wetting solids and using very occlusive wrapping of application.
3. Irritate application site.
4. Abrade application site.
5. Injection of test material (if possible).
6. Proper selection of solvent or suspending system. (See Christensen et al., 1984, for a discussion of the effect of vehicle in the case of even a strong sensitizer.)

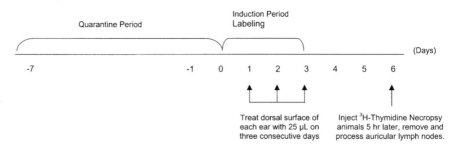

Species: Mouse
Strain: CBA/Ca
Test Group: 6 Animals
Control Group: 6 Vehicle

FIGURE 8.10 Mouse local lymph node assay (ICVAM protocol).

Species: Mouse
Strain: CBA/Ca
Test Group: 6 Animals
Control Group: 6 Vehicle

7. Remove part or all of the ''barrier layer'' (stratum corneum) by tape stripping the application site.
8. Increase the number of induction applications.

Although it is not a factor that increases percutaneous absorption, mildly stimulating the immune system of test animals [e.g., by injecting FCA (or some other adjuvant) alone or FCA blended with the test material] also increases responsiveness to the test system.

Also, it is generally believed that using the highest possible test material concentrations (mildly irritating for inuction, just below irritating for challenge) will guarantee the greatest possible sensitization response and will therefore also serve to universally increase sensitivity. There are reports, however (Gad et al., 1985, for croton oil and Thorne et al., 1987, for isocyanates), that this is not true for all compounds and that a multiple dose (i.e., two or more concentrations) study design would increase sensitivity. Such designs, however, would also significantly increase the cost.

Concurrent or frequent positive and negative controls are essential to guard against test system failure. Any of these test systems should show 0.05% dinitrochlorobenzene (DNCB) in 70% ethanol to be a strong sensitizer.

1. In Vitro Methods

There are actually several approaches available to in vitro evaluation of materials for sensitizing potential. These use cultured cells from various sources, and as end points, look at either biochemical factors (e.g., production of MIF-migration inhibition factor) or cellular events (e.g., as cell migration or cell "transformation").

Milner (1970) reported that lymphocytes from guinea pigs sensitized to dinitrofluorobenzene (DNFB) would transform in culture, as measured by the incorporation of tritiated thymidine, when exposed to epidermal proteins conjugated with DNFB. This work was later extended to guinea pigs sensitized to p-phenylenediamine. He later (Milner, 1971) reported that his method was capable of detecting allergic contact hypersensitivity to DNFB in humans when he used human lymphocytes from sensitized donors and human epidermal extracts conjugated with DNFB.

Miller and Levis (1973) reported the in vitro detection of allergic contact hypersensitivity to DNCB conjugated to leukocyte and erythrocyte cellular membranes. This indicated that reaction was not specifically directed toward epidermal cell conjugates.

Thulin and Zacharian (1972) extended others' earlier work on MIF-induced migration of human peripheral blood lymphocytes to a test for delayed contact hypersensitivity.

None of these approaches has yet been developed as an in vitro predictive test, but work is progressing. Milner (1983) has published a review of the history and state of this field.

Any alternative (in vitro or in vivo) test for sensitization will need to be evaluated against a battery of "known" compounds. The Consumer Product Safety Commission proposed such a battery in 1977. It is shown in Table 8.15.

Gad (1987; 1988) has published comparative data on multiple animal and human test system data for some 72 materials. Such a database should be broadened and developed for other test systems.

IV. APPROACHES

A. Suggested Approaches to Testing

As outlined above, there are numerous assays available to assess the various end points that are relevant to immunotoxicity. Early in the development process, a new compound should be evaluated with regard to various factors that may flag it as a potential immunotoxin, including chemical, structural, or physicochemical properties (e.g., photoallergin) and therapeutic class (i.e., immunomodulators, anti-inflammatories, and antimetabolites). Compounds from therapeutic or struc-

TABLE 8.15 Requested Reference Compounds for Skin
Sensitization Studies (U.S. Consumer Product Safety Commission)

Tribromophylophosphate	Formalin
Ditallow dimethyl ammonium methyl sulfate	Turpentine
Hydroxylamine sulfate	Potassium dichromate
Ethyl amino benzoate	Penicillin G
Todochlorohydroxy quinoline (Clioquinol, Chinoform)	p-Phenylenediamine
	Epoxy systems (ethylenediamine, diethylenetriamine, and diglycidyl ethers)
Nickel sulfate	
Monomethyl methacrylate	Toluene 2,4-diisocyanate
Mercaptobenzothiazole	Oil of Bergamot

tural classes that are known to be potential immunotoxins or immunomodulators should be evaluated for the effects in question on a case-by-case basis. With the exception of immunomodulators, protein products, and products of biotechnology, the majority of pharmaceuticals can be assessed for most forms of immunotoxicity during routine preclinical toxicity tests. In general, a well-conducted preclinical toxicity study can detect most serious immunotoxins in the form of altered clinical, hematologic, or histological end points. For example, possible effects on humoral immunity may be indicated from clinical observation of gastrointestinal or respiratory pathology and changes in serum total protein and globulin, and by histological changes in lymphoid cellularity. Likewise, effects on the cell-mediated response may be observed as increases in infections and tumor incidences and by changes in the T cell compartments of lymphoid tissues. In the case of immunosuppressive drugs such as cyclophosphamide and cyclosporin A, the immune effects seen in rodents are similar to those observed in the clinic (Dean et al., 1987).

If perturbations are observed in any hematologic or histopathologic indicators of immunotoxicity, it is prudent to follow up these findings with one or more of the following:

Use of special immunochemical and cytological assays that can be performed retrospectively on samples taken from the animals in question.
Use of more specific in vitro assays to further assess effects on the pertinent target system and potential mechanism of activity.
Use of more specific in vivo and ex vivo assays to determine toxicological significance.

Inclusion of additional nonroutine parameters for immunotoxicity assessment in subsequent (longer-term) toxicity assays. This can also include additional satellite groups for functional tests that may require coadministration of adjuvants, pathogens, or tumor cells.

B. Suggested Approaches to Evaluation of Results

Several rodent toxicity studies have shown impaired host resistance to infectious agents or tumor cells at exposure levels of drugs that did not cause overt signs of toxicity (Vos, 1977; Dean et al., 1982). One serious limitation to the incorporation of specific immunotoxicological evaluations into general use in safety assessment for pharmaceuticals is a lack of clarity in how to evaluate and use such findings. This problem is true for all new diagnostic techniques in medicine and for all the new and more sensitive tools designed to evaluate specific target organ toxicities. Ultimately, as we have more experience and a reliable database that allows us to correlate laboratory findings with clinical experience, the required course of action will become clearer. Some general suggestions and guidance can be offered, however.

First, it is generally agreed that adverse effects observed above a certain level of severity should be given the same importance as any other life-threatening events when assessing biological significance. These are effects that are so severe that they are detected as part of the routine evaluations made in safety assessment studies. Such findings may include death, severe weight loss, and an early appearance of tumors. Findings such as significantly increased mortalities in a host-resistance assay would also fit into this category.

Second, there are specific end point assays for which an adverse outcome clearly dictates the action to be taken. These end points include either immediate or delayed hypersensitivity reactions, because once the individual is sensitized, a dose-response relationship may not apply.

Third, as with most toxicological effects, toxic effects to the immune system are dependent upon dose to the target site. The dose-response curve can be used to determine no-effect and low-effect levels for immunotoxicity. These levels can then be compared to the therapeutic levels to assess whether or not there is an adequate margin of safety for humans.

If we consider both the specific immunotoxicity assays surveyed earlier in the chapter and the arrays of end points evaluated in traditional toxicology studies, which may be indicative of an immune system effect, these guidelines leave many potential questions unanswered. As additional data on individual end points indicative of immune system responses are collected, the pharmaceutical toxicologist is challenged with various issues regarding assay interpretation and relevance to proposed (or future) clinical trials. For example, what do significant, but non-life-threatening, decreases in antibody response, lymphocyte numbers, macrophage functions, or host resistance in an animal mean about the clinic use of a drug in a patient? The intended patient population is clearly relevant here; if the disease is one in which the immune system is already challenged or incorrectly modulated, any immune system effect other than an intended one should be avoided. There are several additional considerations and questions that should be answered when evaluating the biological and clinical significance of a statistically significant immune response.

1. *Is there a dose response*? The dose response should be evaluated as a dose-related trend in both incidence and severity of the response. If there is a dose-related response, is the lowest dose (preferably plasma level) at which the effect is seen near or below the target clinical dose (plasma level), and is there an adequate therapeutic margin of safety?
2. *Does the finding stand alone*? Is a change observed in only one parameter, or are there correlated findings that suggest a generalized, biologically significant effect? For example, are there changes in lymph node and spleen weights and morphological changes in these tissues to accompany changes in lymphocyte numbers?
3. *Is the effect a measure of function or a single end point measurement*? Functional measures such as host resistance or phagocytosis involve multiple cells and immunocomponents, and therefore are considered to be more biologically relevant than a significant change in a single end point measurement (e.g., T cell number).
4. *Is the effect reversible*? Reversibility of a response is dependent on the drug itself, exposure levels and duration, and factors related to the test animal (metabolic capability, genetic susceptibility, etc.). Most effects produced by immunosuppressive drugs have been shown to be reversible after cessation of therapy, such as those produced during cancer chemotherapy. If a tumor develops before the immune system is restored, however, the effect is not reversible, as is the case of secondary tumors related to chemotherapy.
5. *Is there sufficient systematic toxicity data available at levels that demonstrate adequate exposure*? If a study was designed in such a way that there was insufficient exposure or duration of exposure to potential lymphoid target tissues, the test protocol may not be adequate to demonstrate an adverse effect.

In general, a well-conducted long-term study in two species, with no indication of immunotoxicity and based on the considerations outlined above, should be adequate to evaluate the potential for drug-induced immunotoxicity. If the results from these studies do not produce evidence of immune-specific toxicity after examination of standard and/or additional hematologic, serum chemical, and histopathologic parameters, then additional testing should not be indicated. If there are structure-activity considerations that may indicate a potential for concern, however, or if significant abnormalities are observed that cannot be clearly attributed to other toxicities, then it is important to perform additional tests to fully assess the biological significance of the findings.

V. PROBLEMS AND FUTURE DIRECTIONS

There are some very pressing problems for immunotoxicology, particularly in the context of pharmaceuticals and biological therapeutics and the assessment of their safety. Unlike industrial chemicals, environmental agents, or agricultural chemicals, pharmaceutical products are intended for human exposure, are usually systemically absorbed, and have intentionally biological effects on man—some of which are intentionally immunomodulating (interleukins, growth factors) or immunotoxic (cyclosporin, cyclophosphamide).

Data Interpretation. The first major issue was presented and explored in the preceding section. This is how to evaluate and utilize the entire range of data that current immunotoxicological methodologies provide to determine the potential for immunotoxicity, and how to interpret the biological significance of minor findings.

Appropriate Animal Models. As previously addressed, most routine preclinical toxicology tests are performed with rats and dogs; therefore toxicity, pharmacokinetic, and pharmacology data are most abundant for these species. Most immunological parameters are best characterized and validated with mice, however. In addition, the NTP test battery was developed for the mouse, and some of these assays cannot be readily transferred to the rat. Over the last few years, several laboratories have begun adapting tests to both the rat and dog (Bloom et al., 1985a, b; Thiem et al., 1988); however, efforts need to continue along these lines to further our understanding of the immune responses in these species and how they correlate with other animal models and man.

Indirect Immunotoxic Effects. A problem related to data interpretation is how to distinguish secondary effects that may indirectly result in immunotoxicity from the primary effects of immunotoxicity in preclinic toxicity studies. Various factors may produce pathology similar to that of an immunotoxin, including

   Stress in a chronically ill animal as related to general toxicity, such as lung or liver damage, can result in immune suppression.
   Malnutrition in animals with drug-induced anorexia or malabsorption can trigger immune suppression.
   Infections and/or parasites may also modulate immune parameters.

These indirect factors must be systematically ruled out, and additional mechanistic studies may be necessary to address this problem. The potential for some indirect effects may be assessed through histopathologic evaluation of endocrine organs such as the adrenals and the pituitary.

Hypersensitivity Tests.   Probably the largest immunotoxicity concern in clinical studies is unexpected hypersensitivity reactions. While the available guinea pig- and mouse-based tests for delayed contact hypersensitivity resulting from dermal exposure are generally good predictors, there are currently no well-validated models for either immediate or delayed hypersensitivity responses resulting from either oral ingestion or parenteral administration. These two situations are the largest single cause for discontinuing clinical trials, however.

One assay that may hold some promise for delayed hypersensitivity is an adoptive transfer-popliteal lymph node assay (Klinkhammer et al., 1988). This assay, based on the techniques previously described for the popliteal lymph node assay, allows assessment of hypersensitivity following systemic exposure of the drug. Donor mice are first injected with drug for five consecutive days. After a 4-week latency period, potentially sensitized T cells obtained from the spleen are injected into the footpad of a syngeneic mouse together with a subcutaneous challenge dose of the drug. Two to 5 days after the cell transfer, the popliteal lymph nodes are measured and observed for evidence of a response (enlargement). Once this assay is validated, it should allow for a more relevant assessment of hypersensitivity for drugs that are administered systemically (Gleichman et al., 1989).

Autoimmunity.   Traditional methods for assessing immunotoxicity as part of routine preclinical toxicity tests are primarily geared toward the detection of immunosuppressive effects. Although it is possible to incorporate clinical methods for detecting immune complexes and autoantibodies into the preclinical test protocols, the significance of adverse findings is ambiguous. Since these effects have a genetic component to their expression, the relevance of findings in animals is of questionable significance, particularly since these findings in the clinic do not always correlate with pathological effects.

Functional Reserve Capacity.   As previously discussed, the immune system has a tremendous reserve capacity that offers several levels of protection and backups to the primary response. As a consequence, this functional reserve can allow biologically significant immunotoxic insults to occur without the appearance of morphological changes. Furthermore, adverse effects may remain subclinical until the organism is subjected to undue stress or subsequent challenge. There is thus some concern that routine immunopathological assessments by themselves may not be sufficiently sensitive to detect all immunotoxins, particularly when testing is conducted in a relatively pathogen-free, stress-free laboratory environment.

Significance of Minor Perturbations. Although the immune system has a well-developed reserve capacity, some of these systems may act synergistically rather than independently. For instance, a macrophage can recognize and kill bacteria coated with antibodies more effectively than either the macrophage or antibodies alone. Even minor deficiencies and impairments may thus have some impact on the organism's ability to fend off infection or tumors, particularly if the organism is very young, old, ill, stressed, genetically predisposed to certain cancers, or otherwise immunocompromised. These considerations lead to some additional questions that must be addressed.

What level of immunosuppression will predispose healthy or immunocompromised individuals to increased risk of infection or tumors?

What slight disturbances or immunosuppression lead to a prolonged recovery from viral or bacterial infections?

Will slight up-modulation for extended periods result in autoimmune diseases or increased susceptibility to allergy?

Are individuals that are slightly immunosuppressed at higher risk of developing AIDS after exposure to HIV?

REFERENCES

Adams, D. O. (1983). The biology of the granuloma. In: Pathology of Granulomas (H. L. Ioachim, Ed.). Raven, New York, pp. 1–20.

Anderson, J. M. (1988). Inflammatory response to implants, Trans. Amer. Soc. Art. Int. Organs, 34:101–107.

Arts, J. H. E., Droge, S. C. M., Bloksma, N., and Kuper, C. F. (1996). Local lymph node activation in rats after application of the sensitizers 2,4-dinitrichlorobenzene and trimellic anhydride, Fd. Chem. Toxicol. 34:55–62.

Asherson, G. L., and Ptak, W. (1968). Contact and delayed hypersensitivity in the mouse. I. Active sensitization and passive transfer, Immunology, 15:405–416.

Bach, F. H., and Voynow, N. K. (1966). One-way stimulation in mixed leukocyte cultures, Science, 153:545–547.

Bakke, O. M., Wardell, W. M., and Lasagna, L. (1984). Drug discontinuations in the United Kingdom and United States, 1964–1983: Issues of safety, Clin. Pharm. Ther., 35:559–567.

Basketter, D. A., Scholes, E. W., Kimber, I., Botham, P. A., Hilton, J., Miller, K., Robbins, M. C., Harrison, P. T. C., and Waite, S. J. (1991). Interlaboratory evaluation of the local lymph node assay with 25 chemicals and comparison with guinea pig test data, Toxicol. Methods, 1:30–43.

Battisto, J. R., Claman H. N., and Scott, D. W. (1983). Immunological tolerance to self and nonself, Ann. NY Acad. Sci., 392:1–433.

Bellon, B., Capron, M., Druet, E., Verroust, P., Vial, M.-C., Girard, J. F., Foidart, J. M., Mahieu, P., and Druet, P. (1982). Mercuric chloride induced autoimmune disease in Brown–Norway rats: Sequential search for anti-basement membrane antibodies and circulating immune complexes, Eur. J. Clin. Invest., 12:127–133.

Bick, P. H. (1985). The immune system: Organization and function: In: Immunotoxicology and Immunopharmacology (J. H. Dean, M. I. Luster, A. E. Munson, H. Amos, Eds.). Raven, New York, pp. 1–10.

Bigazzi, P. E. (1985). Mechanisms of chemical-induced autoimmunity. Immunotoxicology and Immunopharmacology (J. H. Dean, M. I. Luster, A. E. Munson, and H. Amos, Eds.). Raven, New York, p. 277.

Bigazzi, P. E. (1988). Autoimmunity induced by chemicals, Clin. Toxicol., 26:125–156.

Black, J. (1981). Rating system for tissues at animal implant sites. In: Biological Performance of Materials, Fundamentals of Biocompatibility, Marcel Dekker, New York, p. 220, Appendix 2.

Bloom, J. C., Thiem, P. A., Sellers, T. S., Deldar, A., and Lewis, H. B. (1985a). Cephalosporin-induced immune cytopenia in the dog—Demonstration of cell associated antibodies, Blood, 66:1232.

Bloom, J. C., Blackmer, S. A., Bugelski, P. J., Sowinski, J. M., and Saunders, L. Z. (1985b). Gold-included immune thrombocytopenia in the dog, Vet. Pathol., 22:492–499.

Bloom, J. C., Thiem, P. A., and Morgan D. G. (1987). The role of conventional pathology and toxicology in evaluating the immunotoxic potential of xenobiotics, Toxicol. Path., 15:283–293.

Buehler, E. V. (1964). A new method for detecting potential sensitizers using the guinea pig, Toxicol. Appl. Pharm., 6:341.

Buehler, E. V. (1965). Delayed contact hypersensitivity in the guinea pig, Arch. Derm., 91: 171–177.

Burkitt, D. S., Barwell, N. J., and Wilson, A. G. M. (1986). Urethral catheter structures, Lancet, 1:688.

Burnet, F. M. (1970). The concept of immunological surveillance, Prog. Exper. Tumor Res., 13:1–27.

CDRH. (1997). Immunotoxicology Testing Framework, draft document.

Christensen, O. B., Christensen, M. B., and Maibach, H. I. (1984). Effect of vehicle on elicitation of DNCB contact allergy in the guinea pig, Contact Dermatitis, 10:166–169.

Clark, W. R. (1983). The Experimental Foundations of Modern Immunology 2nd ed., Wiley, New York, pp. 1–453.

Coombs, R. R. A., and Gell, P. G. H. (1975). Classification of allergic reactions responsible for clinical hypersensitivity and disease. In: Clinical Aspects of Immunology (P. G. H. Gell, R. A. A., Coombs, and D. J. Lachman, Eds.). Blackwell Scientific, Oxford, p. 761.

Cromwell, O., Durham, S. R., Shaw, R. J., Mackay, J. A., and Kay, A. B. (1986). Provocation tests and measurements of mediators from mast cells and basophils in asthma and allergic rhinitis. In: Handbook of Experimental Immunology, 4th ed. (D. M. Weir, L. A. Herzenberg, and C. Blackwell, Eds.). Blackwell, Oxford, pp. 127.1–127-51.

Cronin, E. and Agrup, G. (1970). Contact dermatitis X, Brit. J. Derm, 82:428–433.

Crowle, A. J. (1959a). Delayed hypersensitivity in mice: Its detection by skin tests and its passive transfer, Science, 130:159.

Crowle, A. J. (1959b). Delayed hypersensitivity in several strains of mice studied with six different tests, J. Allergy 30:442–459.

Dean, J. H., Luster, M. I., and Boorman, G. A. (1982). Immunotoxicology. In: Immuno-pharmacology (P. Sirois and M. Rola-Pleszczynski, Eds.). Elsevier Biomedical, Amsterdam, pp. 349–397.

Dean, J. H., Boorman, G. A., Luster, M. I., Adkins, B. J., Lauer, L. D., and Adams, D. O. (1984). Effect of agents of environmental concern on macrophage functions. In: Mononuclear Phagocyte Biology (A. Volkman, Ed.). Marcel Dekker, New York, pp. 473–485.

Dean, J. H., Thurmond, L. M., Lauer, L. D., and House, R. V. (1987). Comparative toxicology and correlative immunotoxicology in rodents. In: Environmental Chemical Exposure and Immune System Integrity (E. J. Burger, R. G. Tardiff, and J. A. Bellanti, Eds.). Princeton Scientific, Princeton, NJ, pp. 265–271.

Descotes, G., and Mazue, G. (1987). Immunotoxicology, Advances Vet. Sci. Comp. Med., 31:95–119.

DeSousa, M. A. B., and Parrott, D. M. V. (1969). Induction and recall in contact sensitivity, changes in skin and draining lymph nodes of intact and thymectomized mice, J. Exp. Med., 130:671–686.

DeSwarte, R. D. (1986). Drug allergy: An overview, Clin. Rev. Allergy, 4:143–169.

DeWeck, A. L. (1983). Immunopathological mechanisms and clinical aspects of allergic reactions to drugs. In: Handbook of Experimental Pharmacology: Allergic Reactions to Drugs (A. L. deWeck and H. Burdgaard, Eds.). Springer-Verlag, New York, pp. 75–133.

Dighiero, G., Lymberi, J., Marie, J. C., Rouyse, S., Butler-Browne, G. S., Whalen, R. G., and Avrameas, S. (1983). Murine hybridomas secreting natural monoclonal antibodies reacting with self antigens, J. Immunol., 135:2267–2271.

Draize, J. H. (1959). The Appraisal of Chemicals in Foods, Drugs and Cosmetics, Association of Food and Drug Officials of the U.S., Austin, TX, pp. 36–45.

Draize, J. H., Woodard, G., and Calvery, H. O. (1944). Methods for the study of irritation and toxicity of substances applied topically to the skin and mucus membranes, J. Pharm. Exp. Ther., 82:377–390.

Druet, P., Bernard, A., Hirsch, F., Weening, J. J., Gengoux, P., Mahieu, P., and Brikenland, S. (1982). Immunologically mediated glomerulonephritis induced by heavy metals, Arch. Toxicol., 50:187–194.

Duke, S. S., Schook, L. B., and Holsapple, M. P. (1985). Effects of N-nitrosodimethylamine on tumor susceptibility, J. Leukocyte Bio., 37:383–394.

Exon, J. H., Koller, L. D., Talcott, P. A., O'Reilly, C. A., and Henningsen, G. M. (1986). Immunotoxicity testing: An economical multiple assay approach, Fund. Appl. Toxicol., 7:387–397.

FDA (Food and Drug Administration), Center for Safety and Applied Nutrition. (1993). Draft: Toxicological principles for the safety assessment of direct food additives and color additives used in food, Fed. Reg., 58:10536.

Gad, S. C. (1987). Scheme for the ranking and prediction of relative potencies of dermal sensitizers, based on data from several test systems, Toxicologist, A343.

Gad, S. C. (1988). A scheme for the ranking and prediction of relative potencies of dermal sensitizers based on data from several test systems, J. Appl. Toxicol, 8:301–312.

Gad, S. C., Darr, R. W., Dobbs, D. W., Dunn, B. J., Reilly, C., and Walsh, R. D. (1986a). Comparison of the potency of 52 dermal sensitizers in the Mouse Ear Swelling Test (MEST), presented at SOT Meetings, March 1986.

Gad, S. C., Dobbs, D. W., Dunn, B. J., Reilly, C., and Walsh, R. D. (1985). Elucidation of the delayed contact sensitization response to Croton Oil, presented at the American College of Toxicology, Washington, DC, Nov. 1985.

Gad, S. C., Dobbs, D. W., Dunn, B. J., Reilly, C., and Walsh, R. D. (1987). Development, validation and transfer of a new test system technology in toxicology. In: New Test Systems in Toxicology, vol. 5 (A. M. Goldberg, Ed.). Mary Ann Liebert, New York, pp. 275–292.

Gad, S. C., Dunn, B. J., and Dobb, D. W. (1985). Development of alternative dermal sensitization test: Mouse Ear Swelling Test (MEST), In Vitro Toxicology, proceedings of 1984 Johns Hopkins Symposium (A. M. Goldberg, Ed.). pp. 539–551.

Gad, S. C., Dunn, B. J., Dobbs, D. W., and Walsh, R. D. (1986b). Development and validation of an alternative dermal sensitization test: The mouse ear swelling test (MEST). Toxicol Appl. Pharm., 84, 93–114.

Garratlz, G. and Petz, L. D. (1975). Drug-induced immune hemolytic anemia, Amerx I. Med., 58:398–407.

Gibson, G. G., Hubbard, R., and Parke, D. U. (1983). Immunotoxicology. Academic, San Diego, CA.

Gleichmann, H. (1989). Testing the sensitization of T cells to chemicals: From murine graft-versus host (GVH) reactions to chemical-induced GVH-like immunological diseases. In: Autoimmunity and Toxicology (M. E. Kammueller, N. Bloksma,and W. Seinen, Eds.). Elsevier, Amsterdam, pp. 263–385.

Gleichmann, E., Kimber, I., and Purchase, I. F. H. (1989). Immunotoxicology: Suppressive and stimulatory effects of drugs and environmental chemicals on the immune system, Arch. Toxicol., 63:257–273.

Godfrey, H. P. and Gell, P. G. H. (1978). Cellular and molecular events in the delayed-onset hypersensitivities, Rev. Physiol. Biochem. Pharm., 84:2.

Golub, E. S. and Green, D. R. (1991). Immunology: A Synthesis, Sinauer, Sunderland, MA, pp. 1–744.

Guillaume, J. C., Roujeau, J. C., and Touraine, R. (1984). Purine analogs as immunomodulators. In: Progress in Immunology IV (Y. Yamamura and T. Tada, Ed.). Academic, London, pp. 1393–1407.

Guillot, J. P. and Gonnet, J. F. (1985). The epicutaneous maximization test, Curr. Prob. Derm. 14:220–247.

Harmon, W. E., Parkman, R., Gavin, P. T., Grupe, W. E., Ingelfunger, J. R., Yunis, E. J., and Levey, R. H. (1982). Comparison of cell-mediated lympholysis and mixed lymphocyte culture in the immunologic evaluation for renal transplantation, J. Immunol., 129:1573–1577.

Hassman, R. A., Lazarus, J. H., Dieguez, C., Weetman, A. P., Hall, R., and McGregor, A. M. (1985). The influence of lithium chloride on experimental autoimmune thyroid disease, Clin. Exp. Immunol., 61:49–57.

Hinton, D. M. (1992). Testing guidelines for evaluation of the immunotoxic potential of direct food additives, Criti. Rev. Food Sci. Nutri., 32:173–190.

Hutchings, P., Nador, D., and Cooke, A. (1985). Effects of low doses of cyclophosphamide and low doses of irradiation on the regulation of induced erythrocyte autoantibodies in mice, Immunol., 54:97–104.

Idsøe, O., Guthe, T., Willcox, R. R., and DeWeck, A. L. (1968). Nature and extent of penicillin side-reactions, with particular reference to fatalities from anaphylactic shock, Bull. WHO, 38:159–188.

Jerne, N. K. and Nordin, A. A. (1963). Plaque formation in agar by single antibody-producing cells, Science, 140:405.

Kimber, I. and Dearman, R. J. (1994). Immune responses to contact and respiratory allergens. In: Immunotoxicology and Immunopharmacology (J. H. Dean, M. I. Luster, E. A. Munson, and I. Kimber, Eds.). Raven, New York, pp. 663–679.

Kimber, I., Mitchell, J. A., and Griffin, A. C. (1986). Development of an immurine local lymph node assay for the determination of sensitizing potential, Food Chem. Toxicol., 24:585–586.

Kimber, I. and Weisenberger, C. (1989). A murine local lymph node assay for the identification of contact allergens: Assay development and results of an initial validation study, Arch. Toxicol, 63:274–282.

Klaus, G. G. B. and Hawrylowicz, C. N. M. (1984). Cell-cycle control in lymphocyte stimulation, Immunol. Today, 5:15–19.

Kleinman, S., Nelson, R., Smith, L., and Goldfinger, D. (1984). Positive direct antiglobulin tests and immune hemolytic anemia in patients receiving procainamide, New Eng. J. Med., 311:809–812.

Kligman, A. M. (1966). The identification of contact allergens by human assay. III. The maximization test. A procedure for screening and rating contact sensitizers, J. Invest. Derm., 47:393–409.

Klinkhammer, C., Popowa, P., and Gleichmann, H. (1988). Specific immunity to the diabetogen streptozotocin: Cellular requirements for induction of lymphoproliferation, Diabetes, 37:74–80.

Koeter, H. B. W. M. (1995). International harmonization of immunotoxicity testing, Human Exp. Toxicol, 14:151–154.

Koller, L. D. (1987). Immunotoxicology today, Toxicol. Path., 15:346–351.

Kumagai, Y., Shiokawa, Y., Medsger, T. A. J., and Rodnan, G. P. (1984). Clinical spectrum of connective tissue disease after cosmetic surgery: Observations of eighteen patients and a review of the Japanese literature. Arth. Rheum., 27:1–12.

Landsteiner, K. and Chase, M. W. (1942). Experiments on transfer of cutaneous sensitivity to simple chemical compounds, Proc. Soc. Exp. Bio. Med., 49:288–390.

Landsteiner, K. and Jacobs, J. (1935). Studies on sensitization of animals with simple chemical compounds, J. Exp. Med., 61:643–656.

Laskin, D. L., Laskin, J. D., Weinstein, I. B., and Carchman, R. A. (1981). Induction of chemotaxis in mouse peritoneal macrophages by phorbolester tumor promoter, Cancer Res., 41:1923.

Logue, G. L., Boyd, A. E., and Rosse, W. F. (1970). Chlorpropamide-induced immune hemolytic anemia, New Eng. J. Med., 283:900–904.

Loveless, S. E., Ladics, G. S., Greberick, G. F., Ryan, C. A., Basketter, D. A., Scholes,

E. W., House, R. V., Hilton, J., Dearman, R. J., and Kimber, I. (1996). Further evaluations of the local lymph node assay in the final phase of the international collaborative trial, Toxicology, 108: 141–152.

Luster, M. I., Munson, A. E., Thomas, P. T., Holsapple, M. P., Fenters, J. D., White, K. L. Jr., Lauer, L. D., Germolec, D. R., Rosenthal, G. L., and Dean, J. H. (1988). Development of a testing battery to assess chemical-induced immunotoxicity: National Toxicology Program's guidelines for immunotoxicity evaluation in mice, Fund. Appl. Toxicol., 10:2–19.

Luster, M. I., Pait, D. G., Portier, C., Rosenthal, G. J., Dermolec, D. R., Comment, C. E., Munson, A. E., White, K., Pollock, P. (1992a). Qualitative and quantitative experimental models to aid in risk assessment for immunotoxicology, Toxicol. Lett., 64/65:71–78.

Luster, M. I., Portier, C., Pait, D. G., White, K. L. Jr., Gennings, C., Munson, A. E., and Rosenthal, G. J. (1992b). Risk assessment in immunotoxicology. I. Sensitivity and predictability of immune tests, Fund. Appl. Toxicol., 18:200–210.

Magnusson, B. (1975). The relevance of results obtained with the guinea pig maximization test. In: Animal Models in Dermatology (H. Maibach, Ed.). Churchill Livingstone, Edinburgh, pp. 76–83.

Magnusson, B. and Kligman, A. M. (1969). The identification of contact allergens by animal assay: The guinea pig maximization test, J. Invest Derma., 52:268–276.

Magnusson, B. and Kligman, A. M. (1970). Allergic Contact Dermatitis in the Guinea Pig: Identification of Contact Allergens, Thomas, Springfield, IL, Chap. 8.

Maguire, H. C. and Chase, M. W. (1967). Exaggerated delayed-type hypersensitivity to simple chemical allergens in the guinea pig, J. Invest. Derm., 49:460–468.

Male. D., Champion, B., and Cooke, A. (1987). Advanced Immunology, Lippincott, Philadelphia.

Marchant, R. E., Miller, K. M., Hiltner, A., and Anderson, J. M. (1985). Selected aspects of cell and molecular biology of in vivo biocompatibility. In: Polymers as Biomaterials (S. W. Shalaby, A. S. Hoffman, B. D. Ratner, and T. A. Horbett, Eds.). Plenum, New York, pp. 209–223.

Marzulli, F. N. and Maibach, H. L. (1996). Dermatotoxicity, 5th ed., Taylor and Francis, Philadelphia.

Matory, Y. L., Chang, A. E., Lipford, E. H., Braziel, R., Hyatt, C. L., McDonald, H. D., and Rosenber, S. A. (1985). Toxicity of recombinant human interleukin-2 in rats following intravenous infusion, J. Biol. Resp. Mod., 4:377–390.

Maurer, T., Thomann, P., Weirich, E. G., and Hess, R. (1975). The optimization test in the guinea pig, Agents Actions, 5:174–179.

Maurer, T., Weirich, E. G., and Hess, R. (1980). The optimization test in the guinea pig in relation to other predictive sensitization methods, Toxicology, 15:163–171.

Merluzzi, V. J. (1985). Comparison of murine lymphokine, activated killer cells, natural killer cells, and cytotoxic T lymphocytes. Cell Immunol., 95:95–104.

Miller, A. E. Jr. and Levis, W. R. (1973). Studies on the contact sensitization of man with simple chemicals, I. Specific lymphocyte transformation in response to dinitrochlorobenzene sensitization, J. Invest. Derm., 61:261–269.

Milner, J. E. (1970). In vitro lymphocyte responses in contact hypersensitivity, J. Invest. Derm, 55:34–38.

Milner, J. E. (1971). In vitro lymphocyte responses in contact hypersensitivity II, J. Invest. Derm., 56:349–352.

Milner, J. E. (1983). In vitro tests for delayed skin hypersensitivity: Lymphokine production in allergic contact dermatisis, Dermatotoxicology (F. N. Marzulli and H. D. Maibach, Eds.). Hemisphere, New York, pp. 185–192.

NAS. (1977). Principles and Procedures for Evaluating the Toxicity of Household Substances, publication 1138, prepared for the Consumer Product Safety Commission, National Academy of Sciences, Washington, DC, pp. 36–39.

Paranjpe, M. S. and Boone, C. W. (1972). Delayed hypersensitivity to simianvirus 40 tumor cells in BALB/c mice demonstrated by a radioisotopic footpad assay, J. Nat. Cancer Inst., 48:563.

Pastan, I., Willingham, M. C., and FitzGerald, D. J. (1986). Immunotoxins, Cell, 47:641–648.

Penn, I. (1977). Development of cancer as a complication of clinical transplantation, Transplant. Proc., 9:1121–1127.

Pennisi, I. (1996). Teetering on the brink of danger, Science, 271:1665–1667.

Riccardi, C., Puccetti, P., Santoni, A., and Herberman, R. B. (1979). Rapid in vivo assay of mouse natural killer cell activity, J. Nat. Cancer Inst., 63:1041–1045.

Roitt, I., Brostoff, J., and Male, D. (1985). Adaptive and innate immunity. In: Immunology (I. Roitt, J. Brostoff, and D. Mabe, Eds.). C. V. Mosby, St. Louis, pp. 1.1–1.10.

Russel, A. S. (1981). Drug-induced autoimmune disease, Clin. Immun. Allergy, 1:57.

Salthouse, T. N. (1982). Biocompatibility in Clinical Practice (D. F. Williams, Ed.). CRC Press, Boca Raton, FL, pp. 18–24.

Spreafico, F. (1988). Immunotoxicology in 1987: Problems and challenges, Fund. Clin. Pharm., 2:353–367.

Sullivan, J. (1989). Immunological alterations and chemical exposure, Clin. Toxicol., 27:311–343.

Tabo, J. D. and Paul, W. E. (1973). Functional heterogeneity of murine lymphoid cells. III. Differential responsiveness of T cells to phytohemaglutinin and concanavalin A for T cell subsets, J. Immunol., 110:362–369.

Talal, N. (1987). Autoimmune mechanisms in patients and animal models, Toxicol. Path., 15:272–275.

TCSA. (1979). Fed. Reg., 44 (145), July 26, Part IV, Proposed EPA Test Standards for Toxic Substances Control Act Test Rules, Part 772.112–26.

Thiem, P. A., Halper, L. K., and Bloom, J. C. (1988). Techniques for assessing canine mononuclear phagocyte function as part of an immunotoxicologic evaluation, Int. J. Immunopharm., 10:765–771.

Thorne, P. S., Hawk, C., Kalizewski, S. D., and Guinez, P. D. (1991). The noninvasive mouse ear swelling assay. I. Refinements for detecting weak contact sensitizers. Fundam. Appl. Toxicol., 17:790–806.

Thorne, P. S., Hillebrand, J. A., Lewis, G. R., and Karol, M. H. (1987). Contact sensitivity by diisocyanates: Potencies and cross-reactivities, Toxicol Appl. Pharm., 87: 155–165.

Thulin, H. and Zacharian, H. (1972). The leukocyte migration test in chromium hypersensitivity, J. Invest. Derm., 58:55–58.

Ueda, S., Wakahim, Y., Takei, I., Mori, T., and Lesato, K. (1980). Autologous immune complex nephritis in gold injected guinea pigs, Nippon Jinzo Gakkai Shi, 22:1221–1230.

Unanue, E. R. (1994). The immune granulomas. In: Textbook of Immunology (E. R. Unanue and B. Benaceraf, Eds.). Williams and Wilkins, Baltimore, pp. 297–306.

U.S. Congress, Office of Technical Assessment. (1991). Identifying & Controlling Immunotoxic Substances—Background Paper. U.S. Government Printing Office, Washington, DC, pp. 1–93.

Volkman, A. (1984). Mononuclear Phagocyte Function, Marcel Dekker, New York.

Vos, J. G. (1977). Immune suppression as related to toxicology, CRC Crit. Rev. Toxicol., 5:67.

Vos, J., Van Loveren, H., Weester, P., and Vathaak, D. (1989). Toxic effects of environmental chemicals on the immune system, TIPS, 10:289–292.

Weening, J. J., Fleuren, G. J., and Hoedemaeker, J. (1978). Demonstration of antinuclear antibodies in mercuric chloride-induced glomerulopathy in the rat, Lab. Invest., 39:405–411.

Weigle, W. O. (1980). Analysis of autoimmunity through experimental models of thyroditis and allergic encephalomyelitis, Adv. Immunol., 30:159–275.

White, K. L. Jr., Sanders, V. M., Barnes, D. W., Shopp, J. G. M., and Munson, A. E. (1985). Immunotoxicological investigations in the mouse: General approach and methods, Drug. Chem. Toxicol., 8:299–331.

Woodward, S. C. and Salthouse, T. N. (1986). The tissue response to implants and its evaluation by light microscopy. In: Handbook of Biomaterials (A. F. von Recum, Ed.). Macmillan, New York, pp. 364–379.

Yoshida, S., Golub, M. S., and Gershwin, M. E. (1989). Immunological aspects of toxicology: Premises not promises, Reg. Toxicol. Pharm., 9:56–80.

9

Implantation Biology and Studies

Implantation studies are a type of assay unique to medical devices and biomaterials, having been specifically devised for those situations in which an exogenous (and usually man-made) construct or material is enclosed in the body or partially entered into it by a breached surface. It is intended to assess the effects of devices (usually polymers or elastomers) that are in direct contact with living tissue (not including the skin). Most commonly (and primarily discussed here) the effects of concern are often a relatively short-term exposure and limited to various indicators of local tissue tolerance. Longer-term studies are conducted for long-term implants, and focus more on broader systemic effects and potential carcinogenicity.

I. USP IMPLANTATION TEST

The USP (USP, 1996) test is designed to evaluate relatively short-term exposures, and it is the normative reference method for both the FDA and ISO (1995).

The implantation test is designed for the evaluation of plastic materials and other polymeric materials in direct contact with living tissue. Of importance are the proper preparation of the implant strips and their proper implantation under aseptic conditions. Prepare for implantation eight strips of the *sample* and four strips of USP negative control plastic reference standard (RS). Each strip should measure not less than 10×1 mm. The edges of the strips should be as smooth as possible to avoid additional mechanical trauma upon implantation. Strips of the specified minimum size are implanted by means of a hypodermic needle (15-

to 19-gauge) with an intravenous point and a sterile trocar. Either use presterilized needles into which the sterile plastic strips are aseptically inserted, or insert each clean strip into a needle, the cannula and hub of which are protected with an appropriate cover, and then subjected to the appropriate sterilization procedure. (*Note*: Allow for proper degassing if agents such as ethylene oxide are used.)

Test Animal.   Select healthy adult rabbits weighing not less than 2.5 kg, whose paravertebral muscles are sufficiently large to allow for implantation of the test strips. Do not use any muscular tissue other than the paravertebral site. The animals may be anesthetized with a commonly used anesthetic agent to a degree deep enough to prevent muscular movements, such as twitching.

Procedure.   Perform the test in a clean area. On the day of the test or up to 20 hr before testing, clip the fur of the animals on both sides of the spinal column. Remove loose hair by means of a vacuum. Swab the skin lightly with diluted alcohol and dry the skin prior to injection.

Implant four strips of the *sample* into the paravertabral muscle on one side of the spine of each of two rabbits, 2.5 to 5 cm from the midline and parallel to the spinal column, and about 2.5 cm apart from each other. In a similar fashion implant two strips of USP negative control plastic RS in the opposite muscle of each animal. Insert a sterile stylet into the needle to hold the implant strip in the tissue while withdrawing the needle. If excessive bleeding is observed after implantation of a strip, place a duplicate strip at another site.

Keep the animals for a period of not less than 120 hr, and sacrifice them at the end of the observation period by administering an overdose of an anesthetic agent or other suitable agents. Allow sufficient time to elapse for the tissue to be cut without bleeding. Examine macroscopically the area of the tissue surrounding the center portion of each implant strip. Use a magnifying lens if necessary. The tissue immediately surrounding the USP negative control plastic RS strips appears normal and entirely free from hemorrhage, film, or encapsulation. The requirements of the test are met if in each rabbit the reaction to not more than one of the four *sample* strips is significantly greater than that to the strips of USP negative control plastic RS.

Observation
  Macroscopically
  Hemorrhage
  Necrosis
  Discolorations
  Infections
  Encapsulation
Histopathology (not required, but generally conducted)
  Connective tissue proliferation
  Mononuclear cell infiltration

TABLE 9.1   Microscopic Examination Findings in Implant Studies

Cell type	Implication
Granulocytes and neutrophils	Cells of acute inflammation: first line of defense against bacteria and absorbable materials. These cells attempt to engulf and digest materials. Their presence implies a bioreactive material.
Monocytes and macrophages	Cells of subacute inflammation: second line of defense and more resistant to damage by breakdown products. Their presence implies a prolongation of the effort to degrade the bioreactive material.
Giant cells	Cells of chronic inflammation: giant cells result from the fusion of monocytes and macrophages. Their presence is indicative of bioreactive materials that are resistant to degradation.
Fibroblasts	These are the cells that encapsulate and isolate foreign particles from surrounding tissue. Their presence implies that the body has surrendered in its effort to rid itself of the foreign material and has chosen to isolate instead.
Lymphocytes	Large densities of lymphocytes are characteristic of immunologic injury. Their presence in large numbers implies an immunologic response to the material.

> Polymorphonuclear cell infiltration
> Muscle degeneration
> Multinucleated giant cell infiltration

Table 9.1 summarizes the most common microscopic findings in an implantation study (Greco, 1994; von Recum, 1998).

II. BRITISH PHARMACOPOEIA

Implantation tests in rabbits are also required for medical devices and plastics, but in this case to evaluate the local effects of direct contact between solid samples and muscle tissue. The British specification (British Standard, 1981a) is for medical devices intended for long-term implantation, such as hip prostheses, and for short-term use within the body or in contact with mucosal surfaces, such as urinary catheters. The USP specification (USP, 1996) is for plastics and other polymers intended for fabricating containers or their accessories, and for use in medical devices, implants, and other materials. The British method is similar but specifies not fewer than three rabbits, additional implantation or positive control strips (such as tin-stabilized polyvinylchloride), a duration of 7 days, and histology of the sites if any macroscopic reaction to the test material is negative. It also advocates a less objective assessment of the results. The anesthetic suggested is pentobarbitone (pentobarbital), but the neuroleptic–analgesic combination of fluanisone and fentanyl citrate is preferable because it is safer in rabbits and reversible.

One problem of the implantation test is a tendency for the strips to migrate from their implantation sites, even to subcutaneous positions, and this often prolongs the search for them. It is nevertheless an effective detection system for toxic ingredients of solid materials that leach in contact with tissue fluid. It is important to recognize the microscopic effects of the standard negative control strips (additive-free polyethylene). These are typical of skeletal muscle in contact for a week with a foreign body and comprise mild mononuclear cell infiltration, multinucleated giant cell formation, fibroplasia, slight dystrophic calcification, muscle fiber atrophy, and centripetal migration of sarcolemmal nuclei. Also, traumatic hemorrhage is common. Positive reactions are similar but more pronounced, and additionally include focal necrosis and education, particularly of heterophils. It is a useful test, not only for finished products, but also to identify unacceptable changes in the formulation or manufacturing process, such as the introduction of chlorinating cycles to remove bloom on latex catheters.

III. ISO 10993 IMPLANTATION TEST

The ISO 10993-mandated test is covered by part 6 of the test guidelines and is specifically intended to test for local effects after implantation. It can be performed for either the short term (from 1 up to 12 weeks) or long term (from 12 to 104 weeks).

The test specimen is implanted into a site and tissue that are appropriate for evaluation of the biological safety of the material. The implant is not intended to be subjected to mechanical or functional loading. The local effects are evaluated by a comparison of the tissue response caused by a test specimen to that caused by materials used in medical devices whose clinical acceptability has been established.

A. Preparation of Specimens for Implantation

1. Solid Specimens (Excluding Powders)

Physical characteristics (i.e., form, density, hardness, surface finish) can influence the character of the tissue response to the test material. Each implant shall be manufactured, processed, cleaned of contaminants, and sterilized by the method intended for the final product. After final preparation and sterilization, the implant specimens shall be handled in such a way as to ensure that they are not scratched, damaged, or contaminated in any way prior to or during insertion.

2. Nonsolid Specimens (Including Powders)

Nonsolid specimens may be liquids, pastes, and particulates, as distinct from the materials covered in Sec. III.A. The components may be mixed before use (e.g., bone cements, dental materials) and set after varying time periods. The materials may be contained in tubes for the purpose of testing for local effects after implantation. Polyethylene (PE), polypropylene (PP), or polytetrafluoroethylene (PTEE) tubes are commonly used for this purpose.

Prior to testing the tubes shall be rinsed with 70% (v/v) ethanol and distilled water and sterilized by autoclaving or other appropriate methods relevant for clinical applications. Materials tested in their freshly mixed state shall be tested for microbiological contamination.

Prepare the test material according to the manufacturer's instructions and insert the material into the tube until it is level with the top. Exercise the utmost care to prevent contamination of the outer surface of the tube by the test material. Avoid entrapment of air in the tube and ensure that the end surfaces of the inserted material in the tube and the tube ends are smooth. (*Note*: PE tubes may be deformed by autoclaving. It is difficult to section PTFE tubes in the microtome, and substitution by PE or PP tubes of the same dimensions may be preferable when the tubes are to remain in the tissue blocks during sectioning.)

3. Control Specimens

The size, shape, and especially the surface condition of the control(s) shall be as similar to that of the implant test specimens as is practically possible. When the test material is contained in a tube, the control shall be a rod of the same material as the tube and with the same diameter as the outer diameter of the tube. The control specimens shall be handled, cleaned, and sterilized in such a manner as to maintain them as acceptable and well-characterized controls.

Selection of control material(s) should be based on their established use in clinical applications similar to those proposed for the candidate test material and is not otherwise restricted.

4. Animals and Tissues

Select an animal species with due consideration of the size of the implant test specimens and the intended duration of the test in relation to the expected life span of the animals, as well as the recognized species differences in biological response in both hard and soft tissues. For short-term testing in subcutaneous tissue and muscle, animals such as mice, rats, guinea pigs, and rabbits are commonly used (Gad and Chengelis, 1994). Select one species among these. For long-term testing in subcutaneous tissue, muscle, and bone, rats, guinea pigs, rabbits, dogs, sheep, goats, pigs, and other animals with a relatively long life expectancy are suitable. Select one species among these.

The specimens of test and control materials shall be implanted under the same conditions in the same species of the same age, sex, and strain in corresponding anatomical sites. The number and size of implants inserted in an animal depends on the size of the species and the anatomical location of the implantation.

B. Test Periods

The local tissue response to implanted materials is assessed in short-term tests up to 12 weeks and in long-term tests exceeding 12 weeks.

Test periods are chosen to ascertain that a steady state has been reached with respect to biological response. The local biological response to implanted materials depends both on the properties of the materials and on the trauma of surgery. The tissue configuration found in the vicinity of an implant changes with the time elapsed after surgery. Usually, at 1-week observation periods, a high cell activity is found, followed by a transitional stage. In muscle and connective tissue, depending on the species, a steady state is seen in the cell population after 9 to 12 weeks. Implantation in bone tissues may need longer observation periods.

Test periods shall be selected from those specified in Table 9.2 for short-term implantation, or from Table 9.3 for long-term implantation.

Depending on the intended use of the test material, not all implantation periods may be necessary. (See ISO, 1995.) An observation period of 104 weeks may be of interest in selected instances. The number of implants per animal and the number of animals per observation period are described in the appropriate sections below. A sufficient number of implants shall be inserted to ensure that the final number of specimens to be evaluated will give valid results.

C. Surgery

Anesthetize the animals. Remove hair from the surgical area by clipping, shaving, or other mechanical means. Wash the area with an antiseptic solution. Ensure that hair does not come in contact with the implants or the wound surfaces.

TABLE 9.2 Selection of Test Periods for Short-Term
Implantation in Subcutaneous Tissue and Muscle

	Implantation period (weeks)				
Species	1	3	4	9	12
Mice	X	X		X	
Rats	X		X		X
Guinea pigs	X		X		X
Rabbits	X		X		X

TABLE **9.3** Selection of Test Periods for Long-Term
Implantation in Subcutaneous Tissue, Muscle, and Bond

Species	Implantation period (weeks)				
	12	26	52	78	104
Rats	X	X	X		
Guinea pigs	X	X	X		
Rabbits	X	X	X	X	
Dogs	X	X	X	X	X
Sheep	X	X	X	X	X
Goats	X	X	X	X	X
Pigs	X	X	X	X	X

The surgical technique may profoundly influence the result of any implantation procedure. The surgery shall be carried out under aseptic conditions and in a manner that minimizes trauma at the implant site. After surgery close the wound, using either wound clips or sutures, taking precautions to maintain aseptic conditions.

D. Postoperative Assessment

Observe each animal at appropriate intervals during the test period and record any abnormal findings, including local, systemic, and behavioral abnormalities.

E. Euthanasia

At the termination of the experimental period, euthanize the animals with an overdose of anesthetic or by some other acceptable humane method. (See ISO, 1995.)

F. Evaluation of Biological Response

Evaluate the biological response by grading and documenting the macroscopic and histopathological test responses as a function of time. Compare the responses to the test material and control material.

Carry out a comparison of the control and the test implants at equivalent locations relative to each implant so that the effect of relative motion between tissue and implant is at a minimum. For a cylindrical specimen the region is midway between ends. With grooved cylindrical implants the center portions between the grooves as well as the flat-top end surfaces of the implant are suitable for evaluation.

For a nonsolid or particulate material incorporated into a tube, the area at the end of the tube is the only available area for evaluation.

G. Macroscopic Assessment

Examine each implant site with the aid of a low magnification lens. Record the nature and extent of any tissue reaction observed.

H. Preparation for Histology: Implant Retrieval and Specimen Preparation

Excise the implant together with sufficient unaffected surrounding tissue to enable evaluation of the local biological response. Process the excised tissue blocks containing test or control implants for histopathological and other studies as appropriate.

When conventional techniques are used, the tissue envelope may be opened before or after exposure to a fixative, and the condition of the implant surface and tissue bed shall be reported. With this technique the tissue layers closest to the implant are usually destroyed, however.

When the implant/tissue surface is to be studied, embedding the intact tissue envelope with the implant in situ using hard plastics is preferred. Appropriate sectioning or grinding techniques are employed for the preparation of histological sections. It shall be demonstrated that the technique of embedding in plastics does not markedly alter the interface tissue.

I. Histological Assessment

The extent of response may be determined by measuring the distance from the implant/tissue interface to unaffected areas with the characteristics of both normal tissue and normal vascularity. Record the section orientation in relation to the implant dimensions. Record the implant orientation, number of sections, and cutting geometry.

The biological response parameters that shall be assessed and recorded include the following:

1. Extent of fibrosis/fibrous capsule and inflammation
2. Degeneration as determined by changes in tissue morphology
3. Number and distribution as a function of distance from the material/tissue interface of the inflammatory cell types, namely polymorphonuclear leukocytes, lymphocytes, plasma cells, eosinophils, macrophages, and multinucleated cells
4. Presence of necrosis as determined by nuclear debris and/or capillary wall breakdown

5. Other parameters, such as material debris, fatty infiltrations, and granu-loma
6. For porous implant materials, the quality and quantity of tissue in-growth

In the case of bone, the interface between the tissue and the material is of special interest. Evaluate the area of bone contact and the amount of bone in the vicinity of the implant as well as the presence of intervening noncalcified tissues. Note the presence of bone resorption and bone formation.

J. Implant Specimens

Description of test and control materials, material condition, fabrication, surface condition, and the shape and size of implants.
Remember to specify the rationale for selection of control material(s).
The surface preparation of the specimens can affect the tissue reaction, therefore the preparation procedure should be noted in the report.
Report the cleaning, handling, and sterilization techniques employed. If not done in-house, this information should be supplied by the manufacturer before the investigation commences.

K. Animals and Implantation

Report the origin, age, sex, and strain of the animals. Report housing conditions, diet, and mass of animals during the study period. The health of the animals shall be evaluated during the study. All observations, including unexpected death, shall be reported.
Report insertion techniques. Report the number of implants inserted per animal, per site, and per observation period.

L. Retrieval and Histological Procedure

The report shall include a description of the retrieval technique. The number of implants retrieved per animal and per observation period shall be recorded. All specimens shall be accounted for and considered as part of the test. The tech-niques for taking histological sections shall be described.

M. Evaluation

Macroscopic observations shall include the observations made on implant as well as the macroscopic appearance of the tissue surrounding the implant. The report shall include the results obtained from each histological examination.

The report shall include a comparative evaluation of the biological responses to test and control materials, as well as a descriptive narrative of the biological response.

IV. TEST METHOD FOR IMPLANTATION IN SUBCUTANEOUS TISSUE

A. Field of Application

This test material is used for assessing the biological response of subcutaneous tissue to an implanted material.

    The study may be used to compare the effect of different surface textures or conditions of the same material or to assess the effect of various treatments or medications or a material.

B. Principle

Insertion of the implants in the subcutaneous tissue of test animals is as per USP (2000). The method compares the biological response to implants of test specimens with the biological response to implants of control specimens made of materials that are established in clinical use.

C. Test Specimens

Common provisions for the preparation of test and control specimens are described in Sec. III. Implant sizes are based on the size of the test animal.

    Specimens made of sheet material shall be 10 mm to 12 mm in diameter and from 0.3 mm to 1 mm in thickness. (*Note*: The subcutaneous site, deep to the panniculus carnosus muscle, is particularly suitable for the evaluation of polymeric sheet material. In an intramuscular site, sheet material may become folded, which makes it difficult to assess the effect of the material per se.)

    Bulk materials shall be fabricated into specimens 1.5 mm in diameter and 5 mm in length, and have radiused ends.

    Grooved specimens shall be 4 mm in diameter and 7 mm in length. (*Note*: Tissue ingrowth into the grooves minimizes tissue irritation caused by interface motion.)

    Nonsolid specimens (including powders) shall be prepared in tubes 1.5 mm in diameter and 5 mm in length.

D. Test Animals and Implant Sites

The implants shall be inserted in the dorsal subcutaneous tissue of adult mice, rats, guinea pigs, or rabbits. Select one species among these.

Use at least three animals and sufficient sites to yield 10 specimens for each material and implantation period.

E. Implantation Procedure

Select one of the procedures described below.

> *Implantation along dorsal midline*: Make an incision of the skin and make one or more subcutaneous pockets by blunt dissection. The base of the pocket shall be more than 10 mm from the line of incision. Place one implant in each pocket. The implants shall not be able to touch one another. (*Note*: Alternatively, the implants may be delivered by a trocar to the desired site.
>
> *Implantation in neck*: In mice, make a 10-mm-long incision above the sacrum and prepare a subcutaneous tunnel by blunt dissection toward the neck. Push one implant through the tunnel to position it at the neck.
>
> In rats, insert one implant of each of the control and candidate materials separately on each side of the neck. The implants should not be able to touch one another.
>
> At some distance from the implant, close the tunnel with stitches of appropriate suture material to prevent the implant from moving.
>
> *Implantation period*: To ensure a steady state of biological tissue response the implantation period(s) shall be as specified in Table 9.2 and Table 9.3.

F. Evaluation of Biological Response

The evaluation shall take into account the items specified earlier.

V. TEST METHOD FOR IMPLANTATION IN MUSCLE

A. Field of Application

This test is used for assessing the biological response of muscle tissue to an implanted material.

B. Principle

The method of insertion of the implant into the muscle of the test animal compares the biological response to implants of test specimens with the biological response to implants of control specimens made of materials that are established in clinical use.

C. Test Specimens

Common provisions for preparation of test and control specimens are described earlier. Implant sizes are based on the size of the muscle group chosen.

For rabbit paravertabral muscles, implants of a width of 1 mm to 3 mm with a length of approximately 10 mm shall be used.

The specimens shall have rounded edges and the ends finished to a full radius.

D. Test Animals and Implant Sites

Insert the implants in the muscle tissue of rabbits or other animals. Ensure that the muscles are of sufficient size to accommodate the implant specimens. Use only one species per test. (*Note*: The paravertabral muscles of rabbits are the preferred implant sites. Alternatively, the gluteal muscles of rats or the thigh muscles of rabbits may be used.)

Use at least three animals and sufficient implant sites to yield eight test specimens and eight control specimens for each implantation period.

In cases in which the control material is expected to elicit more than a minimal response, use two specimens of this control. Implant two additional control specimens, composed of a material known to evoke a minimal tissue reaction, in a location opposite to the test materials.

E. Implantation Procedure

Implantation shall be by hypodermic needle or trocar. For larger implants other appropriate surgical implantation techniques may be used.

Implant test specimens into the body muscle with the long axis parallel to the muscle fibers.

For rabbit paravertabral muscles, implant four specimens of the test materials along one side of the spine, 25 mm to 50 mm from the midline and parallel to the spinal column, and about 25 mm apart from each other. In similar fashion implant four specimens of the control material in the contralateral muscle of each animal.

F. Implantation Period

To ensure a steady state of biological tissue response, the implantation period(s) shall be as specified in Table 9.2 and Table 9.3.

VI. TEST METHOD FOR IMPLANTATION IN BONE

A. Field of Application

This test method is used for assessing the biological response of bone tissue to an implanted material. The study may be used to compare the effect of different surface textures or conditions of the same material, or to assess the effect of various treatments or modifications of a material.

B. Principle

The method compares the biological response to implants of test specimens with the biological response to implants of control specimens made of materials that are established in clinical use.

C. Shape of Implant Specimens

The specimens may be screw-shaped or threaded to provide initial stability of the implants in bone. If preparation of a screw shape is impractical, a cylinder shape may be used.

D. Size of Test Specimens

Implant sizes are based on the size of the test animal and bone chosen. The following dimensions shall be considered:

1. Rabbits: cylindrical implants 2 mm in diameter and 6 mm in length
2. Dogs, sheep, and goats: cylindrical implants 4 mm in diameter and 12 mm in length
3. Rabbits, dogs, sheep, goats, and pigs: 2-mm to 4.5-mm orthopedic bone screw-type implants.

E. Test Animals

The implants shall be inserted into the bone of dogs, sheep, goats, pigs, or rabbits. Select one species among these. Species differences are important in bone physiology, and should be assessed before implantation procedures are initiated. At least four rabbits, or at least two each of other animals, shall be used for each implantation period.

F. Implant Sites

Equivalent anatomical sites shall be used for test and control specimens. The test implants shall be contralateral to the control implants. Select the implant site to minimize the risk of mobility of the implant. (*Note*: The femur and tibia are suitable. Other sites may be considered.)

The number of implant sites shall be as follows:

1. In each rabbit there shall be a maximum of six implant sites: three for test specimens and three for control specimens.
2. In each dog, sheep, goat, or pig, there shall be a maximum of 12 im-

plant sites; six for test specimens and six for control specimens. Do not insert more than 12 specimens in any one animal.

The size, mass, and age of the animal and the implant site chosen should ensure that the implant placement does not cause significant risk of pathological fracture of the test site. In younger animals it is especially important to ensure that the implants avoid the epiphyseal area or other immature bone.

G. Implantation Procedure

Perform bone preparation using a low drilling speed and intermittent drilling with profuse irrigation with physiological saline solution and suction, because overheating will result in local tissue necrosis.

It is important that the diameter of the implant and the implant bed in the bone match well enough to avoid ingrowth of fibrous tissue.

Expose the cortex of each femur or tibia and drill the appropriate number of holes to receive implants. For rabbits, prepare up to three holes; for larger animals prepare up to six holes. Ream to final diameter or tap screw thread before insertion. Insert cylinders by finger pressure to allow press fit. Tighten screw-shaped implants in place with an instrument capable of delivering a predetermined torque. Record the torque.

H. Implantation Period

To ensure a steady state of biological tissue response the implantation period(s) shall be as specified in Table 9.2 and Table 9.3.

VII. CONTROL MATERIALS

A. Response

The biological response to these materials is not defined as to response, but rather the response is used as a reference against which a reaction to another material is compared.

As a porous control material is not available at present, it is acceptable to use a dense control material for comparative purposes.

If the most appropriate control material is expected to elicit a tissue response greater than that normally observed with the control materials cited in this section, samples of these latter materials may be implanted as controls to check the surgical technique.

B. Metallic Control Materials

Stainless steel, cobalt-chromium, titanium, and titanium alloys are used to fabricate control specimens. The biological response to these materials has been well characterized by their extensive use in research and clinical practice. (For further information see ISO 5832, parts 1 to 8.)

C. Polymeric and Ceramic Control Materials

Information on nonmetallic control materials is to be found in ASTM F 748, 763, and 981.

D. Implantation as a Method for Other End Points

Implantation studies can also be conducted to evaluate the longer term (sub-chronic and chronic) potential for devices to elicit systemic toxicity, or to evaluate the carcinogenic potential of devices. Uses for these cases are addressed in Chapters 11 and 12.

VIII. LONG-TERM IMPLANT STUDIES

Chapter 11 will address the issues and considerations involved in evaluating the systemic effects of long-term implant devices, and Chapter 12 the case of evaluation of materials for potential carcinogenicity. There are also local tissue and body/implant interactions that must be evaluated (Leninger et al., 1964). The spectrum of interactions can be thought of in the terms presented in Table 9.4.

Such interactions are assessed in long-term studies that may or may not include the eventual retrieval of the implant itself from the host. Retrieval studies seek to study the biological and device-related performance characteristics under actual conditions of use, and to determine the efficacy, reliability, and biocompatibility (safety) of medical devices.

As such, retrieval studies have seven objects.

1. Enhanced patient management
2. Recognition of complications
3. Device design criteria
4. Evaluation of patient/prosthesis matching
5. Elimination of complications
6. Identification of interactions
7. Elucidation of mechanisms of interactions

Implants can fail for any of six different categories of causes.

1. Thrombosis and thromboembolism
2. Device-assisted infection
3. Inappropriate healing
4. Degradation, fracture
5. Adverse local tissue reaction
6. Adverse systemic reaction

TABLE 9.4   Host/Implant Interactions

Effects of implant on host
  Local
    Blood material interactions
      Protein adsorption
      Coagulation
      Fibrinolysis
      Platelet reactions
      Complement activation
    Blood
      Leukocyte reactions
      Hemolysis
    Toxicity
    Derangements of healing
      Encapsulation
      Foreign body reaction
      Pannus formation
    Infection
    Tumorigenesis
  Systemic
    Embolization
      Thrombus
    Hypersensitivity
    Alteration of lymphatic system
Effects of host on implant
  Physical
    Abrasive wear
    Fatigue
    Stress-corrosion
    Degeneration
    Dissolution
  Biological
    Adsorption of tissue substances
    Enzymatic degradation
    Calcification

ASTM standard practice F981-87 ("Standard Practice for Assessment of Compatibility of Biomaterials [Nonporous] for Surgical Implants with Respect to Effect of Materials on Muscle and Bone") provides a framework for evaluating long-term host/implant interactions.

The practice provides a series of experimental protocols for biological assays of tissue reaction to nonporous, nonabsorbable biomaterials for surgical implants. It assesses the effects of the material on animal tissue in which it is implanted. The specified experimental protocol is not designed to provide a comprehensive assessment of the systemic toxicity, carcinogenicity, teratogenicity, or mutagenicity of the material. It applies only to materials with projected applications in human subjects, in which the materials will reside in bone or soft tissue in excess of 30 days and will remain unabsorbed. Applications in other organ systems or tissues may be inappropriate and are therefore excluded. Control materials will consist of any one of the metal alloys in ASRM specifications F67, F75, F90, F136, F138, or F562, or ultra-high-molecular-weight polyethylene as stated in ASTM specification F648 or USP polyethylene negative control.

Referenced ASTM standards include the following:

F67: Specification for Unalloyed Titanium for Surgical Implant Applications*

F75: Specification for Cast Cobalt-Chromium-Molybdenum Alloy for Surgical Implant Applications†

F86: Practice for Surface Preparation and Marking of Metallic Surgical Implants*

F90: Specification for Wrought Cobalt-Chromium-Tungsten-Nickel Alloy for Surgical Implant Applications†

F136: Specification for Wrought Titanium 7A1-4V ELI Alloy for Surgical Implant Applications*

F138: Specification for Stainless Steel Bars and Wire for Surgical Implants (Special Quality)*

F361: Practice for Assessment of Compatibility of Metallic Materials for Surgical Implants with Respect to Effect of Materials on Tissue†

F469: Practice for Assessment of Compatibility of Nonporous Polymeric Materials for Surgical Implants with Regard to Effect of Materials on Tissue‡

F562: Specification for Wrought Cobalt-Nickel-Chromium-Molybdenum Alloys for Surgical Implant Application*

F648: Specification for Ultra-High-Molecular-Weight Polyethylene Powder and Fabricated Form for Surgical Implants*

F673: Practice for Short-Term Screening of Implant Materials*

The practice describes the preparation of implants; the number of implants and test hosts, test sites, exposure schedule, and implant sterilization techniques; and the methods of implant retrieval and tissue examination of each test site. Histological criteria for evaluating tissue reaction are provided. A test protocol

---

* *Annual Book of ASTM Standards*, vol. 13.01.
† Discontinued. See 1986 *Annual Book of ASTM Standards*, vol. 13.01.
‡ Discontinued. See 1987 *Annual Book of ASTM Standards*, vol. 13.01.

for comparing the local tissue response evoked by biomaterials is specified, from which medical implantable devices might ultimately be fabricated, with the local tissue response elicited by control materials currently accepted for the fabrication of surgical devices. Currently accepted materials are the metals, metal alloys, and polyethylene previously specified that are standardized on the basis of acceptable long-term clinical experience. The controls consistently produce cellular reaction and scar to a degree that has been found to be acceptable to the host.

Rats (acceptable strains such as Fischer 344), New Zealand rabbits, and dogs may be used as test hosts for soft tissue implant response. It is suggested that the rats be age- and sex-matched. Rabbits and dogs may be used as test hosts for bone implants.

The sacrospinalis, paralumbar, gluteal muscles, and femur or tibia can serve as the test site for implants. The same site must be used for test and material implants in all the animal species, however.

Table 9.5 contains a suggested minimum number of study animals and a suggested schedule for the necropsy of animals.

Each implant shall be made in a cylindrical shape with hemispherical ends. (See below for sizes.) If the ends are not hemispherical, this must be reported. Each implant shall be fabricated and finished and its surface cleaned in a manner appropriate for its projected application in human subjects in accordance with ASTM practice F86.

Reference metallic specimens shall be fabricated from materials such as the metal alloys in ASTM specifications F67, F75, F90, F138, or F562, or polymeric polyethylene USP negative control plastic.

Suggested sizes and shapes of implants for insertion in muscle are as follows:

For rats 1-mm diameter by 2-cm-long cylindrical implants.
For rabbits 2-mm diameter by 10–15-mm-long cylindrical implants.
For dogs 6-mm diameter by 18-mm-long cylindrical implants.

TABLE 9.5   Intervals of Sacrifice

Necropsy periods (weeks after insertion of implants)	Number of animals to be necropsied		
	Rat	Rabbit	Dog
12 weeks	4	4	2
26 weeks	4	4	2
52 weeks	4	4	2
104 weeks	—	—	2

If fabrication problems prevent preparing specimens 1 mm in diameter, alternative specimen sizes are 2-mm diameter by 6-mm long for rats and 4-mm diameter by 12-mm long for rabbits. If these alternate dimensions are used, they should be reported and such use justified.

Sizes and shapes of implants for insertion in bone are as follows:

For rabbits 2-mm diameter by 6-mm-long cylindrical implants.
For dogs 4-mm diameter by 12-mm-long cylindrical implants.

If the length of the bone implants needs to be less than that designated because of anatomical constraints, it should be reported.

A. Number of Test and Control Implants

Due to size, there should be two implants in each rat: one each for test and control material implant. Due also to size, there should be six implants in each rabbit: four for test materials and two control material implants. In each dog, there should be 12 implants: eight for test materials and four control material implants.

B. Conditioning

Remove all surface contaminants with appropriate solvents and rinse all test and control implants in distilled water prior to sterilization. It is recommended that the implant materials be processed and cleaned in the same way the final product will be; that is, clean, package, and sterilize all implants in the same way as for human implantation.

After final preparation and sterilization, handle the test and control implants with great care to ensure that they are not scratched, damaged, or contaminated in any way prior to insertion.

Report all details of conditioning in accordance with Section VIII.G.3.

C. Implantation Period

Insert all implants into each animal at the same surgical session so that implantation periods run concurrently. The implantation period is 52 weeks for rats and rabbits and 104 weeks for dogs, with interim sacrifices at 12, 26, and 52 weeks. (See Table 9.5.)

1. Implantation (Muscle)

Place material implants in the paravertebral muscles of the adult rats, rabbits, or dogs in such a manner that they are directly in contact with muscle tissue.

Introduce material implants in dogs by the technique of making an implantation site in the muscle by using a hemostat to separate the muscle fibers. Then insert the implant using plastic-tipped forceps or any tool that is nonabrasive to avoid damage to the implant. Do not insert more than 12 implant materials in each dog.

Introduce material implants in rabbits and rats using a sterile technique. Sterile disposable Luer-lock needles may be used to place the material implants into the paravertebral muscles along the spine. In rats insert a negative control implant on one side of the spine and a test material implant on the other. In rabbits implant one negative control material and two test materials on each side of the spine. If larger-diameter specimens are used, an alternative implantation technique such as that described above should be employed.

2. Implantation (Femur)

Expose the lateral cortex of each rabbit femur and drill three holes 1/16 in. (1.6 mm) through the lateral cortex using the technique and instrument appropriate for the procedure. For dogs, make the holes 1/8 inch (3.2 mm) in diameter; make six holes in each femur. Into each one of these holes, insert one of the implants by finger pressure. Then close the wound.

Caution should be taken to minimize the motion of the implant in the tissue on the desired result.

D. Postoperative Care

Care for the animals in accordance with accepted standards as outlined in the *Guide for the Care and Use of Laboratory Animals*. Carefully observe each animal during the period of assay and report any abnormal findings. Infection or injury of the test implant site may invalidate the results. The decision to replace the animal so that the total number of retrieved implants will be as represented in the schedule should be dependent upon the design of the study.

If an animal dies prior to the expected date of sacrifice, necropsy it to determine the cause of death. Replacement of the animal to the study should be dependent upon the design of the study. Include the animal in the assay of data if the cause of death is related to the procedure or the test material.

E. Sacrifice and Implant Retrieval

Euthanize animals by a humane method at the intervals listed in Table 9.5. The necropsy periods start at 12 weeks because it is assumed that acceptable implant data have been received for earlier periods such as 1, 4, and 8 weeks from short-term implant testing.

At necropsy, record any gross abnormalities of color or consistency observed in the tissue surrounding the implant. Remove each implant with an intact envelope of surrounding tissue. Include in the tissue sample a minimum of a 4-mm-thick layer of tissue surrounding the implant. If less than a 4-mm-thick layer is removed, report such as being the case.

F. Postmortem Observations

Necropsy all animals that are sacrificed for the purposes of the assay or that die during the assay period in accordance with standard laboratory practice. Establish the status of the health of the experimental animals during the period of the assay.

G.   Histological Procedure

1.   Tissue Sample Preparation

Prepare two blocks from each implantation site. Process the excised tissue block containing either a test implant or control implant for histopathological examination and such other studies as are appropriate. Cut the sample midway from end to end into the appropriate size for each study. Record the gross appearance of the implant and the tissue. If special stains are deemed necessary, prepare additional tissue blocks or slides (or both) and make appropriate observations.

2.   Histopathological Observations

Compare the amount of tissue reaction adjacent to the test implant to that adjacent to a similar location on the control implant with respect to thickness of scar, presence of inflammatory or other cell types, presence of particles, and such other indications of interaction of tissue and material as might occur with the actual material under test (Pizzoferrato et al., 1988; Rahn et al., 1982). A suggested method for the evaluation of tissue response after implantation can be found in Turner et al. (1973), as summarized in Table 9.6.

   Pathologists may choose to use this scoring system while comparing the negative control to the test material as an aid in their evaluation. The overall toxicity of the test material as compared to the negative control is to be evaluated independently for all time periods. Table 9.7 provides a suggested format for evaluation and scoring.

3.   Report

The final report shall include the following information:

> All details of implant characterization, fabrication, and conditioning (including cleaning, handling, and sterilization techniques employed)
> Procedures for implantation and implant retrieval
> Details of any special procedure (e.g., an unusual or unique diet fed to test animals)
> The observations of each control and test implant as well as the gross appearance of the surrounding tissue in which the implants were inserted
> The observation of each histopathological examination and the pathologist's evaluation as to the toxicity of the test material provided

TABLE 9.6 Suggested Methods for Tissue
Response Evaluation

Number of elements[a]	Score
0	0
1–5	0.5
6–15	1
16–25	2
26 or more	3
Degree of necrosis	
Not present	0
Minimal present	0.5
Mild degree of involvement	1
Moderate degree of involvement	2
Marked degree of involvement	3
Overall toxicity rating of test samples	
Nontoxic	0
Very slight toxic reaction	1
Mild toxic reaction	2
Moderate toxic reaction	3
Marked toxic reaction	4

[a] Cellular elements to be evaluated based upon the number of elements in high power field (470×), average of five fields.

The ASTM standard practice is based on the research techniques utilized by Cohen (1959) and Laing et al. (1967) in the early 1960s. These studies involved the implantation of metal cylinders in the paravertebral muscle of rabbits. The biological reaction to the cylinders was described as the thickness of the fibrous membrane or capsule formed adjacent to the implant. The thickness of the capsule and the presence of inflammatory cells were used as a measure of the degree of adverse reaction to the test material.

As first published in 1972, practice F361 was a test for the biological response to metallic materials. The scope had been expanded beyond that of the published reports to include bone as well as muscle as an implant test site. To avoid species-specific reactions, the method called for the use of rats and dogs as well as rabbits. Cylindrical test specimens with rounded ends were used to avoid biological reactions associated with sharp corners or other variations in specimen shape.

In 1978, practice F469 was published as a parallel document for the test of polymeric materials. In that the methods are essentially the same, the scope

TABLE 9.7 Suggested Evaluation Format and Scoring Range

Animal number	_____				
Duration of implant (weeks)	_____				
Sample description	_____				
Gross response	_____				
Histopath (number)	_____				
Score	0.5	1	2	3	4
Necrosis	_____				
Degeneration	_____				
Inflammation	_____				
Polymorphonuclear leukocytes	_____				
Lymphocytes	_____				
Eosinophils	_____				
Plasma cells	_____				
Macrophages	_____				
Fibrosis	_____				
Giant cells	_____				
Foreign body debris	_____				
Fatty infiltration	_____				
Relative size of involved area (mm)	_____				
Histopathologic toxicity rating	_____				

of F361 has been expanded to include the testing of specimens made of metallic, polymeric, or ceramic materials, thereby including and superseding F469.

Porous or porous-coated materials are specifically excluded since the response to such material includes ingrowth of tissue into the pores. As a result, the method of tissue fixation and sectioning and the evaluation scheme are substantially different.

Stainless steel, cobalt-chromium, and titanium alloys are used as reference materials since the biological response to these materials has been well characterized by their extensive use in research. The response to these materials is not defined as compatible, but rather the response is used as a reference against which reactions to other materials are compared.

This practice is a modification of the original practice F361 in that it only involved long-term test periods. The short-term response to materials is to be evaluated using practice F763. Special methods exist to reduce the impact of relative motion at the implant/tissue interface (Geret et al., 1980a, b).

This practice was revised in 1987 to allow for alternative specimen dimensions for rats and rabbits for muscle implantation. The original specimen dimensions were intended to be implanted through a needle, which was a change from

F361 and F469. The alternate dimensions restore those specified since 1972, which some members felt were more appropriate for some material types.

IX. CONSIDERATIONS

One problem of the implantation tests is a tendency for the strips or prototype implant devices to migrate from their implantation sites, even to subcutaneous positions, and this often prolongs the search for them. The test is nevertheless an effective detection system for toxic ingredients of solid materials that leach in contact with tissue fluid. It is important to recognize the microscopic effects of the standard negative control strips (such as the USP additive-free polyethylene). These reactions are typical of skeletal muscle in contact for a week or more with a foreign body and comprise mild mononuclear cell infiltration, multinucleated giant cell formation, fibroplasia, slight dystrophic calcification, muscle fiber atrophy, and centripetal migration of sarcolemmal nuclei. Traumatic hemorrhage is also common. Positive reactions are similar but more pronounced and additionally include focal necrosis and exudation, particularly of heterophils. These are useful tests, not only for finished products, but also to identify unacceptable changes in formulation or manufacturing processes, such as the introduction of chlorinating cycles to remove bloom on latex catheters. For materials to be utilized in long-term implants, these tests are the only means of accurately predicting long-term tissue and systemic interactions.

The finished state and handling of all components, but particularly metals, in an implant are critical variables, as the primary tissue/implant interactions revolve around surface effects such as the ionization of metals (Ferguson et al., 1960). Such interactions are so predominantly surface interactions (Kordan, 1967) that the surface conditions of an implant, such as porosity and pore size, are critical (Goldhaber, 1961; 1962). The actual site of implantation in the body also influences the nature of the interaction significantly (Kaminski et al., 1968).

REFERENCES

ASTM F748. Practice for Selecting Generic Biological Test Methods for Materials and Devices.

ASTM F763. Practice for Short-Term Screening of Implant Materials.

ASTM F981. Practice for Assessment of Compatibility of Biomaterials for Surgical Implants with Respect to Effect of Materials on Muscle and Bone.

British Standard. (1981a). No. 5736/2, 5736/3 (1981b), 5736/4 (1981c), 5736/5 (1982). British Standards Institution, London.

Cohen, J. (1959). Assay of foreign-body reaction, J. Bone Joint Surg., 41A:152–166.

Ferguson, A. B. Jr., Laing, P. G., and Hodge, E. S. (1960). The ionization of metal implants in living tissues, J. Bone Joint Surg., 42A:77–90.

Gad, S. V. and Chengelis, C. P. (1994). Animal Models in Toxicology, Marcel Dekker, New York.

Geret, V., Rahan, B. A., Mathys, R., Straumann, F., and Perren, S. M. (1980a). In vivo testing of tissue tolerance of implant materials: Improved quantitative evaluation through reduction of relative motion at the implant tissue interface. In: Current Concepts of Internal Fixation of Fracture (H. K. Uhthoff, Ed.). Springer Verlag, New York.

Geret, V., Rahan, B. A., Mathys, R., Straumann, F., and Perren, S. M. (1980b). A method for testing tissue tolerance for improved quantitative evaluation through reduction of relative motion at the implant-tissue interface. In: Evaluation of Biomaterials (G. D. Winter, J. L. Leray, and K. de Groot, Eds.). Wiley, London.

Goldhaber, P. (1961). The influence of pore size on carcinogenicity of subcutaneously implanted millipore filters, Proc. Amer. Assoc. Cancer Res., 3:228.

Goldhaber, P. (1961). Further observations concerning the carcinogenicity of millipore filters, Proc. Amer. Assoc. Cancer Res., 3:323.

Greco, R. S. (1994). Implantation Biology, CRC Press, Boca Raton, FL.

ISO 10993. (1995). Part 6: Tests for Local Effects after Implantation.

Kaminski, E. J., Oblesby, R. J., Wood, N. K., and Sandrik, J. (1968). The behavior of biological materials at different sites of implantation, J. Biomed. Mat. Res., 2:81–88.

Kordan, H. A. (1967). Localized interfacial forces resulting from implanted plastics as possible physical factors involved in tumor formation, J. Theroret. Bio., 17:1–11.

Laing, P. G., Ferguson, A. B. Jr., and Hodge, E. S. (1967). Tissue reaction in rabbit muscle exposed to metallic implants, J. Biomed. Mat. Res., 1:135–149.

Leninger, R. I., Mirkovitch, V., Peters. A., et al. (1964) Change in properties of plastics during implantation, Trans. Amer. Soc. Art. Int. Organs, 10:320–321.

Pizzoferrato, S., Savarino, L., Stea, S., and Tarabusi, C. (1988). Result of histological grading on 100 cases of hip prosthesis failure, Biomaterials, 9:314–318.

Rahn, B. A., Geret, V., Capaul, C., Lardi, M., and Solothurnmann, B. (1982). Morphometric evaluation of tissue reaction to implants using low cost digitizing techniques. In: Clinical Application of Biomaterials (A. J. C. Lee, T. Albrektsson, and P. I. Branemark, Eds.). Wiley, New York.

Turner, J. E., Lawrence, W. H., and Autian J. (1973). Subacute toxicity testing of biomaterials using histopathologic evaluation of rabbit muscle tissue, J. Biomed. Mat. Res., 7:39–58.

USP. (2000). United States Pharmacopoeia XXIV and NF19, U.S. Pharmacopoeia Convention, Washington, DC.

von Recum, A. R. (1998). Handbook of Biomaterials Evaluation, Taylor & Francis, Philadelphia.

10

Genotoxicity

Genotoxicity encompasses all the potential means by which the genetic material of higher organisms may be damaged, with resulting serious consequences. Most forms of genotoxicity are expressions of mutagenicity—the induction of DNA damage and other genetic alterations, ranging from changes in one or a few of DNA bare pairs (gene mutations) to gross changes in chromosomal structure (i.e., chromosomal aberrations) or in chromosome numbers.

It has been known for several hundred years that exposure to particular chemicals or complex mixtures can lead to cancer in later life (Doll, 1977), and it has been postulated more recently that chemicals can also induce heritable changes in man, leading to diseases in the next generation (ICEMC, 1983). There is cumulative evidence that such changes can arise following damage to DNA and resulting mutations (see, e.g., Bridges, 1976; Brusick, 1987), therefore it has become necessary to determine whether widely used chemicals or potentially useful new chemicals possess the ability to damage DNA. In industry, such information may be used to discard a new chemical if a safer alternative can be found, to control or eliminate human exposure for a mutagenic industrial compound, or for a drug, to proceed with development if the benefits clearly outweigh the risks. Data concerning the mutagenicity of a new material have become part of the basic biocompatibility information package. They are needed for decision making and to reduce risks that might otherwise be unforeseen.

TABLE 10.1 ISO Genotoxicity Guidance

Genotoxic effect to be assessed for conformance with ISO 1099-3	Significance of test	Tests meeting requirements
DNA effects	Damage to DNA (deoxyribonucleic acid) by a chemical or material may result in genotoxic effects such as mutations, which in turn may lead to carcinogenicity. Damage to DNA causes the cell to manufacture new DNA to compensate for the loss or damage. This can be assessed by evaluating the formation of newly synthesized DNA.	Unscheduled DNA synthesis.
Gene mutations	Gene mutations (changes in the sequences of DNA that code for critical proteins or functions) have been correlated to carcinogenicity and tumorigenicity.	Ames assay (4 *Salmonella Typhimurium* bacterial strains and *Escherichia coli*) is a reverse mutation assay. A bacterial mutation event causes the bacteria to become histidine-(a vital amino acid) independent. Normal bacteria will not survive in the absence of histidine. Hypoxanthine guanine phosphoribosyl transferase (HGPRT) is a forward mutation assay. Mammalian cells that have been exposed to a mutagen will survive in the presence of a toxic substance (6-Thioguanine).
Chromosomal aberrations	Physical damage to chromosomes (large ordered stretches of DNA in the nuclei of cells) or clastogenicity can lead to DNA damage, in turn leading to abnormal and/or carcinogenic growth of cells.	Chromosomal aberration assay assesses the potential for physical damage to the chromosomes of mammalian cells by a biomaterial.

Note: ISO 10993-3 (ISO, 1993) states that at least three in vitro tests, two of which use mammalian cells, should be used to test for three levels of genotoxic effects: DNA effects, gene mutations, and chromosomal aberrations. ANSI/AAMI/ISO 10993-3 (ISO, 1993) states that "Suitable cell transformation systems may be used for carcinogenicity prescreening."

ISO 10993-3 (ISO, 1993) sets forth clear guidance on testing requirements, as summarized in Table 10.1.

I. DNA STRUCTURE

With the exception of certain viruses, the blueprint for all other organisms is contained in code by deoxyribonucleic acid (DNA), a giant macromolecule whose structure allows a vast amount of information to be stored accurately. We have all arisen from a single cell, the fertilized ovum containing two sets of DNA (packaged with protein to form chromatin), one set from our mother, resident in the nucleus of the unfertilized ovum, the second set from our father, via the successful sperm. Every cell in the adult has arisen from this one cell and (with the exception of the germ cell and specialized liver cells) contains one copy of these original chromosome sets.

The genetic code is composed of four ''letters''—two pyrimidine nitrogenous bases, thymine and cytosine, and two purine bases, guanine and adenine—which can be regarded functionally as arranged in codons (or triplets). Each codon consists of a combination of three letters; therefore, 4^3 (64) different codons are possible. Sixty-one codons code for specific amino acids (three produce stop signals), and as only 20 different amino acids are used to make proteins, one amino acid can be specified by more than one codon.

The bases on one strand are connected together by a sugar (deoxyribose) phosphate backbone. DNA can exist in a single-stranded or double-stranded form. In the latter state, the two strands are held together by hydrogen bonds between the bases. Hydrogen bonds are weak electrostatic forces involving oxygen and nitrogen atoms. As a strict rule, one fundamental to mutagenesis, the adenine bases on one strand always hydrogen bond to the thymine bases on the sister strand. Similarly, guanine bases pair with cytosine bases. Adenine and thymine form two hydrogen bonds, and guanine and cytosine form three.

Double-stranded DNA has a unique property in that it is able to make identical copies of itself when supplied with precursors, relevant enzymes, and cofactors. In simplified terms, two strands begin to unwind and separate as the hydrogen bonds are broken. This produces single-stranded regions. Complementary deoxyribonucleotide triphosphates then pair with the exposed bases under the control of a DNA polymerase enzyme.

A structural gene is a linear sequence of codons that code for a functional polypeptide (i.e., a linear sequence of amino acids). Individual polypeptides may have a structural, enzymatic, or regulatory role in the cell. Although the primary structure of DNA is the same in prokaryotes and eukaryotes, there are differences between the genes of these two types of organisms in internal structure, numbers, and mechanism of replication. In bacteria, there is a single chromosome, normally a closed circle, which is not complexed with protein, and replication does not require specialized cellular structures. In plant and animal cells, there are many chromosomes, each present as two copies, as mentioned earlier, and the DNA is complexed with protein. Replication and cell division require the proteinaceous spindle apparatus. The DNA of eukaryotic cells contains repeated sequences of some genes. Also, unlike prokaryotic genes, eukaryotic genes have noncoding DNA regions called introns between coding regions called exons. This property means that eukaryotic cells have to use an additional processing step at transcription.

A. Transcription

The relationship between the DNA in the nucleus and proteins in the cytoplasm is not direct. The information in the DNA molecule is transmitted to the protein-synthesizing machinery of the cell via another informational nucleic acid, called messenger RNA (mRNA), which is synthesized by an enzyme called RNA polymerase. Although similar to DNA, mRNAs are single-stranded, and possess the base uracil instead of thymine and the sugar ribose rather than deoxyribose. These molecules act as short-lived copies of the genes being expressed.

In eukaryotic cells, the initial mRNA copy contains homologues of both the intron and exon regions. The intron regions are then removed by enzymes located in the nucleus of the cell. Further enzymes splice the exon regions together to form the active mRNA molecules. In both groups of organisms mature mRNA molecules then pass out of the nucleus into the cytoplasm.

B. Translation

The next process is similar in both eukaryotes and prokaryotes, and involves the translation of mRNA molecules into polypeptides. This procedure involves many enzymes and two further types of RNA: transfer RNA (tRNA) and ribosomal RNA (rRNA). There is a specific tRNA for each of the amino acids. These molecules are involved in the transportation and coupling of amino acids into the resulting polypeptide. Each tRNA molecule has two binding sites, one for the specific amino acid, the other containing a triplet of bases (the "anticodon") that are complementary to the appropriate codon on the mRNA.

Ribosomal RNA is complexed with protein to form a subcellular globular organelle called a ribosome. Ribosomes can be regarded as the "reading head" that allows the linear array of mRNA codons each to base-pair with an anticodon of an appropriate incoming tRNA/amino acid complex. The polypeptide chain forms as each tRNA/amino acid comes into register with the RNA codon and with specific sites on the ribosome. A peptide bond is formed between each amino acid as it passes through the reading head of the ribosome (Venitt and Parry, 1984).

C. Gene Regulation

Structural genes are regulated by a special set of codons, in particular "promoter" sequences. The promoter sequence is the initial binding site for RNA polymerase before transcription begins. Different promoter sequences have different affinities for RNA polymerase. Some sets of structural genes with linked functions have a single promoter, and their coordinate expression is controlled by another regulatory gene called an operator. A group of such genes is called an operon. The activity of the operator is further controlled by a protein called a repressor, since it stops the expression of the whole operon by binding to the operator sequence, preventing RNA polymerase from binding to the promoter. Repressors can be removed by relevant chemical signals or in a time-related fashion.

In the ways described above, only the genes required at a given moment are expressed. This not only helps to conserve the energy of the cell, but also is critical for correct cellular differentiation, tissue pattern formation, and formation of the body plan.

D. DNA Repair

All living cells appear to possess several different major DNA repair processes (reviews: Walker, 1984; Rossman and Klein, 1988). Such processes are needed to protect cells from the lethal and mutating effects of heat-induced DNA hydrolysis, ultraviolet light, ionizing radiation, DNA reactive chemicals, free radicals, and so on. In single-celled eukaryotes, such as the yeast *Saccharomyces cerevisiae*, the number of genes known to be involved in DNA repair approaches 100 (Friedberg, 1988). The number in mammalian cells is expected to be at least equal to this and emphasizes the importance of correction of DNA damage.

1. Excision Repair

Some groups of enzymes (light-independent) are apparently organized to act cooperatively to recognize DNA lesions, remove them, and correctly replace the damaged sections of DNA. The most comprehensively studied of these is the excision repair pathway.

Briefly, the pathway can be described as follows:

1. *Preincision reactions.* UVrA protein dimers are formed that bind to the DNA at a location distant from the damaged site. The UVrB protein then binds to the DNA-UVrA complex to produce an energy-requiring topological unwinding of the DNA via DNA gyrase. This area of unwinding is then translocated, again using adenosine triphosphate (ATP) as an energy source, to the site of the damaged DNA.

2. *Incision reactions.* The UVrC protein binds to the DNA-UVrA,B complex and incises the DNA at two sites—seven bases to the 5′ end and three bases to the 3′ end of the damage.

3. *Excision reactions.* UVrD protein and DNA polymerase 1 excise the damaged bases and then resynthesize the strand, using the sister strand as a template. The UVr complex then breaks down, leaving a restored but nicked strand.

4. *Ligation reaction.* The nick in the phosphate backbone is repaired by DNA ligase. A similar excision repair mechanism exists in mammalian cells. (See, e.g., Cleaver, 1983.) In both cases, the process is regarded as error-free and does not lead to the generation of mutations. This pathway can become saturated with excessive numbers of damaged DNA sites, however, forcing the cell to fall back on other repair mechanisms.

2. Error-Prone Repair

Exposure of *E. coli* to agents or conditions that either damage DNA or interfere with DNA replication results in the increased expression of the so-called SOS regulatory network (review: Walker, 1984). Included in this network is a group of at least 17 unlinked DNA damage-inducible (*din*) genes. The *din* gene functions are repressed in undamaged cells by the product of the *lexA* gene (Little and Mount, 1982) and are induced when the lexA protein is cleaved by a process that requires modified RecA protein (RecA*), which then acts as a selective protease (Little, 1984). The *din* genes code for a variety of functions, including filamentation, cessation of respiration, and so forth. Included are the *umuDC* gene products, which are required for so-called error-prone or mutagenic DNA repair (Kato and Shinoura, 1977). The precise biochemical mechanism by which this repair is achieved is still not fully understood. Bacterial polymerase molecules have complex activities, including the ability to ''proofread'' DNA; that is, to ensure that the base-pairing rules of double-stranded DNA are met. It is hypothesized that Umu proteins may suppress this proofreading activity, so that base mismatches are tolerated (Villani et al., 1978). Recent evidence suggests that DNA lesions are bypassed, and this bypass step required UmuDC proteins and RecA* protein (Bridges et al., 1987). The net result is that random base insertion occurs opposite the lesion, which may result in mutation.

Analogues of the *umuDC* genes can be found in locations other than the bacterial chromosome; for example, plasmid pKM101 (Walker and Dobson, 1979), a derivative of the drug resistant plasmid R46 (Mortelmans and Stocker, 1979), which carried *mucAB* genes (Shanabruch and Walker, 1980). (See pp. 879–880.) Mutagenic repair, as controlled by *umuDC*, is not universal even among enterobacteria (Sedgwick and Goodwin, 1985). For instance, *Salmonella typhimurium* LT2 does not appear to express mutagenic repair (Walker, 1984), thus the usefulness of strains of this species is greatly enhanced by using derivatives containing plasmids with genes coding for error-prone repair (MacPhee, 1973; McCann et al., 1975).

3. Mismatch Repair

Mispairs that break the normal base-pairing rules can arise spontaneously due to DNA biosynthetic errors, events associated with genetic recombination, and the deamination of methylated cytosine (review: Modrich, 1987). With the latter, when cytosine deaminates to uracil, an endonuclease enzyme, N-uracil-DNA glycosylase (Lindahl, 1979), excises the uracil residue before it can pair with adenine at the next replication. 5-methyl cytosine, however, deaminates to form thymine and will not be excised by a glycosylase. As a result, thymine exists on one strand paired with guanine on the sister strand (i.e., a mismatch). This will result in a spontaneous point mutation if left unrepaired. For this reason, methylated cytosines form spontaneous mutation "hot spots" (review: Miller, 1985). The cell is able to repair mismatches by being able to distinguish between the DNA strand that exists before replication and a newly synthesized strand.

The mechanism of strand-directed mismatch correction has been demonstrated in *E. coli*. (See, e.g., Wagner and Meselson, 1976.) In this organism, adenine methylation of d(G-A-T-C) sequences determines the strand on which repair occurs. Parental DNA is thus fully methylated, while newly synthesized DNA is undermethylated, for a period sufficient for mismatch correction. By this means the organism preserves the presumed correct sequence (i.e., that present on the original DNA strand) and removes the aberrant base on the newly synthesized strand. Adenine methylation is achieved in *E. coli* by the *dam* methylase, which is dependent on S-adenosylmethionine. Mutants (*dam*) lacking this methylase are hypermutable, as would be expected by this model (Marinus and Morris, 1974).

4. The Adaptive Repair Pathway

The mutagenic and carcinogenic effects of alkylating agents such as ethyl methane sulphonate are due to the generation of O^6-alkylguanine residues in DNA, which result in point mutations. Bacterial and mammalian cells can repair a limited number of such lesions before DNA replication, thus preventing mutagenic and potentially lethal events taking place.

If *E. coli* are exposed to low concentrations of a simple alkylating agent, a repair mechanism is induced that causes increased resistance to subsequent challenge with a high dose. This adaptation response was first described by Samson and Cairns (1977), and has recently been reviewed by Lindahl et al., (1988). The repair pathway is particularly well understood.

5.   Plasmids

Plasmids are extrachromosomal genetic elements that are composed of circular double-stranded DNA. Some can mediate their own transfer from cell to cell in bacteria by conjugation; that is, they contain a set of *tra* genes coding for tubelike structures, such as pili, through which a copy of plasmid DNA can pass during transfer.

Plasmids range in size from 1.5 to 200 million daltons. The number of copies per cell differs from plasmid to plasmid. Copy number relates to control of replication, and this correlates with size; that is, small plasmids tend to have large copy numbers per cell. This may relate to a lack of replication control genes (Mortelmans and Dousman, 1986).

6.   Plasmids and DNA Repair

Many plasmids are known to possess three properties: (1) increased resistance to the bactericidal effects of UV and chemical mutagens; (2) increased spontaneous mutagenesis; and (3) increased susceptibility to UV and chemically induced mutagenesis. Some plasmids possess all three properties; others may possess just one (e.g., increased susceptibility to mutagenesis) (review: Mortelmans and Dousman, 1986). Often the profile of activity depends on the DNA repair status of the host cell (Pinney, 1980). Plasmid pKM101 carries DNA repair genes and has been widely used in strains used in bacterial mutagenicity tests.

E.   Nature of Point Mutations

The word mutation can be applied to point mutations, which are qualitative changes involving one or a few bases in base sequences within genes, as described below, as well as to larger changes involving whole chromosomes (and thus many thousands of genes), and even to changes in whole chromosome sets (described later under cytogenetics).

Point mutations can occur when one base is substituted for another (base substitution). Substitution of another purine for a purine base or of another pyrimidine for pyrimidine is called a transition, while substitutions of purine for pyrimidine or pyrimidine for purine are called transversions. Both types of base substitutions have been identified within mutated genes. These changes lead to a codon change, which can cause the ''wrong'' amino acid to be inserted into the relevant polypeptide, and are known as missense mutations. Such polypeptides may have dramatically altered properties if the new amino acid is close to the active center of an enzyme or affects the three-dimensional makeup of an enzyme or a structural protein. These changes in turn, can lead to a change or reduction in function, which can be detected as a change in phenotype of the affected cells.

A base substitution can also result in the formation of a new inappropriate terminator (or nonsense) codon, and is thus known as a nonsense mutation. The polypeptide formed from such mutated genes will be shorter than normal and is most likely to be inactive. Owing to the redundancy of the genetic code, about a quarter of all possible base substitutions will not result in an amino acid replacement and will be silent mutations.

Bases can be deleted or added to a gene. As each gene is of a precisely defined length, these changes (if they involve a number of bases that are not multiples of 3) result in a change in the "reading frame" of the DNA sequence and are thus known as frameshift mutations. Such mutations tend to have a dramatic effect on the polypeptide of the affected gene, as most amino acids will differ from the point of the insertion or deletion of bases onwards. Very often a new terminator codon is produced, so again short inactive polypeptides will result.

Both types of mutations result in an altered polypeptide, which in turn can have a marked effect on the phenotype of the affected cell. Much use of phenotypic changes is made in mutagenicity tests.

Base substitutions and frameshift changes occur spontaneously and can be induced by radiations and chemical mutagens. It is apparent that the molecular mechanisms resulting in these changes are different in each case, but the potential hazards associated with mutagens capable of inducing the different types of mutations are equivalent.

1. Suppressor Mutations

In some instances a mutation within one gene can be corrected by a second mutational event at a separate site on the chromosome. As a result, the first defect is suppressed and the second mutation is known as a suppressor mutation. Most suppressor mutations have been found to affect genes encoding for RNAs. Usually the mutation causes a change in the sequence of the anticodon of the tRNA, thus if a new terminator or nonsense codon is formed as the first mutation, this can be suppressed by a second mutation forming a tRNA species that now has an anticodon complementary to a termination codon. The new tRNA species thus will supply an amino acid at the terminator site on the mRNA and allow translation to proceed. Surprisingly, most suppressors of this type do not adversely affect cell growth, which implies that the cell can tolerate translation proceeding through termination signals, producing abnormal polypeptides. An alternative explanation is that the particular DNA sequences surrounding normal terminator codons result in a reduced efficiency of suppressor tRNAs (Bossi, 1985).

Frameshift suppression is also possible. This can be achieved by a second mutation in a tRNA gene such that the anticodon of a tRNA molecule consists of four bases rather than three (e.g., an extra C residue in the CCC anticodon sequence of a glycine tRNA gene). This change will allow correction of a +1 frameshift involving the GGG codon for glycine (Bossi, 1985).

2.   Adduct Formation

The earlier discussion of adaptive repair made reference to the fact that some unrepaired alkylated bases are lethal, owing to interference with DNA replication, while others, such as O^6-methylguanine, lead to mutation if unrepaired. These differences indicate that not all DNA adducts (i.e., DNA bases with additional chemical groups not associated with normal DNA physiology) are equivalent. In fact, some adducts appear not to interfere with normal DNA functions or are rapidly repaired. Others are mutagenic, and yet others are lethal. Chemicals that form electrophilic species readily form DNA adducts. These pieces of information are hard-won, and the reader is encouraged to read reviews of the pioneering work of Brooks and Lawley (review: Lawley, 1989) summarizing work identifying the importance of DNA adduct formation with polycyclic hydrocarbons and the importance of "minor" products of base alkylation such as O^6-methylguanine. Also recommended is the work of Miller and Miller, which link the attack of nucleophilic sites in DNA by electrophiles to mutagenesis and carcinogenesis (Miller and Miller, 1971).

   If a DNA adduct involves the nitrogen or oxygen atoms involved in base pairing and the adducted DNA is not repaired, base substitution can result. Adducts can be small, such as the simple addition of methyl or ethyl groups, or they can be very bulky, owing to reaction with multiringed structures. The most vulnerable base is guanine, which can form adducts at several of its atoms (e.g., N^7, C^8, O^6 and exocyclic N^2) (Venitt and Parry, 1984). Adducts can form links between adjacent bases on the same strand (intrastrand cross-links) and can form interstrand cross-links between each strand of double-stranded DNA.

   The induction of frameshift mutation does not necessarily require covalent adduct formation. Some compounds that have a flat, planar structure, such as particular polycyclic hydrocarbons, can intercalate between the DNA strands of the DNA duplex. The intercalated molecules interfere with DNA repair enzymes or replication and cause additions and deletions of base pairs. The precise mechanism is still unclear, although several mechanisms have been proposed. Hot spots for frameshift mutation often involve sections of DNA where there is a run of the same base (e.g., the addition of a guanine to a run of 6 guanine residues). Such information led to a "slipped mispairing" model for frameshift mutation (Streisinger et al., 1966; Roth, 1974). In this scheme single-strand breaks allow one strand to slip and loop out one or more base pairs, the configuration being stabilized by complementary base pairing at the end of the single-stranded region. Subsequent resynthesis results ultimately in additions or deletions of base pairs (Miller, 1985).

3.   Mutations Due to Insertion Sequences

The subject of mutations due to insertion sequences is reviewed in Cullum (1985). Studies of spontaneous mutation in *E. coli* detected a special class of mutations that were strongly polar, reducing the expression of downstream genes (Jordan et al., 1967). These genes mapped as point mutations and reverted like typical point mutations. Unlike point mutations, however, mutagens did not increase their reversion frequency. Further studies showed that these mutations were due to extra pieces of DNA that can be inserted into various places in the genome. They are not just random pieces of DNA but are "insertion sequences" 0.7 to 1.5 kilobases long that can "jump" into other DNA sequences. They are related to transposons, which are insertion sequences carrying easily detected markers such as antibiotic resistance genes and Mu phages (bacterial viruses).

4. The Link Between Mutation and Cancer

The change in cells undergoing normal, controlled cell division and differentiation to cells that are transformed, dividing without check, and are undifferentiated or abnormally differentiated, does not appear to occur as a single step; that is, transformation is multistage. Evidence for this comes from in vitro studies, animal models, and clinical observations—in particular, the long latent period between exposure to a carcinogen and the appearance of a tumor in the target tissue. There is much evidence for the sequence of events shown in Figure 10.1 (tumor initiation, promotion, malignant conversion, and progression). Such a scheme provides a useful working model but clearly does not apply to all "carcinogens" in all circumstances.

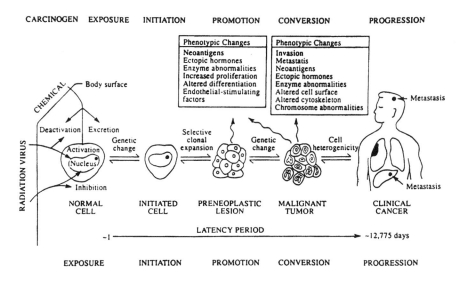

FIGURE 10.1 Schematic representation of events leading to neoplasia. (Adapted from Harris et al., 1987.)

Figure 10.1 shows that there are several points at which genetic change appears to play a role. Such change may occur spontaneously, due to rare errors at cell division such as misreplication of DNA or spindle malfunction, or may be induced by exposure to viruses (e.g., acute transforming retroviruses), ionizing and nonionizing radiations absorbed by DNA (e.g., X rays, UVC), or particular chemical species capable of covalently interacting with either DNA (as discussed earlier) or vital proteins, such as tubulin, that polymerize to form the cell division spindle apparatus.

5. Genotoxic Versus Nongenotoxic Mechanisms of Carcinogenesis

The previous discussions of oncogene activation and human DNA repair deficiencies provide strong evidence for carcinogenesis via genotoxic mechanisms. It has been recognized for many years, however, that cancers can arise without biologically significant direct or indirect interaction between a chemical and cellular DNA. (See, e.g., Gatehouse et al., 1988.) The distinction between nongenotoxic and genotoxic carcinogens has recently been brought into sharper focus following the identification of a comparatively large number of "nongenotoxic" carcinogens by the U.S. National Toxicology Program (Tennant et al., 1987). These include a wide range of chemicals acting via a variety of mechanisms, including augmentation of high "spontaneous" tumor yields, disruption of normal hormonal homeostasis in hormone-responsive tissues, peroxisome proliferation, and proliferation of urothelial cells following damage via induced kidney stones (Clayson, 1989). This author points out that a major effort is under way to determine whether or not many of these compounds can elicit similar effects in humans.

Ashby and Tennant (1988) and Ashby et al. (1989) stress the significance of their observations that 16 tissues are apparently sensitive to genotoxic carcinogens, while a further 13 tissues are sensitive to both genotoxic and nongenotoxic carcinogens (Table 10.2). Also, genotoxic carcinogens tend to induce tumors in several tissues of both males and females in both rats and mice. This contrasts with nongenotoxic carcinogens, which may induce tumors at high doses, in one tissue, of one sex, of one species. Although it is most unlikely that all nongenotoxic carcinogens will prove to be irrelevant in terms of human risk, it appears from the analysis above that a proportion of carcinogens identified by the use of near-toxic levels in rodent bioassays are of dubious relevance to the induction of human cancer. For further discussion, see Butterworth and Slaga (1987).

6. Genetic Damage and Heritable Defects

Concern about the effects of radiation and chemicals on the human gene pool, and the resulting heritable malformations and syndromes, rose steadily during the last century. The recognition that changes in morphology would result from

TABLE 10.2 Tissues Sensitive to Genotoxic and/or
Nongenotoxic Carcinogens

Tissues sensitive primarily to genotoxins	Tissues sensitive to both genotoxins and nongenotoxins
Stomach	Nose
Zymbal gland	Mammary gland
Lung	Pituitary gland
Subcutaneous tissue	Integumentary system
Circulatory system	Kidney
Clitoral gland	Urinary bladder
Skin	Liver
Intestine/colon	Thyroid gland
Uterus	Hematopoietic system
Spleen	Adrenal gland
Tunica vaginalis	Pancreas
Bile duct	Seminal vesicle
Ovary	Urinary tract
Haderian gland	Lymphatic system
Preputial gland	
(Multiple organ sites)	

changes in the hereditary material due to mutations (from the Latin word *mutare*, to change) was adopted by de Vries following observations on the evening primrose, *Oenothera* (de Vries, 1901). Muller went on to demonstrate that X rays could induce mutations in the germ cells of the fruit fly *Drosophila melanogaster* (Muller, 1927).

The human gene pool is known to carry many deleterious genes acquired from preceding generations that result in numerous genetic diseases. It is clear that these arise as a result of DNA changes affecting particular chromosomes or genes. They can be grouped as follows:

1. Chromosome abnormalities, which are small changes in either number or structure.
2. Autosomal dominant gene mutations, in which a change in only one copy of the pair of genes is sufficient for the condition to be expressed.
3. Autosomal recessive gene mutations, in which both copies of a gene must be mutated for the trait to become manifest.
4. Sex-linked conditions, which may also be recessive or dominant, in which the mutant gene is on an X chromosome and will be expressed at high frequency in males (XY) and at a much lower frequency in females (XX) if the gene acts in a recessive manner.

5. Polygenic mutations, in which the condition results from the interaction of several genes and may include an environmental component.

7. Reproductive Effects

If a potent genotoxin is able to cross the placental barrier, it is very likely to interfere with differentiation of the developing embryo and thus possess teratogenic potential. Indeed, many of the better studied teratogens are also mutagenic (Kalter, 1977). Mutagens form only one class of teratogens, and a large proportion of teratogens are not mutagenic, however. Alternative mechanisms of teratogenesis include cell death, mitotic delay, retarded differentiation, vascular insufficiency, and inhibited cell migration (Beckman and Brent, 1986).

It is known that more fetal wastage and many spontaneous abortions arise as a result of the presence of dominant lethal mutations in the developing embryo, many of which appear to be due to major chromosomal damage. In addition, impairment of male fertility is also a consequence of exposure to mutagens.

II. CYTOGENETICS

There are various types of cytogenetic changes that can be detected in chromosomes. These are structural chromosome aberrations (Cas), numerical changes that could result in aneuploidy, and sister chromatid exchanges (SCEs). Chromosome aberration assays are used to detect the induction of chromosome breakage (clastogenesis) in somatic or germinal cells by direct observation of chromosome damage during metaphase analysis, or by indirect observation of micronuclei. Chromosome damage detected in these assays is mostly lethal to the cell during the cell cycle following the induction of the damage. Its presence, however, indicates a potential to induce more subtle chromosome damage that survives cell division to produce heritable cytogenetic changes. Cytogenetic damage is usually accompanied by other genotoxic damage, such as gene mutation.

A. Cytogenetic Damage and Its Consequences

Structural and numerical chromosomal aberrations in somatic cells may be involved in the etiology of neoplasia, and in germ cells can lead to perinatal mortality, dominant lethality, or congenital malformations in the offspring (Chandley, 1981), as well as to some tumors (Anderson, 1990).

Chromosome defects arise at the level of the individual chromosome or at the level of the chromosomal set, thus affecting chromosomal number.

B. Individual Chromosome Damage

Damage to individual chromosomes consists of breakage of chromatids, which must result from a discontinuity of both strands of the DNA in a chromatid. How mutagens produce chromosome breakage is not totally understood, but DNA lesions that are not in themselves discontinuities will produce breakage of a chromosome as a consequence of their interference with the normal process of DNA replication. In haploid micro-organisms and prokaryotes chromosome breaks are usually lethal, but not in diploid eukaryotes. According to Bender et al., (1974), in these organisms chromosome breaks may reconstitute in the same order, probably as a result of an enzyme repair process, resulting in no apparent cytogenetic damage. They may remain unjoined as fragments, which could result in cell death at the next or following mitoses—if, for example, unrejoined fragments are introduced into the zygote via treated germ cells, the embryo may die at a very early stage from a dominant lethal mutation—or they may rejoin in a different order from the original one, producing chromosomal rearrangements. There are various types of chromosomal rearrangements.

Reciprocal translocations can result from the exchange of chromosomal segments between two chromosomes, and depending on the position of the centromeres in the rearranged chromosomes, different configurations will result.

1. Asymmetrical exchanges arise when one of the rearranged chromosomes carries both centromeres and is known as dicentric while the other carries none and is acentric. The cell or zygote carrying this anomaly usually dies, death being caused by segregation difficulties of the dicentric or the loss of the acentric fragment at cell division. Such a translocation contributes to dominant lethality.
2. Symmetrical exchanges occur when each rearranged chromosome carries just one centromere. This allows the zygote to develop normally, but when such heterozygotes form germ cells at meiosis, about half their gametes will be genetically unbalanced, since they have deficiencies and duplications of chromosomal material. The unbalanced gametes that survive produce unbalanced zygotes, resulting either in death shortly before and after birth or congenital malformations.

Centric fusions (Robertsonian translocations) involve the joining together of two chromosomes, each of which has a centromere at or near one end, to produce a single metacentric or submetacentric chromosome. When Robertsonian translocations are produced in a germ cell and result from breakage and rejoining in the short arms of the two chromosomes, a genetic deficiency can result as a consequence of the loss of the derived acentric fragments. Some Robertsonian translocations are able to survive, but others pose a risk. In heterozygotes the two arms of the translocation chromosome may pair with the two separate homologous chromosomes at meiosis but segregate in a disorderly manner. Some of the resultant germ cells lack copies (nullisomy) or carry two copies (disomy) of one of the two chromosomes involved, resulting in monosomic or trisomic embryos. Monosomics die early, but trisomic embryos, which carry three copies of a chromosome, can survive to birth or beyond. If chromosome 21 is involved in the translocation, it can form a translocation trisomy and produce inherited Down's syndrome. (This differs from nondisjunctional Down's syndrome trisomy.)

Deletions and deficiencies are produced when two breaks arise close together in the same chromosome. The two ends of the chromosome join when the fragment between the breaks becomes detached. At the next cell division the unattached piece of chromosome is likely to be lost. Large delections may contribute to dominant lethality. Small delections are difficult to distinguish from point mutations. Deletions may uncover pre-existing recessive genes. If one gene that is essential for survival is uncovered, it can act as a dominant lethal in a homozygote and as a partial dominant in a heterozygote.

Inversions occur when two breaks occur in the same chromosome. The portion between them is detached and becomes reinserted in the opposite way to its original position (i.e., the gene order is reversed). This need not cause a genetic problem, but imbalanced gametes could result in congenital malformation or fetal death.

C. Chromosome Set Damage

Accuracy of chromosome replication and segregation of chromosomes to daughter cells requires accurate maintenance of the chromosome complement of a eukaryotic cell. Chromosome segregation in meiosis and mitosis is dependent upon the synthesis and functioning of the proteins of the spindle apparatus and upon the attachment and movement of chromosomes on the spindle. The kinetochores attach the chromosomes to the spindle and the centrioles are responsible for the polar orientation of the division apparatus. Sometimes such segregation events proceed incorrectly and homologous chromosomes separate, with deviations from the normal number (aneuploidy) into daughter cells or as a multiple of the complete karyotype (polyploidy). When both copies of a particular chromosome move into a daughter cell and the other cell receives none, the event is known as nondisjunction.

Aneuploidy in live births and abortions arises from aneuploid gametes during germ cell meiosis. Trisomy or monosomy of large chromosomes leads to early embryonic death. Trisomy of the smaller chromosomes allows survival but is detrimental to the health of an affected person; for example, Down's syndrome (trisomy 21), Patau syndrome (trisomy 13), and Edward syndrome (trisomy 18). Sex chromosome trisomies (Klinefelter's and XXX syndromes) and the sex chromosome monosomy (XO), known as Turner syndrome, are also compatible with survival.

Aneuploidy in somatic cells is involved in the formation of human tumors. Up to 10% of tumors are monosomic and trisomic for a specific chromosome as the single observable cytogenetic change. Most common among such tumors are trisomy 8, 9, 12, and 21 and monosomy for chromosomes 7, 22, and Y.

D. Test Systems

In vivo and in vitro techniques are available to test mutagenic properties to demonstrate presence or lack of ability of the test material to cause mutation or chromosomal damage or cause cancer, as summarized in Table 10.3. The material intended for intimate contact and long exposure should not have any genotoxic properties. The presence of unpolymerized materials and traces of monomers, oligomers, additives, or biodegration products can cause mutations. Mutation can be a point mutation or chromosomal rearrangement caused by DNA damage, therefore the material's ability to cause point mutation, chromosomal change, or evidence of DNA damage are tested. As we have seen, correlations exist between

TABLE 10.3 Fifteen Common Assays Described by OECD

	In vitro	In vivo
Assays for gene mutations		
Salmonella typhimurium reverse mutation assay (Ames test, bacteria) (OECD 471)	✓	
Escherichia coli reverse mutation assay (bacteria) (OECD 472)	✓	
Gene mutation in mammalian cells in culture (OECD 476)	✓	
Drosophila sex-linked recessive lethal assay (fruit fly) (OECD 477)		✓
Gene mutation in *Saccaromyces cerevisiae* (yeast) (OECD 480)	✓	
Mouse spot test (OECD 484)		✓
Assays for chromosomal and genomic mutations		
In vitro cytogenetic assay (OECD 473)	✓	
In vivo cytogenetic assay (OICD 475)		✓
Micronucleus test (OECD 474)		✓
Dominant lethal assay (OECD 478)		✓
Heritable translocation assay (OECD 485)		✓
Mammalian germ cell cytogenetic assay (OECD 483)		✓
Assays for DNA effects		
DNA damage and repair: unscheduled DNA synthesis in vitro (OECD 482)	✓	
Mitotic recombination in *Saccharomyces cerevisiae* (yeast) (OECD 481)	✓	
In vitro sister chromatid exchange assay (OECD 479)	✓	

mutagenic and carcinogenic properties. Most carcinogens are mutagens, but not all mutagens are human carcinogens.

The Ames salmonella/microsome test is a principal sensitive mutagen screening test. Compounds are tested on the mutants of *Salmonella typhimurium* for reversion from a histidine requirement back to prototrophy. A positive result is seen by the growth of revertant bacteria A microsomal activation system should be included in this assay. The use of all five bacterial test strains are generally required.

Two nonbacterial mutagenicity tests are generally required to support the lack of mutagenic or carcinogenic potential. Some well-known tests include the following:

The L5178Y mouse lymphoma test for mutants at the TK locus
The induction of recessive lethals in *Drosophilia melanogaster*
Metaphase analysis of cultured mammalian cells and of treated animals
Sister chromatid exchange assay
Unscheduled DNA synthesis assay
Cell transformation assay
SOS repair system assay
Gene mutation in cultured mammalian cells such as Chinese hamster V79 cell/HGPRT mutation system.

ISO 10993 specifically requires three genotoxicity assays for all devices. The assays should preferably evaluate DNA effects, gene mutations, and chromosomal aberrations, and two of the assays should preferably use mammalian cells. Guidance for providing tests for selection to meet these needs are the OECD guidelines (OECD, 1983), which include eight in vitro and seven in vivo assays.

E. ISO Test Profile

ISO 10993 Part 3: Tests for Genotoxicity, Carcinogenicity and Reproductive Toxicity (ISO, 1993) suggests that a series of three in vitro assays be conducted, at least two of which should use mammalian cells as a target. The tests should address the three types of genotoxic effects: (1) gene mutations, (2) chromosomal and genomic aberrations, and (3) DNA effects. Three tests that are recommended are shown in Table 10.4. (Note that none of the three recommended tests assays for DNA effects!) In ISO's opinion, a profile of three in vitro genotoxicity tests is considered sufficient to establish safety for most medical devices; in vivo testing need only be done if in vitro tests are positive.

F. ICH Test Profile

The International Conference on Harmonization recommends a rather different profile of genotoxicity tests for drugs. (See Table 10.5.) It wants to see an in vivo test conducted as part of the evaluation.

TABLE 10.4   Genotoxicity Tests Recommended by ISO

Test	Mutation	Cell type	Method
Salmonella reverse mutation assay (OECD 471)	Gene	Bacterial	In vitro
In vitro cytogenetic assay (OECD 473)	Chromosome	Mammalian	In vitro
Gene mutation in mammalian cells (OECD 476)	Gene	Mammalian	In vitro

G. In Vitro Test Systems

The principal tests can be broadly categorized into microbial and mammalian cell assays. In both cases the tests are carried out in the presence and absence of in vitro metabolic activation enzymes, usually derived from rodent liver.

1. In Vitro Metabolic Activation

The target cells for in vitro mutagenicity tests often possess a limited (often overlooked) capacity for endogenous metabolism of xenobiotics. To simulate the complexity of metabolic events that occur in the whole animal, however, there is a critical need to supplement this activity.

2. Choice of Species

A bewildering variety of exogenous systems have been used for one purpose or another in mutagenicity tests. The choice begins with plant or animal preparations. The attraction of plant systems has stemmed from a desire to avoid the use of animals where possible in toxicity testing. In addition, plant systems have particular relevance when certain chemicals are being tested (e.g., herbicides).

If animal systems are chosen, preparations derived from fish (see, e.g., Kada, 1981) and birds (Parry et al., 1985) have been used. By far the most widely used and validated are those derived from rodents, however—in particular, the rat. Hamsters may be preferred as a source of metabolizing enzymes when partic-

TABLE 10.5   Genotoxicity Tests Recommended by ICH

Genotoxicity test—ICH	Mutation	Cell type	Method
A test for gene mutation in bacteria	Gene	Bacterial	In vitro
In vitro cytogenetic assay using mouse lymphomas tk cells	Chromosome	Mammalian	In vitro
In vivo test for chromosomal damage using rodent hematopoietic cells	Gene	Mammalian	In vivo

ular chemical classes are being screened (e.g., aromatic amines, heterocyclic amines, N-nitrosamines and azo dyes) (Prival and Mitchell, 1982; Haworth et al., 1983).

3. Choice of Tissue

The next choice is that of source tissue. Preparations derived from liver are the most useful, as this tissue is a rich source of mixed-function oxygenases capable of converting procarcinogens to genetically active electrophiles. Many extrahepatic tissues (e.g., kidney, lung), however, are also known to possess an important metabolic capacity, which may be relevant to the production of mutagenic metabolites in the whole animal.

4. Cell-Free Versus Cell-Based Systems

Most use has been made of cell-free systems—in particular, crude homogenates such as 9000-gram supernatant (S9 fraction) from rat liver. This fraction is composed of free endoplasmic reticulum, microsomes (membrane-bound packets of ''membrane-associated'' enzymes), soluble enzymes, and some cofactors. Hepatic S9 fractions do not necessarily completely reflect the metabolism of the whole organ in that they mainly possess phase I metabolism (e.g., oxygenases) and are deficient in phase II systems (e.g., conjugation enzymes). The latter are often capable of efficient detoxification, while the former are regarded as ''activating.'' This can be a strength, in that S9 fractions are used in screening tests as a surrogate for all tissues in an animal, some of which may be exposed to reactive metabolites in the absence of efficient detoxification. Many carcinogens are organ-specific in extrahepatic tissues, yet liver S9 fraction will reveal their mutagenicity. The deficiency of S9 fractions for detoxification can also be a weakness, in that detoxification may predominate in the whole animal in such a way that the potential carcinogenicity revealed in vitro is not realized in vivo.

When supplemented with relevant cofactors, cell-free systems are remarkably proficient, despite their crudity in generating reactive electrophiles from most procarcinogens. They provide at best a broad approximation of in vivo metabolism, however, and can either fail to produce a sufficient quantity of a particular reactive metabolite to be detectable by the indicator cells or produce inappropriate metabolites that do not play a role in vivo. (See Gatehouse and Tweats, 1987, for a discussion.)

Some of these problems can be overcome by the use of cell-based systems—in particular, primary hepatocytes. Hepatocytes closely simulate the metabolic systems found in the intact liver and do not require additional cofactors for optimal enzyme activity. Apart from greater technical difficulties in obtaining hepatocytes as opposed to S9 fraction, however, hepatocytes can effectively detoxify particular carcinogens and prevent their detection as mutagens. Despite these difficulties, hepatocytes have a role to play in mutagenicity screening, in both bacterial and mammalian-based systems (Tweats and Gatehouse, 1988).

5. Inducing Agents

The final choice considered here is whether to use "uninduced" liver preparations or those derived from animals pretreated with an enzyme inducer to promote high levels of metabolic activity. If induced preparations are preferred, which inducer should be used?

It appears that uninduced preparations are of limited use in screening assays, as they are deficient in particular important activities, such as cytochrome P-450$_{IA1}$ cytochrome oxygenases. In addition, species and organ differences are most divergent with uninduced enzyme preparations (Brusick, 1987).

The above differences disappear when induced microsomal preparations are used. A number of enzyme inducers have been used, the most popular being Aroclor 1254, which is a mixture of polychlorinated bipheynyls (as described by Ames et al., 1975). Concern about the toxicity, carcinogenicity, and persistence of these compounds in the environment, however, has led to the use of alternatives, such as a combination of phenobarbitone (phenobarbital) and β-naphthoflavone (5,6-benzoflavone). This combination results in the induction of a range of mono-oxygenases similar to that induced by Aroclor 1254. (See, e.g., Ong et al., 1980.) More selective inducers such as phenobarbitone (cytochrome P-450$_{IIa1}$, P-450$_{IIB1}$) or 3-methylcholanthrene (cytochrome P-450$_{IA1}$) have also been used.

In summary, genetic toxicity tests with both bacterial and mammalian cells are normally carried out with rat liver cell-free systems (S9 fraction) from animals pretreated with enzyme inducers. Investigations should not slavishly follow this regimen, however; there may be sound scientifically based reasons for using preparations from different species or different organs or for using whole cells such as hepatocytes.

6. Standard Method of S9 Fraction Preparation

The following method describes the production of hepatic S9 mix from rats induced with a combination of phenobarbitone and β-naphthoflavone, and is an adaptation of the method described by Gatehouse and Delow (1979).

Male albino rats within the weight range from 150 to 250 grams are treated with phenobarbitone sodium 16 mg ml^{-1}, 2.5 ml kg^{-1} in sterile saline, and β-naphthoflavone 20 mg ml^{-1} in corn oil. A fine suspension of the latter is achieved by sonicating for 1 hr. These solutions are dosed by intraperitoneal injection on days 1, 2, and 3.

Phenobarbitone sodium is normally administered between 0.5 and 2 hr prior to β-naphthoflavone.

The animals are killed on day 4 by cervical dislocation and the livers removed as quickly as possible and placed on ice-cold KCl buffer (0.01M Na_2HPO_4 + KCl 1.15%). The liver is cleaned, weighed, minced, and homogenized (in an Ultra Turrx homogenizer) in the above buffer to give a 25% (w/v) liver homogenate. The homogenate is stored at 4°C until it can be centrifuged at 9000 grams for 15 min. The supernatant is decanted, mixed, and divided into 2-ml volumes in cryotubes. These are then snap-frozen in liquid nitrogen. Storage at −196°C for up to 3 months results in no appreciable loss of most P-450 isoenzymes (Ashwood-Smith, 1980).

Quality control of S9 batches is usually monitored by the ability to activate compounds known to require metabolism to generate mutagenic metabolites. This is a rather crude approach, and more accurate data can be obtained by measuring biochemical parameters; for example, protein, cytochrome P-450 total activity (from crude S9), and related enzyme activities (from purified microsomes), such as 7-ethoxyresorufin-*O*-deethylase and 7-methoxycoumarin-*O*-demethylase, to give an indication of S9 batch-to-batch variation and to set standards for rejecting suboptimal batches (Hubbard et al., 1985). For further details on critical features affecting the use and limitations of the S9 fraction, see Gatehouse and Tweats (1987).

7. S9 Mix

The S9 fraction prepared as described above is used as a component in S9 mix, along with buffers and various enzyme cofactors. The amount of S9 fraction in the S9 mix can be varied, but a "standard" level of 0.1 ml ml^{-1} of S9 mix (or 10% S9) is often recommended for general screening.

No single concentration of S9 fraction in the S9 mix will detect all classes of genotoxic carcinogens with equal efficiency (Gatehouse et al., 1990). Some mutagens, including many polycyclic aromatic hydrocarbons, are activated to mutagens by higher than normal levels of S9 fraction in the S9 mix. (See, e.g., Carver et al., 1985.)

The mixed-function oxidases in the S9 fraction require NADPH, normally generated from the action of glucose-6-phosphate dehydrogenase acting on glucose-6-phosphate and reducing NADP, both of which are normally supplied as cofactors. As an alternative, isocitrate can be substituted for glucose-6-phosphate (to be used as a substrate by isocitrate dehydrogenase) (Linblad and Jackim, 1982). Additional cofactors may be added (e.g., flavin mononucleotide), when particular classes of compounds such as azo dyes are being tested (Prival et al., 1984), or acetyl coenzyme A when aromatic amines such as benzidine are being tested (Kennelly et al., 1984).

The composition of a standard S9 mix is given in Table 10.6.

TABLE 10.6   Composition of Standard S9 Mix

Constituent	Final concentration in mix (mM)
Glucose-6-phosphate	5
Nicotinamide adenine dinucleotide phosphate	4
$MgCl_2 6H_2O$ ⎤	8
⎬ Salt solution	
KCl ⎦	33
Phosphate buffer (90.2 mM)	100
Distilled water to make up to the required volume	
S9 fraction added at 0.1 ml per ml of S9 mix	

Note: For assays using cultured mammalian cells, phosphate buffer and distilled water are replaced by tissue culture medium, as high concentrations of Na and K salts are toxic to such cells. The concentration of S9 fraction in the S9 mix varies, depending on the relevant assay. (See individual sections). Once prepared, S9 mix should be used as soon as possible, and should be stored on ice until required. Once thawed, S9 fraction should not be refrozen for future use.

H.   Bacterial Mutation Tests

The study of mutation in bacteria (and bacterial viruses) had a fundamental role in the science of genetics in the twentieth century. In particular, the unraveling of biochemical anabolic and catabolic pathways, the identification of DNA as the hereditary material, the fine structure of the gene, the nature of gene regulation, and so on, have all been aided by bacterial mutants.

As an offshoot of studies of genes concerned with the biosynthesis of amino acids, a range of *E. coli* (see, e.g., Yanofsky, 1971) and *Salmonella typhimurium* strains (see, e.g., Ames, 1971) with relatively well-defined mutations in known genes became available. Bacteria already mutant at an easily detectable locus are thus treated with a range of doses of the test material to determine whether the compound can induce a second mutation that directly reverses or suppresses the original mutations. For amino acid auxotrophs, the original mutation has thus resulted in a loss of ability to grow in the absence of the required amino acid. The second mutation restores prototrophy; that is, the affected cell is now able to grow in the absence of the relevant amino acid if provided with inorganic salts and a carbon source. This simple concept, in fact, underlines the great strength of these assays, for it provides enormous selective power that can identify a small number of the chosen mutants from a population of millions of unmutated cells and cells mutated in other genes. The genetic target (i.e., the mutated DNA bases in the gene in question or bases in the relevant tRNA genes; see the discussion of suppressor mutations) can thus be very small, just one or a few bases in length.

An alternative approach is to use bacteria to detect "forward mutations." Genetic systems detect forward mutations have an apparent advantage in that a wide variety of genetic changes may lead to a forward mutation (e.g., point mutation, deletions, insertions). In addition, forward mutations in a number of different genes may lead to the same change in phenotype; thus, the genetic target is much larger than that seen in most reverse mutation assays. If a particular mutagen causes rare specific changes, however, these changes may be lost against the background of more common events (Gatehouse et al., 1990). Spontaneous mutation rates tend to be relatively high in forward mutation systems. Acquisition of resistance to a toxic chemical (e.g., an amino acid analogue or antibiotic) is a frequently used genetic marker in these systems. For instance, the use of resistance to the antibiotic streptomycin preceded the reversion assays in common use today.

1. Reversion Tests: Background

There are several excellent references describing the background and use of bacteria for reversion tests (Brusick, 1987; Gatehouse et al., 1990). Three different protocols have been widely used: plate incorporation assays, treat and plate tests, and fluctuation tests. These methods are described in detail in the following sections. Fundamental to the operation of these tests is the genetic composition of the tester strains selected for use.

2. Genetic Makeup of Tester Strains

The most widely used strains are those developed by Bruce Ames and colleagues, which are mutant derivatives of the organism *Salmonella typhimurium*. Each strain carries one of a number of mutations in the operon coding for histidine biosynthesis. In each case the mutation can be reverted either by base change or by frameshift mutations. The genotype of the commonly used strains is shown in Table 10.7.

3. The Use of the Plasmid pKM101

Salmonella typhimurium LT2 strains do not appear to possess classic "error-prone" repair as found in *E. coli* strains and some other members of the Enterobacteria (Walker, 1984; Sedgwick and Goodwin, 1985). This is due to a deficiency in *umuD* activity in these *Salmonella* strains (Herrera et al., 1988; Thomas and Sedgwick, 1989). One way to overcome this deficiency and to increase sensitivity to mutagens is to use strains containing plasmid-carrying analogues to the *umu DC* genes.

TABLE 10.7 Genotype of Commonly Used Strains of *Salmonella typhimurium* LT2 and Their Reversion Events

Strain	Genotype	Reversion events
TA1535	hisG$_{46}$ rfa f gal chlD bio uvrB	Subset of base-pair substitution events
TA100	hisG$_{46}$ frfa gal chlD bio uvrB (pKM101)	Subset of base-pair substitution events
TA1537	hisC$_{3076}$ frfa gal chlD bio uvrB	Frameshifts
TA1538	hisD$_{3052}$ frfa gal chlD bio uvrB	Frameshifts
TA98	hisD$_{3052}$ frfa gal chlD bio uvrB (pKM101)	Frameshifts
TA97	hisD$_{6610}$ hisO$_{1242}$ rfa f gal chl^D bio uvrB (pKM101)	Frameshifts
TA102	his$f$ (G)$_{8476}$ rfa galE (pAQ1) (pKM101)	All possible transitions and transversions; small deletions

4. *E. coli* Tester Strains

Ames and colleagues have made an impressive contribution to mutagenicity testing by the development of the *Salmonella*/microsome test, and in particular, its application in the study of environmental mutagens. In genetic terms, *Salmonella* strains are in some ways not the best choice. (See, e.g., Venitt and Croften-Sleigh, 1981.) Unlike the *Salmonella* strains, *E. coli* B strains such as the WP2 series developed by Bridges, Green, and colleagues (Bridges, 1972; Green and Muriel, 1976), possess the *umuDC*$^+$ genes involved in generating mutations; they are also partly rough and thus allow many large molecules to enter the cell.

In addition to being effective general strains for mutagen detection, studies by Wilcox et al. (1990) have shown that a combination of *E. coli* WP2 *trpE* (pKM101), which has a functioning excision repair system for the detection of cross-linking agents, and *E. coli* WP2 *trp E uvrA* (pKM101) can be used as alternatives to *Salmonella* TA102 for the detection of oxidative mutagens. The *E. coli* strains have the advantage of lower spontaneous mutation rates and are somewhat less difficult to use and maintain.

5. Storage and Checking of Tester Strains

Detailed instructions for maintenance and confirmation of the phenotypes of the various tester strains are given in Maron and Ames (1983) and Gatehouse et al. (1990). Permanent master cultures of tester strains should be stored in liquid nitrogen or in dry ice. Such cultures are prepared from fresh nutrient broth cultures, to which DMSO is added as a cryopreservative. These cultures are checked for the various characteristics before storage as described below. Cultures for use in individual experiments should be set up by inoculation from the master culture or from a plate made directly from the master culture, not by passage from a previously used culture. Passage in this way will inevitably increase the number of pre-existing mutants, leading to unacceptably high spontaneous mutation rates (Gatehouse et al., 1990).

The following characteristics of the tester strains should be confirmed at monthly intervals or if the internal controls of a particular experiment fail to meet the required limits, including the following:

Amino acid requirement.
Sensitivity to the lethal effects of the high-molecular-weight dye crystal violet for those strains carrying the *rfaE* mutation.
Increased sensitivity to UV irradiation for those strains carrying the *uvrA* or *uvrB* mutations.
Resistance to ampicillin for strains carrying pKM101 and resistance to tetracycline for strains carrying pAQ1.
Sensitivity to diagnostic mutagens. This can be measured very satisfactorily be testing pairs of strains—one giving a strongly positive response, the partner a weak response.

The importance of these checks, together with careful experiment-to-experiment controls of spontaneous mutation rates and response to both reference mutation rates and response to both reference mutagens cannot be overstressed; failure to apply them can result in much wasted effort.

I. Plate Incorporation Assay

1. Protocol for Dose Ranging and Selection

Before carrying out the main tests, it is necessary to carry out a preliminary toxicity dose-ranging test. This should be carried out following the same basic protocol as the mutation test, except that instead of scoring the number of mutants on, for example, minimal media plates with limiting amounts of a required amino acid, the number of survivors is scored on fully supplemented minimal media. A typical protocol is as follows:

1. Prepare a stock solution of the test compound at a concentration of 50 mg/ml^{-1} in an appropriate solvent. It may be necessary to prepare a lower concentration of stock solution, depending on the solubility of the test compound.
2. Make dilutions of the stock solution.
3. To 2.0 ml aliquots of soft agar overlay medium (0.6% agar and 0.5% sodium chloride in distilled water) containing a trace of histidine and

excess biotin and maintained at 45°C in a dry block, add 100 μl at a solution of the test article. Use only one plate per dilution.

4. Mix and pour onto dried Vogel and Bonner minimal medium plates as in an Ames test, including an untreated control and a solvent control, if necessary. The final concentrations of test compound will be 5000, 1500, 500, 150, and 50 μg plate^{-1}.

5. Repeat step 3, using 0.5 ml of 8% S9 mix per 2.0 ml aliquot of soft agar in addition to the test compound and tester strain. The S9 mix is kept on ice during the experiment.

6. Incubate the plates for 2 days at 37°C and examine the background lawn of growth with a microscope (×8 eyepiece lens, ×10 objective lens). The lowest concentration giving a depleted background lawn is regarded as a toxic dose.

This test will also demonstrate excess growth, which may indicate the presence of histidine or tryptophan or their precursors in the test material, which could make testing for mutagenicity impracticable by this method.

When setting the maximum test concentration, it is important to test into the mg plate^{-1} range where possible (Gatehouse et al., 1990), as some mutagens are only detectable when tested at high concentrations. For nontoxic, soluble mutagens, however, an upper limit of 5 mg plate^{-1} is recommended (DeSerres and Shelby, 1979). For less soluble compounds at least one dose exhibiting precipitation should be included.

2. Ames Salmonella/Plate Incorporation Method

The following procedure is based on that described by Ames and colleagues (Maron and Ames, 1983), with additional modifications.

1. Each selected test strain is grown for 10 hr at 37°C in nutrient broth (oxoid no. 2) or supplemented minimal media (Vogel–Bonner) on an orbital shaker. A timing device can be used to ensure that cultures are ready at the beginning of the working day.

2. 2.0 ml aliquots of soft agar overlay medium are melted just prior to use and cooled to 50°C, and relevant supplements added (i.e., L-histidine, final concentration 9.55 μg ml^{-1}, and D-biotin, 12 μg ml^{-1}). (N.B.: If E. coli WP2 tester strains are used, the only supplement required is tryptophan 3.6 μg ml^{-1}.) The medium is kept semimolten by holding the tubes containing the medium in a hot aluminum dry block held at 45°C. It is best to avoid water baths, as microbial contamination can cause problems.

3. The following additions are made to each tube of top agar: the test article (or solvent control) in solution (10–200 μl), the test strain (100 μl), and where necessary, S9 mix (500 μl). The test is carried out in

the presence and absence of S9 mix. The exact volume of test article or solvent may depend on toxicity or solubility, as described in the preceding section.

4. There should be at least three replicate plates per treatment with at least five test doses plus untreated controls. Duplicate plates are sufficient for the positive and sterility control treatments. The use of twice as many negative control plates as used in each treatment group will lead to more powerful tests from a statistical standpoint (Mahon et al., 1989).

5. Each tube of top agar is mixed and quickly poured onto dried prelabeled Vogel–Bonner basal agar plates.

6. The soft agar is allowed to set at room temperature and the plates are inverted and incubated (within 1 hr of pouring) at 37°C in the dark. Incubation is continued for 2 to 3 days.

7. Before scoring the plates for revertant colonies, the presence of a light background lawn of growth (due to limited growth of nonrevertant colonies before the trace of histidine or tryptophan is exhausted) should be confirmed for each concentration of test article by examination of the plate under low power of a light microscope. At concentrations that are toxic to the test strains, such a lawn will be deplated and colonies may appear that are not true revertants but surviving, nonprototrophic cells. If necessary, the phenotype of any questionable colonies (pseudo-revertants) should be checked by plating on histidine or tryptophan-free medium.

8. Revertant colonies can be counted by hand or with an automatic colony counter. Such machines are relatively accurate in the range of colonies normally observed (although calibration against manual counts is a wise precaution). Where accurate quantitative counts of plates with large numbers of colonies are required, only manual counts will give accurate results.

J. Controls

1. Positive Controls

Where possible, positive controls should be chosen that are structurally related to the test article. This increases the confidence in the results. In the absence of structurally related mutagens, the set of positive controls given in Table 10.8 can be used. The use of such controls validates each test run and helps to confirm the nature of each strain. Pagano and Zeger (1985) have shown that it is possible to store stock solutions of most routinely used positive controls (sodium azide, 2-aminoanthracene, benzo[a]phyene, 4-nitroquinoline oxide) at −20°C to −80°C

TABLE 10.8 Positive Controls for Use in Plate Incorporation Assays

Species	Strain	Mutagen	Concentration (µg plate^{-1})
In the absence of S9 mix			
S. typhimurium	TA1535 TA100	Sodium azide	1–5
	TA1538 TA98	Hycanthone methane sulphonate	5–20
	TA1537	ICR 191	1
E. coli	WP2 uvrA	Nifuroxime	5–15
In the presence of S9 mix			
E. coli	WP2 uvrA (pKM101)		
S. typrhimurium	TA1538 TA1535 TA100 TA90	2-Aminoanthracene	1–10
	TA1537	Neutral red	10–20

Note: The concentrations given above will give relatively small increases in revertant count above the spontaneous level. There is little point in using large concentrations of reference mutagens which invariably give huge increases in revertant counts. This would give little information on the day-to-day performance of the assay.

for several months without any loss of activity. This measure can help reduce potential exposure to laboratory personnel.

2. Untreated/Vehicle Controls

Untreated controls omit the test article, but are made up to volume with buffer. The vehicle control is made up to volume with the solvent used to dissolve the test substance. It is preferable to ensure that each of the treated plates contains the same volume of vehicle throughout.

As detailed by Gatehouse and Tweats (1987), the nature and concentration of solvent may have a marked effect on the test result. Dimethysolphoxide is often used as the solvent of choice for hydrophibic compounds. There may be unforeseen effects, however, such as an increase in the mutagenicity of some compounds (e.g., p-phenylenediamne) (Burnett et al., 1982) or a decrease in the mutagenicity of others, such as simple aliphatic nitrosqamines (Yahagi et al.,

1977). It is essential to use fresh batches of the highest purity grade available and to prevent decomposition/oxidation on storage. The products after such processes as oxidation are toxic and can induce base-pair substitutions in both bacterial and mammalian assays. Finally, DMSO and other organic solvents can inhibit the oxidation of different premutagens by microsomal mono-oxygenases (Wolff, 1977a,b). To reduce the risk of artifactual results, it is essential to use the minimum amount of organic solvent (e.g., <2% w/w) compatible with adequate testing of the test chemical.

It is important to keep a careful check of the number of mutant colonies present on untreated or vehicle control plates. These numbers depend on the following factors:

1. The repair status of the cell (i.e., excision repair-deficient strains tend to have more "spontaneous mutants" than repair-proficient cells).
2. The presence of mutator plasmids. Excision-deficient strains containing pKM101 have a higher spontaneous mutation rate at both base substitution and frameshift loci than excision-proficient strains.
3. The total number of cell divisions that take place in the cells in the supplemented top agar. This is controlled by the supply of nutrients— in particular, histidine. Rat liver extracts may also supply trace amounts of limiting nutrients, resulting in a slight increase in the spontaneous yield of mutants in the presence of S9 mix.
4. The size of the initial inoculum. During growth of the starting culture, mutants will arise, thus if a larger starting inoculum is used, more of these pre-existing mutants will be present per plate. In fact, the "plate mutants" arising as described in point 3 predominate.
5. The intrinsic mutability of the mutation in question. In practice the control mutation values tend to fall within a relatively precise range for each strain. Each laboratory should determine the normal range of revertant colonies per plate for each strain.

Deviations in background reversion counts from the normal range should be investigated. It is possible that cross-contamination, variations in media quality, and so forth have occurred that may invalidate particular experiments.

Frequent checks should also be made on the sterility of S9 preparations, media, and test articles. These simple precautions can prevent the loss of valuable time and resources.

3. Evaluation of Results

At least two independent assays are carried out for each test article. The criterion for a positive response is a reproducible and statistically significant result at any concentration for any strain. When positive results are obtained, the test is repeated, using the strain(s) and concentration range within which the initial posi-tive results were observed. This range may be quite narrow for toxic agents.

Several statistical approaches have been applied to the results of plate incor-poration assays (review: Mahon et al. 1989). These authors make a number of important suggestions to maximize the power of statistical analyses; those that relate to the method of analysis are reproduced below.

1. Unless it is obvious that the test agent has had no effect, the data should be plotted to give a visual impression of the form of any dose response and the pattern of variability.
2. Three methods of analysis—linear regression (see, e.g., Steel and Tor-rie, 1960); a multiple comparison analysis, Dunnett's method (Dunnett, 1955); and a nonparametric analysis, Wahrendorf's method (Wahrend-orf et al., 1985)—can all be recommended. Each has its strengths and weaknesses, and other methods are not excluded.
3. Linear regression assumes that variance across doses is constant and that the dose response is linear. If the variance is not approximately constant, then a transformation may be applied or a weighted analysis may be carried out. If the dose scale tends to plateau, then it may be transformed. If counts decline markedly at high doses, then linear regression is inappropriate.
4. Dunnett's method, perhaps with a transformation, is recommended when counts decline markedly at one or two high doses. When the dose response shows no such decline, however, other methods may be more powerful.
5. Wahrendorf's nonparametric method avoids the complications of transformations of weighting and is about as powerful as any other method. It is inappropriate when the response declines markedly at a high dose, however.

4. Preincubation Tests

Some mutagens are poorly detected in the standard plate incorporation assay, particularly those that are metabolized to short-lived reactive electrophiles (e.g., short-chain aliphatic *N*-nitroso compounds) (Bartsch et. al., 1976). It is also possi-ble that some metabolites may bind to components within the agar. Such com-pounds can be detected by using a preincubation method first described by Yahagi et al. (1975) in which the bacteria, test compound, and S9 mix are incubated together in a small volume at 37°C for a short period (30–60 min) before adding the soft agar and pouring as for the standard assay. In this variation of the test, during the preincubation step the test compound, S9 mix, and bacteria are incu-bated in liquid at higher concentrations than in the standard test, and this may account for the increased sensitivity with relevant mutagens. In the standard method the soluble enzymes in the S9 mix, cofactors, and the test agent may diffuse into the bottom agar. This can interfere with the detection of some mutagens—a problem that is overcome in the preincubation method (Forster et al., 1980; Gatehouse and Wedd, 1984).

The test is carried out as follows:

1. The strains are cultured overnight, and the inocula and S9 mix are prepared as in the standard Ames test.
2. The soft agar overlays are prepared and maintained at 45°C prior to use.
3. To each of three to five tubes maintained at 37°C in a Driblock are added 0.5 ml of S9 mix, 0.1 ml of the tester strain (10–18 hr culture), and a suitable volume of the test compound, to yield the desired range of concentrations. The S9 mix is kept on ice prior to use.
4. The reaction mixtures are incubated for use to 1 hr at 37°C.
5. 2.0 ml of soft agar is added to each tube. After mixing, the agar and reaction mixture are poured onto previously labeled dried Vogel–Bonner plates.
6. Once the agar has set, the plates are incubated for 2 to 3 days before revertant colonies are scored.

The use of controls is as described for the plate incorporation assay. It is crucial to use the minimum amount of organic solvent in this assay, as the total volume of the incubation mixture is small relative to the solvent component.

This procedure can be modified to provide optimum conditions for particular chemical classes. For instance, preincubation times greater than 60 min plus aeration have been found necessary in the detection of allyl compounds (Neudecker and Henschler, 1985).

5. Forward Mutation Tests

Forward mutation is an end point that may arise from various events, including base substitutions, frameshifts, and DNA deletions, as mentioned earlier.

Although bacterial forward mutation systems have not gained the popularity of reverse mutation tests (owing in part to lower sensitivity to some mutagens and lack of specificity), they have proved useful on occasion and have their supporters.

Several forward mutation tests have been devised, and a brief mention of two of the more widely used systems is provided below.

The Ara Forward Mutation Test.   The L-arabinose resistance test with *Salmonella typhimurium* is based on *araD* mutants of the L-arabinose operon (Hera and Pueyo, 1986); *araD* mutants are unable to use L-arabinose as the sole carbon source. The assay scores a change from L-arabinose sensitivity to

L-arabinose resistance, which is defined as the ability to grow in a medium containing L-arabinose plus another carbon source such as glycerol.

This phenotypic change reflects forward mutations in at least three different loci in the arabinose operon (Pueyo and Lopez-Barea, 1979).

Strains have been constructed along the same lines as the recommended Ames strains with mutations to remove excision repair and mutations to increase permeability, and including the mutator plasmid pKM101; that is, *Salmonella typhimurium* BA3 *araD531, hisG46,* ΔuvrB *bio* and BA9 *araD531, hisG46* ΔuvrB, *bio, rfa* (p.KM101).

Protocols for the test have included plate incorporation, preincubation, and treat and plate tests (Hera and Pueyo, 1986). In the latter tests the assay does not have the problem of plate mutants as described for reverse mutation tests in the previous section. The recommended procedure has the following outline protocol:

1. Incubate the test strain of bacteria (10^7–10^8 cells per ml) and the test agent at 37°C in nonselective DM medium with shaking.
2. Wash the cells after a 2-hr exposure period.
3. Plate on a selective medium (DM salts, 2 mg ml^{-1} glycerol, 2 ml ml^{-1} L-arabinose, 20 µg ml^{-1} L-histidine, 12 µg ml^{-1} biotin) containing an additional supplement of D-glucose, 0.5 mg per plate.

For metabolic activation 30 µl of S9 fraction and appropriate cofactors are included in the initial incubation mixture as the standard level. Different concentrations of S9 fraction can be used as required.

The group that developed this test recommend that strain BA9 replace the four strains used in the standard Ames test. For the mutagens tested to date this strain detects the same range of mutagens as the Ames test strains with equal or better sensitivity. The test seems suitable for testing complex mixtures such as red wine (Dorado et al., 1988). The spontaneous background count using the protocol outlined above is over 500 per plate, however. If fewer cells are used, false negative results are obtained (Xu et al., 1984).

K. Eukaryotic Mutation Tests

Prokaryotic systems as described have proven to be quick, versatile, and in many cases surprisingly accurate in identifying potential genetic hazards to man. There are intrinsic differences between eukaryotic and prokaryotic cells in the organization of the genome and the processing of the genetic information, however, thus there is a place for test systems based on mammalian cells for fundamental studies to understand the mutation process in higher cells and for the use of such tests for screening for genotoxic effects.

The early work of Muller showed the usefulness of the fruit fly *Drosophila melanogaster* as a higher system for measuring germ line mutations in a whole animal. The *Drosophila* sex-linked recessive lethal test has yielded much useful information and in the 1970s was a popular system for screening chemicals for mutation. This test failed to perform well in international collaborative trials to study the utility of such tests to detect carcinogens, however, and popularity waned. Another *Drosophila* test devised in the 1980s, the SMART assay (somatic mutation and recombination test) shows much promise and may revive the popularity of *Drosophila* for screening for genotoxic agent.

There are a number of in vivo tests to measure mutation in rodents, such as the mouse specific-locus test. These are very useful for fundamental studies of radiation and chemically induced mutation, but they are rather cumbersome, are used in only a small number of expert laboratories, and are used in special circumstances in which germ-line damage needs to be measured. This situation is rapidly changing as the new technologies of the last 10 to 15 years begin to have an impact in the construction of new model systems to measure mutation in vivo.

In contrast to the situation in vivo there are a number of test systems that use cultured mammalian cells, from both established and primary lines, that now have a large database of tested chemicals in the literature, that are relatively rapid, and that are feasible to use for genetic toxicity screening. These are discussed in the next section.

L. In Vitro Tests for the Detection of Mammalian Mutation

There have been a variety of in vitro mutation systems described in the literature, but only a small number have been defined adequately for quantitative studies (Cole et al., 1990). These are based on the detection of forward mutations in a similar manner to the systems described earlier for bacteria. A defined large number of cells are treated with the test agent, and after a set interval, are exposed to a selective toxic agent so that only cells that have mutated can survive. As cultured mammalian cells are diploid (or near-diploid), normally there are two copies of each gene. Recessive mutations can be missed if a normal copy is present on the homologous chromosome. As mutation frequencies for individual genes are normally very low, an impossibly large population of cells would need to be screened to detect cells in which both copies are inactivated by mutation. This problem is overcome by measuring mutation in genes on the X chromosome in male cells where only one copy of the gene will be present, or using heterozygous genes where two copies of a gene may be present but one copy is already inactive through mutation or deletion.

Many genes are essential for the survival of the cell in culture, and thus mutations in such genes would be difficult to detect. Use has been made, however, of genes that are not essential for cell survival but allow the cell to salvage nucleotides from the surrounding medium. This saves the cell energy, as it does not have to make these compounds from simpler precursors by energy-expensive catabolism. These enzymes are located at the cell membrane. If the cell is supplied with toxic nucleotides, the "normal" unmutated cells will transport these into the cell and kill the cell. If the cells have lost the enzyme as a result of mutation (or chromosomal deletion, rearrangement, etc.), however, they will not be able to "salvage" the exogenous toxic nucleotides and will survive. The surviving mutant cells can be detected by the formation of colonies on tissue culture plates, or in some cases, in the wells of microtitre plates.

One factor to take into account with these tests is that of expression time. Although a gene may be inactivated by mutation, the mRNA existing before the mutational event may decay only slowly, so that active enzyme may be present for some time after exposure to the mutagen. The cells thus have to be left for a period before challenging with the toxic nucleotide; this is the expression time, and differs between systems.

1. Chinese Hamster Lines

Chinese hamster cell lines have given much valuable data over the past 15 years, but their use for screening is limited by their lack of sensitivity, as only a relatively small target cell population can be used, owing to metabolic cooperation. (See Cole et al., 1990.) They are still in use, however, so a brief description follows.

Chinese hamster ovary (CHO) and V79 lines have high plating efficiencies and short generation times (less than 24 hr). These properties make the lines useful for mutagenicity experiments. Both cell lines have grossly rearranged chromosomal complements, which has an unknown effect on their responsiveness to mutagens (Tweats and Gatehouse, 1988). There is some evidence that Chinese hamster lines are undergoing genetic drift in different culture collections (Kirkland, 1992).

2. V79 System

The Chinese hamster V79 line was established in 1958 (Ford and Yerganian, 1958). Publication of the use of the line for mutation studies (by measuring resistance to purine analogues due to mutation of the *Hgprt* locus) occurred 10 years later (Chu and Malling, 1968). The V79 line was derived from a male Chinese hamster, hence V79 cells possess only a single X chromosome.

V79 cells grow as a cell sheet or monolayer on glass or plastic surfaces. If large numbers of cells are treated with a mutagen, cells in close contact can link via intracellular bridges when plated out. These allow the transfer of cellular components between cells such as mRNA. If a cell carries a mutation in the *hgprt* gene resulting in the inactivation of the relevant mRNA, it can thus receive viable mRNA or intact enzyme from adjacent nonmutated cells. When the mutated cell is challenged with a toxic purine, it is therefore lost, owing to the presence of active enzyme derived from the imported mRNA. This phenomenon is termed "metabolic cooperation" and severely limited the sensitivity of lines such as V79 for mutagen detection. This drawback can be overcome to an extent by carrying out the detection of mutant clones in semisolid agar (see, e.g., Oberly et al., 1987) or by using the "respreading technique." (See, e.g., Fox, 1981.)

The preferred expression time for *Hgprt* mutants is 6 to 8 days, although care needs to be taken when testing chemicals well into the toxic range, where the expression time needs to be extended to allow recovery.

3. Preliminary Cytotoxicity Testing

An essential first step is to carry out a preliminary study to evaluate the toxicity of the test material to the indicator cells, under the conditions of the main mutagenicity test. When selecting dose levels, the solubility of the test compound, the resulting pH of the media, and the osmolality of the test solutions all need to be considered. The latter two parameters have been known to induce false positive effects in in vitro mammalian tests. (See, e.g., Brusick, 1986.) The experimental procedure is carried out as follows:

1. Seek T75 plastic tissue culture flasks with a minimum of 2.5×10^6 cells in 120 ml of Eagle's medium containing 20 mM L-glutamine: 0.88 g l^{-1} sodium bicarbonate; 20 mM HEPES; 50 μg ml^{-1} streptomycin sulphate; 50 IU ml^{-1} benzylpenicillin; and 7.5% of fetal bovine serum. The flasks are incubated for 18 to 24 hr at 37°C in a CO_2 incubator to establish monolayer cultures.

2. Prepare treatment medium containing various concentrations of test compound—for example, 19.7 ml of Eagle's medium (without serum) plus 300 μl of stock concentration of compound in a preferred solvent (e.g., water, ethanol, DMSO). The final concentration of solvent other than water should not exceed 1% v/v. Normally a range of 0 to 5000 μg ml^{-1} (final concentration) is covered. For a sparingly soluble compound, the highest concentration will be the lowest at which visible precipitation occurs. Similarly, if a compound has a marked effect on osmolality, concentrations should not be used that exceed 500 milliosmoles (mosm) per kg. In addition, a pH range of 6.5 to 7.5 should not be exceeded.

3. Each cell monolayer is rinsed with a minimum of 20 ml phosphate-buffered saline (PBS) and then 20 ml of treatment medium is carefully added. The flasks are incubated for 3 hr at 37°C in a CO_2 incubator.

4. After treatment, carefully discard the medium from each flask and wash each monolayer twice with PBS. Care needs to be taken to safely dispose of contaminated solutions.

5. 10 ml of trypsin solution (0.025% trypsin in PBS) is added to each flask. Once the cells have rounded up, the trypsin is neutralized by

the addition of 10 ml of complete medium. A cell suspension is obtained by vigorous pipetting to break up cell clumps.

6. The trypsinized cell suspension is counted and diluted in complete media before assessing for survival. For each treatment set up five petri dishes containing 200 cells per dish.
7. Incubate at 37°C in a CO_2 incubator for 7 to 10 days.
8. The medium is removed and the colonies are fixed and stained using 5% Giemsa in buffered formalin. Once the colonies are stained, the Giemsa is removed and the colonies are counted.

The method can be repeated including 20% v/v S9 mix.

To calculate the percentage of survival, the following formula is used:

$$\frac{\text{Cell titre in treated culture}}{\text{Cell titre in control culture}} \times \frac{\text{Mean number of colonies on treated plates}}{\text{Mean number of colonies on control plates}} \times 100$$

The cloning efficiency (CE) of the control culture is calculated as follows:

$$CE = \frac{\text{Mean number of colonies per plate}}{\text{Number of cells per plate (i.e., 200)}} \times 100$$

In the absence of precipitation or effects on pH or osmolality, the maximum concentration of the main mutagenicity study is a concentration that reduces survival to approximately 20% of the control value.

Procedure for the Chinese Hamster V79/Hgprt Assay. The assay usually comprises three test concentrations, each in duplicate, and four vehicle control replicates. Suitable positive controls are ethylmethane sulphonate ($-$S9) and dimethyl benzanthracene ($+$S9). V79 cells with a low nominal passage number should be used from frozen stocks to help minimize genetic drift. The procedure described includes a reseeding step for mutation expression.

Steps 1 through 5 are the same as in the cytotoxicity assay. As before, tests can be carried out in the presence and absence of S9 mix.

6. The trypsinized cultures are counted and a sample is assessed for survival as for the cytotoxicity assay. In addition, an appropriate number of cells are reseeded for estimation of mutation frequency at the day 8 expression time. The cells are transferred to roller bottles (usually 490 cm^2) for this stage. The bottles are gassed with pure CO_2, the tops are tightened, and the bottles are incubated at 37°C on a roller machine (approximate speed 0.5–1.0 rev min^{-1}). Usually 10^6 viable cells are reseeded in 50 ml of Eagle's medium containing serum, but more cells are required at the toxic dose levels.
7. The bottles are subcultured as necessary throughout the expression period to maintain subconfluency. This involves retrypsinization and

determining the cell titre for each treatment. For each culture a fresh roller bottle is reseeded with a minimum of 10^6 cells.

8. On day 8, each culture is again trypsinized, counted, and diluted so that a sample cell population can be assessed for cloning efficiency and a second sample can be assessed for the induction of 6TG-resistant cells.

9. The cell suspension is diluted in complete medium and 2×10^5 cells added per petri dish (10 petri dishes per treatment). 6-Thioguanine is added to the medium at a final concentration of 10 μg ml^{-1}.

10. The petri dishes are incubated for 7 to 10 days and the medium is then removed. The colonies are fixed and stained as previously. The colonies (>50 cells per clone) are then counted.

Mutation frequency in each culture is calculated as

$$\frac{\text{Mean number of colonies on thioguanine plates}}{1000 \times \text{mean number of colonies on survival plates}}$$

Data Analysis. A weighted analysis (see Arlett et al., 1989) of variance is performed on the mutation frequencies, as the variation in the number of mutations per plate usually increases as the mean increases. Each dose of test compound is compared with the corresponding vehicle control by means of a one-sided Dunnett's test, and in addition, the mutation frequencies are examined to see whether or not there is a linear relationship with dose.

The criterion employed for a positive response in this assay is a reproducible statistically significant increase in mutation frequency (weighted mean for duplicate treated cultures) over the concurrent vehicle control value (weighted mean for four independent control cultures). Ideally, the response should show evidence of a dose-response relationship. When a small, isolated significant increase in mutation frequency is observed in only one of the two duplicate experiments, then a third test should be carried out. If the third test shows no significant effects, the initial increase is likely to be a chance result. In cases in which an apparent treated-related increase is thought to be a result of unusually low variability or a low control frequency, comparison with the laboratory historical control frequency may be justified.

Chinese Hamster CHO/Hgprt System. Chinese hamster ovary cells have 21 or 22 chromosomes with one intact X chromosome and a large acrocentric marker chromosome (Natarajan and Obe, 1982). The use of these cells in mammalian mutation experiments was first reported by Hsie et al. (1975), and was refined into a quantitative assay for mutagenicity testing by O'Neill. The performance of this system has been reviewed by the U.S. Environmental Protection Agency (EPA) Gene-Tox Program. The experimental procedure for this assay is similar to the V70/Hgprt system already described, and for more detailed descriptions the reader is referred to Li et al. (1987).

Mouse Lymphoma L5178Y TK$^{+/-}$ Assay. Whereas the Chinese hamster cell systems are regarded as relatively insensitive, the mouse lymphoma L5178Y TK$^{+/-}$ test is undoubtedly more sensitive. Unfortunately, there are persistent doubts regarding its specificity; that is, the ability to distinguish between carcinogens and noncarcinogens. (See, e.g., Tennant et al., 1987.) A great advantage is the ability of these cells to grow in suspension culture in which intracellular bridges do not occur, however. The problems of metabolic cooperation are thus avoided, which allows a large number of cells to be treated for optimum statistical analysis of results.

A candid historical overview of the development of the mouse lymphoma TK$^{+/-}$ mutagenicity assay is given by its originator, Clive (1987). Initially methodologies were developed for producing the three TK genotypes (TK$^{+/+}$ and TK$^{-/-}$ homozygotes and the TK$^{+/-}$ heterozygotes) (Clive et al., 1972). This first heterozygote was lost; however, it was recognized that subsequent heterozygotes produced distinctly bimodal distributions of mutant-colony sizes, owing to differences in growth rate. These were interpreted in terms of single-gene (large-colony mutants) and viable chromosomal mutations (small-colony mutants). A period of diversification of the mouse lymphoma assay followed, along with controversy over the significance of small-colony mutants. (See, e.g., Amacher et al., 1980.)

Following this, a series of cytogenetic studies confirmed the cytogenetic interpretation for small-colony mutants. (See, e.g., Hozier et al., 1982.) Molecular studies showed that most mutations resulting in small-colony mutants involve large-scale deletions (Evans et al., 1986). A current theory states that for many compounds deletion mutants are induced by binding the compound to complexes between topoisomerase II and DNA. (See Clive, 1989.) Topoisomerases are enzymes that control supercoiling via breakage and reunion of DNA strands; it is the latter step that is disrupted, which leads to chromosome damage and deletions. Further molecular studies (Applegate et al., 1990) have shown that a wide variety of genetic events can result in the formation of TK$^{+/-}$ genotype from the heterozygote, including recombinations and mitotic nondisjunction.

The TK$^{+/-}$ line was originally isolated as a spontaneously arising revertant clone from a UV-induced TK$^{-/-}$ clone. The parental TK$^{+/+}$ cell and the heterozygote were then the only TK-competent mouse lymphoma cells that could be maintained in THMG medium (3 μg ml^{-1} thymidine, 5 μg ml^{-1} hypoxanthine, 0.1 μg ml^{-1} methotrexate, and 7.5 μg ml^{-1} glycine) (Clive, 1987). Like most established lines, these cells are thus remote from wild-type cells. The karyotype of the TK$^{+/-}$ −3.7.2C line has a modal chromosome number of 40 like wild type, but has a variety of chromosomal rearrangements and centromeric heteromorphisms (Blazak et al., 1986).

Two main protocols have been devised for carrying out mutation assays with mouse lymphoma L5178Y cells; that is, plating the cells in soft agar or a fluctuation test approach. It is the latter that is described in the following section, based on Cole et al. (1986). The reader is referred to Clive et al. (1987) for a full description of the soft-agar method.

Preliminary Cytotoxicity Assay. The cells are maintained in RPMI 1640 medium containing 2.0 mM glutamine, 20 mM HEPES, 200 μg ml^{-1} sodium pyruvate, 50 IU ml^{-1} benzylpenicillin, 50 μg ml^{-1} streptomycin sulphate, and 10% donor horse serum (heat-inactivated for 30 min at 56°C). This medium is designated CM10. Conditioned medium is CM10 in which cells have grown exponentially for at least 1 day. Treatment medium contains 3% horse serum and 30% conditioned media (CM3). Medium without serum is known as incomplete medium (ICM). If treatment time exceeds 3 hr, treatment is carried out in CM10.

The method is as follows:

1. The cell titre of an exponentially growing culture of cells in CM10 is determined with a Coulter counter. The cell suspension is centrifuged at 70 grams for 5 min and the supernatant is reduced such that 3 ml contains approximately 5×10^6 cells (3 hr treatment) or 2×10^6 (treatment >3 hr).

2a. For tests in the absence of S9 mix, treatment groups are prepared by mixing 3 ml of solution of test compound and 6.9 ml of ICM (3 hr treatment) or 6.9 ml of CM10 (treatment >3 hr).

2b. Tests in the presence of S9 mix are carried out in the same way, except the treatment medium contains 10% v/v S9 mix at the expense of ICM; that is, 3-ml cell suspension, 5.9 ml ICM, 1-ml S9 mix, and 0.1 ml test compound solution/vehicle. The composition of the S9 mix is as described earlier (Table 10.6). It is prepared immediately before required and kept on ice until it is added to the test system. For the vehicle controls, if an organic solvent is used, it should not exceed 1% v/v.

3. After the treatment period, cells are spun down at 70 grams for 5 min and the supernatant is transferred for assessment of pH (pH meter) and osmolality (e.g., using Wescor vapour pressure osmometer). The cell pellet is washed twice in PBS and then resuspended in 10 ml CM10. (All contaminated material and waste should be disposed of safely.)

4. The cell titre of each culture is counted and a sample diluted in CM10 for assessment of posttreatment survival. For this two 96-well microtitre plates are charged with 200 μl of a diluted cell suspension using a multichannel pipette such that each well contains on average one cell.

5. Plates are incubated for 7 to 8 days at 37°C and 5% CO_2 in 95 ± 3% relative humidity.

6. The plates are removed from the incubator and 20 μl of MTT [3-(4,5-dimethylthiazol-2-yl)-2,5-diphenyltetrazolium bromide] at 5 mg ml^{-1} (in PBS) is added to each well with a multichannel pipette. The plates are left to stand for 1 to 4 hr and then scored for the presence of colonies with a Titertek mirror box, which allows direct viewing of the bottom surface of the plates.

7. Cytotoxicity can also be determined posttreatment as follows: T25 flasks are set up after treatment containing 0.75×10^5 cells per ml in 5 ml CM10. Flasks are incubated with loose lids at 37°C with 5% CO_2 in 95 ± 3% relative humidity. Two days later the cell titre of each culture is determined with a Coulter counter.

8. Following this procedure, various calculations are carried out to aid selection of dose levels for the main mutation assay.

   a. *Cloning efficiency.* In microtitre assays calculations are based on the Poisson distribution; that is

   $$P(o) = \frac{\text{Number of wells without a colony}}{\text{Total number of cells}}$$

   b. *Relative survival.* Relative survival (S) is calculated as follows:

   $$S = \frac{\text{CE of treated group}}{\text{CE of control group}}$$

   c. *Growth.* Growth in suspension (SG) is calculated as follows:

   $$SG = \frac{\text{Cell count after 3 days}}{0.75 \times 10^5}$$

   Relative suspension growth (RSG) is calculated as follows:

   $$RSG = \frac{\text{SG of treated group}}{\text{SG of control group}} \times 100\%$$

4. Selection of Dose Levels

The highest test concentration is selected from one of the following options, whichever is lowest:

A concentration that reduces survival to about 10–20% of the control value.
A concentration that reduces RSG to 10–20% of the control value.
The lowest concentration at which visible precipitation occurs.
The highest concentration that does not increase the osmolality of the me-

dium to greater than 400 mmol kg^{-1} or 100 mmol above the value for the solvent control.

The highest concentration that does not alter the pH of the treatment medium beyond the range of 6.8 to 7.5.

If none of these conditions is met, 5 mg ml^{-1} should be used.

Lower test concentrations are selected as fractions of the highest concentration, usually including one dose that causes 20–70% survival and one dose that causes >70% survival.

5.   Main Mutation Assay

The assay normally comprises three test concentrations, a positive control, and a vehicle control. All treatment groups are set up in duplicate. The expression time is 2 days, unless there are indications that the test agent inhibits cell proliferation, where an additional or possibly alternative expression time should be employed.

Stock cultures are established from frozen ampules of cells that have been treated with thymidine, hypoxanthine, methotrexate, and glycine for 24 hr, which purges the culture of preexisting TK$^{-/-}$ mutants. This cell stock is used for a maximum of 2 months.

Treatment is normally carried out in 50-ml centrifuge tubes on a roller machine. During the expression time the cells are grown in T75 plastic tissue culture flasks. For estimation of cloning efficiency and mutant induction, cells are plated out in 96-well microtitre plates. Flasks and microtitre plates are incubated at 37°C in a CO$_2$ incubator as in the cytotoxicity assays.

Cell titres are determined by diluting the cell suspension in Isoton and counting an appropriate volume (usually 0.5 ml) with a Coulter counter. Two counts are made per suspension.

The experimental procedure is carried out as follows:

1.   On the day of treatment stock solutions for the positive control and the various concentrations of test compound (selected as per the previous selection) are prepared.

2.   Treatment is carried out in 30% conditioned media. The serum concentration is 3% (3 hr treatment) or 10% (treated >3 hr).

3.   Cell suspensions of exponentially growing cells are prepared as in the cytotoxicity assay, except that 6 ml of media required for each treatment culture contains 10^7 cells (3 hr treatment) or 3 × 10^6 cells (>3 hr treatment). The number of cells per treatment may be increased if marked cytotoxicity is expected to allow enough cells to survive (e.g., if 20% survival or less is expected, 2 × 10^7 cells may be treated).

4.   For tests in the absence of S9 mix, 6 ml of cell suspension, 0.2 ml

test compound/vehicle, and 13.8 ml ICM (3 hr treatment) or 13.8 ml CM10 (treatment >7 hr) are mixed in the presence of S9 mix, and 0.2 ml of test compound/vehicle are prepared.

5. After treatment the cells are centrifuged at 70 grams for 5 min, the supernatant is discarded, and the cell pellet is resuspended in PBS (pH 7). This washing procedure is repeated twice, and finally the cell pellet is resuspended in CM10.
6. Each culture is counted so that a sample of cells can be assessed for posttreatment survival, and the remaining cell population assessed for estimation of mutation frequency.
7. For survival estimation, cells are placed into 96-well microtitre trays at a cell density of 1 cell per well as per the cytotoxicity assay.
8. For mutation estimation, the cells are diluted to a cell density of 2×10^5 cells per ml with CM10 in tissue culture flasks, and the culture is incubated at 37°C in a CO_2 incubator. On day 1 each culture is counted and diluted with fresh medium to a cell density of 2×10^5 cells per ml in a maximum of 100 ml of medium.
9. On day 2 each culture is counted again and an aliquot of cells taken so that
    a. A sample of the cell population can be assessed for cloning efficiency. Plates are incubated at 37°C in a CO_2 incubator for 7 days.
    b. A sample of the cell population can be assessed for the induction of TFT-resistant cells (mutants). For this 2×10^3 cells are plated per well in 200 µl CM10 containing 4 µg ml^{-1} TFT. TFT and TFT-containing cultures must not be exposed to bright light, as the material is light-sensitive. The plates are incubated for 10 to 12 days at 37°C in a CO_2 incubator.
10. At the end of incubation 20 µl MTT is added to each well. The plates are left to develop for 1 to 4 hr at 37°C and then scored for colony-bearing wells. Colonies are scored by eye and are classified as small or large.

The calculation for cloning efficiency is made as for the cytotoxicity assay.

Relative total growth (RTG) is a cytotoxicity parameter that considers growth in suspension during the expression time and the cloning efficiency of the end of the expression time as follows:

$$\text{Suspension growth (SG)} = \frac{\text{24-hr cell count}}{2 \times 10^4} \times \frac{\text{48-hr cell count}}{2 \times 10^5}$$

$$\text{RTG} = \frac{\text{SG treated culture}}{\text{SG control culture}} \times \frac{\text{CE of treated culture}}{\text{CE of control culture}}$$

Mutation frequency (MF) is calculated as follows:

$$MF = \frac{InP_o \text{ for mutation plates}}{\text{Number of cells per well} \times CE/100}$$

6. Data Analysis

Data from the fluctuation test described above are analyzed by an appropriate statistical method as described in Robinson et al. (1989). Data from plate assays are analyzed as described in Arlett et al. (1989) for treated and plate tests.

7. Status of Mammalian Mutation Tests

At present the only practical assays for screening new chemical entities for mammalian mutation are the mammalian cell assays described above. The protocols are well defined, and mutant selection and counting procedures are simple and easily quantified. In general, the genetic end points are understood and relevant to deleterious genetic events in humans. For these reasons the assays are still regarded as valuable in safety evaluation (Li et al., 1991). It is recognized, however, that there are still unknown factors and molecular events that influence test results. This can be illustrated by the conclusions of the third United Kingdom Environmental Mutagen Society (UKEMS) collaborative trial, which focused on tests with cultured mammalian cells. The following points were made:

> The number of cells to be cultured during expression imposes a severe limitation in the use of surface attached cells.
> A careful determination of toxicity is important.
> S9 levels may need to be varied.
> The aromatic amine benzidine is mutagenic only at the TK locus in L5178Y TK$^{+/-}$ cells. The most disturbing finding was that benzidine (detectable without metabolism by S9 mix) did not produce detectable DNA adducts (as shown by ^{32}P-post-labeling) in L5178Y cells, thus the mechanism for mutagenesis in L5178Y cells benzidine remains to be elucidated (Arlett and Cole, 1990).

M. In Vivo Mammalian Mutation Tests

Mammalian mutation studies of chemicals in the whole animal have provided fundamental information on mutation parameters in germ cells, such as dose response, dose fractionation, and sensitivity of various stages in gametogenesis, just as is known for ionizing radiation (Russell, 1989). This has led to estimations of the possible impact chemical mutagens may have on heritable malformation, inborn errors of metabolism, and so on. Today germ cell studies are still required when estimating the heritable damage a mutagen may inflict on exposed human populations.

The existing tests tend to be cumbersome and are not used for routine genetic toxicology screening, and thus only brief descriptions will follow. Reviews of existing data, particularly by Holden (see, e.g., Holden, 1982; Adler and Ashby, 1989), have indicated that most if not all germ cell mutagens also induce DNA damage in somatic cells, as detected by well-established assays such as the rodent micronucleus test. The converse is not true; that is, some mutagens/clastogens can induce somatic cell damage but do not induce germ cell changes, which probably reflects the special protection afforded to the germ cells, such as that provided by the blood-testis barrier. In other words, it appears that germ cell mutagens are a subset of somatic cell mutagens.

In vivo mammalian mutation tests are not restricted to germ cell tests. The mouse spot test described below is again a test used first for studying radiation-induced mutation but has also been used for screening chemicals for in vivo mutagenic potential. This test has had several proponents but compared with in vivo chromosomal assays is not widely used.

1. The Mouse Specific Locus Test

The mouse somatic spot test is a type of specific locus test. The classic specific locus test was developed independently by Russell at Oak Ridge in the late 1940s (Russell, 1951; 1989) and Carter in Edinburgh (Carter et al., 1956). The test consists of treatment of parental mice homozygous for a wild-type set of marker loci. The targets for mutation are the germ cells in the gonads of the treated mice. These are mated with a tester stock that is homozygous recessive at the marker loci. The F_1 offspring that result are normally heterozygous at the marker loci and thus express the wild-type phenotype. In the event of a mutation from the wild-type allele at any of these loci, the F_1 offspring express the recessive phenotype.

The test marker strain (T) developed by Russell uses seven recessive loci; namely, a (nonagouti), b (brown), c^{ch} (chinchilla), d (dilute), p (pink-eyed dilution), s (piebald), and se (short-ear). As for the mouse spot test, these genes control coat pigmentation, intensity, or pattern, and for the se gene, the size of the external ear.

As the occurrence of mutation is rare even after mutagen treatment, the specific locus test is the ultimate study of mutation, requiring many thousands of offspring to be scored, plus significant resources of time, space, and animal husbandry. Because of these constraints it is often difficult to define a negative result, as insufficient animals are scored or not all stages of spermatogenesis are covered. Of the 25 compounds tested in the assay as reviewed by Ehling et al. (1986), 17 were regarded as "inconclusive" and eight as positive. The scale studies can reach is illustrated by the test of ethylene oxide described by Russell (1984), in which exposures of 101,000 and 150,000 ppm per hr were used over 16 to 23 weeks. A total of 71,387 offspring were examined. The spermatogonial stem-cell mutation rate in the treated animals did not differ significantly from the historical control frequency!

With regard to the design of the test, mice are mated when 7 to 8 weeks old. By this age all germ cell stages are present. The test compound is normally administered by the ip route to maximize the likelihood of germ cell exposure. The preferred dose is just below the toxic level as long as fertility is not compromised. One lower dose should also be included.

In males spermatogonia are most at risk, but it is also desirable that later stages also be exposed. The mice are thus mated immediately after treatment to two to four females. This is continued each week for 7 weeks. The first group has then completed its rearing of the first set of offspring and is remated. This cycle can be continued for the lifetime of the males. Tests can also be carried out by dosing females, when treatment is carried out for 3 weeks to cover all stages of ogenesis.

The offspring are examined immediately after birth for identification of malformations (dominant visibles) and then at weaning for the specific locus mutations. Presumptive mutant mice are checked by further crosses to confirm their status (Searle, 1984).

Comparison of mutation frequencies is made with the historical database. For definition of a positive result the same principles are recommended as for the mouse spot test (Selby and Olson, 1981). A minimum size of 18,000 offspring per group is recommended by those authors for definition of a negative result.

III. IN VITRO CYTOGENETIC ASSAYS

The in vitro cytogenetic assay is a short-term mutagenicity test for detecting chromosomal damage in cultured mammalian cells.

Cultured cells have a limited ability metabolically to activate some potential clastogens. This can be overcome by adding an exogenous metabolic activation system such as S9 mix to the cells (Ames et al., 1975; Natarajan et al., 1976; Maron and Ames, 1983; Madle and Obe, 1980).

Observations are made in metaphase cells arrested with a spindle inhibitor such as colchicine or colcemid to accumulate cells in a metaphaselike stage of mitosis (c-metaphase) before hypotonic treatment to enlarge cells and fixation with alcohol/acetic acid solution. Cells are then dispersed onto microscope slides and stained, and the slides are randomized, coded, and analyzed for chromosome aberrations with high-power light microscopy. Details of the procedure are given in Dean and Danford (1984) and Preston et al. (1981; 1987). The UKEMS guidelines (Scott et al., 1990) recommend that all tests be repeated regardless of the outcome of the first test and that if a negative or equivocal result is obtained in the first test, the repeat should include an additional sampling time. In the earlier version of the guidelines (Scott et al., 1983), a single sampling at approximately 1.5 normal cycle times (-24 hr for a 1.5-cell cycle) from the beginning of treatment was recommended, provided that a range of concentrations was used that induced marginal to substantial reductions in the mitotic index, usually an indicator of mitotic delay. Ishidate (1988a), however, reported a number of chemicals that gave negative responses with a fixation time of 24 hr but that were positive at 48 hr. This was when a Chinese hamster fibroblast line (CHO) with a doubling time of 15 hr was used. It would appear, therefore, that there are chemicals that can induce extensive mitotic delay at clastogenic doses and may be clastogenic only when cells have passed through more than one cell cycle since treatment (Thust et al., 1980). A repeat test should include an additional sample approximately 24 hr later, but it may only be necessary to score cells from the highest dose at this later fixation time. When the first test gives a clearly positive result, the repeat test need only utilize the same fixation time. The use of other sampling times is in agreement with other guidelines (European Community EEC directive—OECD, 1983; American Society for Testing and Materials—Preston et al., 1987; Japanese guidelines—JMHW, 1984; Joint Directives, 1987; Ishidate, 1988b).

A. Cell Types

Established cell lines, cell strains, or primary cell cultures may be used. The most often used are Chinese hamster cell lines and human peripheral blood lymphocytes. The merits of these two cell lines have been reported (Ishidate and Harnois, 1987; Kirkland and Garner, 1987). The cell system must be validated and consistently sensitive to known clastogens.

B. Chinese Hamster Cell Lines

Chinese hamster cell lines have a small number of large chromosomes (11 pairs). Chinese hamster ovary cells in which there has been an extensive rearrangement of chromosome material and in which the chromosome number may not be constant from cell to cell, are frequently used. Polyploidy, endoreduplication, and high spontaneous chromosome aberration frequencies can sometimes be found in these established cell lines, but careful cell culture techniques should minimize such effects. Cells should be treated in exponential growth when cells are in all stages of the cell cycle.

C. Human Peripheral Blood Lymphocytes

Blood should be taken from healthy donors not known to be suffering from viral infections or receiving medication. Any staff members handling blood should be immunized against hepatitis B, and regular donors should be shown to be hepatitis B antigen negative. Donors and staff should be aware of AIDS implications, and blood and cultures should be handled at containment level 2 (Advisory Committee on Dangerous Pathogens, 1984).

Peripheral blood cultures are stimulated to divide by the addition of a T cell mitogen such as phytohaemagglutinin (PHA) to the culture medium. Mitotic activity is at a maximum at about 3 days but begins at about 40 hr after PHA stimulation, and the chromosome constitution remains diploid during short-term culture (Evans and O'Riordan, 1975). Treatments should commence at about 44 hr after culture initiation. This is when cells are actively proliferating and cells are in all stages of the cell cycle. They should be sampled about 20 hr later. In a repeat study the second sample time should be about 92 hr after culture initiation. Morimoto et al. (1983) report that the cycle time for lymphocytes averages about 12 to 14 hr except for the first cycle.

Female donors can give higher yields of chromosome damage (Anderson et al., 1989).

D. Positive and Negative Controls

When the solvent is not the culture medium or water, the solvent, liver enzyme activation mixture and solvent, and untreated controls are used as negative controls.

Since cultured cells are normally treated in their usual growth medium, the solubility of the test material in the medium should be ascertained before testing. Extremes of pH can be clastogenic (Cifone et al., 1987), so the effect of the test material on pH should also be determined, but buffers can be utilized.

Various organic solvents are used, such as dimethyl sulfoxide (DMSO), dimethylformamide, ethanol, and acetone. The volume added must not be toxic to cells. Greater than 10% water v/v can be toxic because of nutrient dilution and osmolality changes.

A known clastogen should always be included as a positive control. When metabolic activation is used, a positive control chemical known to require metabolic activation should also be used to ensure that the system is functioning properly. Without metabolic activation, a direct-acting positive control chemical should be used. A structurally related positive control can also be used. Appropriate safety precautions must be taken in handling clastogens (IARC, 1979; MRC, 1981).

Positive control chemicals should be used to produce relatively low frequencies of aberrations so that the sensitivity of the assay for detecting weak clastogens can be established (Preston et al., 1987).

Aberration yields in negative and positive controls should be used to provide a historical database.

E. Treatment of Cells

When an exogenous activation system is employed, short treatments (about 2 hr) are usually necessary because S9 mix is often cytotoxic when used for extended lengths of time. Cells may be treated with chemicals either continuously up to harvest time, however, or for a short time followed by washing and the addition of fresh medium to allow cell cycle progression. Continuous treatment avoids centrifugation steps required with washing of cells and optimizes the endogenous metabolic capacity of the lymphocytes.

When metabolic activation is used, S9 mix should not exceed 1–10% of the culture medium by volume. It has been shown that the S9 mix is clastogenic in CHO cells and mouse lymphoma cells (Cifone et al., 1987; Kirkland et al., 1984) but not in human lymphocytes, where blood components can inactivate active oxygen species that could cause chromosome damage. When S9 mix from animals treated with other enzyme-inducing agents such as phenobarbitone/beta-naphthoflavone is used, clastogenesis may be minimized (Kirkland et al., 1984).

Prior to testing, it is necessary to determine the cytotoxicity of the test material in order to select a suitable dose range for the chromosome assay both with and without metabolic activation. The range most commonly used determines the effect of the agent on the mitotic index (MI); that is, the percentage of cells in mitoses at the time of cell harvest. The highest dose should inhibit mitotic activity by approximately 50% (EEC Annex V) or 75% (UKEMS: Scott et al., 1990) or exhibit some other indication of cytotoxicity. If the reduction in MI is too great, insufficient cells can be found for chromosome analysis. Cytotoxicity can also be assessed by making cell counts in the chromosome aberration test when using cell lines. In the lymphocyte assay total white cell counts can be used in addition to MI. A dose that induces 50–75% toxicity in these assays should be accompanied by a suitable reduction in MI.

If the test material is not toxic, it is recommended by, for example, the EEC (Annex V) that it be tested up to 5 mg ml^{-1}. The UKEMS recommends that chemicals be tested up to their maximum solubility in the treatment medium and not just their maximum solubility in stock solutions.

For highly soluble nontoxic agents, concentrations above 10 mM may produce substantial increases in the osmolality of the culture medium, which could be clastogenic, by causing ionic imbalance within the cells (Ishidate et al., 1984; Brusick, 1987). At concentrations exceeding 10 mM the osmolality of the treatment media should be measured and if the increase exceeds 50 mmol kg^{-1}, clastogenicity resulting from high osmolality should be suspected, and according to the UKEMS, is unlikely to be of relevance to human risk. The UKEMS also does not recommend the testing of chemicals at concentrations exceeding their solubility limits as suspensions or precipitate.

A minimum of three doses of the test material should be used—the highest chosen as described above, the lowest on the borderline of toxicity, and an intermediate one. Up to six doses can be managed satisfactorily, and this ensures that any dose response is detected and that a toxic range is covered. Mitotic indexes are as required for the preliminary study (at least 1000 cells per culture). It is also useful to score endoreduplication and polyploidy for historical data. Cells from only three doses need to be analyzed.

The range of doses used at the repeat fixation time can be those that induce a suitable degree of mitotic inhibition at the earlier fixation time, but if the highest dose reduces the MI to an unacceptably low level at the second sampling time, the next highest dose should be chosen for screening.

A complete assay requires the test material to be investigated at a minimum of three doses together with a positive (untreated) and solvent-only control (which can be omitted if tissue culture medium is used as a solvent). When two fixation times are used in repeat tests, the positive control is necessary at only one time, but the negative or solvent control is necessary at both times.

Duplicates of each test group and quadruplicates of solvent or negative controls should be set up. The sensitivity of the assay is improved with larger numbers scored in the negative controls (Richardson et al., 1989).

F. Scoring Procedures

Prior to scoring, slides should be coded, randomized, and then scored ''blind.'' Metaphase analysis should only be carried out by an experienced observer. Metaphase cells should be sought under low-power magnification, and those with well-spread (i.e., nonoverlapping) clearly defined nonfuzzy chromosomes examined under high power with oil immersion. It is acceptable to analyze cells that have total chromosome numbers or that have lost one or two chromosomes during processing. In human lymphocytes ($2n - 46$) 44 or more centomeres and in CHO cells ($2n = 22$; range 21–24) 20 or more centromeres can be scored. Chromosome numbers can be recorded for each cell to give an indication of aneuploidy. Only cells with increases in numbers (above 46 in human lymphocytes and 24 in CHO cells) should be considered in this category, since decreases can occur through processing.

Recording microscope coordinates of cells is necessary and allows verification of abnormal cells. A photographic record of cells with aberrations is also useful. Two hundred cells (100 from each of two replicates) should be scored per treatment group. When ambiguous results are obtained, there may be further blind reading of these samples.

G. Data Recording

The classification and nomenclature of the International System for Human Cytogenetic Nomenclature (ISCN, 1985) as applied to acquired chromosome aberrations is recommended. Score sheets giving the slide code, microscope scorer's name, date, cell number, number of chromosomes, and aberration types should be used. These should include chromatid and chromosome gaps, deletions, and exchanges. A space for the Vernier reading for comments and a diagram of the aberration should be available.

From the score sheets, the frequencies of various aberrations should be calculated, and each aberration should be counted only once. To consider a break as one event and an exchange as two events is not acceptable, since unfounded assumptions are made about the mechanisms involved (Revell, 1974).

H.   Presentation of Results

The test material, test cells used, method of treatment, harvesting of cells, cytotoxicity assay, and so on, should be clearly stated as well as the statistical methods used. Richardson et al. (1989) recommend that comparison be made between the frequencies in control cells and at each dose level using Fisher's exact test.

In cytogenetic assays the absence of a clear positive dose-response relationship at a particular time frequently arises. This is because a single common sampling time may be used for all doses of a test compound. Chromosome aberration yields can vary markedly with posttreatment sampling time of an asynchronous population, and increasing dosages of clastogens can induce increasing degrees of mitotic delay (Scott et al., 1990). Additional fixation times should clarify the relationship between dose and aberration yield.

Traditionally gaps are excluded from quantification of chromosome aberration yields. Some gaps have been shown to be real discontinuities in DNA (e.g., Heddle and Bodycote, 1970). Where chromosome aberration yields are on the borderline of statistical significance above control values, the inclusion of gaps could be useful. Further details on this approach may be found in the UKEMS guidelines (Scott et al., 1990).

Since chromosome exchanges are relatively rare events, greater biological significance should be attached to their presence than to gaps and breaks.

Chemicals that are clastogenic in vitro at low doses are more likely to be clastogenic in vivo than those in which clastogenicity is detected only at high concentrations (Ishidate et al., 1988a,b). Negative results in well-conducted in vitro tests are a good indication of a lack of potential for in vivo clastogenesis, since almost all in vivo clastogens have given positive results in vitro when adequately tested (Thompson, 1986; Ishidate et al., 1988a,b).

IV.   IN VIVO CYTOGENETIC ASSAYS

Damage induced in whole animals can be detected in in vivo chromosome assays in either somatic or germinal cells by examination of metaphases or the formation of micronuclei. The micronucleus test can also detect whole chromosome loss or aneuploidy in the absence of clastogenic activity and is considered comparable in sensitivity to chromosome analysis (Tsuchimoto and Matter, 1979).

Rats and mice are generally used for in vivo studies, with the mouse being employed for bone marrow micronucleus analysis and the rat for metaphase analysis, but both can be used for either. Mice are cheaper and easier to handle than rats, and only a qualitative difference in response has been found between the species (Albanese et al., 1987). Chinese hamsters are also widely used for metaphase analysis because of their low diploid chromosome number of 22. There are few other historical toxicological data for this species, however.

A. Somatic Cell Assays

1. Metaphase Analysis

Metaphase analysis can be performed in any tissue with actively dividing cells, but bone marrow is the tissue most often examined. Cells are treated with a test compound and are arrested in metaphase by the administration of colcemid or colchicine at various sampling times after treatment. Preparations are examined for structural chromosome damage. Because the bone marrow has a good blood supply, the cells should be exposed to the test compound or its metabolites in the peripheral blood supply, and the cells are sensitive to S-dependent and S-independent mutagens (Topham et al., 1983).

Peripheral blood cells can be stimulated to divide even though the target cell is relatively insensitive (Newton and Lilly, 1986). It is necessary to stimulate them with a mitogen since the number of lymphocytes that are dividing at any one time is very low. Cells are in G_0 when exposure is taking place, so they may not be sensitive to cell cycle stage-specific mutagens and any damage might be repaired before sampling.

2. Micronuclei

The assessment of micronuclei is considered simpler than the assessment of metaphase analysis. This assay is most often carried out in bone marrow cells, in which polychromatic erythrocytes are examined. Damage is induced in the immature erythroblast and results in a micronucleus outside the main nucleus, which is easily detected after staining as a chromatid-containing body. When the erythroblast matures, the micronucleus, whose formation results from chromosome loss during cell division or from chromosome breakage forming centric and acentric fragments, is not extruded with the nucleus. Micronuclei can also be detected in peripheral blood cells (MacGregor et al., 1980). In addition, they can be detected in a liver (Tates et al., 1980; Braithwaite and Ashby, 1988) after partial hepatectomy or stimulation with 4-acetylaminofluorene, or they can be detected in any proliferating cells.

B. Germ Cell Assays

The study of chromosome damage is highly relevant to the assessment of heritable cytogenetic damage. Many compounds that cause somatic cell damage have not produced germ cell damage (Holden, 1982), and so far all germ mutagens have also produced somatic damage.

Germ cell data, however, are needed for genetic risk estimation, and testing can be performed in male or female germ cells. The former are most often used, owing to the systemic effects in females. Testing in the male is performed in mitotically proliferating premeiotic spermatogonia, but chromosomal errors in such cells can result in cell death or prevent the cell from passing through meiosis. Damage produced in postmeiotic cells, the spermatids, or sperm are more likely to be transmitted to the F_1 progeny (Albanese, 1987). In females it is during early fetal development of the ovary that oocyte stage is the most commonly tested. To test other stages during the first or second meiotic divisions demands the use of oocytes undergoing ovulation that occur naturally or are hormone-stimulated. It is thus more difficult technically to test female germ cells.

C. Heritable Chromosome Assays

Damage may be analyzed in the heritable translocation test, which involves the examination in male F_1 animals if diakinesis metaphase 1 spermatocytes for multivalent association fall within the acceptable range for the laboratory for a substance to be considered positive or negative under the conditions of the study.

D. Germ Cell Cytogenetic Assays

Either mouse or rat can be used, but the mouse is generally the preferred species. Normally such assays are not conducted for routine screening purposes.

Spermatogonial metaphases can be prepared by the air-drying technique of Evans and O'Riordan (1975) for the first and second meiotic metaphase (MI and MII) in the male mouse. This method is not as suitable for rat and hamster. The numbers of spermatogonial metaphases can be boosted if prior to hypotonic treatment the testicular tubules are dispersed in trypsin solution (0.25%). At least 1 month between treatment and sample should be allowed to pass in the mouse to allow treated cells to reach meiosis. Brook and Chandley (1986) established that 11 days and 4 hr were required for spermatogonial cells to reach preleptotene and 8 days and 10 hr to reach zygotene. It takes 4 hr for cells to move from MI to MII, but test compounds can alter this rate. A search for multivalent formation can be made at MI for the structural rearrangements induced in spermatogonia. Cawood and Breckon (1983) examined the synaptonemal complex at pachytene using electron microscopy. Errors of segregation should be searched for at the first meiotic division in the male mouse, MII cells showing 19 (hypoploid) and 21 (hyperploid) chromosomes (Brook and Chandley, 1986). Hansmann and El-Nahass (1979), Brook (1982), and Brook and Chandley (1985) describe assays in the female mouse and procedures used for inducing ovulation by hormones and treatment of specific stages of meiosis.

V. SISTER CHROMATID EXCHANGE ASSAYS

Sister chromatid exchanges are reciprocal exchanges between sister chromatids. They result in a change in morphology of the chromosome Breakage and reunion are involved, although the exact mechanism is unclear. They are thought to occur at homologous loci.

In 1958 Taylor demonstrated SCEs, using autoradiographic techniques to detect the disposition or labeled DNA following incorporation of [³H]-thymidine. 5-Bromo-2′-deoxyuridine (drdU) has now replaced [³H]-thymidine, and various staining methods have been used to show the differential incorporation of BrdU between sister chromatids: fluorescent—Hoechst 33258 (Latt, 1973), combined fluorescent and Giemsa (Perry and Wolff, 1974), and Giemsa (Korenberg and Freedlander, 1974). The fluorescent plus Giemsa procedure is recommended in view of the fact that stained slides can be stored and microscope analysis is simpler.

In order for SCEs to be seen at metaphase, cells must pass through the S phase (Kato, 1973; 1974; Wolff and Perry, 1974). Sister chromatid exchange assays appear to occur at the replication point, since SCE induction is maximal at the beginning of DNA synthesis but drops to zero at the end of the S phase (Latt and Loveday, 1978).

For SCE analysis in vitro any cell type that is replicating or can be stimulated to divide is suitable. The incorporation of BrdU into cells in vivo allows the examination of a variety of tissues (Latt et al., 1980). Edwards et al. (1993) suggest that is necessary to standardize protocols measuring SCE since different responses can be obtained depending on the extent of simultaneous exposure of test compound and BrdU.

A. Relevance of SCE in Terms of Genotoxicity

Sister chromatid exchanges do not appear to be related to other cytogenetic events, since potent clastogens such as bleomycin and ionizing radiation induce low levels of SCE (Perry and Evans, 1975). The mechanisms involved in chromosome aberrations and SCE formation are dissimilar (e.g., Galloway and Wolff, 1979). There is not evidence that SCEs are in themselves lethal events, since there is little relationship to cytotoxicity (e.g., Bowden et al., 1979). It was suggested by Wolff (1977a, b) that they relate more to mutational events due to a compatibility with cell survival. There are examples of agents that induce significant SCE increases in the absence of mutation (Bradley et al., 1979), however, as well as the converse (Connell, 1979; Connell and Medcalf, 1982).

The SCE assay is particularly sensitive for alkylating agents and base analogues, agents causing single-strand breaks in DNA, and compounds acting through DNA binding (Latt et al., 1981). The most potent SCE inducers are S-phase-dependent. Painter (1980) reports that agents such as X irradiation, which inhibits replicon initiation, are poor SCE inducers, whereas mitomycin C, which inhibits replication fork progression, is a potent SCE inducer.

B. Experimental Design

Established cell lines and primary cell cultures of rodents may be used. Detailed information on in vitro and in vivo assays may be obtained in reviews of SCE methods by Latt et al. (1977; 1981), Perry and Thompson (1984), and Perry et al. (1984). The in vitro methods will be briefly explored here.

Monolayer or suspension cultures can be employed, as well as human lymphocytes. Human fibroblasts are less suitable because of their long cell cycle duration.

The concentration of organic solvents for the test compound should not exceed 0.8% v/v, as higher concentrations could lead to slight elevations in the SCE level (Perry et al., 1984).

For monolayer cultures, the cultures are set up the day before BrdU treatment so that the cells will be in exponential growth before the addition of BrdU or the test compound. After BrdU addition the cells are allowed to undergo the equivalent of two cell cycles before cell harvest. A spindle inhibitor such as colchicine or colcemid is introduced for the final 1 to 2 hr of culture to arrest cells in metaphase, after which the cells are harvested and chromosome preparations are made by routine cytogenetic techniques.

In the absence of metabolic activation, BrdU and the test agent can be added simultaneously and left for the duration of BrdU labeling. Shorter treatments should be used in the presence of metabolic activation or to avoid synergistic effects with BrdU, in which cells can be pulse treated (e.g., 1 hr before BrdU addition). (See Edwards et al., 1993.)

Peripheral blood cultures are established in medium containing BrdU and PHA. Cocemid is added 1 to 2 hr before harvest and the cells are harvested between 60 and 70 hr post-PHA stimulation. Cell harvest and slide preparations are conducted according to routine cytogenetic methods.

Heparinized blood samples may be stored at 4°C for up to 48 hr without affecting the SCE response (Lambert et al., 1982). If the test agent is known to react with serum or red blood cells, the mononuclear lymphocytes may be isolated by use of a Ficoll/Hypaque gradient (Boyum, 1968).

If metabolic activation is not required, treatment is best conducted over the whole of the final 24 hr of culture, or if metabolic activation is required, a pulse exposure may be employed to treat cultures at the first S phase at around 24 to 30 hr, or at 48 hr for an asynchronous population.

Exposure of cells to fluorescent light during the culture period leads to photolysis of BrdU-containing DNA and a concomitant increase in SCE frequency (Wolff and Perry, 1974). Consequently, SCE cultures should be kept in the dark and manipulated under subdued light conditions such as yellow safe light. Furthermore, media used in SCE assays should be stored in the dark, since certain media components produce reactive SCE-inducing intermediates on exposure to fluorescent light (Monticone and Schneider, 1979).

Coded and randomized slides should be read. All experiments should be repeated at least once (Perry et al., 1984) with higher and lower concentrations of S9 mix if a negative response is achieved. Even for an apparently unambiguous positive response with a greater than twofold increase in SCEs over the background level at the highest dose, and with at least two consecutive dose levels with an increased SCE response, a repeat study is necessary to show a consistent response.

The quality of differential staining will determine the ease and accuracy of SCE scoring, and to eliminate variation, results from different observers should occasionally be compared. Furthermore, to avoid observer bias, scorers should have slides from different treatment groups equally distributed among them, as with all cytogenetic studies.

REFERENCES

Adler, I. D. and Ashby, J. (1989). The present lack of evidence for unique rodent germ-cell mutagens, Muta. Res., 212:55–66.

Albanese, R. (1987). Mammalian male germ cell cytogenetics, Mutagenesis, 2:79–85.

Amacher, D. E., Paillet, S. C., Turner, G. N., Ray, V. A., and Salsburg, D. S. (1980). Point mutations at the thymidine kinase locus in L5178Y mouse lymphoma cells. 2. Test validation and interpretation, Muta. Res., 72:447–474.

Ames, B. N. (1971). The detection of chemical mutagens with enteric bacteria. In: Chemical Mutagens, Principles and Methods for Their Detection, vol. 1 (A. Hollaender, Ed.). Plenum, New York, pp. 267–282.

Ames, B. N., McCann, J., and Yamasaki, E. (1975). Methods for detecting carcinogens and mutagens with the Salmonella/mammalian-microsome mutagenicity test, Muta. Res. 31:237–364.

Anderson, D. (1990). Male mediated F_1 abnormalities, Muta. Res. 229:103–246.

Applegate, M. L., Moore, M. M., Broder, C. B. et al. (1990). Molecular dissection of mutations at the heterozygous thymidine canise locus in mouse lymphoma cells. Proceed. Natl. Acad. Sci. USA, 87:51–55.

Arlett, C. F. and Cole, J. (1990). The third United Kingdom Environmental Mutagen Society collaborative trial: Overview, a summary and assessment, Mutagenesis, 5 (suppl):85–88.

Arlett, C. F., Smith, D. M., Clark, G. M., Green, J. H. L., Cole, J., McGregor, D. B., and Asquith, J. C. (1989). Mammalian cell assays based upon colony formation. In: UKEMS Subcommittee on Guidelines for Mutagenicity Testing. Report Part III: Statistical Evaluation of Mutagenicity Test Data (D. J. Kirkland, Ed.). Cambridge University Press, Cambridge, pp. 66–101.

Ashby, J. and Tennant, R. W. (1988). Chemical structure, Salmonella mutagenicity and extent of carcinogenicity as indices of genotoxic carcinogens among 222 chemicals tested in rodents by the US NCI/NTP, Muta. Res., 204:17–115.

Ashby, J., Tennant, R. W., Zeiger, E., and Stasiewiczs, S. (1989). Classification according to chemical structure, mutagenicity to Salmonella and level of carcinogenicity of a further 42 chemicals tested for carcinogenicity by the U.S. National Toxicology Program, Muta. Res., 223:73–104.

Ashwood-Smith, M. J. (1980). Stability of frozen microsome preparations for use in the Ames Salmonella mutagenicity assay, Muta. Res., 69:199–200.

Bartsch, H., Camus, A.-M., and Malaveille, C. (1976). Comparative mutagenicity of N-nitrosamines in a semi-solid and in a liquid incubation system in the presence of rat or human tissue fractions, Muta. Res., 37:149–162.

Beckman, D. A. and Brent, R. L. (1986). Mechanism of known environmental teratogens: Drugs and chemicals, Clin. Perinatol., 13:649–687.

Bender, M. A., Griggs, H. G., and Bedford, J. S. (1974). Mechanisms of chromosomal aberration production. III. Chemicals and ionizing radiation, Muta. Res., 23:197–212.

Blazak, W. F., Steward, B. E., Galperin, I., Allen, K. L., Rudd, C. J., Mitchell, A. D., and Caspary, W. J. (1986). Chromosome analysis of triflourothymidine-resistant L5178Y mouse lymphoma cells colonies, Environ. Mutagen., 8:229–240.

Bossi, L. (1985). Information suppression. In: Genetics of Bacteria (J. Scaife, D. Leach, and A. Galizzi, Eds.). Academic, New York, pp. 49–64.

Bowden, G. T., Hsu, I. C., and Harris, C. C. (1979). The effect of caffeine on cytotoxicity, mutagenesis and sister chromatid exchanges in Chinese hamster cells treated with dihydrodiol epoxide derivatives of benzo(a)pyrene, Muta. Res., 63:361–370.

Boyum, A. (1968). Separation of lymphocytes and erythrocytes by centrifugation, Scand. J. Clin. Invest., 21:77–85.

Bradley, M. O., Hsu, I. C., and Harris, C. C. (1979). Relationships between sister chromatid exchange and mutagenicity, toxicity and DNA damage, Nature, 282:318–320.

Braithwaite, I. and Ashby, J. (1988). A non-invasive micronucleus assay in rat liver, Muta. Res., 203:23–32.

Bridges, B. A. (1972). Simple bacterial systems for detecting mutagenic agents, Lab. Prac., 21:413–419.

Bridges, B. A. (1976). Short-term screening tests for carcinogens, Nature, 261:195–200.

Bridges, B. A., Woodgate, R., Ruiz-Rubio, M., Sharif, F., Sedgwick, S. G., and Hubschere, U. (1987). Current understanding of UV-induced base pair substitution mutation in E. coli with particular reference to the DNA polymerase III complex, Muta. Res., 181:219–226.

Brook, J. D. (1982). The effect of 4CMB on germ cells of the mouse, Muta. Res., 100:305–308.

Brook, J. D. and Chandley, A. C. (1985). Testing of 3 chemical compounds for aneuploidy induction in the female mouse, Muta. Res., 157:215–220.

Brook, J. D. and Chandley, A. C. (1986). Testing for the chemical induction of aneuploidy in the male mouse, Muta. Res., 164:117–125.

Brusick, D. (1986). Genotoxic effects in cultures mammalian cells produced by low pH treatment conditions and increased ion concentrations, Environ. Mutagen., 8:879–886.

Brusick, D. (1987). Genotoxicity produced in cultures mammalian cell assays by treatment conditions (special issue), Muta. Res., 189:1–80.

Brusick, D. (1987). Principles of Genetic Toxicology, 2nd ed., Plenum, New York.

Burnett, C., Fuchs, C., Corbett, J., and Menkart, J. (1982). The effect of dimethylsulphoxide on the mutagenicity of the hair-dye, p-phenylenediamine, Muta. Res., 103:1–4.

Butterworth, B. E. and Slaga, T. J. (1987). Nongenotoxic Mechanisms in Carcinogenesis, Banbury report no. 25, Cold Spring Harbor Laboratory, Cold Spring Harbor, NY.

Carter, T. C., Lyon, M. F., and Philips, R. J. S. (1956). Induction of mutations in mice by chronic gamma irradiation: Interim report, Brit. J. Radiol., 29:106–108.

Carver, J. H., Machado, M. L., and MacGregor, J. A. (1985). Petroleum distillates suppress in vitro metabolic activation: Higher (S9) required in the Salmonella/microsome mutagenicity assay, Environ. Mutagen., 7:369–380.

Cawood, A. D. and Breckon, G. (1983). Synaptonemal complexes as indicators of induced structural change in chromosomes after irradiation of spermatogonia, Muta. Res., 122:149–154.

Chandley, A. C. (1981). The origin of chromosomal aberrations in man and their potential for survival and reproduction in the adult human population, Ann. Genet., 24:5–11.

Chu, E. H. Y. and Malling, H. U. (1968). Mammalian cell genetics. II. Chemical induction of specific lucus mutations in Chinese hamster cells in vitro, Proc. Nat. Acad. Sci. USA, 61:1306–1312.

Cifone, M. A., Myhr, B., Eiche, A., and Bolisfodi, G. (1987). Effect of pH shifts on the mutant frequency at the thymidine kinase locus in mouse lymphoma L5178Y TK$^{+/-}$ cells, Muta. Res., 189:39–46.

Clayson, D. B. (1989). ICPEMC publication No. 17: Can a mechanistic rationale be provided for non-genotoxic carcinogens identified in rodent bioassays? Muta. Res., 221:53–67.

Cleaver, J. E. (1983). Xeroderma pigmentosum. In: The Metabolic Basis of Inherited Disease (J. B. Stanbury, J. B. Wyngaarden, D. S. Fredrickson, J. C. Goldstein, and M. S. Brown, Eds.). McGraw-Hill, New York, pp. 1227–1248.

Clive, D. (1989). Mammalian cell genotoxicity: A major role for non-DNA targets? Muta. Res., 223:327–328.

Clive, D. (1987). Historical overview of the mouse lymphoma TK$^{+/-}$ mutagenicity assay. In: Mammalian Cell Mutagenesis (M. M. Moore, D. M. Demarini, F. J. De Serres, and K. R. Tindall, Eds.). Banbury report 28. Cold Spring Harbor Laboratory, Cold Spring Harbor, NY, pp. 25–36.

Clive, D., Caspary, W., Kirkby, P. E., Krehl, R., Moore, M., Mayo, J., and Oberly, T. J. (1987). Guide for performing the mouse lymphoma assay for mammalian cell mutagenicity, Muta. Res., 189:145–146.

Clive, D., Flamm, W. G., and Patterson, J. B. (1972). A mutational assay system using the thymidine kinase locus in mouse lymphoma cells, Muta. Res., 16:77–87.

Cole, J., Fox, M., Garner, R. C., McGregor, D. B., and Thacker, J. (1990). Gene mutation assays in cultured mammalian cells. In: UKEMS Subcommittee on Guidelines for Mutagenicity Testing: Report Part I Revised (D. J. Kirkland, Ed.). Cambridge University Press, Cambridge, pp. 87–114.

Cole, J., Muriel, W. J., and Bridges, B. A. (1986). The mutagenicity of sodium fluoride to L5178Y (wildtype and TK$^{+/-}$ 3.7.2c) mouse lymphoma cells, Mutagenesis, 1: 157–167.

Connell, J. R. (1979). The relationship between sister chromatid exchange, chromosome aberration and gene mutation induction by several reactive polycyclic hydrocarbon metabolites in cultured mammalian cells, Int. J. Cancer, 24:485–489.

Connell, J. R. and Medcalf, A. S. (1982). The induction of SCE and chromosomal aberrations with relation to specific base methylation of DNA in Chinese hamster cells by N-methyl-n-nitrosourea and dimethyl sulphate, Carcinogenesis, 3:385–390.

Dean, B. J. and Danford, N. (1984). Assays for the detection of chemically-induced chromosome damage in cultures mammalian cells. In: Mutagenicity Testing: A Practical Approach (S. Venitt and J. M. Parry, Eds.). IRL Press, Oxford, pp. 187–232.

DeSerres, F. J. and Shelby, M. D. (1979). Recommendations on data production and analysis using the Salmonella/microsome mutagenicity assay, Muta. Res., 64:159–165.

deVries, J. H. (1901). The Mutation Theory, Verlag von Veit, Leipzig.

Doll, R. (1977). Strategy for detection of cancer hazards to man, Nature, 265:589–596.

Dorado, G., Ariza, R. R., and Pueyo, C. (1988). Mutagenicity of red wine in the L-arabinose resistance test with Salmonella typhimurium, Mutagenesis, 3:497–502.

Dunnett, C. W. (1955). A multiple comparison procedure for comparing several treatments with a control, J. Amer. Stat. Assoc., 50:1096–1121.

Edwards, A. J., Moon, E. Y., Anderson, D., and McGregor, D. B. (1993). The effect of simultaneous exposure to bromodeoxyuridine and methyl methansulphonate on sister chromatid exchange frequency in culture human lymphocytes and its mutation research, Muta. Res., 247:117–125.

Ehling, U. H., Chu, E. H. Y., DeCarli, L., Evans, H. J., Hayashi, M., Lambert, B., Neubert, D., Thilly, W. G., and Vainio, H. (1986). Report 8: Assays for germ-cell mutations in mammals. In: Long-term and Short-term Assays for Carcinogens: A Critical Appraisal (R. Montesano, H. Bartsch, H. Vainio, J. Wilbourn, and H. Yamasaki, Eds.). IARC Scientific Publications, no. 83, Lyon, France, pp. 245–265.

Evans, H. H., Mencl, J., Horng, M. F., Ricanti, M., Sanchez, D., and Hozier, J. (1986). Lucus specificity in the mutability of L5178Y mouse lymphoma cells: The role of multilocus lesions, Proc. Nat. Acad. Sci. USA, 83:4379–4385.

Evans, H. J. and O'Riordan, M. L. (1975). Human peripheral blood lymphocytes for the analysis of chromosome aberrations in mutagen tests, Muta. Res., 31:135–148.

Ford, D. K. and Yerganian, G. (1958). Observations on the chromosomes of Chinese hamster cells in tissue culture, J. Natl. Cancer Inst., 21:393–425.

Forster, R., Green, M. H. L., and Priestley, A. (1980). Optimal levels of S9 fraction in Ames and fluctuation tests: Apparent importance of diffusion of metabolites from top agar, Carcinogenesis, 2:1081–1085.

Fox, M. (1981). Some quantitative aspects of the response of mammalian in vitro to induced mutagenesis. In: Cancer Biology Reviews, vol. 3 (J. J. Marchelonis and M. G. Hanna, Eds.). Marcel Dekker, New York, pp. 23–62.

Friedberg, E. C. (1988). DNA repair in the yeast Saccharomyces cerevisiae, Microb. Rev., 52:70–102.

Galloway, S. M. and Wolff, S. (1979). The relation between chemically induced SCE's and chromatid breakage, Muta. Res., 61:297–307.

Gatehouse, D. G. and Delow, G. F. (1979). The development of a ''Microtitre®'' fluctuation test for the detection of indirect mutagens and its use in the evaluation of mixed enzyme induction of the liver, Muta. Res., 60:239–252.

Gatehouse, D. G. and Tweats, D. J. (1987). Letter to the editor, Mutagenesis, 1:307–308.

Gatehouse, D. and Wedd, D. J. (1984). The differential mutagenicity of isoniazid in fluctuation assays and Salmonella plate tests, Carcinogenesis, 5:391–397.

Gatehouse, D. G., Wedd, D. J., Paes, D., Delow, G., Burlinson, B., Pascoe, S., Brice, A., Stemp, G., and Tweats, D. J. (1988). Investigations into the genotoxic potential of Ioxtidine, a long-acting H_2-receptor antagonist, Mutagenesis, 3:57–68.

Gatehouse, D. G., Wilcox, P., Forster, R., Rowland, I. R., and Callander, R. D. (1990). Bacterial mutation assays. In: Basic Mutagenicity Tests: UKEMS Recommended Procedures (D. J. Kirkland, Ed.). Cambridge University Press, Cambridge, pp. 13–61.

Green, M. H. L. and Muriel, W. J. (1976). Mutagen testing using TRP$^+$ reversion in E. coli, Muta. Res., 38:3–32.

Hansmann, I. and El-Nahass, E. (1979). Incidence of non-disjunction in mouse öocytes, Cytogenet. Cell Genet., 24:115–121.

Harris, C. C., Weston, A., Willey, J. C., Trivers, G. E., and Mann, D. L. (1987). Biochemical and molecular epidemiology of human cancer. Indicators of carcinogen exposure, DNA damage and genetic predisposition, Environ. Health Perspect., 75:109–119.

Haworth, S., Lawlor, T., Mortelmanns, K., Speck, W., and Zeiger, E., (1983). Salmonella mutagenicity results for 250 chemicals, Environ. Mutagen. (suppl.), 1:3–142.

Heddle, J. A. and Bodycote, D. J. (1970). On the formation of chromosomal aberrations, Muta. Res., 9:117–126.

Hera, C. and Pueyo, C. (1986). Conditions for optimal use of the L-arabinose-resistance mutagenesis test with Salmonella typhimurium, Mutagenesis, 1:267–274.

Herrera, G., Urios, A., Alexandre, V., and Blanco, M. (1988). UV light induced mutability in Salmonella strains containing the umu DC or the muc AB operon: Evidence for a umu C function, Muta. Res., 198:9–13.

Holden, H. E. (1982). Comparison of somatic and germ cell models for cytogenetic screening, J. Appl. Tox., 2:196–200.

Hozier, J., Sawger, D., Clieve, D., and Moore, M. (1982). Cytogenetic distinction between the TK$^+$ and TK$^-$ chromosomes in L5178Y/TK$^{+/-}$-3.7.2.C mouse lymphoma cell line, Muta. Res., 105:451–456.

Hsie, A. W., Brimer, P. A., Mitchell, T. J., and Gosslee, D. G. (1975). The dose-response relationship for ethyl methane sulfonate-induced mutation at the hypoxanthine-guanine phosphoribosyl transferase locus in Chinese hamster ovary cells, Somat. Cell Genet., 1:247–261.

Hubbard, S. A., Brooks, T. M., Gonzalez, L. P., and Bridges, J. W. (1985). Preparation and characterization of S9-fractions. In: Comparative Genetic Toxicology (J. M. Parry and C. F. Arlett, Eds.). Macmillan, London, pp. 413–438.

IARC. (1979). Handling Chemical Carcinogens in the Laboratory; Problems of Safety, Scientific Publications, no. 33, International Agency for Research on Cancer, Lyons, France.

ICEMC. (1983). Committee and final report: Screening strategy for chemicals that are potential germ-cell mutagens in mammals, Muta. Res., 114:117–177.

ISCN. (1985). An International System for Human Cytogenetic Nomenclature. In: Report of the Standing Committee on Human Cytogenetic Nomenclature (D. G. Harnden and H. P. Klinger, Eds.). Karger, Basel, Switzerland.

Ishidate, M. Jr. (1988a). Data Book of Chromosomal Aberration Tests in Vitro, Elsevier, Amsterdam.

Ishidate, M. Jr. (1988b). A proposed battery of tests for the initial evaluation of the mutagenic potential of medicinal and industrial chemicals, Muta. Res., 205:397–407.

Ishidate, M. Jr. and Harnois, M. C. (1987). The clastogenicity of chemicals in mammalian cells, letter to the editor, Mutagenesis, 2:240–243.

Ishidate, M. Jr., Sofuni, T., Yoshikawa, K., et al. (1984). Primary mutagenicity screening of food additives currently used in Japan, Fd. Chem. Toxicol., 22:623–636.

ISO. (1993). Biological Evaluation of Medical Devices—Part 3: Tests for Genotoxicity, Carcinogenicity, and Reproductive Toxicity, ISO 10993-3.

JMHW. (1984). Guidelines for Testing of Drugs for Toxicity, Pharmaceutical Affairs Bureau, notice no. 118, Ministry of Health and Welfare, Japan.

Joint Directives of the Japanese Environmental Protection Agency. (1987). Japanese Ministry of Health and Welfare and Japanese Ministry of International Trade and Industry, March 31.

Jordan, E., Saedler, H., and Starlinger, P. (1967). Strong polar mutations in the transferase gene of the galactose operon in E. coli, Molec. Gen. Genet., 100:296–306.

Kada, T. (1981). The DNA damaging activity of 42 coded compounds in the Rec-assay. In: Evaluation of Short-term Tests for Carcinogens—Report of the International Collaborative Program (F. de Serres and J. Ashby, Eds.). Elsevier/North Holland, Amsterdam, pp. 175–182.

Kakunaga, T. and Yamasaki, H. eds. (1984). Transformation Assays of Established Cell Lines: Mechanisms and Application, Proceedings of a Workshop Organized by IARC in Collaboration with the U.S. National Cancer Institute and the U.S. Environmental Protection Agency, Lyon, France, Feb. 15–17, IARC scientific publication no. 67.

Kalter, K. (1977). Correlation between teratogenic and mutagenic effects of chemicals in mammals. In: Chemical Mutagens: Principles and Methods for Their Detection, vol. 6 (A. Hollaender, Ed.). Plenum, New York, pp. 57–82.

Kato, H. (1973). Induction of sister chromatid exchanges by UV light and its inhibition by caffeine, Exptl. Cell Res., 82:383–390.

Kato, H. (1974). Induction of sister chromatid exchanges by chemical mutagens and its possible relevance to DNA repair, Exptl. Cell Res., 85:239–247.

Kato, T. and Shinoura, Y. (1977). Isolation and characterization of mutants of Escherichia coli deficient in induction of mutation by ultraviolet light, Molec. Gen. Genet., 156: 121–132.

Kennelly, J. C., Stanton, C., and Martin, C. N. (1984). The effect of acetyl-CoA supplementation on the mutagenicity of benzidines in the Ames assay, Muta. Res., 137: 39–45.

Kirkland, D. (1992). Chromosomal aberration tests in vitro: problems with protocol design and interpretation of results, Mutagenesis, 7:95–106.

Kirkland, D. J. and Garner, R. C. (1987). Testing for genotoxicity-chromosomal aberrations in vitro—CHO cells or human lymphocytes? Muta. Res., 189:186–187.

Korenberg, J. R. and Freedlender, E. F. (1974). Giesma technique for the detection of sister chromatid exchanges, Chromasoma, 48:355–360.

Lambert, B., Lindblad, A., Holmberg, K., and Francesconi, D. (1982). The use of sister chromatid exchange to monitor human populations for exposure to toxicologically harmful agents. In: Sister Chromatid Exchange (S. Wolff, Ed.). Wiley, New York, pp. 149–182.

Latt, S. A. (1973). Microfluorometric detection of deoxyribonucleic acid replication in human metaphase chromosomes, Proceed. Nat. Acad. Sci. USA, 770:3395–3399.

Latt, S., Allen, J. W., Bloom, S. E., et al. (1981). Sister chromatid exchanges: A report of the gene-tox program, Muta. Res., 87:17–62.

Latt, S. A., Allen, J. W., Rogers, W. E., and Jurgens, L. A. (1977). In vitro and in vivo analysis of sister chromatid exchange formation. In: Handbook of Mutagenicity Test Procedures (B. J. Kilbey, M. Legator, W. Nichols, and C. Ramel, Eds.). Elsevier, Amsterdam, pp. 275–291.

Latt, S. A. and Loveday, K. S. (1978). Characterization of sister chromatid exchange induction by 8-methoxypsoralen plus UV light, Cytogen. Cell Genet., 21:184–200.

Latt, S. A., Schreck, R. R., Loveday, K. S., Dougherty, C. P., and Shuler, C. F. (1980). Sister chromatid exchanges, Adv. Human Genet., 31:291–298.

Lawley, P. (1989). Mutagens as carcinogens: Development of current concepts, Muta. Res., 213:3–26.

Li, A. P., Aaron, C. S., Aueltta, A. E., Dearfield, K. L., Riddle, J. C., Slesinski, R. S., and Stankowski, L. F. Jr. (1991). An evaluation of the roles of mammalian cell mutation assays in the testing of chemical genotoxicity, Reg. Toxicol. Pharmacol., 14:24–40.

Li, A. P., Carver, J. H., Choy, W. N., Bupta, R. S., Loveday, K. S., O'Neill, J. P., Riddle, J. C., Stankowski, L. F., and Yang, L. C. (1987). A guide for the performance of the Chinese hamster ovary cell/hypoxanthine guanine phosphoribosyl transferase gene mutation assay, Muta. Res., 189:135–141.

Linblad, W. J. and Jackim, E. (1982). Mechanism for the differential induction of mutation by kS9 activated benzo(a)pyrene employing either a glucose-6-phosphate dependent NADPH-regenerating system or an isocitrate dependent system, Muta. Res., 96:109–118.

Lindahl, T. (1979). DNA glycosylases, endonucleases for apurinic/apyrimidinic sites and base excision repair, Proc. Nucl. Acid Res. Mol. Bio., 22:109–118.

Lindahl, T., Sedwick, B., Sekiguchi, M., and Nakabeppu, Y. (1988). Regulation and expression of the adaptive response to alkylating agents, Ann. Rev. Biochem., 57:133–157.

Little, J. W. (1984). Autodigestion of lex A and phage T repressors, Proc. Nat. Acad. Sci. USA, 81:1375–1379.

Little, J. W. and Mount, D. W. (1982). The SOS regulatory system of Escherichia coli, Cell, 29:11–22.

MacGregor, J. T., Wehr, C. M., and Gould, D. H. (1980). Clastogen-induced micronuclei in peripheral blood erythrocytes: The basis of an improved micronucleus test, Environ. Mutagen., 2:509–514.

MacPhee, D. G. (1973). Salmonella typhimurium hisG46 (R-Utrecht): Possible use in screening mutagens and carcinogens, Appl. Microbio., 26:1004–1005.

Madle, S. and Obe, G. (1980). Methods for the analysis of the mutagenicity of indirect mutagens/carcinogens in eukaryotic cells, Human Genet., 56:7–20.

Mahon, G. A. T., Green, M. H. L., Middleton, B., Mitchell, I. DeG., Robinson, W. D., and Tweats, D. J. (1989). Analysis of data from microbial colon assays. In: Statistical Evaluation of Mutagenicity Test Data (D. J. Kirkland, Ed.). Cambridge University Press, Cambridge, pp. 26–65.

Marinus, M. G. and Morris, R. N. (1974). Biological function for the 6-methyladenine residues in the DNA of Escherichia coli K12, J. Molec. Bio., 85:309–322.

Maron, D. M. and Ames, B. N. (1983). Revised methods for the Salmonella mutagenicity test, Muta. Res., 113:173–215.

McCann, J., Choi, E., Yamasaki, E., and Ames, B. N. (1975). Detection of carcinogens as mutagens in the *Salmonella typhimurium* test assay of 300 chemicals, Proc. Natl. Acad. Sci. USA, 72:5135–5139.

Miller, E. C. and Miller, J. A. (1971). The mutagenicity of chemical carcinogens: Correlations, problems and interpretations. In: Chemical Mutagens, Principles and Methods for Their Detection, vol. 1 (A. Hollaender, Ed.). Plenum, New York, pp. 83–120.

Miller, J. H. (1985). Pathways of mutagenesis revealed by analysis of mutational specificity. In: Genetics of Bacteria (J. Scaife, D. Leach, and A. Galizzi, Eds.). Academic, New York, pp. 25–40.

Modrich, P. (1987). DNA mismatch correction, Ann. Rev. Biochem., 56:435–466.

Monticone, R. E. and Schneider, E. L. (1979). Induction of SCEs in human cells by fluorescent light, Muta. Res., 59:215–221.

Morimoto, K., Sato, M., and Koizumi, A. (1983). Proliferative kinetics of human lymphocytes in culture measure by autoradiography and sister chromatid differential staining, Epithel. Cell Res., 145:249–356.

Mortelmans, K. E. and Dousman, L. (1986). Mutagenesis and plasmids. In: Chemical Mutagens, Principles and Methods for Their Detection vol. 10 (F. J. de Serres, Ed.). Plenum, New York, pp. 469–508.

Mortelmans, K. E. and Strocker, B. A. D. (1979). Segregation of the mutator property of plasmid R46 from its ultraviolet-protecting property, Molec. Gen. Genet., 167:317–328.

MRC. (1981). Guidelines for Work with Chemical Carcinogens in Medical Research Council Establishments, Medical Research Council, London.

Muller, H. J. (1927). Artificial transmutation of the gene, Science, 66:84–87.

Natarajan, A. T. and Obe, G. (1982). Mutagenicity testing with cultured mammalian cells: Cytogenetic assays. In: Mutagenicity: New Horizons in Genetic Toxicology (J. A. Heddle, Ed.). Academic, New York, pp. 172–213.

Neudecker, T. and Henschler, D. (1985). Allyl isothiocyanate is mutagenic in Salmonella typhimurium, Muta. Res., 30:143–148.

Newton, M. F. and Lilly, L. J. (1986). Tissue specific clastogenic effects of chromium and selenium salts in vivo, Muta. Res., 169:61–69.

Oberly, T. J., Bewsey, B. J., and Probst, G. S. (1987). A procedure for the CHO/HGPRT mutation assay involving treatment of cells in suspension culture and selection of mutants in soft agar, Muta. Res., 182:99–111.

OECD. (1983). OECD Guidelines for the Testing of Chemicals, no. 475: Genetic toxicology: In vivo mammalian bone marrow cytogenetic test—chromosomal analysis. adopted April 4, 1984, Geneva, Switzerland.

Ong. T., Mukhtar, M., Wolf, C. R., and Zeiger, E. (1980). Differential effects of cytochrome P450-inducers on promutagen activation capabilities and enzymatic activities of S-9 from rat liver, J. Environ. Path. Toxicol., 4:55–65.

Pagano, D. A. and Zeiger, E. (1985). The stability of mutagenic chemicals tested in solution, Environ. Mutagen., 7:293–302.

Painter, R. B. (1980). A replication model of sister-chromatid exchange, Muta. Res., 70: 337–341.

Parry, J. M., Arlett, C. F., and Ashby, J. (1985). An overview of the results of the in vivo and in vitro test systems used to assay the genotoxicity of BZD, DAT, DAB and CDA in the second UKEMS study. In: Comparative Genetic Toxicology: The Second UKEMS Collaborative Study (J. M. Parry, and C. F. Arlett, Eds.). Macmillan, London, pp. 597–616.

Perry, P. E. and Evans, H. J. (1975). Cytological detection of mutagen/carcinogen exposure by sister chromatid exchange, Nature, 258:121–125.

Perry, P., Henderson, L., and Kirkland, D. (1984). Sister chromatid exchange in cultured cells. In: UKEMS Subcommittee on Guidelines for Mutagenicity Testing. Report Part IIA, pp. 89–121.

Perry, P. E. and Thomson, E. J. (1984). Sister chromatid exchange methodology. In: Handbook of Mutagenicity Test Procedures (B. J. Kilbey, M. Legator, W. Nichols, and C. Ramel, Eds.). Elsevier, Amsterdam, pp. 495–529.

Perry, P. E. and Wolff, S. (1974). New Giemsa method for the differential staining of sister chromatids, Nature, 251:156–158.

Pinney, R. J. (1980). Distribution among incompatibility groups of plasmids that confer UV mutability and UV resistance, Muta. Res., 72:155–159.

Preston, R. J., Au, W., Bender, M., et al. (1981). Mammalian in vivo and in vitro cytogenetic assays, Muta. Res., 87:143–188.

Preston, R. J., San Sebastian, J. R., and McFee, A. F. (1987). The in vitro human lymphocyte assay for assessing the clastogenicity of chemical agents, Muta. Res., 189: 175–183.

Prival, M. J., Bell, S. J., Mitchell, V. D., Peiperi, M. D., and Vaughn, V. L. (1984). Mutagenicity of benzidine and benzidine-congener dyes and selected monoazo dyes in a modified Salmonella assay, Muta. Res., 136:33–47.

Prival, M. J. and Mitchell, V. D. (1982). Analysis of a method for testing azo-dyes for mutagenic activity in S. typhimurium in the presence of FMN in hamster liver S9, Muta. Res., 97:103–116.

Pueyo, C. and Lopez-Barea, J. (1979). The L-arabinose-resistance test with Salmonella typimurium strain SV3 selects forward mutations at several ara genes, Muta. Res., 64:249–258.

Revell, S. H. (1974). The breakage-and-reunion theory and the exchange theory for chromosome aberrations induced by ionizing radiations: A short history. In: Advances in Radiation Biology, vol. 4 (J. T. Lett and M. Zelle, Eds.). Academic, New York, pp. 367–415.

Richardson, C., Williams, D. A., Allen, J. A., Amphlett, G., Changer, D. O., and Phillips,

B. (1989). Analysis of data from in vitro cytogenetic assays. In: UKEMS Sub-committee on Guidelines for Mutagenicity Testing. Report. Part III. Statistical Evaluation of Mutagenicity Test Data (D. J. Kirkland, Ed.). Cambridge University Press, Cambridge, pp. 141–154.

Robinson, W. D., Green, M. H. L., Cole, J., Healy, M. J. R., Garner, R. C., and Gatehouse, D. (1989). Statistical evaluation of bacterial mammalian fluctuation tests. In: Statistical Evaluation of Mutagenicity Test Data (D. J. Kirkland, Ed.). Cambridge University Press, Cambridge, pp. 102–140.

Rossman, T. G. and Klein, C. B. (1988). From DNA damage to mutation in mammalian cells: A review, Environ. Molec. Mutagen., 11:119–133.

Roth, J. R. (1974). Frameshift mutations, Ann. Rev. Genet., 8:319–346.

Russell, L. B. (1984). Procedures and evaluation of results of the mouse spot test. In: Handbook of Mutagenicity Test Procedures (B. J. Kilbey, M. Legator, W. Nichols, and C. Ramel, Eds.). Elsevier, Amsterdam, pp. 393–403.

Russell, W. L. (1951). X-ray induced mutations in mice, Cold Spg. Harb. Symp. Quant. Bio., 16:327–336.

Russell, W. L. (1989). Reminiscences of a mouse specific-locus addict, Environ. Molec. Mutagen., 14 (suppl. 16):16–22.

Samson, L. and Cairns, J. (1977). A new pathway for DNA repair in E. coli, Nature, 267: 281–282.

Scott, D., Dean, B. J., Danford, N. D., and Kirkland, D. J. (1990). Metaphase chromosome aberration assays in vitro. In: UKEMS Subcommittee on Guidelines for Mutagenicity Testing, Report. Part I: Revised Basic Mutagenicity Tests, UKEMS Recommended Procedures (D. J. Kirkland, Ed.). Cambridge University Press, Cambridge, pp. 63–86.

Searle, A. G. (1984). The specific locus test in the mouse. In: Handbook of Mutagenicity Test Procedures (B. J. Kilbey, M. Legator, W. Nichols, and C. Ramel, Eds.). Elsevier, Amsterdam, pp. 373–391.

Sedgwick, S. G. and Goodwin, P. A. (1985). Differences in mutagenic and recombinational DNA repair in enterobacteria, Proceed. Nat. Acad. Sci. USA, 82:4172–4176.

Selby, P. B. and Olson, W. H. (1981). Methods and criteria for deciding whether specific-locus mutation-rate data in mice indicates a positive, negative or inconclusive result, Muta. Res., 83:403–418.

Shanabruch, W. G. and Walker, G. C. (1980). Localization of the plasmid (pKM101) gene(s) involved in recA$^+$lexA$^+$-dependent mutagenesis, Molec. Gen. Genet., 129: 289–297.

Steel, R. G. D. and Torrie, J. H. (1960). Principles and Procedures of Statistics, McGraw-Hill, New York.

Streisinger, G., Okada, T., Emrich, J., et al. (1966). Frameshift mutations and the genetic code, Cold Spg. Harb. Symp. Quant. Bio., 31:77–84.

Tates, A. D., Neuteboom, I., Hofker, M., and den Engelese, L. (1980). A micronucleus technique for detecting clastogenic effects of mutagens/carcinogens (DEN,DMN) in hepatocytes of rat liver in vivo, Muta. Res., 74:11–20.

Tennant, R. W., Margolin, B. H., Shelby, M. D., Zeiger, E., Haseman, J. K., Spalding, J., Caspary, W., Resnick, M., Stasiewicz, S., Anderson, B., and Minor, R. (1987).

Prediction of chemical carcinogenicity in rodents from in vitro genetic toxicity assays, Science, 236:933–941.

Thomas, S. M. and Sedgwick, S. G. (1989). Cloning of Salmonella typimurium DNA encoding mutagenic DNA repair, J. Bacteriol., 171:5776–5782.

Thompson, E. D. (1986). Comparison of in vivo and in vitro cytogenetic assay results, Environ. Mutagen., 8:753–767.

Thust, R., Mendel, J., Schwarz, H., and Warzoki, R. (1980). Nitrosated urea pesticide metabolites and other nitrosamides: Activity in clastogenicity and SCE assays, and aberration kinetics in Chinese hamster V79-E cells, Muta. Res., 79:239–248.

Topham, J., Albanese, R., Bootman, J., Scott, D., and Tweats, D. (1983). In vivo cytogenetic assays. In: Report of UKEMS Sub-committee on Guidelines for Mutagenicity Testing. Part I (B. Dea, Ed.). pp. 119–141, Swansea, UK.

Tsuchimoto, T. and Matter, B. E. (1979). In vivo cytogenetic screening methods for mutagens with special reference to the micronucleus test, Arch. Toxicol., 42:239–248.

Tweats, D. J. and Gatehouse, D. G. (1988). Discussion forum: Further debate of testing strategies, Mutagenesis, 3:95–102.

Venitt, S. and Crofton-Sleigh, C. (1981). Mutagenicity of 42 coded compounds in a bacterial assay using Escherichia coli and Salmonella typhimurium. In: Evaluation of Short-term Tests for Carcinogens. Report of the International Collaborative Program. Progress in Mutational Research, vol. 1 (F. J. de Serres and J. Ashby, Eds.). Elsevier, New York, pp. 351–360.

Venitt, S. and Parry, J. M. (1984). Background to mutagenicity testing. In: Mutagenicity Testing: A Practical Approach (S. Venitt and J. M. Parry, Eds.). IRL Press, Oxford, pp. 1–24.

Villani, G., Boiteux, S., and Radman, M. (1978). Mechanisms of ultraviolet-induced mutagenesis: Extent and fidelity of in vitro DNA synthesis on irradiated template, Proc. Nat. Acad. Sci. USA, 75:3037–3041.

Wagner, R. and Meselson, M. (1976). Repair tracts in mismatched DNA heteroduplexes, Proc. Nat. Acad. Sci. USA, 73:4135–4139.

Wahrendorf, J., Mahon, G. A. T., and Schumacher, M. (1985). A non-parametric approach to the statistical analysis of mutagenicity data, Muta. Res., 147:5–13.

Walker, G. C. (1984). Mutagenesis and inducible responses to deoxyribonucleic acid damage in Escherichia coli, Microbio. Rev., 48:60–93.

Walker, G. C. and Dobson, P. P. (1979). Mutagenesis and repair deficiencies of Escherichia coli umu C mutants are suppressed by the plasmid pKM101, Proc. Gen. Genet., 172:17–24.

Wilcox, P., Naidoo, A., Wedd, D. J., and Gatehouse, D. G. (1990). Comparison of Salmonella Typhimurium TA102 with Escherichia coli WP2 tester strains, Mutagenesis, 5:285–291.

Wolff, S. (1977a). Lesions that lead to SCEs are different from those that lead to chromosome aberrations, Muta. Res., 46:164.

Wolff, S. (1977b). In vitro inhibition of mono-oxygenase dependent reactions by organic solvents, International Conference on Industrial and Environmental Xenobiotics, Prague. Czechoslovakia.

Wolff, S. and Perry, P. (1974). Differential staining of sister chromatids and the study of sister chromatid exchange without autoradiography, Chromosomes, 48:341–353.

Xu, L., Whong, W. Z., and Ong, T. M. (1984). Validation of the Salmonella (SV50)/L-arabinose-resistant forward mutation assay with 26 compounds, Muta. Res., 130: 79–86.

Yahagi, T., Degawa, M., Seino, Y., et al. (1975). Mutagenicity of carcinogen azo dyes and their derivatives, Cancer Lett., 1:91–96.

Yahagi, T., Nagao, M., Seino, Y., Matsushima, T., Sugimura, T., and Okada, M. (1977). Mutagenicities of N-nitrosamines in Salmonella, Muta. Res., 48:120–130.

Yanofsky, C. (1971). Mutagenesis studies with Escherichia coli mutants with known amino acid and base-pair changes. In: Chemical Mutagens, Principles and Methods for Their Detection, vol. 1 (A. Hollaender, Ed.). Plenum, New York, pp. 283–287.

11

Subchronic and Chronic Toxicity and Reproductive and Developmental Toxicity

This chapter addresses a group of studies that (1) are intended to predict longer-term effects that occur after repeated exposure to an agent and (2) are only performed on a small subset of devices and the materials used to make them.

Subchronic and chronic studies for medical devices are generally in the range of being hybrids between what we are used to regarding as subchronic studies and the simple implant studies. The studies are performed using only one route—implantation—with "dose" being determined in terms of how many devices (or much material) are implanted. In their simplest forms these subchronic and chronic studies are conducted as nothing more than very long implantation studies with only the limited set of local issue tolerance indicators in the region of the implants being evaluated. It should also be kept in mind that it is frequent practice to combine such biocompatibility studies with evaluations of efficacy and/or device performance.

I. OBJECTIVES

As with any scientific study or experiment (but especially for those in safety assessment), the essential first step is to define and understand the reason(s) for the conduct of the study—that is, its objectives. There are three major (scientific) reasons for conducting subchronic studies, but a basic characteristic of all but a few subchronic studies needs to be understood. The subchronic study is (as are most other studies in whole animal toxicology) a broad screen. It is not focused on a specific end point; rather, it is a broad exploration of the cumulative biological effects of the administered agent over a range of doses. It is so broad an exploration, in fact, that it can be called a "shotgun" study. The objectives of the typical subchronic device study fall into two categories. The first is to broadly define the toxicity of prolonged exposure to a medical device or medical device material in an animal model (most commonly, the rabbit). The second objective is one of looking forward to later studies. The subchronic study must provide sufficient information to allow a prudent setting of doses for later, longer studies (including, ultimately, carcinogenicity studies). At the same time, the subchronic study must also provide guidance for the other (than dose) design features of longer-term studies (e.g., what parameters to measure and when to measure them, how many animals to use, and how long to conduct the study). These objectives are addressed by the usual subchronic study.

Chronic studies (those that last 6 months or a year) may also be conducted for the above purposes but are primarily done to fulfill registration requirements for drugs that are intended for continuous long-term (lifetime) use or frequent intermittent use.

II. REGULATORY CONSIDERATIONS

Much of what is done (and how it is done) in repeat-dose studies is a response to a number of regulations. Three of these have very broad impact. These are the good laboratory practices (GLPs) requirements, Animal Welfare Act requirements, and regulatory requirements that actually govern study design.

A. Good Laboratory Practices

Since 1978, the design and conduct of preclinical safety assessment studies for pharmaceuticals in the United States (and indeed, internationally) have been governed and significantly influenced by GLPs. Strictly speaking, these regulations cover qualifications of staff and facilities, training, record keeping, documentation, and actions required to ensure compliance with and the effectiveness of these steps. Though the initial regulations were from the U.S. FDA (Food and Drug Administration, 1983), they have always been extended to cover studies performed overseas (Food and Drug Administration, 1988). Most other countries have adopted similar regulations. A discussion of these regulations is beyond the scope of the current chapter, but several aspects are central to this effort. Each technique or methodology to be employed in a study (e.g., animal identification, weighting and examination, blood collection, and data recording) must be adequately described in the standard operating procedure (SOP) before the study begins. Those who are to perform such procedures must be trained in them beforehand. The actual design of the study, including start date and how it is to be ended and analyzed, plus the principal scientists involved (particularly the study director), must be specified in a protocol that is signed before the study commences. Any changes to these features must be documented in amendments once the study has begun. It is a good idea that the pathologist who is to later perform or oversee histopathology be designated before the start of the study, and that the design be a team effort involving the best efforts of the toxicologist and pathologist.

B. Animal Welfare Act

Gone are the days in which the pharmaceutical scientist could conduct whatever procedures or studies that were desired using experimental animals. The Animal Welfare Act (APHIS, 1989) (and its analogues in other countries) rightfully requires careful consideration of animal usage to ensure that research and testing uses as few animals as possible in as humane a manner as possible. As a start, all protocols must be reviewed by an institutional animal care and use committee. Such review takes time, but should not hinder good science. When designing a study or developing a new procedure or technique, the following points should be kept in mind:

1. Will the number of animals used be sufficient to provide the required data yet not constitute excessive use? (It ultimately does not reduce animal use to utilize too few animals to begin with and then have to repeat the study.)
2. Are the procedures employed the least invasive and traumatic available? This practice is not only required by regulations, but is also sound scientific practice, since any induced stress will produce a range of responses in test animals that can mask or confound the chemically induced effects.

C. Regulatory Requirements for Study Design

The first consideration in the construction of a study is a clear statement of its objectives, which are almost always headed by meeting regulatory requirements to support device development and registration. Accordingly, the relevant regulatory requirement must be analyzed, which is complicated by the fact that new drugs are no longer developed for registration and sale in a single-market country. The expense is too great, and the potential for broad international sales too appealing. Chapter 2 should be consulted for the broad overview of such regulation.

D. Study Design and Conduct

1. Animals

In all but a few rare cases, medical devices are evaluated for subchronic and chronic biocompatibility in only a single species. This is most often the rabbit, although the rat, dog, and hamster have also been used. The factors that should and do govern species selection are reviewed in detail in Gad and Chengelis (1992).

Except in rare cases, the animals used are young, healthy adults in the logarithmic phase of their growth curve. (The FDA specifies that rodents be less than 6 weeks of age at the initiation of dosing.)

The numbers of animals to be used in each dose group of a study are presented in Table 11.1. Although the usual practice is to use three different dose groups and at least one equal-sized control group, this number is not fixed and should be viewed as a minimum. There must be as many control animals as are in the largest-size test group.

Animals are assigned to groups (test and control) by one or another form of statistical randomization. Prior to assignment, animals are evaluated for some period of time after being received in house (usually at least 1 week for rodents and 2 for nonrodents) to ensure that they are healthy and have no discernible abnormalities. The randomization is never pure; it is always "blocked" in some form or another (by initial body weight, at least) so that each group is not (statistically) significantly different from the others in terms of the "blocked" parameters (usually initial body weight).

Proper facilities and care for test animals are not only a matter of regulatory compliance (and a legal requirement), but also essential for a scientifically sound and valid study. Husbandry requires clean cages of sufficient size and continuous availability of clean water and food (unless the protocol requires some restriction on their availability). Environmental conditions (temperature, humidity, and

TABLE 11.1 Number of Animals for Chronic and Subchronic Study per Test Group

Study length	Rats per sex	Dogs per sex	Rabbits per sex
Two–4 weeks	5	3	4
Three months	20	6	8
Six months	30	8	8
One year	50	10	10

Note: Starting with 13-week studies, one should consider adding animals (particularly to the high-dose group) to allow evaluation of reversal (or progression) of effects.

light–dark cycle) must be kept within specified limits. All of these must in turn be detailed in the protocols of studies. The limits for these conditions are set forth in relevant National Institutes of Health (NIH) and United States Department of Agriculture (USDA) publications.

2. Setting Doses

Setting doses for longer-term toxicity studies is one of the most difficult tasks in study design. The doses administered must include one that is devoid of any adverse effect (preferably of *any* effect) and yet still high enough to "clear" the projected clinical dose by the traditional or regulatory safety factors (10× for rodents, 5× for nonrodents), and a second that presents the actual "dose" of clinical exposure. The resulting dose response curve should establish the following:

> The *no adverse effect level* (NOEL)—the maximum dose that an animal can tolerate over a defined period of time without showing any adverse effects; above this dose, adverse effects are observed.
> The *maximum implantable dose* (MID)—the maximum amount of implant material (dose) that a test animal can tolerate without any adverse physical or mechanical effects. (Note: To avoid unnecessary morbidity in animals on a long-term test, preliminary testing may be necessary.)

Dose for devices and implant materials is usually evaluated in terms of exposed surface area per body mass except for the case of absorbable sutures where it is considered in terms of weight/body mass.

Traditionally, studies include three or more dose groups to fulfill these two objectives. Based on earlier results (generally, single-dose or 2-week studies), doses are selected. Also, it is generally an excellent idea to observe the "decade rule" in extrapolation of results from shorter to longer studies; that is, do not try to project doses for more than an order-of-magnitude-longer study (thus the traditional progression from single-dose to 14-day to 90-day studies). In addition, one should not allow the traditional use of three dose groups plus a control to limit designs. If there is a great deal of uncertainty, it is much cheaper in every way to use four or five dose groups in a single study than to have to repeat the entire study. Finally, remember that different doses may be appropriate for each sex.

III. PARAMETERS TO MEASURE

As was stated earlier, subchronic studies are usually shotgun in nature; that is, they are designed to look at a very broad range of end points with the intention of screening as broadly as indications of toxicity. Meaningful findings are rarely limited to a single end point; rather, what typically emerges is a pattern of findings. This broad search for components of a toxicity profile is not just a response to regulatory guidelines intended to identify potentially unsafe drugs. An understanding of all indicators of biological effect can also frequently help one to understand the relevance of findings, to establish some as unrepresentative of a risk to humans, and even to identify new therapeutic uses of an agent.

Parameters of interest in the repeat-dose study can be considered as sets of measure, each with its own history, rationale, and requirements. It is critical to remember, however, that the strength of the study design as a scientific evaluation lies in the relationships and patterns of effects that are seen not in simply looking at each of these measures (or groups) as independent findings, but rather as integrated profiles of biological effects.

A. Body Weight

Body weight (and the associated calculated parameter of body weight gain) is a nonspecific broad screen for adverse systemic toxicity. Animals are initially assigned to groups based on a randomization scheme that includes having each group vary insignificantly from one another in terms of body weight. Weights are measured prior to the initial dose, then typically 1, 3, 5, 7, 11, and 14 days thereafter. The frequency of measurement of weights goes down as the study proceeds. After 2 weeks, weighting is typically weekly through 6 weeks, then every other week through 3 months, and monthly thereafter. Because the animals used in these studies are young adults in the early log phase of their growth, decreases in the rate of gain relative to control animals is a very sensitive (albeit nonspecific) indicator of systemic toxicity.

B. Food Consumption

Food consumption is typically measured with one or two uses in mind. First, it may be explanatory in the interpretation of reductions (either absolute or relative) in body weight. In cases in which administration of the test compound is via diet, it is essential to be able to adjust dietary content to accurately maintain dose levels. Additionally, the actual parameter itself is a broad and nonspecific indicator of systemic toxicity. Food consumption is usually measured over a period of several days, first weekly and then on a once-a-month basis. Water consumption, which is also sometimes measured, is similar in interpretation and use.

C. Clinical Signs

Clinical signs are generally vastly underrated in value, probably because insufficient attention is paid to care in their collection. Two separate levels of data collection are actually involved here. The first is the morbidity and mortality observation, which is made twice a day. This generally consists of a simple cage-side visual assessment of each animal to determine if it is still alive, and if so, whether or not it appears in good (or at least stable) health. Historically, this regulatorily required observation was intended to ensure that tissues from intoxicated animals were not lost for meaningful histopathologic evaluation due to autolysis (Arnold et al., 1990).

The second level of clinical observation is the detailed hands-on examination analogous to the human physical examination. It is usually performed against a checklist (see Gad and Chengelis, 1998, for an example), and evaluation is of the incidence of observations of a particular type in a group of treated animals compared to controls. Observations range from being indicative of nonspecific systemic toxicity to fairly specific indicators of target organ toxicity. These more detailed observations are typically taken after the first week of a study and on a monthly basis thereafter.

Ophthalmologic examinations are typically made immediately prior to initiation of a study (and thus serve to screen out animals with pre-existing conditions) and toward the end of a study.

TABLE 11.2 Number of Animals for Chronic and Subchronic Study per Test Group

Clinical chemistry	Hematology	Urinalysis
Albumin	Erythrocyte count (RBC)	Chloride
Alkaline phosphatase (ALP)	Hemaglobin (HGB)	Bilirubin
Blood urea nitrogen (BUN)	Hematocrit (HCT)	Glucose
Calcium	Mean corpuscular hemo-	Ketone
Chloride	globin (MCH)	Osmolality
Creatine	Mean corpuscular volume	Occult blood
Creatine phosphokinase (CPK)	(MCV)	pH
Direct bilirubin	Platelet count	Phosphorus
Gamma glutamyl transferase	Prothrombin time	Potassium
(GGT)	Reticulocyte count	Protein
Globulin	White cell count (WBC)	Sodium
Glucose	White cell differential count	Specific gravity
Lactic dehydrogenase (LDH)		Volume
Phosphorus		
Potassium		
Serum glutamic-oxaloacetic transaminase (SGOT)		
Serum glutamic-pyruvic trans- aminase (SGPT)		
Sodium		
Total bilirubin		
Total cholesterol		
Total protein		
Triglycerides		

TABLE 11.3 Association of Changes in Biochemical Parameters with Actions at Particular Target Organs

Parameter	Blood	Heart	Lung	Kidney	Liver	Bone	Intestine	Pancreas	Notes
Albumin				↓	↓				Produced by the liver. Very significant reductions indicate extensive liver damage.
ALP (alkaline phosphatase)				↑	↑	↑	↑		Elevations usually associated with cholestasis. Bone alkaline phosphatase tends to be higher in young animals.
Bilirubin (total)	↑				↑				Usually elevated due to cholestasis either due to obstruction or hepatopathy.
BUN (blood urea nitrogen)				↑	↓				Estimates blood-filtering capacity of the kidneys. Doesn't become significantly elevated until kidney function is reduced 60–75%.
Calcium				↑					Can be life-threatening and result in acute death.
Cholinesterase				↑					Found in plasma, brain, and RBC.
CPK (creatinine phosphokinase)		↑			↓				Most often elevated due to skeletal muscle damage but can also be produced by cardiac muscle damage. Can be more sensitive than histopathology.
Creatine				↑					Also estimates blood-filtering capacity of kidney as BUN does. More specific than BUN.

Parameter	Change	Comments
Glucose	↑	Alterations other than those associated with stress are uncommon and reflect an effect on the pancreatic islets or anorexia.
GGT (gamma glutamyl transferase)	↑	Elevated in cholestasis. This is a microsomal enzyme and levels often increase in response to microsomal enzyme induction.
HBDH (hydroxybutyric dehydrogenase)	↑	Most prominent in cardiac muscle tissue.
LDH (lactic dehydrogenase)	↑	Increase usually due to skeletal muscle, cardiac muscle, and liver damage. Not very specific unless isozymes are evaluated.
Protein (total)	↑	Absolute alterations are usually associated with decreased production (liver) or increased loss (kidney).
SGOT (serum glutamic-oxaloacetic transaminase; also called AST (aspirate amino transferase);	↑	Present in skeletal muscle and heart and most commonly associated with damage to these.
SGPT (serum glutamic-pyruvic transaminase; also called ALT (alanide amino transferase);	↑	Elevations usually associated with hepatic damage or disease.
SDH (sorbitol dehydrogenase)	↑ or ↓	Liver enzyme that can be quite sensitive but is fairly unstable. Samples should be processed as soon as possible.

TABLE 11.4 Some Probable Conditions Affecting Hematological Changes

Parameter	Elevation	Depression

Red blood cells	1. Vascular shock
	2. Excessive diuresis
	3. Chronic hypoxia
	4. Hyperadrenocorticism
		1. Anemias
		  a. Blood loss
		  b. Hemolysis
		  c. Low RBC production

Hematocrit	1. Increased RBC
	2. Stress
	3. Shock
	  a. Trauma
	  b. Surgery
	4. Polycythemia
		1. Anemias
		2. Pregnancy
		3. Excessive hydration

Hemoglobin	1. Polycythemia (increase in production of RBC)	1. Anemias 2. Lead poisonings
Mean cell volume	1. Anemias 2. B-12 deficiency	1. Iron deficiency
Mean corpuscular hemoglobin	1. Reticulocytosis	1. Iron deficiency
White blood cells	1. Bacterial infections 2. Bone marrow stimulation	1. Bone marrow depression 2. Cancer chemotherapy 3. Chemical intoxication 4. Splenic disorders
Platelets		1. Bone marrow depression 2. Immune disorder
Neutrophilis	1. Acute bacterial infections 2. Tissue necrosis 3. Strenuous exercise 4. Convulsions 5. Tachycardia 6. Acute hemorrhage	1. Viral infections
Lymphocytes	1. Leukemia 2. Malnutrition 3. Viral infections	
Monocytes	1. Protozoal infections	
Eosinophils	1. Allergy 2. Irradiation 3. Pernicious anemia 4. Parasitism	
Basophils	1. Lead poisoning	

Particularly when the agent under investigation either targets or acts via a mechanism likely to have a primary effect on a certain organ for which functional measures are available, an extra set of measurements of functional performance should be considered. The organs or organ systems that are usually of particular concern are the kidneys, liver, cardiovascular, nervous, and immune. Special measures (e.g., creatinine clearance as a measure of renal function) are combined with other data already collected (organ weights, histopathology, clinical pathology, etc.) to provide a focused ''special'' investigation or evaluation of adverse effects on the target organ system of concern.

D. Clinical Pathology

Clinical pathology covers a number of biochemical and morphological evaluations based on invasive and noninvasive sampling of fluids from animals that are made periodically during the course of a subchronic study. These evaluations are sometimes labeled as clinical (as opposed to anatomical) pathology determinations. Table 11.2 presents a summary of the parameters measured under the headings of clinical chemistry, hematology, and urinalysis, using samples of blood and urine collected at predetermined intervals during the study. Conventionally, these intervals are typically at three points evenly spaced over the course of the study, with the first being 1 month after study initiation and the last being immediately prior to termination of the test animals. For a 3-month study, this means that samples of blood and urine would be collected at 1, 2, and 3 months after study initiation (i.e., after the first day of dosing the animals). There are some implications of these sampling plans that should be considered when the data are being interpreted. Many of the clinical chemistry (and some of the hematologic) markers are really the result of organ system damage that may be transient in nature. (See Table 11.3 for a summary of interpretations of clinical chemistry findings and Table 11.4 for a similar summary for hematological findings.) The samples on which analysis is performed are from fixed points in time, which may miss transient changes (typically, increases) in some enzyme levels.

IV. HISTOPATHOLOGY

Histopathology is generally considered the single most significant portion of data to come out of a repeat-dose toxicity study. It actually consists of three related sets of data (gross pathology observations, organ weights, and microscopic pathology) that are collected during the termination of the study animals. At the end of the study, a number of tissues are collected during termination of all surviving animals (test and control). Organ weights and terminal body weights are recorded at study termination, so that absolute and relative (to body weight) values can be statistically evaluated.

TABLE **11.5**   Tissues for Histopathology

Adrenals[a]
Body and cervix
Brain, all three levels[a]
Cervical lymph nodes
Cervical spinal cord
Duodenum
Esophagogastric junction
Esophagus
Eyes with optic nerves
Femur with marrow
Heart
Ileum
Kidneys[a]
Large bowel
Larynx with thyroid and parathyroid
Liver[a]
Lungs[a]
Mainstream bronchi
Major salivary gland
Mesenteric lymph nodes
Ovaries and tubes
Pancreas
Pituitary
Prostate
Skeletal muscle from proximal hind limb
Spleen[a]
Sternbrae with marrow
Stomach
Testes with epididymides[a]
Thymus and mediastinal contents[a]
Thyroid with parathyroid[a]
Trachea
Urinary bladder
Uterus, including horns

[a] Organs to be weighed.

These tissues, along with the organs for which weights are determined, are listed in Table 11.4. All tissues collected are typically processed for microscopic observation, but only those from the high-dose and control groups are necessarily evaluated microscopically. If a target organ is discovered in the high-dose group, then successively lower-dose groups are examined until a "clean" (devoid of effect) level is discovered (Haschek and Rousseaup, 1991).

In theory, all microscopic evaluations should be performed blind (without the pathologist knowing from which dose group a particular animal came), but this is difficult to do in practice, and such an approach frequently degrades the quality of the evaluation. Like all the other portions of data in the study, proper evaluation benefits from having access to all data that address the relevance, severity, timing, and potential mechanisms of a specific toxicity. Blind examination is best applied in peer review or consultations on specific findings.

In addition to the "standard" set of tissues specified in Table 11.5, observations during the course of the study or in other or previous studies may dictate that additional tissues be collected or that special examinations (e.g., special stains, polarized light or electron microscopy, immunocytochemistry, or quantitative morphometry) be undertaken to either evaluate the relevance of or understand the mechanisms underlying certain observations.

Histopathology testing is a terminal procedure, and therefore sampling of any single animal is a one-time event (except in the case of a tissue collected by biopsy). Because it is a regulatory requirement that the tissues from a basic number of animals be examined at the stated end of the study, an assessment of effects at any other time course (most commonly, to investigate recovery from an effect found at study termination) requires that satellite groups of animals be incorporated into the study at start-up. Such animals are randomly assigned at the beginning of the study, and otherwise treated exactly the same as the equivalent treatment (or control) animals.

For devices, the tissue list may either be limited to or augmented by the addition of specific examination of the tissues at the site(s) of implantation as follows:

Section, stain, and examine implant and other sites showing gross pathology.
Score lesions on a numerical scale from normal to extreme (1 to 5).
Criteria for implant site.
Acute inflammatory response
Inflammatory cells (PMNs)
Necrosis
Hemorrhage
Fibrin or serum

  Subacute/chronic response
    Mononuclear inflammatory cells (lymphocytes, macrophages, eosino-
      phils, plasma cells)
    Epithelial cells
    Giant cells
    Fibroblasts
  Components of subacute or chronic response.
    Mononuclear inflammatory cells (lymphocytes, macrophages, plasma
      cells)
    Epithelioid or giant cells
    Fibroplasia or fibrosis
  Measure width of reactive zone.
  Score on a scale of 0 (not present) to 5 (extreme).
  Components of acute inflammatory response.
    Inflammatory cells (polymorphonuclear leukocytes)
    Necrosis
    Hemorrhage
    Fibrin/serum

V. STUDY INTERPRETATION AND REPORTING

For a successful repeat-dose study, the bottom line is the clear demonstration of a no-effect level, characterization of a toxicity profile (providing guidance for any clinical studies), and at least a basic understanding of the mechanisms involved in any identified pathogenesis. The report that is produced as a result of the study should clearly communicate these points, along with the study design and experimental procedures and the summarized data and their statistical analysis, and it should be GLP-compliant, suitable for FDA submission format.

  Interpretation of the results of a study should be truly scientific and integrative. It is elementary to have the report state only each statistically and biologically significant finding in an orderly manner. The meaning and significance of each in relation to other findings, as well as the relevance to potential human effects, must be evaluated and addressed.

  The author of the report should ensure that it is accurate and complete, but also that it clearly tells a story and concludes with the relevant (to clinical development) findings.

VI. REPRODUCTIVE AND DEVELOPMENTAL TOXICITY

Reproductive toxicity tests for medical devices should normally be considered for the following:

1. Intrauterine devices (IUDs) or any other long-term contact devices likely to come into direct contact with reproductive tissues or the embryo/fetus
2. Energy-depositing devices
3. Resorbable or leachable materials and devices

There is no need for testing resorbable devices or devices containing leachable moieties where there is adequate and reassuring data from absorption, metabolism, and distribution and on the reproductive toxicity of all major components identified in extracts. Individual compounds known to cause reproductive toxicity should not be present as significant components of extracts of materials or devices.

Such tests are intended and should be adequate to evaluate the potential effects of devices, materials, and/or extracts on reproductive function, embryonic development (developmental toxicity tenatagenicity), and prenatal and early postnatal development.

A. Introduction

The goal of testing the developmental and reproductive toxicity of candidate devices and device material in laboratory animals is to predict which agent would adversely affect pregnancy and reproduction in humans.

The types of developmental and reproductive toxicity studies performed prior to 1993 and the methods used have been extensively documented. (See Palmer, 1981; Christian, 1983; Heinrichs, 1985; Heywood and James, 1985; Persaud, 1985; Schardein, 1988; Tyl, 1988; Christian and Hoberman, 1989; Khera, 1985; Manson and Kang, 1989.) Since June 20, 1979, the FDA has required that these studies be conducted according to GLP regulations. (See Food and Drug Administration, 1983; 1988.) The conduct of these studies had been complicated by the need to satisfy worldwide regulatory guidelines that varied from country to country. As a result, studies were conducted for regulatory purposes that, from a scientific viewpoint, were redundant, superfluous, and/or unnecessarily complex. This situation was changed in 1993 when the International Conference on Harmonization of Technical Requirements for the Registration of Pharmaceuticals for Human Use (ICH) standardized worldwide requirements in the guideline "Detection of Toxicity to Reproduction for Medicinal Products." ISO is likewise working on guidelines for medical devices.

B. ICH Study Designs

The new ICH guideline allows for various combinations of studies. (Note: the complete guideline is included in the appendix of this volume.) The studies conducted must include evaluation of the following components:

1. Male and female fertility and early embryonic development to implantation
2. Embryo–fetal development
3. Pre- and postnatal development, including maternal function

These components would normally be evaluated in a rodent species (preferably rats), and in addition, embryo–fetal development would be evaluated in a second species, typically the rabbit. The "most probable option" was considered in the ICH guideline to be the case in which three rodent studies would be conducted that separately addressed each of the components listed above. These study designs are described below. The day of insemination or detection of evidence of mating is considered day 0 of gestation and the day of birth is considered postpartum and postnatal day 0.

1. Male and Female Fertility and Early Embryonic Development to Implantation

The purpose of this component is to assess the effects that result from treatment during maturation of gametes, during cohabitation, and in females, during gestation up through the time of embryo implantation (typically last dose on day 6 of gestation). Assuming that the findings from a toxicity study of at least 1 month in duration do not contraindicate, the treatment period begins in males 4 weeks before male/female cohabitation, and in females, 2 weeks prior to cohabitation. A group size of 16 to 24 litters would generally be considered acceptable. (The author recommends mating 26 males with 26 females.)

Minimal in-life observations include the following:

1. Clinical signs and mortality daily
2. Body weight twice weekly
3. Food consumption weekly
4. Vaginal cytology daily during cohabitation
5. Valuable target effects seen in previous toxicity studies

Females are sacrificed after the middle of the gestation period. Males are sacrificed at any time after the end of the cohabitation period, but it is generally advisable to retain the males until after the outcome of the first mating is known to ensure that a repeat cohabitation with untreated females will not be needed to determine if an observed effect on mating performance is a male effect. Males are treated until termination. Terminal examination of adults includes the following:

1. Necropsy
2. Preservation of organs with gross changes and sufficient control organs for comparison
3. Preservation of testes, epididymides, ovaries, and uteri
4. Sperm count and sperm viability

5. Count of corpora lutea and implantation sites
6. Count of live and dead conceptuses

Among the study designs conducted before the ICH guidelines, the segment I fertility study conducted according to Japanese guidelines is most similar to this ICH study design. The major differences are the shortening of the treatment period of males prior to cohabitation from the duration of spermatogenesis (60 to 80 days) to 4 weeks and the addition of sperm evaluation. The justifications given for shortening the treatment period of males are as follows:

1. Careful organ weight and histopathological evaluation of testes in general toxicity studies will detect most testicular toxins.
2. Fertility is an insensitive measure of testicular effects.
3. Compounds known to affect spermatogenesis generally exert their effects during the first 4 weeks of treatment.

Sperm counts can be performed with sperm from either the testis or the epididymis. Sperm motility is commonly treated as a measure of sperm viability. The addition of sperm evaluation greatly increases the sensitivity of the study to detect effects on sperm maturation, and the new study design will likely detect more male effects than the previous design even though the treatment period has been shortened.

2. Embryo–Fetal Development

The purpose of this component is to detect anatomical effects on the developing conceptus by treating during the period of organogenesis from implantation to closure of the secondary palate. The study design is very similar to the previous segment II developmental toxicity study. A group size of 16 to 24 litters would generally be considered acceptable. The author recommends the following:

	Rat	Rabbit	Mouse
Treatment period (gestational days)	6–17	6–18	6–15
Group size (mated or inseminated)	25	20	25

Minimal in-life observations include the following:

1. Clinical signs and mortality daily
2. Body weight twice weekly
3. Food consumption weekly
4. Valuable target effect seen in previous toxicity studies

Females are sacrificed at the end of the gestation period, about 1 day prior to parturition (day 20 or 21 for rats, day 28 or 29 for rabbits, and day 17 or 18 for mice). Terminal examinations include the following:

1. Necropsy
2. Preservation of organs with gross changes and sufficient control organs for comparison
3. Count of corporea lutea and live and dead implantations
4. Fetal body weight
5. External, visceral, and skeletal examinations of fetuses
6. Gross evaluation of placenta

A minimum of 50% of fetuses are to be examined for visceral alterations and a minimum of 50% for skeletal abnormalities. When a fresh microdissection technique is being used for the visceral examination of rabbit fetuses, all fetuses should be examined for both visceral and skeletal abnormalities.

3. Pre- and Postnatal Development

The purpose of this component is to detect effects of treatment from implantation through lactation on the pregnant and lactating female and on the development of the conceptus and offspring through sexual maturity. The study design is similar to the previous segment III study design except that dosing begins on day 6 of gestation instead of day 15. A group size of 16 to 24 litters would generally be considered acceptable. (The author recommends 25 mated females.)

Minimal in-life observations for parental (F0 generation) females include the following:

1. Clinical signs and mortality daily
2. Body weight twice weekly
3. Food consumption weekly
4. Valuable target effects seen in previous toxicity studies
5. Length of gestation
6. Parturition

Parental females are sacrificed after weaning of the F1 generation. The age of sacrifice of the F1 generation animals is not specified in the ICH guideline and varies among laboratories. Typically, they are sacrificed intermittently with some laboratories reducing litter size on postnatal day 0, 3, or 4, on postnatal day 21 or at weaning, at male/female cohabitation to produce an F2 generation, and the terminal sacrifice, after production of the F2 generation. Terminal examinations for maternal animals and offspring include the following:

1. Necropsy of all parental and F1 adults
2. Preservation of organs with gross changes and sufficient control organs for comparison
3. Count of implantations

Additional observations of the F1 generation include the following:

1. Abnormalities
2. Live and dead offspring at birth
3. Body weight at birth
4. Pre- and postnatal survival, growth, maturation, and fertility
5. Physical development, including vaginal opening and preputial separation
6. Sensory function, reflexes, motor activity, learning, and memory

C. Single-Study and Two-Study Designs for Rodents

Except for the embryo–fetal development component in rabbits, the components described above can be combined into fewer, larger studies instead of conducting each component separately. Acceptable alternatives include the ''single-study design'' and ''two-study design.''

In the single-study design, all of the above components are combined into one study. The dosing period, extending from before mating through lactation, is a combination of that for the fertility study together with that for the pre- and postnatal development study. Subgroups of animals are terminated at the end of gestation for fetal examination.

There are a variety of possible two-study designs. One is to conduct the single study described above except that instead of having subgroups for fetal examination, a separate embryo–fetal development study in rodents is conducted. Another two-study design consists of combining the embryo–fetal development study with the pre- and postnatal development study in such a way that the two studies to be conducted would be (1) the fertility study and (2) the pre- and postnatal development study with subgroups terminated at the end of gestation for fetal examination. A third two-study design is to combine the fertility study with the embryo–fetal development study. In the first study, treatment would extend through the end of organogenesis, and then, at termination at the end of gestation, there would be a complete fetal examination. The second study would be the pre- and postnatal development study.

For all the options described above, the effects on male and female fertility can be evaluated separately by conducting separate studies in which only one sex is treated. The treatment periods are the same, but the treated animals are cohabited with untreated animals of the opposite sex. In the male fertility study, the untreated females are terminated after the middle of gestation and terminal observations include embryo survival and possibly external examination of fetuses (if terminated at the end of gestation; see Tanimura, 1990). The advantage of conducting separate male and female studies is that if there are effects, it is clear which sex was affected by treatment. Often when effects are seen in a combined male and female study, additional work is required to resolve which sex was affected. Either a second cohabitation of the treated males with untreated females is added or studies with only one sex treated must then be conducted.

With the possible exception of combining the female fertility component with the embryo–fetal development component, the combined-study approach is not likely to be used often. The female fertility and embryo–fetal development components are needed to support clinical trials in women of childbearing potential in most countries and thus will be conducted early in the development of a drug. Since the pre- and postnatal development component is not routinely required for clinical studies of women of childbearing potential and represents a large commitment of resources, however, it will not generally be conducted until late in the drug development process.

D. Dose and Sample Preparation

In the case of energy-depositing devices, whole-body irradiation of the animals with a multiple of the dose to be expected in humans should be applied. When possible, IUDs, resorbable devices, or devices containing leachable moieties shall be tested in their ''ready-to-use'' form, otherwise a suitably formed implant shall be made of the test material. The MID of a material or device should be applied. Where possible this dose should be expressed as a multiple of the worst case human exposure (in mg per kg).

E. Methodological Issues

1. Control of Bias

As in any study, an important element to consider when designing developmental and reproductive toxicity studies is the control of bias. For example, animals should be assigned to groups randomly and preferably balanced by body weight. This can be accomplished by first ranking the animals in order of body weight and then, starting with the lightest or heaviest, assigning them by rank to groups based on a list of sets or random permutations of numbers (e.g., 1, 2, 3, and 4 if there are four groups, where 1 represents the control group, 2 represents the low-dose group, etc.). Housing of the treatment groups should also be unbiased. This can be by ''Latin square'' design, in which each block of four cages (if there are four groups) includes an animal from each group. It is often an acceptable compromise to have animals from different groups in alternating vertical columns with all the animals in a column from the same group. This provides equal vertical balancing for all groups.

The order of sacrifice on the day of cesarean sectioning should be balanced by group (again using random permutations), since fetuses continue to grow during the day and an unbalanced time of sacrifice would bias fetal weights, particularly for rodents. Alternatively, all animals can be killed at about the same time in the morning and the fetuses stored for examination later the same day. Fetal examinations should be conducted blind; that is, without knowledge of the treatment group.

2. Diet

It is known that rodents require a diet relatively rich in protein and fats for successful reproduction (Zeman, 1967; Chow and Rider, 1973; Turner, 1973; Mulay et al., 1982), consequently rodents are fed high-protein, high-fat diets ad lib for reproductive toxicity studies and also generally as a maintenance diet for all toxicity studies. Female rats fed in this manner begin to show decreases in fertility, litter size, and the incidence of normal estrus cycling at the age of 6 months (Matt et al., 1986; 1987). The disadvantage of this feeding practice is that the animals more quickly acquire age-related diseases and sexual dysfunctions and die sooner than if they were fed a restricted amount of calories. (For a review, see Weindruch and Walford, 1988.) In relatively short-term studies (e.g., the standard ICH studies), this rapid aging does not present a problem. For male breeding colonies or multigeneration studies with multiple litters per generation, however, it could be advantageous to restrict caloric intake, at least when the animals are not being bred. Restriction of food intake fails to achieve adverse effect on male rat reproduction (Chapin et al., 1991), although it does affect reproduction in mice (Gulati et al., 1969) and female rats (Chapin et al., 1991).

It is thus desirable to improve the assessment of toxicity in range-finding studies in pregnant animals. Complete histopathologic examination is too impractical. It is often feasible, however, to perform hematologic and serum biochemical analyses that can significantly increase the chances of detecting significant toxicity and provide important information for selecting an appropriate highest dosage level for the embryo–fetal developmental toxicity study.

Body weight effects most often provided the basis for selection of dosage levels in the segment II study. There have been cases in which clinical pathology was or would have been useful to justify dosage selection, however. For example, the nonsteroidal anti-inflammatory drug diflunisal caused a decrease in erythrocyte count from 6.0 (million/mm^3) to 2.9 at a dosage level (40 mg kg^{-1} day^{-1}) that caused only a 1% decrease in body weight in pregnant rabbits. The severe hemolytic anemia caused by this excessively high dosage level in turn caused secondary axial skeletal malformations in the fetuses (Clark et al., 1984). Also, the angiotensin-converting enzyme (ACE) inhibitor enalapril caused an increase in serum urea nitrogen from 16 mg dl^{-1} to 46 mg dl^{-1} (highest value = 117) at a dosage level (10 mg kg^{-1} day^{-1}) that had no apparent effect on body weight but caused a significant ($p < 0.05$) increase in resorptions. Serum urea nitrogen concentration was used to select dosage levels for a subsequent ACE inhibitor, lisinopril.

The routine use of clinical pathology in range-finding studies has previously been proposed (Wise et al., 1988). The animals can be bled on the day after the last dose or sooner to detect transient effects or to allow an evaluation of the data prior to cesarean section.

F. Gravid Uterine Weights

The effects of treatment on maternal body weight gain are commonly evaluated as indicators of maternal toxicity. Maternal body weight gain, however, is influenced by fetal parameters such as live fetuses per litter and fetal body weight, thus effects indicative of developmental toxicity could contribute to decreased maternal body weight gain and confound the interpretation of maternal toxicity. In addition, other maternal but pregnancy-related parameters, such as volume of intrauterine fluid, could be affected by treatment and contribute to effects on overall body weight gain.

In an attempt to correct this complication, some laboratories weigh the gravid uterus at cesarean section and then subtract the weight of the gravid uterus from the body weight gain to obtain an adjusted weight gain that is more purely maternal. This adjustment may be imprecise but not inappropriate for rats for which gravid uterine weight is correlated with and generally substantially less than maternal body weight change during gestation. The subtraction of gravid uterine weight from maternal weight gain is an overadjustment for rabbits, however. The maternal body weight gain of rabbits during gestation is generally less than the weight of the gravid uterus. Moreover, gravid uterine weight is correlated with maternal body weight change in some but not all studies, thus subtracting the gravid uterine weight from the maternal weight gain is not always appropriate. A preferred method for adjusting maternal body weight gain for possible developmental effects is to test, and if appropriate, use gravid uterine weight as a covariate (J. Antonello, personal communication, 1990). This method can be used for both rats and rabbits and for body weight change intervals in addition to those ending at study termination.

Alternatively, to avoid weighing the uterus (or if the analysis is being performed retrospectively and uterine weights are unavailable) or if a more purely fetal adjustment is desired, one can use the sum of the live fetal weights within the litter (total live fetal weight) as the covariate instead of gravid uterine weight. As one would expect, total live fetal weight is very highly correlated with gravid uterine weight in control animals ($r = 0.99$ in control rats and 0.95 in control rabbits (J. Antonello, personal communication, 1990), thus in general, using either gravid uterine weight or total live fetal weight as the covariate will yield similar results. If treatment was to have an effect on gravid uterine weight that was not reflected in total live weight (e.g., if the volume of amniotic, extracoelomic, or intrauterine fluid was affected), however, then total live fetal weight may not be highly correlated with gravid uterine weight, and hence not interchangeable as a covariate. In that case, only weighing the gravid uterus would allow the detection of these effects not revealed by total live fetal weight.

1. Implant Counts and Determination of Pregnancy

Two observations suggest that the remnants of embryos that die soon after implantation are not apparent at gross examination of the uterus near term. First, embryos that were observed to be resorbing at laparotomy early in gestation left no readily visible trace near term (Staples, 1971). Second, occult implantation sites can be revealed near term by staining the uterus with ammonium sulfide or sodium hydroxide (Salewski, 1964; Yamada et al., 1988). It is not known if the uterine-staining techniques reveal all implantation sites. It is clear, though, that when uterine-staining techniques are not used, very early resorptions may not be included in what is termed the "resorption rate" but instead may contribute to the apparent "preimplantation loss," or if no implantation sites were detected, the rate of "nonpregnant" animals.

In normal circumstances, probably very few implantation sites are not detected without staining. Cases have occurred in which probable treatment effects were detected only as a result of uterine staining, however.

2. Fetal Examinations

Many fetal anomalies, such as cleft palate, exencephaly, ectrodactyly, and missing vertebra, are discrete and therefore easy to recognize objectively. Some anatomical structures, though, occur along a continuous gradation of size and shape and are only considered anomalous if the deviation from the typical exceeds a somewhat arbitrarily selected threshold. These anomalies are observed in all examination types and include, for example, micrognathia, reduced gallbladder, enlarged heart, distended ureter, wavy rib, and incomplete ossification at many sites. In many cases, it cannot be said with certainty if a specific degree of variation from normal would have resulted in an adverse consequence to the animal and should therefore be considered abnormal. In the absence of certainty about outcome, the best approach is to uniformly apply a single criterion within a study (and preferably among studies) so that all treatment groups are examined consistently. The subjectivity (and hence fetus-to-fetus variability) of the examination can be minimized by having the criteria be as clear and objective as possible. For example, when examining for incompletely ossified thoracis centra or supraoccipitals, it can be required that the ossification pattern be absent (unossified), unilateral, or bipartite (which are objective observations) before recording and observation. Subjective criteria such as being dumbbell- or butterfly-shaped would not be applied. Additional comments about specific examination types follow.

Examination of External Genitalia. One aspect of external anatomy that is largely overlooked in the examination of offspring exposed in utero to test agents is the external genitalia, even though major malformations can occur in those structures. For example, hypospadias is a malformation in the male in which the urethra opens on the underside of the penis or on the perineum. Hypospadias can occur in the male rat following in utero exposure to antiandrogens, testosterone synthesis inhibitors (e.g., Bloch et al., 1971), or finasteride, a 5 α-reductase inhibitor (Clark et al., 1990b). It is impractical to detect hypospadias in fetuses or young pups, however. Although the genital tubercle of the normal male rat fetus is grossly distinguishable from that of the normal female as early as day 21 of gestation (the female has a groove on the ventral side), the difference is very subtle, and partial feminization of the male genital tubercle would be very difficult to ascertain. Routine histological examination is obviously too labor-intensive to be considered. Hypospadias can be readily determined, though, by expressing and examining the penis of the adult. It is thus recommended that adult F_1 males be examined for hypospadias. If the timing of the separation of the balano-preputial membrane is being included in the pre- and postnatal development study as a developmental sign (see Korenbrot et al., 1977), the examination of the penis for hypospadias can be conducted at the same time.

The critical period for the induction of hypospadias by finasteride in rats is day 16 to 17 of gestation (Clark et al., 1990a). It is unlikely that other agents would have a much earlier critical period since testosterone synthesis, which is required for the development of the penile urethra, begins in the rat on day 15 of gestation (Habert and Picon, 1984). If treatment in the embryo–fetal development study terminates on day 15 of gestation (as is done in some laboratories), it is thus doubtful that hypospadias could be induced. Hypospadias could be induced in the pre- and postnatal development study, however. Since the formation of the penile urethra in the rat is not completed until day 21 of gestation (Anderson and Clark, 1990), it could be argued that "major organogenesis" continues until that time.

One parameter that is readily and commonly measured as an indicator of effects on differentiation of the external genitalia in rodent fetuses is the sexually dimorphic distance between the anus and the genital tubercle (anogenital distance). It should not be assumed that anogenital distance is synonymous with hypospadias, however, since effects on anogenital distance are not necessarily predictive of hypospadias. Finasteride caused both hypospadias and the decreased anogenital distance in male offspring but with very different dose-response relationships and only a slight tendency for animals with hypospadias to have a shorter anogenital distance (Clark et al., 1990b). Also, the effects on anogenital distance in male rat fetuses on day 20 of gestation did not affect the development of the genital tubercle and did not cause hypospadias (Wise et al., 1990a). Decreased anogenital distance per se thus does not necessarily indicate a serious congenital anomaly.

When evaluating the effects of treatment on fetal anogenital distance, it is obviously important to correct for effects on fetal weight. One approach is to calculate ''relative'' anogenital distance, the ratio between anogenital distance and another linear measure, for example, biparietal diameter (head width). The cube root of fetal weight simulates a linear measure (Wise et al., 1990b) and can also be used to normalize anogenital distance. Another approach is to compare the anogenital distance in a weight-reduced treatment group to that in a weight-matched control group at a younger age.

Visceral Fetal Examinations. The examination of the abdominal and thoracic viscera of fetuses is performed either fresh without fixation (''Staples technique'') or after Bouin's fixation by making freehand razor blade sections (''Wilson's technique'') (Wilson, 1965). Both techniques have advantages. The fresh examination technique, which may require less training for proficiency, provides a more easily interpreted view of heart anomalies. The examination must be performed on the day the dam is terminated, though, so having a large number of litters to examine in one day requires that a large team of workers be committed to the task.

With both techniques, the heads of one-half of the fetuses can be fixed in Bouin's fixative for subsequent freehand sectioning and examination. A common artifact induced by fixation in rabbit fetal heads is retinal folding.

Skeletal Fetal Examination. There is variability in the development of the fetal skeleton, including numbers of vertebrae and ribs, patterns of sternebral ossification, alignment of ribs with sternebrae, and alignment of ilia with lumbar and sacral vertebrae. There is also extensive plasticity in the development of the skeleton beyond the fetal stage. For example, it is known that markedly wavy ribs in fetuses can resolve so that the ribs in the adult are normal (Saegusa et al., 1980) and supernumerary ribs can be resorbed (Wickramaratne, 1988). This variability and plasticity complicates the classification of anomalies as true malformations as opposed to variations of normal. There is no unanimity on terminology, but in general a variation tends to be an alteration that occurs at a relatively high spontaneous incidence (>1%), is often reversible, and has little or no adverse consequence for the animal.

When tabulating and interpreting fetal skeleton data, a distinction is made between alterations in the pattern of development and simple delays in development that are considered to be less serious. A delay in skeletal development is usually apparent as a delay in ossification, as evidenced by an increased incidence of specific, incompletely ossified sites or decreases in counts of ossified bones in specific regions (e.g., sacrocaudal vertebrae). These delays are normally associated with decreases in fetal weight and commonly occur at dosage levels of the test agent that also cause decreased maternal body weight gain.

When determining the criteria for recording skeletal alterations, particularly sites of incomplete ossification, it is legitimate to consider the resulting incidences. For example, including an unossified fifth sternebra in the criteria for recording incomplete sternebra ossification may increase the control incidence to a very high proportion (over 95%) of fetuses affected, which would then reduce the sensitivity for detecting treatment effects. The additional effort expended in recording the extra observations due to sternebra 5 would be wasted. In addition, recording high incidences of complete ossification at many sites is not worth the effort involved. The ossification at various sites is highly correlated, so recording at multiple sites is redundant. In some cases, the incidences can be reduced to reasonable levels (1–20% of control fetuses) and the criteria simultaneously made more objective by requiring that the bone be entirely unossified before recording.

3. Developmental Signs

The postnatal evaluation of F_1 pups includes the observation of developmental signs in two or more pups per sex per litter. In general, the acquisition of these developmental landmarks, including anatomical changes (e.g., ear pinna detachment, incisor eruption, hair growth, and eye opening) and reflexes (negative geotaxis, surface righting, and free-fall righting), are highly correlated with body weight, but as indicators of developmental toxicity they are not as sensitive as body weight (Lochry et al., 1984; Lochry, 1987) and thus have minimal value. Possible exceptions to this generality are the ontogeny of the auditory startle reflex and the markers of sexual maturation (vaginal patency, testes descent, and balano-preputial separation in males).

The examinations for developmental signs can be performed daily starting before and continuing until criterion is achieved. Alternatively, the examinations can be conducted on animals on preselected postnatal days. For example, 3 days can be selected—one when only a few control animals will achieve criterion, one when approximately one-half of the control animals will achieve criterion, and one when nearly all control animals will achieve criterion. The latter method has the advantages of requiring less time and assuring that all examined animals have the same testing experience (so as not to bias subsequent tests).

The separation of the balano-preputial membrane of the penis (occurring at postnatal week 6 to 7) (Korenbrot et al., 1977) is becoming the preferred landmark of sexual maturation in males. The timing of testes descent is more variable and very dependent on the achievement criteria used. Another advantage of determining the time of balano-preputial separation is that anomalies of the penis may be observed at the same time (as noted above).

4. Behavioral Tests

The trend within reproductive toxicology is to move from simple determinations of developmental landmarks and reflexes to more sophisticated and sensitive behavioral tests. This process was accelerated by the Environmental Protection Agency (EPA), which issued guidelines requiring a ''developmental neurotoxicity'' study of compounds that meet any of several broad criteria. The behavioral tests to be performed in this study are extensive and rigidly defined. As laboratories become equipped and trained to meet these guidelines, they are adding such tests to their evaluations of pharmaceuticals. The suggestions for routine testing made below are considered reasonable for pre- and postnatal development studies intended as routine screens. It is suggested that testing be conducted on one or two adults per sex per litter, keeping the range of actual ages as tight as possible.

Measurement of motor activity is commonly performed in the dark in cages or plastic boxes (open field) or residential mazes in which movement is quantitated by infrared detectors or by recording the interruption of light beams as the test subject moves through a horizontal grid of light beams. Possible parameters to evaluate include horizontal activity (light beams interrupted), number of movements, and time spent in the middle of the cage. The test period is selected to be long enough (normally 30 to 50 min) to allow the activity of the animals to decrease to an approximately constant level (asymptote). Testing of young pups (e.g., 13 days of age) is not recommended, as their activity level is fairly constant during the test period and young, unweaned pups should not be separated from their mothers for extended periods of time.

Another test paradigm for detecting treatment effects on brain functioning in F1 offspring measures auditory startle habituation. In this test, the animal is placed in a chamber with a floor that detects movement. The animal is exposed to a sequence of 50 to 60 auditory stimuli, each at 110 to 120 decibels for 20 to 50 msec and separated by 5 to 20 sec. The gradual diminution of the animal's movement response is indicative of normal habituation.

There is not a consensus about the procedures to use to test for effects on learning and memory. The two most commonly used techniques are the water-filled maze, which is preferred for measuring learning, and passive avoidance, which is preferred for measuring memory. (See Buelke-Sam et al., 1985.) Retention is tested in a repeat test conducted approximately 1 week later.

5. Detecting Effects on Male Reproduction

Male fertility studies with typical group sizes (15 to 30 male per group) are very insensitive for detecting effects on male fertility. If the control fertility rate is 80%, even a group size of 30 will only detect (at the 5% significance level) a

38% decrease in fertility 80% of the time and a 50% decrease 95% of the time (J. Antonello, personal communication, 1990). To detect slight effects on male fertility would require enormous group sizes. Mating each male with more than one female provides a more precise estimate of the reproductive capacity of each male but does not greatly increase statistical power. If multiple matings are to be done, it is recommended that the cohabitations with multiple females be sequential rather than concurrent.

Not only is it difficult to detect effects on male fertility because of group-size considerations, effects on male fertility mediated by decreased sperm production are also difficult to detect because of the normally huge excess of sperm included in a rat ejaculate. Sperm production can be decreased by up to 90% without effect on fertility (either pregnancy rate or litter size) in the rat. This is not the case for men, so the sperm excess in the rat represents a serious flaw in the rat model. (See Working, 1988.) To address this deficiency and improve the sensitivity of the model, it is advisable to determine the effects of the test agent on testes weights, testicular spermatid counts, and histopathology of the testes (preferably plastic sections) in the male fertility study and/or the 14-week toxicity study. In some cases, these parameters may be more predictive of possible effects on male fertility in humans than the fertility rate in rats.

G. Data Interpretation

1. Use of Statistical Analyses

Statistical analysis is a very useful tool for evaluating the effects of treatment on many developmental and reproductive toxicity parameters. For some parameters, such as maternal body weight changes, fetal weight, and horizontal activity in an open field, the comparison to the concurrent control is the primary consideration, and assuming adequate group size, the investigator relies heavily on the results of appropriate statistical analyses to interpret differences from control.

For other parameters, though, statistical analysis is just one of several considerations that include historical control data and other relevant information about the test agent and related test agents. For example, statistical analysis of a low incidence of an uncommon fetal malformation will usually not be significant ($p > 0.05$) even if treatment-related, due to the low power for detecting such effects with typical group sizes. In such cases, examination of the historical control data becomes paramount. If two fetuses with a particular malformation occur in separate litters only in a high-dose group, the finding is of much more concern if it is a very rare malformation than if recent historical control groups have had a few fetuses with that malformation.

Other known effects of the test agent or related agents also sometimes contribute to data interpretation. For example, a low incidence of a malformation may be considered treatment-related if it is at the low end of a typical dose-response curve or if it is in a high-dose group and that malformation is an expected effect of the test agent. In general, though, a single occurrence of a fetal malformation in a treatment group (with none in control) is not cause for alarm, since this occurs in almost every study (together with occurrences of some malformations only in the control group).

Statistical methods exist to appropriately analyze most developmental and reproductive toxicity parameters. Exceptions to this are the "r/m" litter parameters in which for each litter there is a number affected divided by the number in the litter. These parameters include preimplantation loss ($r =$ corpora lutea-implants, $m =$ corpora lutea), resorption rate ($r =$ resorptions, $m =$ implants), and the family of alteration rates ($r =$ affected fetuses, $m =$ fetuses). There are two factors complicating the statistical analysis of these data that have heretofore been inadequately handled (Clark et al., 1989). One is that almost all of these parameters have a strong dependence on m. For example, both preimplantation loss and resorption rate are normally higher at both the low and high extremes of m. In contrast, supernumerary rib tends to occur at higher incidences in average-size litters. The second factor that complicates the statistical analysis of r/m data is that affected implants tend to occur in clusters within litters ("litter effects"); that is, the intralitter correlation is greater than the interlitter correlation. For example, the total number of litters affected with anasarca, missing vertebra, and supernumerary rib is much less than would be expected by chance based on the number of affected fetuses.

These problems have recently been resolved for analysis of resorption rate (and preimplantation loss) in Sprague–Dawley rats using a three-step process (Sopor and Clark, 1990). First, based on an analysis of data from 1379 control rat litters examined since 1978, a likelihood score was derived for each (r,m) couplet based on the incidence of that couplet given that value of m. These scores were approximately equal to r. Second, an analysis of 136 litters from groups with slight effects on resorption rate revealed that at low-effect doses of embryocidal test agents the increases in resorptions tended to occur as increased proportions of affected litters. To maximize the difference in scores between control and affected litters, the scores for controllike litters ($r = 1, 2,$ or 3) were downgraded from r (1, 2, and 3) to 0.4, 1, and 2.4, respectively. Third, to arrive at the final score for each litter, the modified r score for each litter was divided by the expected control value for that value of m. This last step makes the litter score immune to spontaneous or treatment-related effects on m. The final "robust" scores have more power for detecting effects than various other measures (raw r/m, affected litters/litters, r, $\Sigma r/\Sigma n$, and the likelihood score) and has a lower false positive rate with fluctuations in m.

Covariance analysis (Snedecor and Cochran, 1967) can be used to reduce variability in a parameter and thereby increase sensitivity. For example, much of the variability in fetal weight data is due to variable litter size, and for rats, litters being sacrificed at different times during the workday. The variability due to these sources can be reduced by using litter size and time of sacrifice as potential covariates. Similarly, litter size and length of gestation can be used as covariates for neonatal pup weights, and body weight at the beginning of treatment can be used as a covariate for maternal body weight changes during the treatment period of an embryo–fetal development study.

A useful technique for determining if there is an effect of treatment on any toxicological parameter is the NOSTASOT method (Tukey et al., 1985; Antonello et al., 1993). This test is based on the principle that a possible toxicological effect of interest occurs with a normal dose response; that is, there is an increasing effect with increasing dosage. The data to be analyzed should be examined first to confirm that this principle is not violated. In this method, regression analysis is used to determine if there is an increased or decreased response in a parameter with increasing dosage. This method can be visualized as a plot of response versus dosage in which the analysis determines if the slope of the plotted line deviates significantly from zero.

This method can be used for essentially all parameters. Three analyses are performed, each with different spacing between dosage levels. The spacing in the first analysis is based on the arithmetic values of the dosage levels. The spacing in the second, referred to as the ordinal scaling, has equal spacing between dosage levels; that is, the control through high-dosage levels are assigned values of 0, 1, 2, and 3. In the third analysis, the log of the dosage level is used. Since the log of zero is impractical, the control group is assigned a value based on the spacing between the low- and middle-dosage levels according to a formula that assigns a log scale value to the control such that the ratio of the difference between the control and low-dose groups and the difference between the low- and middle-dose groups is equal both in absolute values and in log scale values. This places the control group at a reasonable distance from the low-dosage group. The lowest p value among the three analyses—arithmetic, ordinal, and logarithmic— is taken as the p value of the overall analysis based on the assumption that, if there is a dosage-related effect, the method of analysis yielding the lowest value is the best model for that dosage response. A correction for the multiplicity of analyses can be applied. If none of the three analyses is significant at the 0.5 level, the analysis is complete and the high-dosage level is referred to as the NOSTASOT dose. If there is a significant trend through the high-dosage level, the data from the high-dosage level is deleted and the trend test repeated. This process is repeated until a NOSTASOT dose is determined. Effects at dosage levels above the NOSTASOT dose are then considered to be statistically significant.

There are two major benefits of the NOSTASOT method. One is that spurious statistically significant results only at the low- and/or middle-dosage levels are eliminated, resulting in a reduction in false positives. A second benefit is that in some cases there may be real effects at multiple dosage levels that at any single dosage level are not statistically significant but will nevertheless result in a significant trend, thus providing increased sensitivity and halving the false negative rate.

2. Associations Between Developmental and Maternal Toxicity

The developmental toxicity of many pharmaceuticals occurs only at maternally toxic dosages (Khera, 1984; 1985; Schardein, 1987). Also, there are several compounds for which there is evidence that their developmental toxicity is secondary to their maternal toxicity. The decreased uterine blood flow associated with hydroxyurea treatment of pregnant rabbits may account for the embryotoxicity observed. The teratogenicity of diphenylhydantoin in mice may be secondary to decreased maternal heart rate (Watkinson and Millicovsky, 1983), as supported by the amelioration of the teratogenicity by hyperoxia and the dependence on maternal genotype in genetic crosses between sensitive and resistant strains (Johnston et al., 1979). The hemolytic anemia caused in pregnant rabbits by diflunisal was severe enough to explain the concomitant axial skeletal malformations (Clark et al., 1984). Acetazolamide-induced fetal malformations in mice are apparently related to maternal hypercapnia (Weaver and Scott, 1984a, b) and hypokalemia (Ellison and Maren, 1972). The increased resorption rate induced in rabbits by the antibiotic norfloxacin depends on exposure of the maternal gastrointestinal tract (Clark et al., 1986).

In addition, various treatments that simulate effects that can result from pharmaceutical treatment have been shown to cause developmental toxicity. Food deprivation can cause embryo–fetal toxicity and teratogenicity in mice (Szabo and Brent, 1975; Hemm et al., 1977) and rats (Ellington, 1980) and fetal death, decreased fetal weight, and abortions in rabbits (Matsuzawa et al., 1981; Clark et al., 1986). Treatments that result in maternal hypoxia, such as hypobaric exposure (Degenhardt and Kladetzky, 1955) and blood loss (Grote, 1969), have been shown to be teratogenic. Also, the results from testing with numerous agents suggest that supernumerary rib in mice is caused by maternal stress (Kavlock et al., 1985; Beyer and Chernoff, 1986).

In any case in which developmental toxicity occurs at dosage levels with only moderate to severe maternal toxicity, the possibility of the developmental toxicity being secondary to the maternal toxicity can thus be considered. That is not to say, however, that it can be concluded that the developmental toxicity is secondary any time there is coincident maternal toxicity. To the contrary, it is usually very difficult to establish a causal relationship. Superficially similar types of maternal toxicity do not always cause the same pattern of developmental toxicity. (See Chernoff et al., 1990.) This may be because the developmental toxicity is secondary to maternotoxicity, but since typical developmental toxicity studies include only a very cursory evaluation of maternal toxicity, the developmental toxicity may be secondary to an aspect of maternotoxicity that is not even being measured.

To demonstrate that a developmental effect is secondary to a particular parameter of maternal toxicity, it is necessary but not sufficient to show that all mothers with developmental toxicity also had maternal toxicity and that the severity of the developmental effect was correlated with the maternal effect. Other examples in which this approach has been used to evaluate the relationship between maternal and developmental toxicity include: (1) the negative correlation between resorption rate and maternal body weight change in norfloxacin-treated rabbits (Clark et al., 1986), supporting the contention that the developmental toxicity was secondary; and (2) the lack of correlation between the embryotoxicity and maternal body weight change in pregnant mice treated with caffeine and L-phenylisopropyladenosine (Clark et al., 1987), suggesting no causal relationship. In many cases, additional studies specifically designed to address the relationship between developmental and maternal toxicity may be required.

3. In Vitro Alternatives

The area of developmental toxicology actually is one of the earliest to have alternative models suggested for it, and has one of the most extensive and oldest literatures. This is, of course, partly owing to such models originally being used to elucidate the essential mechanisms and process of embryogenesis.

Because of the complicated and multiphasic nature of the developmental process, it has not been proposed that any of these systems be definitive tests, but rather that they serve as one form or another of a screen. As such, these test systems would either preclude or facilitate more effective full-scale evaluation in one or more of the traditional whole-animal test protocols.

The literature and field are much too extensive to review comprehensively here. There are a number of extensive review articles and books on the subject (Wilson, 1978; Clayton, 1981; Kochhar, 1981; Saxen, 1984; Homburger and Goldberg, 1985; Faustman, 1988; Daston and D'Amato, 1989), which should be consulted by those with in-depth interest.

The existing alternative test systems fall into six broad classes: (1) lower organisms; (2) cell culture systems; (3) organ culture systems; (4) submammalian embryos; (5) mammalian embryos; (6) others.

Table 11.6 provides an overview of the major representatives of these six groups, along with at least one basic reference to the actual techniques involved and the system components for each.

The comparative characteristics of these different classes of test systems are presented in Table 11.6. The key point is that these systems can be used for a wide range of purposes, only one of which is to screen compounds to determine the degree of concern for developmental toxicity.

TABLE 11.6 Alternative Developmental Toxicity Test Systems

Category	Test system	Model	References
I: Lower organisms	Sea urchins	Organism	Kotzin and Baker (1972)
	Drosophila	Intact and embryonic cells	Abrahamson and Lewis (1971)
	Trout	(Fish species)	MacCrimmon and Kwain (1969)
	Planaria	Regeneration	Best et al. (1981)
	Brine Shrimp	Disruption of elongation: DNA and protein levels in *Artemia nauplii*	Kerster and Schaeffer (1983); Sleet and Brendel (1985)
II: Cell culture	Protein synthesis of cultured cells	Pregnant mouse and chickens' epithelial cells	Clayton (1979)
	Avian neural crest	Differentiation of cells	Sieber-Blym (1985)
	Neuroblastoma	Differentiation of cells	Mummery et al. (1984)
	Lectin-mediated attachment	Tumor cells	Braun and Horowicz (1983)
III: Organ culture	Frog limb	Regeneration	Bazzoli et al. (1977)
	Mouse embryo limb bud	Inhibition of incorporation of precursor and of DNA synthesis	Kochhar and Aydelotte (1974)
	Metanephric kidney organ cultures	From 11-day mouse embryos	Saxen and Saksela (1971)
IV: Submammalian embryo	Chick embryo		Gebhardt (1972)
V: Mammalian embryo	Frog embryo	*Xenopus laevis*	Davis et al. (1981)
	Rat embryo culture	Whole postimplantation embryos	Brown and Fabro (1981); Cockroft and Stelle (1989)
	Chernoff	Mouse embryo short test	Chernoff and Kavlock (1980)
	"Micromass cultures"	Rat embryo midbrain and limb	Flint and Orton (1984)
VI: Other	Structure-activity relationships (SAR)	Mathematical correlations of activity with structural features	Einslein et al. 1983
			Gombar et al. (1990)

TABLE 11.7 Developmental Toxicity Test System Considerations

Possibility	In vivo	Organ culture	Cell structure	Lower organisms	Mammalian embryo culture	Submammalian embryos	Other
To study maternal organ factors	Yes	No	No	No	No/yes	No/yes	NA
To study embryogenesis as a whole	Yes	No	No	No	Yes	Somewhat	NA
To eliminate maternal confounding factors (nutrition, etc.)	No	Yes	Yes	No	Yes	Yes	NA
To eliminate placental factors (barrier differences)	No	Yes	Yes	No	Yes	No	NA
To study morphogenetic events	Difficult	Yes	No	Maybe	Yes	Yes	NA
To create controllable, reproducible conditions	Difficult	Yes	Yes	Yes	Yes	Yes	NA
For exact exposure and timing	Difficult	Yes	Yes	Yes	Yes	Yes	NA
For microsurgical manipulations	Difficult	Yes	No	Maybe	Yes	Yes	NA
For continuous registration of the effects	Difficult	Yes	Yes	No	Yes	Yes	NA
To collect large amounts of tissue for analysis	Yes	Difficult	Yes	No	Yes	No	NA
To use human embryonic tissue for testing	No	Yes	Yes	No	No	No	NA
Screening	Expensive	Yes	Yes	Yes	Yes	Yes	Yes

Note: NA = not available.

The utility of these systems for screening is limited by the degree of dependability in predicting effects primarily in people and secondarily in the traditional whole-animal test systems. Determining the predictive performance of alternative test systems requires the evaluation of a number of compounds for which the "true" (human) effect is known. In 1983 a consensus workshop generated a so-called gold standard set of compounds of known activity (Smith et al., 1989). The composition of this list has been open to a fair degree to controversy over the years (Flint, 1989; Johnson, 1989; Johnson et al., 1989). An agreed-upon gold standard set of compounds of known activity, however, is an essential starting point for the validation of any single test system or battery of test systems because of the multitude of mechanisms for developmental toxicity. It is unlikely that any one system will be able to stand in place of segment II studies in two species, much less to accurately predict activity in humans. Their use as general screens or as test systems with little potential for extensive or intended human exposure will, however, probably be appropriate. Table 11.7 presents the relative merits and utility of these test systems.

REFERENCES

Abrahamson, S. and Lewis, E. B. (1971). The detection of mutations in Drosophila melanogaster. In: Chemical Mutagens: Principles and Methods of Their Detection, vol. 2 (A. Hollaender, Ed.). Plenum, New York, pp. 461–488.

Anderson, C. and Clark, R. L. (1990). External genitalia of the rat: Normal development and the histogenesis of 5α-reductase inhibitor-induced abnormalities, Teratology, 42:483–496.

Antonello, J. M., Clark, R. L., and Heyse, J. F. (1993). Application of the Tukey trend test procedure to assess developmental and reproductive toxicity. I. Measurement data, Fund. Appl. Tox., 21:52–58.

Arnold, D. L., Grice, H. C., and Krawski, D. R. (1990). Handbook of In Vivo Toxicity Testing. Academic Press, San Diego, CA.

Bazzoli, A. S., Manson, J., Scott, W. J., and Wilson, J. B. (1977). The effects of thalidomide and two analogues on the regenerating forelimb of the newt, J. Embryol. Exptl Morphol., 41:125–135.

Best, J. B., Moritia, M., Ragin, J., and Best, J. Jr. (1981). Acute toxic responses of the freshwater planarian, Dugesia dorothocephala, to methylmercury, Bull. Environ. Contam. Toxicol., 27:49–54.

Beyer, P. E. and Chernoff, N. (1986). The induction of supernumerary ribs in rodents: The role of maternal stress, Teretog. Carcinog. Utag., 6:419–429.

Bloch, E., Lew, M., and Klein, M. (1971). Studies on the inhibition of fetal androgen formation: Inhibition of testosterone synthesis in rat and rabbit fetal testes with observations on reproductive tract development, Endocrinology, 89:16–31.

Braun, A. G. and Horowicz, P. B. (1983). Lectin-mediated attachment assay for teratogens: Results with 32 pesticides, J. Toxicol. Environ. Health, 11(2):275–286.

398

Brown, N. A. and Fabro, S. (1981). Quantitation of rat embryonic development in vitro: A morphological scoring system, Teratology, 24:65–78.

Buelke-Sam, J., Kimmel, C. A., and Adams, J. (1985). Design considerations in screening for behavioral teratogens: Results of the collaborative behavioral teratology study, Teratology, 29:240–254.

Chapin, R. E., Gulati, D. R., and Barnes, L. H. (1991). The effects of dietary restriction on reproductive endpoints in Sprague–Dawley rats, Toxicologist, 11:112.

Chernoff, N. and Kavlock, R. J. (1980). A potential in vivo screen for the determination of teratogenic effects in mammals, Teratology, 21:33A–34A.

Chernoff, N., Setzer, R. W., Miller, D. B., Rosen, M. B., and Rogers, J. M. (1990). Effects of chemically induced maternal toxicity on prenatal development in the rat, Teratology, 42:651–658.

Chow, B. F. and Rider, A. A. (1973). Implication of the effects of maternal diets in various species, J. Anim. Sci., 36:167–173.

Christian, M. S. (1983). Assessment of reproductive toxicity: State of the art. In: Assessment of Reproductive and Teratogenic Hazards (M. S. Christian, M. Galbraith, P. Voytek, and M. A. Mehlman, Eds.). Princeton Scientific, Princeton, NJ, pp. 65–76.

Christian, M. S. and Hoberman, A. M. (1989). Current in vivo reproductive toxicity and developmental toxicity (teratology) test methods. In: A Guide to General Toxicology, 2nd ed. (J. A. Marquis and A. W. Hayes, Eds.). S. Karger, Basel, Switzerland, pp. 91–100.

Clark, R. L., Robertson, R. T., Minsker, D. H., Cohen, S. M., Toco, D. J., Allen, H. L., James, M. L., and Bokelman, D. L. (1984). Diflunisal-induced maternal anemia as a cause of teratogenicity in rabbits, Teratology, 30:319–332.

Clark, R. L., Robertson, R. T., Peter, C. P., Bland, J. A., Nolan, T. E., Oppenheimer, L., and Bokelman, D. L. (1986). Association between adverse maternal and embryo–fetal effects in norfloxacin-treated and food-deprived rabbits, Fund. Appl. Toxicol., 7:272–286.

Clark, R. L., Eschbach, K., Cusick, W. A., and Heyse, J. F. (1987). Interactions between caffeine and adenosine agonists in producing embryo resorptions and malformation in mice, Fund. Appl. Toxicol., 8:116–124.

Clark, R. L., Antonello, J. M., Soper, K. A., Bradstreet, T. E., Heyse, J. F., and Ciminera, J. L. (1989). Statistical analysis of developmental toxicity data, Teratology, 39: 445–446.

Clark, R. L., Anderson, C. A., Prahalada, S., Leonard, Y. M., Stevens, J. L., and Hoberman, A. M. (1990a). 5α-Reductase inhibitor-induced congenital abnormalities in male rat external genitalia, Teratology, 41:544.

Clark, R. L., Antonello, J. M., Grossman, J. T., Wise, L. D., Anderson, C., Bagdon, W. J., Prahalada, S., MacDonald, J. S., and Robertson, R. T. (1990b). External genitalia abnormalities in male rats exposed in utero to finasteride, a 5α-reductase inhibitor, Teratology, 42:91–100.

Clayton, R. M. (1979). In: Alternatives in Drug Research (A. N. Rowan and C. J. Stratmann, Eds.). Macmillan, London, p. 153.

Clayton, R. M. (1981). An in vitro system for teratogenicity testing. In: The Use of Alternatives in Drug Research (A. N. Rowan and C. J. Stratmann, Eds.). University Park Press, Baltimore, pp. 153–173.

Cockroft, D. L. and Steele, C. E. (1989) Postimplantation embryo culture and its application to problems in teratology. In: In Vitro Methods in Toxicology (C. K. Atterwill and C. E. Steele, Eds.). Cambridge University Press, New York, pp. 365–389.

Daston, D. L. and D'Amato, R. A. (1989). In vitro techniques in teratology. In: Benchmarks: Alternative Methods in Toxicology (M. Mehlman, Ed.). Princeton Scientific, Princeton, NJ, pp. 79–109.

Davis, K. R., Schultz, T. W., and Dumont, J. N. (1981). Toxic and teratogenic effects of selected aramatic amines on embryos of the amphibian Xenopus laevis, Arch. Environ. Contam. Toxicol., 10:371–391.

Degenhardt, K. and Kladetzky, J. (1955). Spinal deformation and chordal attachment, Z. Menschl. Vererb. Konstitutionsl., 33:151–192.

Ellington, S. (1980). In vivo and in vitro studies on the effects of maternal fasting during embryonic organogenesis in the rat, J. Repro. Fertl. 60:383–388.

Ellison, A. C. and Maren, T. H. (1972). The effect of potassium metabolism on acetazolamide-induced teratogenesis, Teratology, 15:84–110.

Enslein, K., Lander, T. R., and Strange, J. L. (1983b). Teratogenesis: A statistical structure-activity model, Terat. Carcin Mutagen, 3:289–309.

Faustman, E. M. (1988). Short-term tests for teratogens, Mutat. Res., 205:355–384.

Flint, O. P. (1989). Reply to letter to the editor, Toxicol. Appl. Pharm., 99:176–180.

Flint, O. P. and Orton, T. C. (1984). An in vitro assay for teratogens with cultures of rat embryo midbrain and limb bud cells, Toxicol. Appl. Pharma., 76:383–395.

Food and Drug Administration. (1983). Good laboratory practices for nonclinical laboratory studies, CFR 21 part 58, March.

Food and Drug Administration. (1988). Good laboratory practices, CFR 21 part 58, April.

Gad, S. C. and Chengelis, C. P. (1992). Animal Models in Toxicology, Marcel Dekker, New York.

Gebhardt, D. O. E. (1972). The use of the chick embryo in applied teratology. In: Advances in Teratology, vol. 5 (D. H. M. Woollam, Ed.). Academic, London, pp. 97–111.

Gombar, V. K., Borgstedt, H. H., Enslein, K., Hart, J. B., and Blake, B. W. (1990). A QSAR model of teratogenesis, Quant. Struc. Activ. Rel., 10:306–332.

Grote, W. (1969). Trunk skeletal malformations following blood loss in gravid rabbits, Z. Anat. Entwicklungsgesch., 128:66–74.

Habert, R. and Picon, R. (1984). Testosterone, dihydrostestosterone and estadiol-17 β levels in maternal and fetal plasma and in fetal testes in the rat, J. Steroid Biochem., 21:183–198.

Haschek, W. M. and Rousseaup, C. G. (1991). Handbook of Toxicology Pathology, Academic, San Diego, CA.

Heinrichs, W. L. (1985). Current laboratory approaches for assessing female reproductive toxicity. In: Reproductive Toxicology (R. L. Dixon, Ed.). Raven, New York, pp. 95–108.

Hemm, R., Arslanoglou, L., and Pollock, J. (1977). Cleft palate following prenatal food restriction in mice: Association with elevated maternal corticosteroids, Teratology, 15:243–248.

Heywood, R. and James, R. W. (1985). Current laboratory approaches for assessing male reproductive toxicity: Testicular toxicity in laboratory animals. In: Reproductive Toxicology (R. L. Dixon, Ed.). Environ. Health Perspect., 147–160.

Homburger, F. and Goldberg, A. M. (1985). In Vitro Embryotoxicity and Teratogenicity Tests, Kraeger, Geneva, Switzerland.

Johnson, E. M. (1989). Problems in validation of in vitro developmental toxicity assays, Fund. Appl. Toxicol., 13:863–867.

Johnson, E. M., Gorman, R. M., Gabel, B. E. C., and George, M. E. (1982). The Hydra attenuata system for detection of teratogenic hazards. Terat. Carcin. Mutagen, 2: 263–276.

Johnson, E. M., Newman, L. M., and Fu, L. (1989) Letter to the editor, Toxicol. Appl. Pharm. 99:173–176.

Johnston, M. C., Sulik, K. K., and Dudley, K. H. (1979). Genetic and metabolic studies of the differential sensitivity of A/J and C57BL/6J mice to phenytoin ("Dilantin")-induced cleft lip, Teratology, 19:33A.

Kavlock, R. J., Chernoff, N., and Rogers, E. H. (1985). The effect of acute maternal toxicity on fetal development in the mouse, Terat. Carcin. Mutagen, 5:3–13.

Kerster, H. W. and Schaeffer, D. J. (1983). Brine shrimp (Artemia salina) Nauplia as a teratogen test system, Ecotoxicol. Environ. Safety, 7:342–349.

Khera, K. S. (1984). Maternal toxicity—A possible factor in fetal malformations in mice, Teratology, 29:411–416.

Khera, K. S. (1985). Maternal toxicity: A possible etiological factor in embryo–fetal deaths and fetal malformations of rodent–rabbit species, Teratology, 31:129–153.

Kochhar, D. M. (1981). Embryo explants and organ cultures in screening of chemicals for teratogenic effects. In: Developmental Toxicology (C. A. Kimmel and J. Buelbe-Saw, Eds.). Raven, New York, pp. 303–319.

Kochhar, D. M. and Aydelotte, M. B. (1974). Susceptible stages and abnormal morphogenesis in the developing mouse limb, analyzed in organ culture after transplacental exposure to vitamin A (retinoic acid), J. Embryol. Exptl. Morphol., 31:721–734.

Korenbrot, C. C., Huhtaniemi, I. T., and Weiner, R. I. (1977). Preputial separation as an external sign of pubertal development in the male rat, Bio. Repro., 17:298–303.

Kotzin, B. L. and Baker, R. F. (1972). Selective inhibition of genetic transcription in sea urchin embryos, J. Cell. Bio. 55:74–81.

Lochry, E. A., Hoberman, A. M., and Christian, M. S. (1984). Positive correlation of pup body weight with other commonly used developmental landmarks, Teratology, 29: 44A.

Lochry, E. A. (1987). Concurrent use of behavioral/functional testing in reproductive and developmental toxicity screen: Practical considerations, J. Amer. Coll. Toxicol., 6: 433–439.

MacCrimmon, H. R. and Kwain, W. H. (1969). Influences of light on early development and meristic characters in the rainbow trout (Salmo gairdneri Richardson), Can. J. Zool., 47:631–637.

Manson, J. M. and Kang, Y. J. (1989). Test methods for assessing female reproductive and developmental toxicology. In: Principles and Methods of Toxicology, 2nd ed. (A. W. Hayes, Ed.). Raven, New York, pp. 311–359.

Matt, D. W., Lee, J., Sarver, P. L., Judd, H. L., and Lu, J. K. H. (1986). Chronological changes in fertility, fecundity, and steroid hormone secretion during consecutive pregnancies in aging rats, Bio. Repro. 34:478–487.

Matt, D. M., Sarver, P. L., and Lu, J. K. H. (1987). Relation of parity and estrous cyclicity to the biology of pregnancy in aging female rats, Bio. Repro., 37:421–430.

Matsuzawa, T., Nakata, M., Goto, I., and Tsushima, M. (1981). Dietary deprivation induces fetal loss and abortions in rabbits, Toxicology, 22:255–259.

Mulay, S., Varma, D. R., and Soloman, S. (1982). Influence of protein deficiency in rats on hormonal status and cytoplasmic glucocorticoid receptors in maternal and fetal tissues, J. Endocrin., 95:49–58.

Mummery, C. L., van den Brink, C. E., van der Saag, P. T., and de Loat, S. W. (1984). A short-term screening test for teratogens using differentiating neuroblastoma cells in vitro, Teratology, 29:271–279.

Palmer, A. K. (1981). Regulatory requirements for reproductive toxicology: Theory and practice. In: Developmental Toxicology (C. A. Kimmel and J. Buelke-Sam, Eds.). Raven, New York, pp. 259–287.

Persaud, T. V. N. (1985). Teratogenicity testing. In: Basic Concepts in Teratology (T. V. N. Persaud, A. E. Chudley, and R. G. Skalko, Eds.). Alan R. Liss, New York, pp. 155–181.

Saegusa, T., Kaneko, Y., Sato, T., Nrama, I., and Segima, Y. (1980). BD40A-induced wavy ribs in rats, Teratology, 22:14A.

Salewski, V. E. (1964). Färbethode zum makroskopischen Nachweis von Implantationsstellen am Uterus der Ratte. Nauyn-Schmiedebergs. Arch. Exp. Path. U. Pharmak., 247:367.

Saxen, L. (1984). Tests in vitro for teratogenicity. In: Testing for Toxicity (J. W. Gorrod, Ed.) Taylor and Francis, London, pp. 185–197.

Saxen, L. and Saksela, E. (1971). Transmission and spread of embryonic induction. II. Exclusion of an assimilatory transmission mechanism in kidney tubule induction, Exptl. Cell Res., 66:369–377.

Schardein, J. (1987). Approaches to defining the relationship of maternal and developmental toxicity, Terat. Carcin. Mutagen, 7:255–271.

Schardein, J. (1988). Teratologic testing: Status and issues after two decades of evolution, Rev. Environ. Contam. Toxicol. 102:1–78.

Sieber-Blum, M. F. (1985). Differentiation of avian neural crest cells in vitro (quail, chick, rodent), Crisp Data Base, HD15311-04.

Sleet, R. B. and Brendel, K. (1985). Homogenous populations of Artemia nauplii and their potential use for in vitro testing in developmental toxicology, Terat. Carcin. Mutagen, 5(1):41–54.

Smith, M. K., Kimmel, G. L., Kochhar, D. M., Shepard, T. H., Spielberg, S. P., and Wilson, J. C. (1989). A selection of candidate compounds for in vitro teratogenesis test validation, Terat. Carcin. Mutagen, 3:461–480.

Snedecor, G. W. and Cochran, W. G. (1967). Statistical Methods, 6th ed., Iowa State University Press, Ames, Chapter 10.

Sopor, K. A. and Clark, R. L. (1990). Exact permutation trend tests for fetal survival data, Proc. Biopharm. Section Amer. Stat. Assoc., 263–268.

Staples, R. E. (1971). Blastocyst transplantation in the rabbit. In: Methods in Mammalian Embryology (J. C. Daniel, Jr., Ed.). Freeman, San Francisco, pp. 290–304.

Szabo, K., and Brent, R. (1975). Reduction of drug-induced cleft palate in mice, Lancet (June):1296–1297.

Tanimura, T. (1990). The Japanese perspectives on the reproductive and developmental toxicity evaluation of pharmaceuticals, J. Amer. Coll. Toxicol., 9:27–38.

Tukey, J. W., Ciminera, J. L., and Heyse, J. F. (1985). Testing the statistical certainty of a response to increasing doses of a drug, Biometrics, 41:295–301.

Turner, J. R. (1973). Perinatal mortality, growth, and survival to weaning in offspring of rats reared on diets moderately deficient in protein, Brit. J. Nutr., 29:139–147.

Tyl, R. W. (1988). Developmental toxicity in toxicological research and testing. In: Perspectives in Basic and Applied Toxicology (B. Ballantyne, Ed.). Butterworth, London, pp. 206–241.

Watkinson, W. P. and Millocovsky, G. (1983). Effect of phenytoin on maternal heart rate in A/J mice: Possible role in teratogenesis, Teratology, 28:1–8.

Weaver, T. E. and Scott, W. J. (1984a). Acetazolamide teratogenesis: Association of maternal respiratory acidosis and ectrodactyly in C57BL/6J mice, Teratology, 30:187–193.

Weaver, T. E. and Scott, J. J. (1984b). Acetazolamide teratogenesis: Interaction of maternal metabolic and respiratory acidosis in the induction of ectrodactyly in C57BL/6J mice, Teratology, 30:195–202.

Weindruch, R. and Walford, R. L. (1988). The Retardation of Aging and Disease by Dietary Restriction, Charles C. Thomas, Springfield, ILL.

Wickramaratne, G. A. de S. (1988). The post-natal fate of supernumerary ribs in rat teratogenicity studies, J. Appl. Toxicol., 8:91–94.

Wilson, J. G. (1978). Review of in vitro systems with potential for use in teratogenicity screening, J. Dev. Biol., 2:149–167.

Wilson, J. (1965). Methods for administering agents and detecting malformations in experimental animals. In: Teratology, Principles and Techniques (J. J. Wilson and J. Warkany, Eds.). University of Chicago Press, Chicago, pp. 262–277.

Wise, L. D., Clark, R. L., Minsker, D. H., and Robertson, R. T. (1988). Use of hematology and serum biochemistry data in developmental toxicity studies, Teratology, 37:502–503.

Wise, L. D., Clark, R. L., Rundell, J. O., and Robertson, R. T. (1990a). Examination of a rodent limbbud micromass assay as a prescreen for developmental toxicity, Teratology, 41:341–351.

Wise, L. D., Vetter, C. M., Anderson, C., Antonello, J. M., and Clark, R. L. (1990b). Reversible effects on external genitalia in rats exposed in vitro to triamcinolone acetonide, Teratology, 41:600.

Working, P. K. (1988). Male reproductive toxicology: Comparison of the human to animal models, Environ. Health Perspec., 77:37–44.

Yamada, T., Ohsawa, K., and Ohno, H. (1988). The usefulness of alkaline solutions for clearing the uterus and staining implantation sites in rates, Exp. Anim. (Tokyo), 37:325–332.

Zeman, F. J. (1967). Effect on the young rat of maternal protein restriction, J. Nutr., 93:167–173.

12

Carcinogenicity

This chapter studies the potential tumorigenicity and carcinogenicity of devices and biomaterials with prolonged human exposure.

Carcinogenicity studies are infrequently required for medical devices (ASTM, 1981). The tables in Chapter 1 cite each of the general cases, although these do not catch all the nuances. Under ISO 10993-11, for example, carcinogenicity tests are to be performed for

Devices introduced in the body >30 days cumulative contact.
Devices or materials with positive genotoxicity tests.
Resorbable materials and devices.
In those cases in which carcinogenicity testing is required but no effects have occurred in genotoxicity tests, clinical testing may be performed concurrently with carcinogenicity testing.
Where implantation does not represent the most appropriate route of exposure, scientifically justified alternatives should be considered.

Even then, the ISO standard states that ''carcinogenicity studies should be conducted only if there are suggestive data from other sources.'' Where implantation does not represent the most appropriate, or there is a more practical, route of exposure, scientifically justified alternative routes should be considered (Henry, 1985). The intent of such testing is to determine the carcinogenic (''tumorigenic'') potential of devices, materials, and/or multiple exposures over a period of the total life span of the test animal. Such tests may be designed to evaluate both the chronic toxicity and the tumorigenicity in a single study. These studies are the longest and most expensive of the preclinical (nonhuman) studies typically conducted on any new device or device material. These studies are important because, as noted by the International Agency for Research on Cancer (1987), "in the absence of adequate data on humans, it is biologically plausible and prudent to regard agents for which there is sufficient evidence of carcinogenicity in experimental animals as if they presented a carcinogenic risk to humans." The best established risks of carcinogenicity have to do with the effects of metals leading from long-term implants.

I. ANIMAL MODEL

Unlike pharmaceuticals and agrichemicals only one species is required to be evaluated in a carcinogenicity assay for a device or device material. The Sprague–Dawley-derived rat is by far the most commonly used with other strains of rats (Wistar, Long Evans, CFE, and Fischer 344) seeing only rare use. On very rare occasions dogs have been used [besides other concerns, a dog tumorigenial study is required to run 7 years (as opposed to 2 for a rat) to be valid], but this is now so infrequent we will concentrate on the case of the rat study in this section. The use of a single species is unlikely to adversely effect the overall ability to detect potential risks (Zbinden, 1993).

The choice of species and strain to be used in a carcinogenicity study is based on various criteria, including susceptibility to tumor induction, incidence of spontaneous tumor survival, existence of an adequate historical database, and availability (Cameron et al., 1985; Arnold et al., 1990; Gad and Chengelis, 1992).

Susceptibility to tumor induction is an important criterion. There would be little justification for doing carcinogenicity studies in an animal model that did not respond when treated with a "true" carcinogen. Ideally, the perfect species/strain would have the same susceptibility to tumor induction as the human. Unfortunately, this information is usually unavailable, and the tendency has been to choose animal models that are highly sensitive to tumor induction to minimize the probability of false negatives.

The incidence of spontaneous tumors is also an important issue. Rodent species and strains differ greatly in the incidence of various types of spontaneous tumors. The Sprague–Dawley stock, although preferred, has a very high incidence of mammary tumors in aging females, which results in substantial morbidity during the second year of a carcinogenicity study. If one chooses the Fischer 344 (F344) strain, the female mammary tumor incidence will be lower but the incidence of testicular tumors will be higher (close to 100%) than in Sprague–Dawley rats.

A high spontaneous tumor incidence can compromise the results of a carcinogenicity study in two ways. If a compound induces tumors at a site that already has a high spontaneous tumor incidence, it may be impossible to detect an increase above the high background "noise." Conversely, if a significant increase above levels is demonstrated, one may question the relevance of this finding to humans on the basis that the species is "highly susceptible" to tumors of this type (Hajian, 1983).

Such considerations are further compounded by the "Oppenheimer effect" (Turner, 1941; Oppenheimer et al., 1948; 1952; 1953; 1955; 1958; 1961; 1964). This is the occurrence of parenchymal tumors produced after long-lasting periods in which smooth-surfaced solids are implanted. Such solids have included everything from plastics to marble chips. This is a well-established phenomenon in rodents that has not been demonstrated in nonrodents or humans. These tumors are thought to be due to an epigenetic mechanism, and no sex differences in response have been seen. About 80% of the resulting tumors are fibrosarcomas (Alexander and Horning, 1959; Brand et al., 1975; 1976; Ecanow et al., 1977; Brand and Brand, 1982; Memol, 1986). Particulate "generation" by the degradation of device components increases the degree of problems.

From these early investigations, one can derive a number of characteristics for the phenomenon termed solid-state carcinogenesis. The major ones are as follows:

1. Composition of the material per se appears to be of little importance (unless it contains leachable carcinogens) because a wide variety of materials elicits a similar response.
2. A continuous, impermeable surface is important since perforations, weaves, or powders tend to reduce or abolish tumorigenicity of the material (Bates and Klein, 1966; Bischoff and Bryson, 1964; Dukes and Mitchley, 1962; Goldhaber, 1961; 1962).
3. The implant must be of at least a minimum ("critical") size.
4. The implant must remain in situ for a minimum period of time. The studies of Oppenheimer et al. (1958) found the presarcomatous changes occurred when the material was in place for about 6 months, although tumors may not appear for many more months.

The ability of a species/strain to survive for an adequate period is essential for a valid assessment of carcinogenicity. Poor survival has caused regulatory problems for pharmaceutical companies (PMA, 1988), and is therefore an important issue for medical devices. The underlying concept is that animals should be exposed to the drug for the greater part of their normal life span to make a valid assessment of carcinogenicity. If animals in the study die from causes other than drug-induced tumors, they may not have been at risk long enough for tumors to have developed. The sensitivity of the bioassay would be reduced, and the probability of a false negative result would be increased.

The availability of an adequate historical database is often cited as an important criterion for species/strain selection. Historical control data can sometimes be useful in evaluating the results of a study. Although such data are not considered equal in value to concurrent control data, they can be helpful if there is reason to believe that the concurrent control data are "atypical" for the species/strain.

The advantages of the Sprague–Dawley rat are (1) a large historical database, including various routes of exposure, (2) demonstrated susceptibility to known carcinogens, (3) generally good survival until recently (see below), and (4) ease of handling compared with certain other stocks. Disadvantages include (1) moderate to high incidence of spontaneous tumors, especially mammary and pituitary, (2) old rat nephropathy, and (3) marked genetic variability in stocks obtained from different suppliers (Chu et al., 1981; Sher et al., 1982).

There has recently been a reduction in survival of Sprague–Dawley rats and rats of other strains [Food and Drug Administration]. This reduction may be the result of ad libitum feeding, as preliminary results suggest that caloric restriction may improve survival. Leukemia appears to be the major cause of decreasing survival in the F344 rat. The problem of reduced survival may necessitate a re-evaluation of the survival requirements for carcinogenicity studies by regulatory agencies. Also, there is now a significant body of data that suggest that switching from the long favored ad libitum feeding of animals in bioassays can both extend their life span and decrease the incidences of some background tumors (Rao and Huff, 1990)

II. DOSE SELECTION

A. Number of Dose Levels

There will ordinarily be two dose levels, the maximum implantable dose (MID), and a fraction thereof (usually one-half of the MID). The controls will generally include polyethylene implants or other materials whose lack of carcinogenic potential is documented in a comparable form and shape.

In carcinogenicity testing on rodents, the MID of a material or device should be applied. Where possible, this dose should be expressed as a multiple of the worst-case human exposure in milligrams per kilogram.

B. Group Size

The minimum number of animals assigned to each dose group in implant carcinogenicity studies is 50 of each sex. Most companies, however, use more than the minimum number, and some use up to 80 animals per sex per group. The most important factor in determining group size is the need to have an adequate number of animals for a valid assessment of carcinogenic activity at the end of the study. Larger group sizes are also used when the carcinogenicity study is combined with a chronic toxicity study in the rat. In this case, serial sacrifices are performed at 6 and 12 months to evaluate potential toxic effects of the device.

In the final analysis, the sensitivity of the bioassay for detecting carcinogens is directly related to the sample size. Use of the maximum tolerated dose (MTD) has often been justified based on the small number of animals at risk compared to the potential human population, in spite of the difficulties inherent in extrapolating effects at high doses to those expected at much lower clinical doses. A reasonable compromise may be the use of doses lower than the MTD combined with a larger group size than the 50 per sex minimum accepted by regulatory agencies.

C. Route of Administration

Device carcinogenicity studies are conducted with the device or material being implanted into the test animals. Prior to implantation the samples are prepared. Whenever possible, the device shall be tested in its "ready-to-use" form, otherwise a suitably formed implant shall be made of the test material, with appropriate consideration of potential solid state carcinogenicity.

Treated animals typically receive single implants in a flank by making an incision, opening a pouch, inserting the sample, and closing the pouch. Dose groups are achieved by implanting variable numbers of devices in multiple flanks. Controls are generally untreated in the sense that no device is implanted—only the surgical procedure is performed.

D. Study Duration

The duration of carcinogenicity studies for rats is 2 years. Occasionally, rat studies are extended to 30 months. When hamsters are used, the study duration is limited to 18 months, a period that is consistent with the survival characteristics of this species.

Irrespective of the intended duration of the study, the most important consideration is that adequate numbers of animals survive long enough to allow for a valid assessment of carcinogenic activity. When survival is problematic, the duration of the study may be modified accordingly. The effect of survival on study duration is discussed in the next section.

E. Survival

As stated earlier, adequate survival is of primary importance in carcinogenicity studies because animals must be exposed to a drug for the greater part of their life span to increase the probability that late-occurring tumors can be detected. Early mortality, resulting from causes other than tumors, can jeopardize the validity of a study because dead animals cannot get tumors.

In general, the sensitivity of a carcinogenicity bioassay is increased when animals survive to the end of their natural life span, because weak carcinogens may induce late-occurring tumors. The potency of a carcinogen is often inversely related to the time to tumor development. By analogy, as the dose of a carcinogen is reduced, the time to tumor occurrence is increased (Littlefield et al., 1979; DePass et al., 1986).

Why do we not allow all animals on a carcinogenicity study to live until they die a natural death if by so doing we could identify more drugs as carcinogens? In fact, the sensitivity of a bioassay may not be improved by allowing the animals to live out their natural life span because the incidence of spontaneous tumors tends to increase with age. Depending on the tumor type, the ability of the bioassay to detect a device-related increase in tumor incidence may thus actually decrease rather than increase with time. The optimum duration of a carcinogenicity study is therefore that which allows late-occurring tumors to be detected but does not allow the incidence of spontaneous tumors to become excessive.

Reduced survival in a carcinogenicity study may or may not be device-related. Sometimes the MTD is exceeded and increased mortality occurs at the highest dose level, and occasionally at the middose level as well. This situation may not necessarily invalidate a study; in fact, the protocol may be amended to minimize the impact of the device-induced mortality. For example, cessation of drug treatment may enhance the survival of the animals in the affected groups, and allow previously initiated tumors to develop. As shown by Littlefield et al. (1979) in the NCTR ED01 study, liver tumors induced by 2-acetylaminofluorene, which appeared very late in the study, were shown to have been induced much earlier and not to require the continuous presence of the carcinogen to develop. By contrast, bladder tumors that occurred in the same study were dependent on the continued presence of the carcinogen.

Whether treatment is terminated or not, device-related toxicity may also be managed by performing complete histopathology on animals in the lower-dose groups rather than on high-dose and control animals only. If there is no increase in tumor incidence at a lower-dose level that is not compromised by reduced survival, the study may still be considered valid as an assessment of carcinogenicity.

When reduced survival is related to factors other than excessive toxicity, the number of animals at risk for tumor development may be inadequate, and the validity of the study may be compromised even in the absence of a device's effect on survival. Obviously, the adjustments described above for excessive drug-related toxicity are not relevant to this situation.

There is no unanimity of opinion among regulatory agencies as to the minimum survival required to produce a valid carcinogenicity study or as to the best approach for dealing with survival problems. Even within a single agency such as the FDA, different opinions exist on these issues. For example, the recently issued

FDA Redbook II Draft Guidelines requires that rats, mice, or hamsters be treated for 24 months. Early termination due to decreased survival is not recommended. The EEC guidelines differ in that they suggest termination of the study when survival in the control group reaches 20%, while Japanese guidelines suggest termination at 25% survival in the control or low-dose groups (Speid et al., 1990). These provisions make good sense in that they do not request termination of the study when device-related mortality may be present only at the highest dose.

F. Parameters Evaluated

In a pure carcinogenicity study the chief parameters measured are survival and the occurrence of tumors (Table 12.1).

Also measured are typically urinalysis parameters on samples collected prior to study start, at 6-month intervals during the study, and just prior to the final sacrifice, as presented in Table 12.2.

Clinical pathology and hematology measurements are made on blood samples collected at the same intervals with parameters measured in Table 12.2.

G. Statistical Analysis

Irrespective of the specific protocols used, all carcinogenicity studies end with a statistical comparison of tumor proportions between treated and control groups. This analysis is necessary because the control incidence of most tumor types is rarely zero. In the unlikely case that a type of tumor is found in treated animals but not in concurrent or appropriate historical controls, it is reasonable to conclude that the tumor is treatment-related without statistical analysis (Haschek and Rousseaup, 1991).

Most companies analyze tumor data using mortality-adjusted methods (PMA, 1988). Peto/International Agency for Research on Cancer (IARC) methodology is most commonly used, perhaps because this method is currently favored by the FDA (Peto et al., 1980). The use of life-table methods is most appropriate for "lethal" tumors; that is, those that cause the death of the animals. Various statistical methods are available for analyzing the incidence of lethal and nonlethal tumors (e.g., Gart et al., 1979; 1986; Dinse and Lagokos, 1983; McKnight, 1988; Portier and Bailer, 1989). These methods are especially useful when there are drug-related differences in mortality rates. When there is no drug effect of survival, unadjusted methods will generally give the same results.

As a general approach, most pharmaceutical statisticians begin by testing for the presence of a dose-related trend in tumor proportions. If the trend test is significant—that is, the p value is less than or equal to 0.05—pairwise comparisons are performed between the treated and control groups. Trend and pairwise analyses may be adjusted for mortality as stated earlier, or performed without mortality adjustment using such simple methods as chi-square or Fisher's exact tests.

TABLE 12.1 Lifetime Carcinogenicity Study (Implant) Organs and Sites to Be Examined

Adrenals (2)
Brain (3 levels: forebrain, mid-, and hindbrain, including brainstem)
Eyes (2)
Gastrointestinal tract
  Esophagus
  Stomach (glandular and nonglandular)
  Duodenum
  Jejunum
  Ileum
  Cecum
  Colon
  Rectum
Gonads
  ovaries with oviducts (2)
  testes with epididymids (2)
Harderian glands (2)
Heart
Kidneys (2)
Larynx
Liver (2 lobes)
Lung (2 coronal sections, including all lobes and mainstem bronchi)
Lymph node (mesenteric)
Mammary region (males and females)
Pancreas
Pituitary
Prostate
Salivary gland (submaxillary)
Sciatic nerve
Seminal vesicles
Skeletal muscle (thigh)
Spleen
Spinal cord (cervical)
Skin (dorsal)
Sternum/bone marrow
Thymic region
Thyroid/parathyroid
Trachea
Urinary bladder
Uterus
Implant site (4 sections of subcutaneous site and contiguous per-formal region)
Any other grossly abnormal tissues or organs

TABLE 12.2 Urinalysis Parameters
Measured

Appearance (color)
pH
Ketones
Urobilinogen
Specific gravity (refractive index)
Albumin
Glucose
Occult blood
Urinary sediment
Volume
Bilirubin

Although in most cases the use of trend tests is appropriate since most biological responses are dose-related, there are exceptions to this rule. Certain drugs, especially those with hormonal activity, may not produce classic dose responses and may even induce inverse dose-response phenomena. In these cases, a pairwise comparison may be appropriate in the absence of a significant positive trend.

Most companies use one-tailed comparisons, and a substantial number use two-tailed methods. Since regulatory agencies are primarily interested in identifying carcinogenic drugs, as opposed to those that inhibit carcinogenesis, the use of one-tailed tests is generally considered more appropriate. Some companies prefer two-tailed comparisons because in the absence of a true carcinogenic effect there is an equal probability of seeing significant decreases as well as significant increases by chance alone.

One of the most important statistical issues in the analysis of carcinogenicity data is the frequency of false positives, or type I errors. Because of the multiplicity of tumor sites examined and the number of tests employed, there is concern that noncarcinogenic devices may be erroneously declared carcinogens. If any $p < 0.05$ increase in tumor incidence is automatically regarded as a biologically meaningful result, then the false positive rate may be as high as 47–50% (Haseman et al., 1986).

Several statistical procedures designed to correct for the multiplicity of significance tests have been published (Haseman, 1990). One approach to the problem of multiple tumor site/type testing is a procedure attributed to Tukey by Mantel (1980). This method is used to adjust a calculated p value based on the number of tumor types/sites for which there are a minimum number of tumors in the particular study. The reasoning here is that for most tumor sites the number of tumors found is so small that it is impossible to obtain a significant result for that tumor site no matter how the tumors might have been distributed among the dose groups. Only those sites for which a minimum number of tumors is present can contribute to the false positive rate for a particular study.

A method proposed by Schweder and Spjotvoll (1982) is based on a plot of the cumulative distribution of observed p values. Farrar and Crump (1988) have published a statistical procedure designed not only to control the probability of false positive findings, but also to combine the probabilities of a carcinogenic effect across tumor sites, sexes, and species.

Another approach to controlling the false positive rate in carcinogenicity studies was proposed by Haseman (1983). Under this "rule," a compound would be declared a carcinogen if it produced an increase significant at the 1% level in a common tumor or an increase significant at the 5% level in a rare tumor. A rare neoplasm was defined as a neoplasm that occurred with a frequency of less than 1% in control animals. The overall false positive rate associated with the decision rule was found to be no more than 7–8%, based on control tumor incidences from National Toxicology Program (NTP) studies in rats and mice. This false positive rate compares favorably with the expected rate of 5%, which is the probability at which one would erroneously conclude that a compound was a carcinogen. This method is notable for its simplicity, and deserves serious consideration by pharmaceutical statisticians and toxicologists. Without resorting to sophisticated mathematics, this method recognizes the fact that tumors differ in their spontaneous frequencies and therefore in their contribution to the overall false positive rates in carcinogenicity studies. False positive results are much less likely to occur at tissue sites with low spontaneous tumor incidences than at those with high frequencies.

As a final point that has special relevance to pharmaceutical carcinogenicity studies, one may question whether the corrections for multiple comparisons and their effect on the overall false positive rate are appropriate for all tumor types. For example, if a compound is known to bind to receptors and produce pharmacological effects in a certain organ, is it justified to arbitrarily correct the calculated p value for the incidence of tumors in that organ, using the methods described above? It is difficult to justify such a correction, considering that the basis for correcting the calculated p value is that the true probability of observing an increased incidence of tumors at any site by chance alone may be much higher than the nominal alpha level (usually 0.05). It is reasonable to expect that when a drug has known pharmacological effects on a given organ the probability of observing an increased tumor incidence in that organ by chance alone is unlikely to be higher than the nominal 5% alpha level.

Although most pharmaceutical statisticians and toxicologists agree on the need to control the probability of false positive results, there is no consensus as to which method is most appropriate or most acceptable to regulatory agencies. The FDA and other such agencies will accept a variety of statistical procedures but will often reanalyze the data and draw their own conclusions based on their analyses.

III. INTERPRETATION OF RESULTS

A. Criteria for a Positive Result

There are three generally accepted criteria for a positive result in a carcinogenicity study. The first two are derived directly from the results of the statistical analysis: (1) a statistically significant increase in the incidence of a common tumor and (2) a statistically significant reduction in the time to tumor development. The third criterion is the occurrence of very rare tumors; that is, those not normally seen in control animals, even if the incidence is not statistically significant.

B. Use of Historical Controls

When the study is over, the data analyzed, and the p values corrected as appropriate, one may find that one or more tumor types increased in drug-treated groups relative to concurrent control group(s) but that they are comparable to or lower than the historical incidence. Occasionally, a small number of tumors may be found in a treated group and the incidence may be significant because of the absence of this tumor in the concurrent controls. A review of appropriate historical control data may reveal that the low tumor incidence in the treated group is within the "expected" range for this tumor.

The role of historical control data in interpreting carcinogenicity findings depends on the "quality" of the historical data. Ideally, the data should be derived from animals of the same age, sex, strain, and supplier. The animals should be housed in the same facility, and the pathology examinations should have been performed by the same pathologist or using the same pathological criteria for diagnosis. Since genetic drift occurs even in animals of a given strain and supplier, recent data are more useful than older data. The value of historical control data is directly proportional to the extent to which these conditions are fulfilled.

Although methods are available for including historical control data in the formal statistical analysis (Tarone, 1982; Dempster et al., 1983), this is usually not done—and for good reason. The heterogeneity of historical data requires that they be used qualitatively and selectively to aid in the final interpretation of the data after completion of the formal statistical analysis.

REFERENCES

Alexander, P. and Horning, E. S. (1959). Observations on the Oppenheimer method of inducing tumors by subcutaneous implantation of plastic films. In: Ciba Foundation

Symposium on Carcinogenesis, Mechanisms of Action (G. E. W. Wolstenholme and M. O'Conner, Eds.). Little, Brown, Boston, pp. 12–25.

Arnold, D. L., Grice, H. C., and Krawski, D. R. (1990). Handbook of in Vivo Toxicity Testing, Academic, San Diego, CA.

ASTM. (1981). Performance of lifetime bioassay for the tumorigenic potential of implant materials: Designation F1439-92. In: ASTM Standards Book, vol. 13, ASTM, Philadelphia, pp. 761–765.

Bates, R. R. and Klein, M. (1966). Importance of a smooth surface in carcinogenesis by plastic film, J. Nat. Cancer Inst., 37:145–151.

Bischoff, F. and Bryson, G. (1964). Carcinogenesis through solid state surfaces, Prog. Exper. Tumor Res., 5:85–113.

Brand, G. G., Johnson, K. H., and Buoen, L. C. (1976). Foreign Body, Tumorigenesis, CRC Crit. Rev. Toxicol, Oct.: 353.

Brand, K. G., Buoen, L. C., Johnson, K. H., et al. (1975). Foreign body in foreign body tumorigenesis: A review, Cancer Res., 35:279–286.

Brand, L. and Brand, K. G. (1980). Testing of implant materials for foreign body carcinogenesis. In: Biomaterials (G. D. Winter, D. G. Gibbons, and H. Plenk Jr., Eds.). Advances in Biomaterials, vol. 13, Wiley, New York, 1982, p. 819.

Cameron, T. P., Hickman, R. L., Kornreich, M. R., and Tarone, R. E. (1985). History, survival, and growth patterns of B6C3F1 mice and F344 rats in the National Cancer Institute Carcinogenesis Testing Program, Fund. Appl. Toxicol., 5:526–538.

Chu, K., Cueto, C., and Ward, J. (1981). Factors in the evaluation of 20 NCI carcinogenicity bioassays, J. Toxicol. Environ. Health, 8:251–280.

Dempster, A. P., Selivyn, M. R., and Weeks, B. J. (1983). Combining historical and randomized controls for assessing trends in proportions, J. Amer. Stat. Assoc., 78:221–227.

DePass, L. R., Weil, C. S., and Ballentyne, B. (1986). Influence of housing conditions for mice on results of a dermal oncogenicity bioassay, Fund. Appl. Toxicol., 7: 601–608.

Dinse, G. E. and Lagokos, S. W. (1983). Regression analysis of tumor prevalence data, Appl. Stat., 32:236–248.

Dukes, C. E. and Mitchley, B. C. V. (1962). Polyvinyl sponge implants: Experimental and clinical observations, Brit. J. Plas. Surg., 15:225–235.

Ecanow, B., Gold, B. H., and Sadove, M. (1977). The role of inert foreign bodies in the pathogenesis of cancer, Brit. J. Cancer, 36:397.

Farrar, D. B. and Crump, K. S. (1988). Exact statistical tests for any carcinogenic effect in animal bioassays, Fund. Appl. Toxicol., 11:652–663.

Gad, S. C. and Chengelis, C. P. (1992). Animal Models in Toxicology, Marcel Dekker, New York.

Gart, J. J., Chu, K. C., and Tarone, R. E. (1979). Statistical issues in interpretation of chronic bioassay tests for carcinogenicity, J. Nat. Cancer Inst., 62:957–974.

Gart, J. J., Krewski, D., Lee, P. A., Tarone, R. E., and Wahrendorf, J. (1986). Statistical Methods in Cancer Research, Vol. III. The Design and Analysis of Long-term Animal Experiments, IARC Scientific Publication no. 79, International Agency for Research on Cancer, Lyon.

Goldhaber, P. (1961). The influence of pore size on carcinogenicity of subcutaneously implanted Millipore filters, Proc. Amer. Assoc. Cancer Res., 3:228.

Goldhaber, P. (1962). Further observations concerning the carcinogenicity of Millipore filters, Proc. Amer. Assoc. Cancer Res, 3:323.

Hajian, G. (1983). Statistical issues in the design and analysis of carcinogenicity bioassays, Toxicol. Path., 11:83–89.

Haschek, W. M. and Rousseaup, C. G. (1991). Handbook of Toxicology Pathology, Academic, San Diego, CA.

Haseman, J. K. (1983). A reexamination of false-positive rates for carcinogenicity studies, Fund. Appl. Toxicol., 3:334–339.

Haseman, J. K. (1990). Use of statistical decision rules for evaluating laboratory animal carcinogenicity studies, Fund. Appl. Toxicol., 14:637–648.

Haseman, J. K., Winbush, J. S., and O'Donnell, M. W. (1986). Use of dual control groups to estimate false positive rates in laboratory animal carcinogenicity studies, Fund. Appl. Toxicol., 7:573–584.

Henry, T. J., ed. (1985). HIMA Report 85-1, Guidelines for the Preclinical Safety Evaluation of Materials Used in Medical Devices, Health Industry Manufacturers Association, Washington, DC.

International Agency for Research on Cancer. (1987). IARC Monographs on the Evaluation of Carcinogenic Risks to Humans—Preamble, IARC Internal. Technical Report 87/001, IARC, Lyon.

ISO. (1995). ISO10993—3: Carcinogenicity.

Littlefield, N. A., Farmer, J. H., Taylor, D. W., and Sheldon, W. G. (1979). Effects of dose and time in a long term, low-dose carcinogenicity study. In: Innovations in Cancer Risk Assessment (EDOI Study) (J. A. Staffer and M. A. Shellman, Eds.). Pathtox, IL, pp. 17–34.

Mantel, N. (1980). Assessing laboratory evidence for neoplastic activity, Biometrics, 36:381–399.

McKnight, B. (1988). A guide to the statistical analysis of long-term carcinogenicity assays, Fund. Appl. Toxicol., 10:355–364.

Memol, V. (1986). Malignant neoplasms associated with orthopedic implant materials in rats, J. Orthoped. Res. 4:346–355.

Oppenheimer, B. S., Oppenheimer, E. T., and Stout, A. P. (1948). Sarcomas induced in rats by implanting cellophane, Proc. Soc. Exp. Bio. Med., 67:33–34.

Oppenheimer, B. S., Oppenheimer, E. T., and Stout, A. P. (1952). Sarcomas induced in rodents by imbedding various plastic films, Proc. Soc. Exp. Bio. Med., 79:66–369.

Oppenheimer, B. S., Oppenheimer, E. T., and Stout, A. P., et. al. (1953). Malignant tumors resulting from embedding plastics in rodents, Science, 118:305–306.

Oppenheimer, B. S., Oppenheimer, E. T., and Danishefsky, I., et al. (1955). Further studies of polymers as carcinogenic agents in animals, Cancer Res., 15:333–340.

Oppenheimer, B. S., Oppenheimer, E. T., Stout, A. P., et al. (1958). The latent period in carcinogenesis by plastic in rats and its relation to the presarcomatous stage, Cancer, 11:204–213.

Oppenheimer, E. T., Willhite, M., Danishefsky, I., et al. (1961). Observations on the effects of powdered polymer in the carcinogenic process, Cancer Res., 21:32–136.

Oppenheimer, E. T., Willhite, M., Stout, A. P., et al. (1964). A comparative study of the effects of imbedding cellophane and polystyrene films in rats, Cancer Res., 24:379–387.

Peto, R., Pike, M. C., Day, N. E., Gray, R. G., Lee, P. N., Parish, S., Peto, J., Richards, S., and Wahrendorf, J. (1980). Guidelines for Simple, Sensitive Significance Tests for Carcinogenic Effects in Long-Term Animal Experiments, IARC Monographs on the Evaluation of the Carcinogenic Risk of Chemicals to Humans, International Agency for Research on Cancer, Lyon.

PMA. (1988). Results of a Questionnaire Involving the Design and Experience with Carcinogenicity Studies, Pharmaceutical Manufacturers Association (now PhRMA), Washington, DC.

Portier, C. J. and Bailer, A. J. (1989). Testing for increased carcinogenicity using a survival-adjusted quantal response test, Fund. Appl. Toxicol., 12:731–737.

Rao, G. N. and Huff, J. (1990). Refinement of long-term toxicity and carcinogenesis studies, Fund. Appl. Toxicol, 15:33–43.

Schweder, T. and Spjotvoll, E. (1982). Plots of p-values to evaluate many test simultaneously, Biometrika, 60:493–502.

Sher, S. P., Jensen, R. D., and Bokelman, D. L. (1982). Spontaneous tumors in control F344 and Charles River CD rats and Charles River CD-1 and B6C3F1 mice, Toxicol. Lett., 11:103–110.

Speid, L. H., Lumlez, C. F., and Walker, S. R. (1990). Harmonization of guidelines for toxicity testing of pharmaceuticals by 1992, Res. Toxicol. Pharm., 12:179–211.

Tarone, R. E. (1982). The use of historical control information in testing for a trend in proportions, Biometrics, 38:215–220.

Turner, F. C. (1941). Sarcomas at sites of subcutaneously implanted Bakelite disks, J. Nat. Cancer Inst., 2:81–83.

Zbinden, G. (1993). The concept of multispecies testing in industrial toxicology, Reg. Toxicol. Pharm., 17:84–94.

13

Sterility, Sterilization, and Heavy Metals

I. STERILITY

Medical devices may be sold and used in two different states in terms of their bioburden (i.e., the number of viable micro-organisms present on the device)—either sterile or nonsterile. If they are intended to be used in the sterile state, the actual act of sterilization may be performed either by the manufacturer or by the user (although the latter is commonly the case only for reusable devices and instruments, such as surgical instruments). If the manufacturer is to sterilize the instruments, then this is specified in the DMF (and in product-related literature), along with the means for achieving a suitable degree of sterilization and specification of a program for assuming performance of the process. ANSI/AAMI ST60 (AAMI, 1997) provides standards for indications of adequate sterilization of device products. The FDA sets standards for actual sterilization results (FDA, 1982).

The sterility assurance level (SAL) is the statistical probability of a device's not being sterile after going through an established sterilization cycle. Residual micro-organisms are usually measured as colony-forming units (CFUs), with the amount of sterilization required to reduce the number of CFUs by an order of magnitude for a specific device being termed the D_{10} (the dose to produce a tenfold reduction in bioburden). Doses here are both a concentration (or, for radiation, a power level) and the time internal the device (or material) is exposed to that dose (Prince and Rubino, 1984; AAMI, 1995).

There are four major means employed for sterilizing medical instruments, each of which has advantages and drawbacks.

Heat (steam) is effective and inexpensive but can only be used for relatively small-volume materials that are not degraded or deformed by it. Accordingly, it is typically useful only for smaller metal devices and cannot be used for plastics and such. It is most commonly used for reusable instruments and glassware. ISO 11134 sets forth requirements for the use of moist heat.

Steam sterilization by autoclaving has traditionally been the most widely used method for medical instruments. Today, prevacuum, high-temperature steam sterilization is considered to be the safest and most practical means of sterilizing the majority of surgical instruments, surgical dressings, fluids, fabrics, and other absorbent materials. The process should be used with caution while sterilizing polymers and composites, as both heat and steam can drastically alter the properties of these materials. The main deleterious effect arising due to steam sterilization of polymeric materials is when hydrolysis of the polymer takes place, leading to undesirable contaminants. Under prolonged steam autoclaving, 3 to 5 ppb of methylene dianiline has been detected (Mazzu and Smith, 1984) in the aqueous extract of methyl diisocyanate (MDI)-based polyurethane, which was attributed to the hydrolysis of the polymer. Habermann and Waitzova (1985) observed the release of contaminating substances, whose structure was not elucidated, when polyvinyl chloride (PVC)-containing aqueous suspensions were autoclaved. Repeated autoclaving of PVC intended for biomedical applications was found to increase the mechanical properties of PVC of both covered and uncovered PVC samples. The change in the mechanical properties was attributed to the rearrangements in the PVC macromolecular chains giving rise to branches of varied lengths. Repeated autoclaving of uncovered PVC samples for 150 min was seen to induce higher leaching of the plasticizer.

Seemingly stable polymers can also undergo changes in the surface morphology, especially if the glass transition temperature of the polymer is exceeded while autoclaving. This may cause changes in the biocompatibility or blood-contacting properties of the material. Oligomers or other inadvertent contaminants introduced subsequent to steam sterilization may have significant effect on the biocompatibility and the performance of the polymers. A scanning electron microscopy study of different types of arterial prostheses made from Dacron found that all the prostheses were coated with a layer of oligomers on autoclaving. The Cooley knitted Dacron grafts show the maximal amount of oligomer crystals, which was progressively increased with each successive resterilization. This coating of oligomers also resulted in increased hemolysis. Berger and Sauvage (1981) also noted late fiber deterioration in 493 Dacron arterial prostheses that had been implanted for 3 to 15 years. One of the contributing factors to this deterioration was believed to be due to autoclaving.

Commercial poly (ethyleneterephthalate) (PET) is known to contain cyclic and linear oligomers as natural impurities, which are formed as a by-product during polymerization and texturing. Cyclic trimer is a major oligomer component, and the content of cyclic trimer is actually a criterion for the quality of PET. Study of the effect of steam sterilization on PET has shown that oligomers, and in particular, the cyclic trimer, increases in PET on repeated autoclaving. Studies (Nair, 1995) of the PET materials indicated increased values of heat of fusion and percentage crystallinity, which suggested reorganization of the amorphous phase. Generation of new crystalline regions was ruled out as there was no increase in the intensity of the infrared peak of 973 cm^{-1}, which indicates crystallinity. Chain scission of amorphous regions, resulting in the formation of new amorphous regions, was therefore believed to be the reason for the increased values of crystallinity. The changes of the molecular weights of M_n and M_w suggested that although degradation would take place on autoclaving for 15 min, subsequent sterilization of 30 min results in solid-state polymerization or cyclization reactions. These cyclization reactions were responsible for the formation of fresh cyclic trimer molecules, which could migrate to the surface. As moisture and air enhance oxidation and hydrolysis reactions, subsequent autoclaving for 60 min would result in more degradation of amorphous regions. The increased temperature could also facilitate the easy migration of the cyclic trimer to the surface.

Chemical sterilants include ethylene oxide, glutaraldehyde, and formaldehyde. These can all be used for most devices that do not have any readily reactive (degradable) components. Ethylene oxide (ETO) is the most widely used, but is a mutagen, carcinogen, and neurotoxic, and causes hypersensitivity responses in some individuals (Crammer et al., 1984; Chapman et al., 1986; Rockel et al., 1986). The concern with all of the chemical sterilants is residuals left on and (permeated) in devices. If any of the chemical sterilants are used, residual levels must be determined and kept below (or brought below by allowing the devices to "off gas") certain established limits (HIMA, 1981). Table 13.1 states the ISO standards (ISO 11135) for allowable ETO residuals.

Ethylene oxide, ECH, and ethylene glycol residual levels must all typically be determined. Ethylene oxide is an effective bactericide active at temperatures

TABLE 13.1 ISO 10993-7: Ethylene Oxide Sterilization Residuals

Residue	Average delivered dose of EO and ECH (mg/day)		
	Permanent contact (>30 days)	Prolonged exposure (1 to 30 days)	Limited exposure (<24 hr)
Ethylene oxide	0.1[a]	2	20[b]
Ethylene chlorohydrin	2	2	12

[a] Intraocular devices $\leq$ 0.5 µg/day.
[b] Extracorporeal blood purification setups $\leq$ 20 mg/d and 60 mg/ml; blood oxygenators and blood separators, $\leq$ 60 mg.

as low as 60°C. As ETO can easily diffuse into materials to be sterilized, it is possible to sterilize heat- or moisture-sensitive materials, even through sealed plastic wrapping. One of the disadvantages of this method for polymeric materials is that they retain varying amounts of ETO. Residual ETO in sterilized plastic tubing has been reported to cause hemolysis of blood in heart–lung surgery. Adverse hemolytic reactions were also caused when blood was exposed to plastics that retained significant quantities of residual ETO. Ethylene oxide also possesses toxic properties and is a strong alkylating agent. As the ETO consists of two carbon atoms and an oxygen atom linked together in an unstable three-membered ring, it can react with various functional groups as follows:

H_2C—CH_2 \ / O	+HSR	→	CH_2OHCH_2SHR
	+HNHR	→	CH_2OHCH_2NHR
	+HOCOR	→	CH_2OHCH_2OCOR
	+COOH	→	CH_2OCH_2COOH

These are the sulfhydryl, amino, carboxyl, and hydroxyl groups of proteins and nucleic acids. The lethal effect of the ETO arises from its alkylating effect on these susceptible molecules. Due to the reactivity of the gas with such functional groups, however, this type of sterilization should only be carried out at room temperature with materials such as polyurethanes, polyesters, and other polymers with potentially reactive groups. Several of the composite polymeric materials used these days, such as albuminated Dacron grafts or heparinized grafts, are liable to lose the beneficial effect extended by the albumin coating or heparin coating by subjecting these materials to ETO sterilization. Ethylene oxide sterilization of heparinized polymers reduces their nonthrombogenic properties (Bruck, 1971), while Guidoin et al. (1985) reported that ETO sterilized albuminated polyester grafts have a slower rate of healing when implanted in comparison to a similar graft sterilized by irradiation. Although retention of residual ETO is believed to be the cause for this slower rate of healing, it is likely that the alkylating action of ETO could denature the albuminated surface, forming products that delay the healing process.

Most manufacturers of ETO sterilizer equipment routinely recommend at least 3 and preferably 5 days aeration for ETO sterilized plastic tubings. The time for aeration is dependent on the material sterilized, however. Highly porous materials such as cellulose, paper, and natural rubber show very high values of ETO solubility and low diffusion coefficients. A study (Vink and Pleijsier, 1986) of residual ETO content in different polymers revealed that for a number of materials, the residual content was well above the levels that are currently considered to be safe even after aeration for 15 days. For a reliable determination of aeration times after ETO sterilization of medical devices, the type of the material from which the device is made, and in particular its thickness, should be considered.

Another point worth noting on the subject of adequate deaeration is the procedure for estimation of residual ETO. In a project involving the interlaboratory comparisons of the procedures for the estimation of ETO, it was observed (Marlowe et al., 1987) that the average estimated total coefficient ranged from 8–22%, even when following the same standard procedure of residual ETO estimation, emphasizing the need for standard and reliable procedures for estimating the residual ETO content. The concern with all of the chemical sterilants is residuals left on and (permeated) in devices. If any of the chemical sterilants are used, residual levels must be determined and kept below (or brought below by allowing the devices to vent or off gas) certain established limits.

Radiation provides the third means of sterilization. Gamma radiation or ultraviolet light are both used, with the former being very predominant on the industrial scale. Radiation's advantages are that it can be used on sealed packages of material, leaves no residues, and can be used for large volumes of material. At the same time, there is a significant capital investment involved, safety precautions must be vigorously enforced, and some polymers are degraded (although this usually translates only to being discolored) by the absorbed energy in a gamma field. ISO 1137 sets requirements for radiation sterilization. Additionally, if a ^{60}Co source is used, the sterilization time is long (AAMI, 1982). Biological indicator systems are typically used to ensure adequate sterilization performance (Prince, 1980).

Irradiation of high polymers results in either cross-linking or degradation, depending on the chemical nature of the system. Although the accepted dose for radiation sterilization is 2.5 Mrad, it is known that certain species require up to 6 Mrads for complete destruction. The effects of irradiation at increased doses or multiple sterilization are assumed to be cumulative. Polymers that tend to cross-link show a steady increase in their molecular weights with increasing dose and with the formation of branches until a three-dimensional network is formed, while polymers that undergo degradation exhibit chain scission, the molecular weight steadily decreases with increasing radiation dose, and mechanical properties of the system simultaneously undergo changes. These properties include tensile strength, elastic modulus, shear strength, elongation, and occasionally color.

Though cross-linking and chain scission processes may occur simultaneously, usually one or the other predominates. In the case of vinyl polymers, if the carbon atoms of the main chain carry at least one hydrogen atom, the polymer tends to cross-link, whereas if the carbon atoms are fully substituted, the polymer tends to degrade. There is a correlation between cross-linking tendency and the heats of polymerization, showing that polymers that exhibit high heats of polymerization (above approximately 16 kcals/mole) cross-link, while polymers that exhibit low heats of polymerization (less than 16 kcal/mole) degrade. Irradiation of polymers can also result in gas evolution, double bond formation, and the production of trapped free radicals. The presence of impurities can accelerate the degradation process with the possibility of producing irritants or other undesirable products. Free radicals produced in polymers by irradiation in air convert to peroxidic radicals. Additionally, the irradiation process may result in discoloration of polymeric products.

While general effects of irradiation on polymeric materials have been extensively studied (Chapiro, 1962), relatively small changes in physicochemical, mechanical, and biological properties may be tolerable in the short term, whereas similar changes may lead to catastrophic failures in long-term application. Besides, seemingly unchanged materials may also suffer some minor damages that affect their biological and mechanical performance. An example is the reported stability of cellulosic polymers up to 20 Mrad; however, when the regenerated cellulose membranes are sterilized by radiation, Takesawa et al. (1987) have observed reduction of vitamin B_{12} clearance and hydraulic permeability of the membranes increased if the sterilization was carried out in the wet condition. Similarly, Rose et al. (1984) have observed that the wear of polyethylene exposed to γ irradiation increased with dosage and contact stress, becoming measurable in many cases only after a critical dose or stress was exceeded. The most significant effect noted was that the pressure dependence of the wear rate appeared to be a combination of chain scission and oxidation, suggesting that the radiation should be carried out in an inert atmosphere.

Studying the effects of aging of γ radiation-sterilized isotactic polypropylene revealed that though both cross-linking and degradation occur simultaneously during irradiation, branching in addition to postirradiation takes place during aging. A dose of 2.5 Mrads was sufficient to introduce changes in crystallinity. These changes were attributed to the semicrystalline nature of the polymer and were observed to be different for the covered and uncovered samples. Additionally, the transitions between short- and long-range order and short- and long-duration stiffness in both covered and uncovered samples were affected by the formation of branches in the backbone of the polymer. A higher degree of branching was observed in covered samples, resulting in greater long-duration stiffness in the transition between short- and long-duration stiffness. The higher degree of branching in the covered samples was attributed to the high diffusion of energized oxygen into the polymer matrix when compared to the uncovered samples.

Used extensively in biomedical applications, PET has been believed to withstand radiation sterilization without significant degradation. Study of PET fibers, however, revealed that a single dose of 2.5 Mrads was sufficient to induce chemical changes that were reflected in the changes of crystallinity and breaking load of the fibers. These changes were attributed to the degradation of PET in the amorphous regions and the recombination of degraded aliphatic segments. Baquey et al. (1987) and Takesawa et al. (1987) report the increased stability of Dacron or PET fabrics coated with albumin on irradiation, but the results of the investigation also indicate a leakage of albumin on irradiation. The amount of albumin released was found to be dependent upon the nature of fabric used. The migration of chicken embryonic cells was also observed to be decreased for the irradiated fabrics.

Another group of polymers used extensively in biomedical applications are the polyurethanes. Gamma irradiation of polyurethanes based on 4,4′ diphenyl MDI have been reported (Shinatari and Nakamura, 1989) to produce the carcinogen 4,4′ methylene aniline with simultaneous detection of polyurethane oligomers.

The γ irradiation of poly(DL-lactide/glycolide)-type microspheres has been reported to result in decreased molecular weights with the degradation continuing on storage. An inadvertent effect is the change in the release pattern of the drug loaded in the microspheres. Higher-molecular-weight polyglycolide sutures that were initially more resistant to enzymatic degradation become more prone to enzymatic attack as a consequence of the altered physical and chemical structure obtained on γ irradiation. Melberg et al. (1988) also report that the irradiation of PVC catheters of an external insulin pump produced chemical transformation products and damaged the insulin solution. Bacterial endotoxins were found to be unaffected by γ irradiation, and hence gloves and software sterilized by irradiation have been observed (Shumnes and Darby, 1984) to contain significant amounts of bacterial endotoxin. As another inadvertent effect, it was also observed that the endotoxin levels were increased when the bacterial counts were elevated, in some cases leading to contact dermatitis (Shumnes and Darby, 1984). The γ irradiation of intraocular lens, however, decreased the inflammatory reactions observed on implantation of an ETO-sterilized lens. Ludwig et al. (1988) attributed this decreased response not only to less absorption of the toxic agent, but also to polymerization of any residual monomeric methylmethacrylate. Gamma radiation or ultraviolet light are both used, with the former being very predominant on the industrial scale.

Radiation has significant advantages, but there is a significant capital investment involved, safety precautions must be vigorously enforced, and some polymers are degraded (though this usually translates only to being discolored) by the absorbed energy in a gamma field.

Dry heat is an additional available method, but one limited to use with metals and ceramics. It is the simple use of heat without any moisture present. There are a number of new sterilization technologies available—variable pressure hydrogen peroxide, peracetic acid plasma, hydrogen peroxide plasma, ozone, intense pulsed light, and chlorine dioxide.

The USP provides guidance on tests for verifying that devices have achieved the desired level of sterilization. These are sterility tests.

A. Sterility Tests

The following procedures are applicable for determining whether or not a pharmacopoeial article purporting to be sterile complies with the requirements set forth in the individual monograph with respect to the test for *sterility*. In view of the possibility that positive results may be due to faulty aseptic techniques or environmental contamination in testing, provisions are included under Sec. B below for two stages of testing.

Alternative procedures may be employed to demonstrate that an article is sterile, provided that the results obtained are at least of equivalent reliability. Where a difference appears or in the event of a dispute, when evidence of microbial contamination is obtained by the procedure given in this pharmacopoeia, the result so obtained is conclusive of failure of the article to meet the requirements of the test. Similarly, failure to demonstrate microbial contamination by the procedure given in this pharmacopoeia is evidence that the article meets the requirements of the test.

The following considerations apply to sterilized devices manufactured in lots, each consisting of a number of units. Special considerations apply to sterile devices manufactured in small lots or in individual units in which the self-destructive nature of the sterility test renders the conventional sterility test impracticable. For these articles, appropriate and acceptable modifications to the sterility test must be made.

For articles of such size and shape as to permit complete immersion in not more than 1000 ml of culture medium, test the intact article, using the appropriate media, and incubate as directed under USP (USP, 2000). Proceed as directed under Liquids, beginning with "Examine the media visually."

For devices having hollow tubes, such as transfusion or infusion assemblies, or where the size of an item makes immersion impracticable and where only the fluid pathway must be sterile, flush the lumen of each of 20 units with a sufficient quantity of fluid thioglycollate medium and the lumen of each of 20 units with a sufficient quantity of soybean-casein digest medium to yield a recovery of not less than 15 ml of each medium, and incubate with not less than 100 ml of each of the two media as directed under USP (USP, 2000). For devices in which the lumen is so small that fluid thioglycollate medium will not pass through, substitute alternative thioglycollate medium for fluid thioglycollate medium, but incubate the medium anaerobically.

Where the entire intact article, because of its size and shape, cannot be tested for sterility by immersion in not more than 1000 ml of culture medium, expose that portion of the article most difficult to sterilize, and test that portion, or where practicable remove two or more portions each from the innermost portion of the article. Aseptically transfer these portions of the article to the specified number of vessels of appropriate media in a volume of not more than 1000 ml and incubate as directed under General Procedure in the USP. Proceed as directed under Liquids, beginning with "Examine the media visually."

Where the presence of the test specimen in the medium interferes with the test because of bacteriostatic or fungistatic action, rinse the article thoroughly with a minimal amount of rinse fluid. (See under Diluting and Rinsing Fluids.) Recover the rinse fluid, and test as directed for *devices* under Test Procedures Using Membrane Filtration (USP, 2000).

1. Sterile Empty or Prefilled Syringes

Sterility testing of prefilled syringes is performed by employing the same techniques used in testing sterile products in vials or ampules. The direct transfer technique may be employed if the *bacteriostasis and fungistasis* determination has indicated no adverse activity under the test conditions. Where appropriate, the membrane filtration procedure may be employed. For prefilled syringes containing a sterile needle, flush the contained produce through the lumen. For syringes packaged with a separate needle, aseptically attach the needle, and expel the product into the appropriate media. Pay special attention to demonstrating that the outside of the attached needle (that portion that will enter the patient's tissues) is sterile. For empty sterile syringes, take up sterile medium or diluent into the barrel through the needle if attached, or if not attached, through a sterile needle attached for the purpose of the test, and express the contents into the appropriate media.

Devices that are purported to contain sterile pathways may be tested for sterility by the membrane filtration technique as follows.

Aseptically pass a sufficient volume of *fluid D* through each of no fewer than 20 devices so that not less than 100 ml is recovered from each device. Collect the fluids in aseptic containers and filter the entire volume collected through membrane filter funnel(s).

Where the devices are large and lot sizes are small, test an appropriate number of units as described for similar cases in the section Sterilized Devices, under Test Procedures for Direct Transfer to Test Media (USP, 2000).

B. Interpretation of Sterility Test Results

1. First Stage

At the prescribed intervals during and at the conclusion of the incubation period, examine the contents of all of the vessels for evidence of microbial growth, such as the development of turbidity and/or surface growth. If no growth is observed, the article tested meets the requirements of the test for sterility.

If microbial growth is found but a review in the sterility testing facility of the monitoring, materials used, testing procedure, and negative controls indicates that inadequate or faulty aseptic technique was used in the test itself, the *first stage* is declared invalid and may be repeated.

If microbial growth is observed but there is no evidence invalidating the *first stage* of the test, proceed to the *second stage*.

2. Second Stage

The minimum number of specimens selected is double the number tested in the *first stage*. The minimum volumes tested from each specimen and the media and incubation periods are the same as those indicated for the *first stage*. If no microbial growth is found, the article tested meets the requirements of the test for sterility. If, however, it can be demonstrated that the *second stage* was invalid because of faulty or inadequate aseptic technique in the performance of the test the *second stage* may be repeated. [*Note*: Where sterility testing is used as part of an assessment of a production lot or batch or as one of the quality control criteria for release of such lot or batch, see USP *Sterilization and Sterility Assurance of Compendial Articles* (1211).]

II. HEAVY METALS

Leachable heavy metals are a concern both in devices per se (for the possible potential hazard they present to patients) and in devices and their packaging (both of which end up in landfills) for their potential pollution of the environment, with subsequent potential harm to man and wildlife.

Traditionally the heavy metals are defined as all those metals with atomic weights greater than sodium (23) that form soaps on reaction with fatty acids. In practice, the metals of concern are lead, aluminum, selenium, nickel, cadmium, zinc, chromium, arsenic, mercury, tin, antimony, and iron. The USP presents specific methods in sections 231, 241, 251, 161, 291, and 211. Extractors are performed in purified water, and great care must be taken to avoid contamination of the test apparatus and material due to the ubiquitous presence of the heavy metals—particularly lead—in the industrialized environment.

Other pharmacopoeias also prescribe methods for analysis, but these are all severely limited (Anon, 1995).

The present pharmacopoeial heavy metals test by sulfide precipitation is about 100 years old. Today, instrumental analytical techniques, such as atomic absorption spectrometry (AAS), X-ray fluorescence spectrometry (SRFS), and inductively coupled plasma-optical emission spectrometry (ICP-OES), are widely used in the pharmaceutical and food industry as well as in other industrial branches for the specific determination of metal traces. Scientific publications on heavy metals contamination and pollution are based exclusively on such modern instrumental techniques.

A. History and Objectives of Compendial Heavy Metals Tests

Over the hundreds of years of their history, pharmacopoeias have evolved from compendia on drug selection and manufacture (compounding) into compendia for device and drug testing. One of the first analytical tests introduced in the early phase of this development (at the turn of the twentieth century) was the test for heavy metals.

USP VIII (1905) included the first general test for heavy metals, *Time-Limit Test for Heavy Metals*. The aim of this test was defined as follows: "This test is to be used to detect the presence of undesirable metallic impurities in official chemical substances or their solutions; these should not respond affirmatively within the stated time."

The test had two steps: (1) sulfide precipitation in a strongly acidic range, and (2) sulfide precipitation in an ammonia–alkaline medium.

The metals listed as undesirable were antimony, arsenic, cadmium, copper, iron, lead, and zinc. A general test for the separate specific determination of arsenic had already appeared in *USP VI* (1893).

In *USP XII* (1942), there was a change to determination in an acetic–acid medium. Simultaneously, a comparison solution for lead was also introduced, and it was the "darkness" of this solution that was to serve as a permissible limit.

The Swiss and German pharmacopoeias (*Ph. Helvetica, Deutsches Arznei-buch*) underwent a very similar but to some extent more delayed development.

In addition to testing for heavy metals in general, pharmacopoeias also require specific testing for a number of individual heavy metals, such as nickel (in polyols and hardened fats), iron (in diverse substances), and lead (in sugars).

An analysis of the history of the pharmacopoeial heavy metals testing shows that the following objectives were pursued.

In the nineteenth century and the early part of the twentieth century, a number of heavy metal compounds considered to have medicinal value were commonly used in pharmaceutical products. The test was therefore originally very broad in scope (detection of all colored and dark sulfides precipitated in acidic and alkaline solutions) to prevent the use of mislabeled products or products containing inadvertent admixtures of heavy metal compounds.

The later restriction to dark sulfides precipitated from weakly acid solution, with lead as a comparison standard, and the additional specific tests for individual elements such as arsenic and iron, imply a fundamental change of perspective. Clearly, the purpose now was to detect contamination caused by toxicologically significant heavy metals coming from manufacturing equipment and processes. The conditions of detection chosen show that the focus of interest was on lead and copper, two elements formerly widely used in factory equipment (e.g., in water pipes, in copper and brass kettles, and in the lead chamber process used in the manufacture of sulfuric acid, an essential basic chemical substance used in numerous synthetic processes).

This historical review leads to the conclusion that the heavy metals test in its present form was clearly neither designed to be a universal test nor meant to be understood as one, and it clearly does not allow for such an interpretation.

B. Scope and Limitations of the Present Pharmacopeial Heavy Metals Test

The test in its present form—sulfide precipitation in a weakly acidic medium and comparison against a lead comparison solution at a concentration (usually) of 10 ppm—is theoretically suitable for the determination of bismuth, copper, gold, lead, mercury, ruthenium, silver (*I*), and tin (*II*). In practice, however, this method has several serious limitations (Gerney and Moine, 1989).

> Such elements as cadmium, antimony, and arsenic are not covered by this test because of the different colors of their respective sulfides (the test is suitable for black or dark brown sulfides only) are only partially covered in the presence of very high concentrations without providing reliable information about the true amount of impurity present (source for wrong conclusions).
>
> Frequently a substance must be ignited before it is tested for heavy metals. In most cases, this leads to a considerable loss of analyte, a loss that is matrix-dependent, as shown in the average recovery rates found by Blake for hydroxypropyl methylcellulose (HPMC).
>
> Important metals used in modern production equipment or as catalysts, such as iron, chromium, and nickel, are missed completely.
>
> It is virtually impossible to differentiate between highly toxic and less toxic metals. The test is nonselective and barely semiquantitative.

A unified and updated international approach is currently being pursued by ISO (Blake, 1989).

REFERENCES

AAMI. (1982). Process Control Guidelines for Radiation Sterilization of Medical Devices, AAMI Recommended Practice, Association for the Advancement of Medical Instrumentation, Arlington, VA.

AAMI. (1997). ANSI/AAMI ST60—Sterilization of Health Care Products—Chemical Indicators. Part 1: General Requirements. AAMI, Washington, DC.

Anon. (1995). Determination of Metal Traces—A Critical Review of the Pharmacopeial Heavy Metals Test, Pharmaco. Forum, 21:1638–1640.

Baquey, C., Sigot-Luizard, M. F., Friede, R. E., Proud'hom, R. E., and Guidoin, R. G. (1987). Radiosterilization of albuminated polyester prostheses, Biomat., 8:185–189.

Berger, K. and Sauvage, L. R. (1981). Late fiber deterioration in dacron arterial grafts, Ann. Surg., 193(4):477–491.

Blake, K. (1989). Harmonization of the USP, EP, and JP heavy metals testing procedures, Pharm. Forum, 21(6).

Bruck, S. D. (1971). Sterilization problems of synthetic biocompatible materials, J. Biomed. Mat. Res., 5:139–158.

Chapiro, A. (1962). Radiation Chemistry of Polymeric Systems, Wiley-Interscience, New York.

Chapman, J., Lee, W., Youkilis, E., and Martis, L. (1986). Animal model for ethylene oxide (ETO) associated hypersensitivity reactions, Trans. Amer. Soc. Art. Int. Organs, 32:482–484.

Crammer, L. C., Roberts, M., Nicholis, A. J., Platts, M. M., and Patterson, R. (1984). IgE against ethylene oxide-altered human serum albumin in patients who have had acute dialysis reactions, J. Allergy Clin. Immunol., 74:544–546.

FDA. (1982). Sterilization of medical devices, program 7378.008A. In: FDA Program Guidance Manual, FDA, Rockville, MD.

Gerney, G. and Moine, J. (1989). Reflexions sur l'essai des metaux lourds. Pharmeuropa, 1(5).

Guidoin, R., Snyder, J., King, M., et al. (1985). A compound arterial prosthesis: The importance of the sterilization procedure on the healing and stability of albuminate dipolyester grafts, Biomat., 6(2):122–128.

Habermann, V. and Waitzova, D. (1985). On the early evaluation of extracts from synthetic polymers used in medicine, Arch. Toxicol., Suppl., 8:458–460.

HIMA. (1981). Guidelines for Evaluating the Safety of Materials Used in Medical Devices—Sensitization Studies, HIMA document no. 10., vol. 3, Washington, DC.

ISO. (1993). ISO 10993-7: Ethylene Oxide Sterilization Residues.

Ludwig, K., Scheiffarth, O. F., and Von-Meyer, L. (1988). Reducing the amount of monomers in intraocular lenses through sterilization by gamma radiation, Ophthal. Res., 20(5):304–307.

Marlowe, D. E., Lao, N. T., Eaton, A. R., Page, B. F., and Lao, C. S. (1987). Interlaboratory comparison of analytical methods for residual ethylene oxide in medical device materials, J. Pharm. Sci., 76(4):333–337.

Mazzu, A. L. and Smith, C. P. (1984). Degradation of extractable methylene dianiline in thermoplastic polyurethanes by HPLC, J. Biomed. Mat. Res., 18(8):961–968.

Melberg, S. G., Havelund, S., Villumsen, J., and Brange, J. (1988). Insulin compatibility with polymer materials used in external pump infusion systems, Diabetic Med., 5(3):243–247.

Nair, P. D. (1995). Currently practiced sterilization methods—Some inadvertent consequences, J. Biomat. Appl., 10:121–135.

Prince, H. N. (1980). Characterization of biological indicators for gamma irradiation. In: Proceedings of the Third PMA Seminar on Validation of Sterile Manufacturing

Processes: Biological Indicators, Pharmaceutical Manufacturers Association, Washington, DC.

Prince, H. N. and Rubino, J. R. (1984). Bioburden dynamics: The viability of microorganisms on devices before and after sterilization, Med. Dev. Diag. Ind., July.

Rockel, A., Wahn, V., Hertel, J., and Fiegel, P. (1986). Ethylene oxide hypersensitivity reactions in dialysis patients, *Lancet*, 1:382–383.

Rose, R. M., Goldfarb, E. V., Ellis, E., and Crugnola, A. N. (1984). Radiation sterilization and the wear rate of polyethylene, J. Orthoped. Res., 2:393–400.

Shinatari, H. and Nakamura, A. (1989). Analysis of a carcinogen 4,4' emthylene dianiline from thermosetting polyurethane during sterilization, J. Anal. Toxicol., 13:354–357.

Shumnes, E. and Darby, T. (1984). Contact dermatitis due to endotoxin in irradiated latex gloves, Cont. Dematitis, 10:240–244.

Takesawa, S., Ohmi, S., and Konna, Y. (1987). Varying methods of sterilization and their effects on the structure and permeability of dialysis membranes, Nephral. Dial. Transplant, 1(4):254–257.

USP. (2000a). Heavy Metals. In: United States Pharmacopoeia XXIV and NF 19, U.S. Pharmacopeial Convention, Rockville, MD.

USP. (2000b). Sterility Tests. In: United States Pharmacopoeia XXIV and NF 19, U.S. Pharmacopeial Convention, Rockville, MD, pp. 1483–1488.

Vink, P. and Pleijsier, K. (1986). Aeration of ethylene oxide-sterilized polymers, Biomaterials, 7:30–48.

14

Combination Devices

I. COMBINATION PRODUCTS

Recent years have seen a vast increase in the number of new therapeutic products that are not purely drug, device, or biologic, but rather a combination of two or more of these. Classic examples are implanted drug delivery systems (whose primary function is drug delivery) and drug-impregnated devices (in which drug delivery is an adjunct to the device function). Congress first acknowledged the need for specific regulation of such combination products in the 1990 Safe Medical Device Act.

A. Historical Background

The history of this category includes a variety of product–types, dating at least from the perfection of the hypodermic needle (1855). There are many modern examples of implanted delivery systems, such as the insulin pump (1980). One fundamental driving force for delivery systems has been the growth of new pharmaceutical products, especially since the dramatic expansion of drug research after 1945.

That research has led to the synthesis and testing of millions of compounds for pharmacological and antimicrobial properties. Indeed, today much of that development is performed in automated computer-controlled systems, leading to an even greater acceleration of the process. The continued emergence of a stream of novel and more complex combination products has blurred any distinguishing lines of regulatory authority and has complicated product designation and regulation. The issue of products combing a device and a drug, such as an asthma inhaler, has received considerable scrutiny over the past several years, but products combining a device and a biologic, such as organ replacement or assist devices, have received less attention. Recent trends, however, suggest that device and biologic combination products are quickly moving into the spotlight. A 1998 survey conducted by FDA identified hardware and tissue-engineered combination products as a rapidly growing trend in medical device technology (Herman et al., 1998). Table 14.1 presents a partial list of currently approved combination products.

Even less than drug and device combinations, device and biologic products—which include cellular and tissue implants, infused or encapsulated cells, artificial and replacement organs, heart valves and pumps, and cardiac, neural, and neuromuscular stimulation devices—do not fit neatly into existing regulatory paradigms. For example, as part of the question of regulation, FDA must take into account the possibility of tissue contamination and other hazards involved in using animal-derived tissues.

What has resulted to date is a developing regulatory process. The written guidelines are fixed, but the day-to-day process is in flux (Merrill, 1994; March, 1998; Segal, 1999).

B. Future Trends

Table 14.2 presents anticipated developments leading to new clinical products in the device combination product category over both 5- and 10-year periods (Herman et al., 1998). Three types of developments are generally expected. First are new products designed for implanted delivery of insulin and other drugs. These include implanted pumps, and possibly intelligent devices with improved biosensors to monitor concentrations in body fluids and make dynamic adjustments in delivery rates. Also, there is the likely development of new polymeric timed-release devices that could improve the delivery of long-acting pharmaceuticals at optimized locations and rates.

Second, new developments in drug-impregnated devices are expected. Examples included new types of cardiac implants with antithrombogenic drugs, as well as orthopedic implants with bacteriostatic coatings.

Finally, new developments are underway in drug delivery systems to simplify reliable use by unsophisticated patients in home settings, including the growing elderly population. Examples included nasal and inhalation products.

This leads to a problem of deciding which of the three centers shall have ultimate jurisdiction. If a product is part drug and part device, for example, should its sponsor submit a new drug application (NDA), a premarket approval application (PMA), or both? Which FDA center will review the application(s), the Center for Drug Evaluation and Research (CDER), the Center for Devices and Radiological Health (CDRH), or both? The answers to these questions can have significant

TABLE 14.1 Examples of Existing Device/Drug Combination Products

Cardiac output catheter	Heparin	As device in UK
Extracorporeal sets	Heparin	As device in UK
Viscose/rayon dressings	Povidone iodine	As drug in UK
Cardiovascular oxygenator	Heparin	As drug in UK defoamer reservoir
Paste bandages	Clioquinol, coal tar, calamine	As drug in UK (if they have ichthammaol ancillary action)
Medicated tulle dressings	Chlorhexidine	As drug in UK
Antimicrobial drape	Iodophore	As device in UK
Antiseptic wipes	Chlorhexidine, centrimide, alcohol	As drug in UK
Cardiovascular guidewires	Heparin	As device in Spain
Guidewires	Heparin	As device in Spain, Switzerland, UK
Antibiotic bone cement	Antibiotic (e.g., Gentamicin sulphate), colistin sulphomethate, sodium, erythromycin	As drug (but soon to be regulated as device)
Extracorporeal cardiotomy reservoirs and filters	Heparin	As devices in Spain, Benelux, Italy
Extracorporeal venous reservoirs and filters	Heparin	As devices in Spain, Benelux, Italy
Bacteriostatic urological catheters	Silver	As devices in three Benelux countries
Antiseptic island dressing	Chlorhexidine digluconate	As device in Italy
Spermicidal condoms	Nonoxynol-9	As device in Germany
Pacemaker lead with a porous tip (seulte)	Dexamethasone	As device
Pacemaker lead with protector mannitol capsule (Sweet Tip)	Mannitol	As device
Biomedicus centrifugal pump	Heparin	Not applicable
Peripheral vascular cannulae	Heparin	Not applicable
Surgical gauzes or nonwoven fabrics impregnated with iodophore	Iodophore	Not applicable
Surgical gauzes or nonwoven fabrics impregnated with alginates and Clioquinol	Clioquionol (NaCa alignates, clauden powder)	As device in Germany
Vascular prosthesis	Collagen, albumen	As devices in UK

TABLE 14.2 High Likelihood New Combination Device Drug Technologies

Biosensors	Biosensors, genetic diagnostics, laser diagnosis and treatment, minimally invasive devices
Blood vessel prosthetics	Genetic therapy, tissue engineered devices
Bone prosthetics/growth	Artificial organs, tissue engineered devices
Cardiac stimulation	Intelligent devices, microminiaturized devices
Cartilage prosthetics	Tissue engineered device
Computer-aided clinical labs	Computer-aided diagnosis, networks of devices
Drug-impregnated devices	Device/drug/biological products
Endoscopy	Minimally invasive devices, telemedicine, virtual reality
Genetics—cancer	Genetic diagnostics, genetic therapy
Hearing aids	Intelligent devices, microminiaturized devices, nonimplanted sensory aids
Heart pumps	Artificial organs
Heart valves	Artificial organs, tissue engineered devices, device/drug/biological products
Home diagnostics	Home/self-monitoring and diagnosis
Image contrast agents	Medical imaging
Imaging: functional, content	Medical imaging, minimally invasive devices, networks of devices
Implanted drug	Biosensors, device/drug/biological products, delivery systems, home/self-therapy, intelligent devices, robotic devices
Integrated patient medical information systems	Computer-aided diagnosis, networks of devices, telemedicine
Kidney prosthetics	Artificial organs, home/self-therapy, tissue engineered devices
Laser surgery	Laser diagnosis and treatment
Liver prosthetics	Artificial organs, tissue-engineered devices
Minimum invasive cardiology	Minimally invasive devices, vascular surgery
Minimum invasive neurosurgery	Minimally invasive devices
MRI	Medical imaging
Nanotechnology	Microminiaturized devices
Nerve regeneration	Tissue engineered devices
Neural stimulation	Artificial organs, electrical stimulation, intelligent devices
Neuromuscular stimulation	Electrical stimulation, home/self-therapy
Ocular prosthetics	Artificial organs, electrical stimulation, intelligent devices

TABLE 14.2 Continued

Pancreas prosthetics	Artificial organs, tissue engineered devices
Patient smart cards	Computer-aided diagnosis, networks of devices, telemedicine
PET imaging	Medical imaging
Robotic surgery	Microminiaturized devices, robotic devices
Skin prosthetics	Tissue engineered devices
Telemedicine—home use	Home/self-monitoring and amp, diagnosis, telemedicine
Telemedicine—radiology	Telemedicine
Virtual reality—education	Virtual reality

effects on the time it takes to bring a product to market and how much it will cost.

Traditionally the FDA responded to such questions on an ad hoc basis. Prophylaxis pastes containing fluoride are regulated as drugs, although prophylaxis pastes without fluoride are considered medical devices. Bone cement, however, is treated as a device, regardless of whether or not it is combined with an antibiotic drug.

Although both extracorporeal and peritoneal dialysis systems are regulated as devices, dialysate concentrate for use with the former is a device, but prepackaged dialysate for use with the latter is a drug. Sometimes consistency was elusive even when there was no combination, but just a single product. For example, in vitro diagnostics for detecting antibodies to HIV are regulated as biologics when they are used for screening the blood supply, but as medical devices when used for diagnostic or other screening purposes. When the FDA decided quickly and unequivocally on the regulatory status of a product, whether it was deemed a single product or was in combination with another product, there was relatively little objection to the agency's decisions about how to regulate combination products and products whose status was uncertain. In the case of blood devices, the EU has affirmed this process (Anon, 2000)

In two situations, however, the agency's decisions were troublesome to sponsors. When the FDA required two separate approvals, one for the device and one for the drug element of the product—as it did with the drug ursodiol for use with lithotripters—the agency created difficulty and delay in getting the products licensed so they could be used together. Similarly, the FDA's indecisiveness in this area made it particularly difficult for companies such as Robertson Resources. Robertson marketed Revital, a medical protein hydrolysate that came in both powder and gel forms; it was used for wound exudate removal. In 1978, the company received a letter from the Bureau of Medical Devices stating that its product was substantially equivalent to another device on the market prior to

May 20, 1976. In 1981, however, the FDA told Robertson the product was not a device but was an unapproved new drug. A year later, the FDA decided the product was a medical device again and reinstated its 510(k) (CDRH and CDER have clarified this point) (CDER, 1994). In the meantime, of course, Robertson had been the subject of intense enforcement attention (Chapekar, 1996).

In the Safe Medical Devices Act of 1990 (SMDA), Congress took these issues in hand and amended the Federal Food, Drug and Cosmetic Act (FDCA) to make it easier for the FDA to regulate combination products in a rational fashion. The new provisions altered the substantive provisions of the FDCA only in minor respects. The main thrust of the new law was managerial, directing the FDA to make decisions about which center would have ''primary jurisdiction'' over a combination product, based on the agency's understanding of the primary mode of action of the product.

For these products, center jurisdiction turns on the primary mode of action. If it is that of a drug, then CDER has primary jurisdiction; if it is that of a device, jurisdiction is with CDRH; if it is that of a biological product, the Center for Biologics Evaluation and Research (CBER) has jurisdiction. As the statute prescribed, the regulations go on to state that the center with primary jurisdiction may consult with other agency components.

Although neither the statute nor the regulations explain what primary jurisdiction means, it seems clear that the FDA intends it to mean that the center that has primary jurisdiction will review the combination product and ordinarily give it just one approval, that is, an NDA, PMA, or biologic license application (BLA), as appropriate. Section 3.4(b) makes it clear, however, that the FDA's designation of one agency component as having primary jurisdiction does not preclude in appropriate cases the requirement for separate application; for example, a 510(k) and a BLA. When separate applications are required, both can be reviewed by the lead center, but ''exceptional'' cases may involve a second application to be reviewed by a different center. To facilitate this, the agency published new delegations giving officials in each of the three centers the authority to clear devices and to approve devices, drugs, biologics, or any combination of two or more of them (FDA, 1991).

Contemporaneous with publication of the new regulations, the FDA made public three new intercenter agreements among CDRH and CBER, CDRH and CDER, and CDER and CBER. They describe the allocations of responsibility for numerous categories of specific products, both combination and noncombination. According to the regulations, these intercenter agreements are not binding; they are intended to ''provide useful guidance to the public,'' and as a practical matter, to FDA staff as well.

The intercenter agreements are a treasure trove of information. In addition to explicit guidance about which center has the lead with respect to particular products and whether one center or two will work on particular issues, they contain information and hints about whether or not the FDA believes it can regulate certain products at all, and if so, how (Pilot and Waldeermann 1998; Adams et al., 1997).

The regulations and intercenter agreements do not answer every question however, and the regulations recognize a role for the sponsor in cases of uncertainty. When the identity of the center with primary jurisdiction is unclear or in dispute or a sponsor believes its combination product is not covered by the intercenter agreements, a sponsor can request a designation from the FDA's product jurisdiction officer. A sponsor ''should'' file a request for designation with the product jurisdiction officer before submitting its application for marketing approval or an investigational notice. In practice, though, disputes or lack of clarify may not become evident until well into the review process, and it seems likely that the FDA would, if necessary, entertain requests for designation submitted at a later time.

Section 3.7(c) of the regulations lists the information to be included in the request, all of which must fit on 15 pages or less, including the identity of the sponsor, detailed information on the product, where the developmental work stands, the product's known modes of action and its primary mode of action, and most important, the sponsor's recommendation for which center should have primary jurisdiction and the reasons for the recommendation.

The FDA promises to check the request for designation for completeness within 5 working days of receipt, and to issue a letter of designation within 60 days of receipt of a complete request. If the FDA does not meet the 60-day time limit, then the sponsor's recommendation for the appropriate lead center is honored.

The agency's letter of designation can be changed only with the sponsor's written consent, or if the sponsor does not consent, ''to protect the public health or for other compelling reasons.'' A sponsor must be given prior notice of any proposed nonconsensual change, and must be given an opportunity to object in writing and at a ''timely'' meeting with the product jurisdiction officer and appropriate center officials.

The CDRH is designated the center for major policy development and for the promulgation and interpretation of procedural regulations for medical devices under the act. The CDRH regulates all medical devices, inclusive of radiation-related devices, that are not assigned categorically or specifically to CDER. In addition, CDRH will independently administer the following activities (references to ''sections'' are the provisions of the act):

1. A. Small business assistance programs under Section 10 of the amendments. (See PL 94-295.) Both CDER and CDRH will identify any unique problems relating to medical device regulation for small business;

B. Registration and listing under Section 510 including some CDER administered device applications. The CDER will receive printouts and other assistance, as requested;

C. Color additives under Section 706, with review by CDER, as appropriate;

D. Good Manufacturing Practices (GMPs) Advisory Committee. Under Section 520(f) (3), CDER will regularly receive notices of all meetings, with participation by CDER, as appropriate; and

E. Medical Device Reporting. The manufacturers, distributors, importers, and users of all devices, including those regulated by CDER, shall report to CDRH under Section 519 of the act as required. The Center for Devices and Radiological Health will provide monthly reports and special reports as needed to CDER for investigation and follow-up of those medical devices regulated by CDER.

Table 14.3 presents the primary product responsibilities of CDER and CBER.

TABLE 14.3 Product Class Review Responsibilities

Center for Drug Evaluation and Review
    Natural products purified from plant or mineral sources
    Products produced from solid tissue sources (excluding procoagulants, venoms, blood products, etc.)
    Antibiotics, regardless of method of manufacture
    Certain substances produced by fermentation
    Disaccharidase inhibitors
    HMG-CoA inhibitors
    Synthetic chemicals
    Traditional chemical synthesis
    Synthesized mononuclear or polynuclear products including antisense chemicals
    Hormone products
Center for Biologics Evaluation and Review
    Vaccines, regardless of manufacturing method
    In vivo diagnostic allergenic products
    Human blood products
    Protein, peptide, and/or carbohydrate products produced by cell culture (other than antibiotics and hormones)
    Immunoglobulin products
    Products containing intact cells or microorganisms
    Proteins secreted into fluids by transgenic animals
    Animal venoms
    Synthetic allergens
    Blood banking and infusion adjuncts

II. DEVICE PROGRAMS THAT CDER AND CBRH WILL ADMINISTER

Both CDER and CDRH will administer and, as appropriate, enforce the following activities for medical devices assigned to their respective centers (references to "sections" are the provisions of the act):

1. A. Surveillance and compliance actions involving general controls violations, such as misbranded or adulterated devices under Sections 301, 501, and 502;
   B. Warning letters, seizures, injunctions, and prosecutions under Sections 302, 303, and 304;
   C. Civil penalties under Section 303(f) and administrative restraint under Section 304(g);
   D. Nonregulatory activities, such as educational programs directed at users, participation in voluntary standards organizations, etc.;
   E. Promulgation of performance standards and applications of special controls under Section 514;
   F. Premarket Notification, Investigational Device Exemptions including Humanitarian Exemptions, Premarket Approval, Product Development Protocols, Classification, Device Tracking, Petitions for Reclassification, postmarket surveillance under Sections 510(k), 513, 515, 519, 520(g) & (m), and 522, and the advisory committees necessary to support these activities;
   G. Banned devices under Section 516;
   H. FDA-requested and firm-initiated recalls whether under Section 518 or another authority, and other Section 518 remedies such as recall orders;
   I. Exemptions, variances, and applications of CGMP regulations under Section 520(f);
   J. Government-Wide Quality Assurance Program; and
   K. Requests for export approval under Sections 801(e) and 802.

A. Coordination

The centers will coordinate their activities in order to assure that manufacturers do not have to independently secure authorization to market their product from both centers unless this requirement is specified in Section VII.

B. Submissions

Submissions should be made to the appropriate center, as specified herein, at the addresses provided below:

Address update:

Food and Drug Administration
Center for Drug Evaluation and Research
Central Document Room (Room #2–14)
12420 Parklawn Drive
Rockville, Maryland 20852

or

Food and Drug Administration
Center for Devices and Radiological Health
Document Mail Center (HFZ-401)
1390 Piccard Drive
Rockville, Maryland 20850

For submissions involving medical devices and/or drugs that are not clearly addressed in this agreement, sponsors and referred to the product jurisdiction regulations (21 CFR Part 3). These regulations have been promulgated to facilitate the determination of regulatory jurisdiction but do not exclude the possibility for a collaborative review between the centers.

C. Center Jurisdiction

The following subsections provide details concerning status, market approval authority, special label/regulatory considerations, investigational options, and intercenter consultations for the categories of products specified. Section VII provides the general criteria that CDRH and CDER will apply in reaching decisions as to which center will regulate a product.

> A. 1. (a) Device with primary purpose of delivering or aiding in the delivery of a drug that is distributed without a drug (i.e., unfilled).
> *Examples*
> Devices that calculate drug dosages
> Drug delivery pump and/or catheter infusion pump for implantation iontophoreses device
> Medical or surgical kit (e.g., tray) with reference in instructions for use with specific drug (e.g., local anesthetic)
> Nebulizer
> Small particle aerosol generator (SPAG) for administering drug to ventilated patient
> Splitter block for mixing nitrous oxide and oxygen
> Syringe; jet injector; storage and dispensing equipment

Status: Device and drug, as separate entities.

Market Approval Authority: CDRH and CDER, respectively, unless the intended use of the two products, through labeling, creates a combination product.

Special Label/Regulatory Considerations: The following specific procedures will apply, depending on the status of the drug delivery device and drugs that will be delivered with the device:

(i) It may be determined during the design or conduct of clinical trials for a new drug that it is not possible to develop adequate performance specifications data on those characteristics of the device that are required for the safe and effective use of the drug. If this is the case, then drug labeling cannot be written to contain information that makes it possible for the user to substitute a generic, marketed device for the device used during developments to use with the marketed drug. In these situations, CDER will be the lead center for regulation of the device under the device authorities.

(ii) For a device intended for use with a category of drugs that are on the market, CDRH will be the lead center for regulation for the device under the device authorities. The effects of the device use on drug stability must be addressed in the device submission, when relevant. An additional showing of clinical effectiveness of the drug when delivered by the specific device will generally not be required. The device and drug labeling must be mutually conforming with respect to indication, general mode of delivery (e.g., topical, IV), and drug dosage/schedule equivalents.

(iii) For a drug delivery device and drug that are developed for marketing to be used together as a system, a lead center will be designated to be the contact point with the manufacturer(s). If a drug has been developed and marketed and the development and studying of device technology predominates, the principle mode of action will be deemed to be that of the device, and CDRH would have the lead. If a device has been developed and marketed and the development and studying of drug predominates, then, correspondingly, CDER would have the lead. If neither the drug nor the device is on the market, the lead center will be determined on a case-by-case basis.

Investigation Options: IDE or IND, as appropriate.

Inter-Center Consultation: CDER, when lead center, will consult with CDRH if CDER determines that a specific device is required as part of the NDA process. CDRH as lead center will consult with CDER if the device is intended for use with a marketed drug and the device creates a significant change in the intended use, mode of delivery (e.g., topical, IV), or dose/schedule of the drug.

        (b)   Device with primary purpose of delivering or aiding in the delivery of a drug and distributed containing a drug (i.e., "prefilled delivery system")

            Examples

            Nebulizer

            Oxygen tank for therapy and OTC emergency use

            Prefilled syringe

            Transdermal patch

Status: Combination Product

Market Approval Authority: CDER using drug authorities and device authorities, as necessary.

Special Label/Regulatory Considerations: None

Investigation Options: IND

Inter-Center Consultations: Optional

        2.   Device incorporating a drug component with the combination product having the primary intended purpose of fulfilling a device function.

            Examples

            Bone cement containing antimicrobial agent

            Cardiac pacemaker lead with steroid-coated tip

            Condom, diaphragm, or cervical cap with contraceptive or antimicrobial agent (including virucidal) agent

            Dental device with fluoride

            Dental wood wedge with hemostatic agent

            Percutaneous cuff (e.g., for a catheter or orthopedic pin) coated/impregnated with antimicrobial agent

            Skin closure or bandage with antimicrobial agent

            Surgical or barrier drape with antimicrobial agent

            Tissue graft with antimicrobial or other drug agent

            Urinary and vascular catheter coated/impregnated with antimicrobial agent

            Wound dressing with antimicrobial agent

Status: Combination Product

Market Approval Authority: CDRH using device authorities.

Special Label/Regulatory Considerations: These products have a drug component that is present to augment the safety and/or efficacy of the device.

Investigation Options: IDE

Inter-Center Consultation: Required if a drug or the chemical form of the drug has not been legally marketed in the United States as a human drug for the intended effect.

    3. Drug incorporating a device component with the combination product having the primary intended purpose of fulfilling a drug function.

        Examples

        Skin-prep pads with antimicrobial agent

        Surgical scrub brush with antimicrobial agent

Status: Combination Product

Market Approval Authority: CDER using drug authorities and, as necessary, device authorities.

Special Label/Regulatory Considerations: Marketing of such a device requires a submission of an NDA with safety and efficacy data on the drug component or it meets monograph specifications as generally recognized as safe (GRAS) and generally recognized as effective (GRAE). Drug requirements (e.g., CGMPs, registration and listing, experience reporting) apply to products.

Investigation Options: IND

Inter-Center Consultation: Optional

    4. (a) Device used in the production of a drug either to deliver directly to a patient or for the use in the producing medical facility (excluding use in a registered drug manufacturing facility).

            Examples

            Oxygen concentrators (home or hospital)

            Oxygen generator (chemical)

            Ozone generator

Status: Device

Market Approval Authority: CDER, applying both drug and device authorities

Special Label/Regulatory Consideration: May also require an NDA if the drug produced is a new drug. Device requirements (e.g., CGMPs, registration and listing, experience reporting) will apply to products.

Investigation Options: IDA or NDA, as appropriate

Inter-Center Consultation: Optional

      (b) Drug/device combination product intended to process a drug into a finished package form.

Examples

Device that uses drug concentrates to prepare large volume parenterals

Oxygen concentrator (hospital) output used to fill oxygen tanks for use within that medical facility

Status: Combination product

Market Approval Authority: CDER, applying both drug and device authorities.

Special Label/Regulatory Considerations: Respective drug and device requirements, e.g., CGMPs, registration and listing, experience reporting will apply.

Investigation Options: IDE or NDA, as appropriate

Inter-Center Consultation: Optional, but will be routinely obtained.

B.   Device used concomitantly with a drug to directly activate or to augment drug effectiveness.

Examples

Biliary lithotriptor used in conjunction with dissolution agent

Cancer hyperthermia used in conjunction with chemotherapy

Current generator used in conjunction with an implanted silver electrode (drug) that produces silver ions for an antimicrobial purpose

Materials for blocking blood flow temporarily to restrict chemotherapy drug to the intended site of action

UV and/or laser activation of oxsoralen for psoriasis or Cutaneous T-Cell Lymphoma

Status: Device and drug, as separate entities

Market Approval Authority: CDRH and CDER, respectively

Special Label/Regulatory Considerations: The device and drug labeling must be mutually conforming with respect to indications, general mode of delivery (e.g., topical, IV), and drug dosage/schedule equivalence. A lead center will be designated to be the contact point with the manufacturer. If a drug has been developed and approved for another use and the development and studying of device technology predominates, then CDRH would have lead. If a device has been developed and marketed for another use and the development and studying of drug action predominates, then CDER would have lead. If neither the drug nor the device is on the market, the lead center will be determined on a case-by-case basis. If the labeling of the drug and device create a combination product, as defined in the combination product regulations, then the designation of the lead center for both applications will be based upon a determination of the product's primary mode of action.

Investigation Options: IDE or IND, as appropriate.

Inter-Center Consultations: Required.

2. Device kits labeled for use with drugs that include both device(s) and drug(s) as separate entities in one package with the overall primary intended purpose of the kit fulfilling a device function.
   Examples
   Medical or surgical kit (e.g., tray) with drug component

Status: Combination Product

Market Approval Authority: CDRH, using device authorities is responsible for the kit if the manufacturer is repackaging a market drug. Responsibility for overall packaging resides with CDRH. CDER will be consulted as necessary on the use of drug authorities for the repackaged drug component.

Special Label/Regulatory Consideration: Device requirements (e.g., CGMPs, registration and listing, experience reporting) apply to kits. Device manufacturers must assure that manufacturing steps do not adversely affect drug components of the kit. If the manufacturing steps do affect the marketed drug (e.g., the kit is sterilized by irradiation), and ANDA or NDA would also be required with CDRH as lead center.

Investigation Options: IDA or IND, as appropriate.

Inter-Center Consultation: Optional if ANDA or NDA not required.

C. Liquids, gases, or solids intended for use as devices (e.g., implanted, or components, parts, or accessories to devices).
   Examples
   Dye for tissues used in conjunction with laser surgery, to enhance absorption of laser light in target tissue
   Gas mixtures for pulmonary function testing devices
   Gases used to provide "physical effects"
   Hemodialysis fluids
   Hemostatic devices and dressings
   Injectable silicon, collagen, and Teflon
   Liquids functioning through physical action applied to the body to cool or freeze tissues for therapeutic purposes
   Liquids intended to inflate, flush, or moisten (lubricate) indwelling device (in or on the body)
   Lubricants and lubricating jellies
   Ophthalmic solutions for contact lenses
   Organ/tissue transport and/or perfusion fluid with antimicrobial or other drug agent, i.e., preservation solutions
   Powders for lubricating surgical gloves
   Sodium hyaluronate or hyaluronic acid for use as a surgical aid
   Solution for use with dental "chemical drill"
   Spray on dressings not containing a drug component

Status: Device
Market Approval Authority: CDRH
Special Label/Regulatory Considerations: None
Investigation Options: IDE
Inter-Center Consultation: Required if the device has direct contact with the body and the drug or the chemical form of the drug has not been legally marketed as a human drug.
D.   Products regulated as drugs.
     Examples
     Irrigation solutions
     Purified water or saline in prefilled nebulizers for use in inhalation therapy
     Skin protectants (intended for use on intact skin)
     Sun screens
     Topical/internal analgesic-antipyretic
Status: Drug
Market Approval Authority: CDER
Special Label/Regulatory Considerations: None
Investigation Options: IND
Inter-Center Consultations: Optional
E.   Ad Hoc Jurisdictional Decisions.

Examples	*Status*	*Center*
Motility marker constructed of radiopaque plastic	Device	CDRH
Brachytherapy capsules, needles, etc., that are radioactive and may be removed from the body after radiation therapy has been administered	Device	CDRH
Skin markers	Device	CDRH

Status: Device or drug.
Market Approval Authority: CDRH or CDER as indicated.
Special Label/Regulatory Considerations: None
Investigation Options: IDE or IND, as appropriate
Inter-Center Consultation: Required to assure agreement on drug/device status.
General Criteria Affecting Drug/Device Determination.
     The following represent the general criteria that will apply in making device/drug determinations.
A.   Device Criteria:.
     1.   A liquid, powder, or other similar formulation intended only to serve as a component, part, or accessory to a device with a primary mode of action that is physical in nature will be regulated as a device by CDRH.

2. A product that has the physical attributes described in 201(h) (e.g., instrument, apparatus) of the act and does not achieve its primary intended purpose through chemical action within or on the body, or by being metabolized, will be regulated as a device by CDRH.

3. The phrase ''within or on the body'' as used in 201(h) of the act does not include extra corporeal systems or the solutions used in conjunction with such equipment. Such equipment and solutions will be regulated as devices by CDRH.

4. An implant, including an injectable material, placed in the body for primarily a structural purpose even though such an implant may be absorbed or metabolized by the body after it has achieved its primary purpose, will be regulated as a device by CDRH.

5. A device containing a drug substance as a component with the primary purpose of the combination being to fulfill a device function is a combination product and will be regulated as a device by CDRH.

6. A device (e.g., machine or equipment) marketed to the user, pharmacy, or licensed practitioner that produces a drug will be regulated as a device or combination product by CDER. This does not include equipment marketed to a registered drug manufacturer.

7. A device whose labeling or promotional materials make reference to a specific drug or generic class of drugs unless it is prefilled with a drug ordinarily remains a device regulated by CDRH. It may, however, also be subject to the combination products regulation.

B. Drug Criteria

1. A liquid, powder, tablet, or other similar formulation that achieves its primary intended purpose through chemical action within or on the body, or by being metabolized, unless it meets one of the specified device criteria, will as regulated as a drug by CDER.

2. A device that serves as a container for a drug or a device that is a drug delivery system attached to the drug container where the drug is present in the container is a combination product that will be regulated as a drug by CDER.

3. A device containing a drug substance as a component with the primary purpose of the combination product being to fulfill a drug purpose is a combination product and will be regulated as a drug by CDER.

4. A drug whose labeling or promotional materials make reference to a specific device or generic class of devices ordinarily remains a drug regulated by CDER. It may, however, also be subject to the combination products regulation.

REFERENCES

Adams, D. G., Cooper, R. M., and Kahan, J. S. (1997). Fundamentals of Law and Regulation: An In-Depth Look at Therapeutic Products, FDLI, Washington, DC.

Anon. (2000). EU Nations Agree that Directive Will Cover Human Blood Devices, Eur. Drug Dev. Rep., 10(14):1–21.

CDER. (1994). Premarket notifications: 510 (K) regulatory requirements for medical devices. HHS FDA 1990:4158.

Chapekar, M. S. (1996). Regulatory concerns in the development of biologic–biomaterials combination, J. Biomed. Mat. Res., 33:199–203.

FDA. (1991). Assignment of agency component for review of premarket applications: Final rule, 56 Fed. Reg. 58,754 (Nov. 21).

Herman, W. A., Marlowe, D. F., and Harvey, R. (1998). Future trends in medical device technology, Biomed. Market Newsl., 8:19.

March, E. (1998). Combination products: Who's regulating what and how—Part I, Pharmaceut. Eng., July/Aug. 34–38.

Merrill, R. (1994). Regulation of drugs and devices: An evolution, Health Aff., 13:47–69.

Pilot, L. and Waldeermann, D. (1998). Food and Drug Modernization Act of 1997: Medical device provisions, Food Drug Law J., 53:267–295.

Segal, S. A. (1999). Device and biologic combination products—Understanding the evolving regulation, Med. Dev. Diag. Ind., Jan. 180–184.

15

Clinical Studies for Medical Devices

Clinical studies, once rare for devices other than Class III devices, are becoming much more frequently required and performed. Since 1991, ODE has taken actions for imposing more stringent requirements on clinical studies used to support device PMA applications. Clinical studies are also being required more often to support performance claims in 510(k) premarket notifications. The ODE focus on requiring carefully designed clinical trials is based in part on the *Final Report of the Committee for Clinical Review*, also known as the Temple report.

The Temple committee reviewed a sample of PMA applications, IDEs, and 510(k) notices and found numerous deficiencies in the design, conduct, and analysis of clinical trials performed by sponsors in support of their applications. According to the committee, the fundamental problem leading to inadequate data in most device applications was a lack of attention to basic study design. Specifically, the committee's report enumerated the following design deficiencies in the submissions examined:

1. Failure to specify a clear hypothesis to be tested and to develop a clear plan to test it
2. Failure to enroll a sufficient number of patients to answer the primary study questions
3. Failure to adequately specify requirements for patients entering studies
4. Failure to identify a control group
5. Failure to properly assess the comparability of patients in the treatment and control groups
6. Failure to clearly and precisely define end points

449

7. Failure to implement blinded evaluation of end points, especially when end points are subjective in nature

Recent findings support that FDA's bioresearch monitoring program (BIMO) for devices continues to have problems (Anon, 2000). In this volume, of course, we are only concerned specifically with the aspects of clinical studies involved in evaluating device safety. General considerations of device clinical study design, execution, and analysis will be briefly considered to provide a context for this consideration, but those interested in broader issues should consult Spilker (1995) or Kahan (1994).

I. DESIGN CONSIDERATIONS

For any clinical study of a device conducted under an IDE, the sponsor is required to submit an investigational plan, including a protocol for the proposed study to ODE. The plan should describe three fundamental clinical trial areas: study design, study conduct, and data analysis. Each of these three elements needs to be carefully thought out in advance, long before the first patient is recruited into the study.

In planning a device clinical trial, a sponsor must formulate a specific hypothesis to be tested (or question to be answered) in the study, and design a study that will answer the question. Once the main hypothesis has been formulated, however, a number of other questions naturally arises, such as the following:

With what treatment (control) should results in the investigational device be compared?

Is the objective of the study to show that the new device performs better or equivalently to an alternative therapy?

How many patients (sample size) will be required to detect a clinically meaningful difference between the treatment and control groups with adequate statistical power, or ensure an acceptable degree of similarity?

What is the diagnostic criterion by which to select study subjects?

How will patients be assigned to the treatment and control groups?

What baseline characteristics (characteristics of patients at the time of entry into the study) are important to prognosis?

What will be the primary end point(s) of the study?

What are the individual patient success/failure criteria?

Will the patient, physician, or another person be responsible for treatment administered?

What follow-up information is important to collect?

How will the safety of the device be established?

These questions, as well as others, must be addressed when planning a clinical study, rather than after the study has begun or the data collected. The methodology for responding to many of these questions is described in the following discussion of clinical study design parameters.

A. Study Hypothesis

The FDA's ultimate regulatory question in evaluating whether or not to clear a device to market is whether it is safe and effective (PMA review) or whether it is substantially equivalent to a predicate product [510(k) review]. These questions are, however, too nonspecific to be used to develop a clinical protocol intended to be pivotal in the regulatory clearance process for a device.

The rationale for conducting a clinical trial is to determine whether or not an intervention such as a medical device has a particular postulated clinical effect. In designing a clinical trial, a clear statement regarding the objectives of the study should thus be made, and a specific hypothesis should be formulated indicating what proposition will be tested to determine if the investigational device is safe and effective.

Consider, for example, a percutaneous transluminal coronary angioplasty (PTCA) device intended to open obstructed coronary vessels. The hypothesis could focus on whether the investigational device is as effective as a marketed device in achieving postoperative patency of all occluded vessels in a patient or whether the investigational device is more effective than a predicate device in achieving both chronic patency (e.g., at 6 months postprocedure) and acute patency.

The first and key question for any study is thus the hypothesis to be tested. The FDA and the device sponsor should always agree on the hypothesis before the first patient is enrolled. As noted in the Temple report, a flawed hypothesis will lead to a flawed clinical trial, in which the data will not be sufficient to support a marketing application.

In drafting the study hypothesis, the sponsor should always focus on the claims that will form the basis for marketing the device. Most marketing claims cannot be made for a class III device without some foundation in the clinical study, therefore the study hypothesis and the design must be part of the company's overall strategy in determining what marketing claims are necessary to have a commercially viable device.

B. Control Groups

The Temple report makes it clear that some type of control is essential to the conduct of a device clinical study. Having a control group permits the conclusion at the end of the study that observed differences in outcome and changes between the treatment group and control group are due to the device being studied and not to other factors.

The Temple committee noted that several device companies whose applications were reviewed failed to identify any control group when one was plainly needed to assess the safety and effectiveness of the device. Other companies, in the view of the committee, failed to use the most appropriate control group or used poorly defined historical controls. For example, the committee cited a submission for a defibrillator that was implanted in more than 300 patients in which results were reported without reference to any control group or any historical controls. While it appeared that survival for patients using the investigational defibrillator might have been similar to that reported in the literature for other devices, the agency had little information on which to make an assessment of efficacy.

The literature on the clinical evaluation of medical devices is much smaller than that for most medicines. The quality of reported clinical trials varies enormously, and most trials suffer from lack of a control patient group that received a comparison medical device. Studies commonly describe a group of patients who received a device and present before and after values for certain tests and parameters. There is usually no adequate control. One reason for this failure may be that the sponsors of most of these trials (i.e., device manufacturers) often do not wish to compare their device directly against a competitor's. In addition, it is rarely ethical to include a placebo or sham-operated group as a control. Placebo controls are often not necessary or possible in testing certain medical devices. Many situations in which class II and III devices are used are not suitable for observation of a placebo effect (e.g., the patient may be unconscious or the interaction between patient and device may be minimal or nonexistent). There are several types of comparisons that may be used to evaluate medical devices (Table 15.1), and there are special considerations for designing protocols (Table 15.2) that illustrate the differences between medical devices and medicines.

The need of many patients for a class III medical device is often certain (e.g., heart valve replacement, hip replacement). In such cases it is generally unethical to consider including a placebo treatment group in a clinical trial. Clinical trials therefore depend heavily on the patient's baseline values to evaluate the effects of the device. When open-label trials are conducted and no blinding is used, greater reliance should be placed on objective measures of change (e.g.,

TABLE 15.1 Types of Comparisons That May Be Made in Trials of Medical Devices

1. Device A versus device B; usually performed single-blind
2. Device A versus medicine B; usually performed single-blind
3. Device A versus surgery B
4. Device A versus no treatment
5. Device A versus placebo device; preferably performed double-blind
6. Device A versus other treatment modality (e.g., radiation)

TABLE 15.2 Special Considerations in Designing Protocols for Medical Devices

1. In a double-blind trial it may be necessary to blind the identity of the device used: This may be done by disguising its outside appearance or by having the device inserted by one physician and having the patient evaluated by another physician.
2. Describe all increased risks that patients may experience in the trial: Indicate how these risks will be minimized.
3. Label all devices appropriately, including the phrase, "CAUTION: INVESTIGATIONAL DEVICE LIMITED BY FEDERAL LAW TO INVESTIGATIONAL USE."
4. Indicate appropriate methods of disposition of both used and unused devices.
5. Describe all functional tests of range of motion, correction of deformity, relief of symptoms, and other criteria of improvement.
6. Provide written instructions for use of the device, plus warnings, hazards, and contraindications.[a]

Note: These points are in addition to relevant considerations for designing protocols for medicine trials.
[a] Evaluate the clarity of the instructions and their comprehension by potential users.

ejection fraction) or semiobjective measures (e.g., the distance the patient can walk without pain in a given period). Subjective parameters (e.g., quality-of-life measures) are usually more susceptible to influence by a placebo effect than are objective measures. Use of subjective measures should therefore be de-emphasized whenever possible unless they are validated parameters or there is no other choice. When one product is compared with another the parameters evaluated must be comparable.

Simply put, it will be very difficult in the near future to rely on historical controls for device clearance. If a sponsor feels historical controls are appropriate, detailed discussions with FDA are essential, especially concerning the issue of matching controls with active patients. If the control group will be one described in the literature, FDA and the sponsor must agree on whether or not the literature provides sufficient detail on the control patients to provide an adequate basis for comparison. In summary, reliance on historical controls at this point is discouraged by ODE and will require a clear explanation to ODE on why randomized concurrent controls are not feasible.

C. Eligibility Criteria

Eligibility criteria characterize the study population, and thereby impact on the study design, ability to recruit patients, and ability to generalize study results.

Development of clear, unambiguous inclusion and exclusion criteria is essential in planning a clinical trial.

It is necessary that the patients actually enrolled in the study form a subset of the general population defined by the eligibility criteria, and the results of a study can legitimately be generalized to other patients similar to those enrolled in the study. For example, if the only patients enrolled are adult males or post-menopausal females, it may be difficult to generalize any results to pediatric patients or young adult females.

Formulation of eligibility criteria should be guided by a sponsor's desire to demonstrate efficacy and its concern for patient safety. Patients who could benefit from the device are obvious candidates. Patients in whom hypothesized results of the device can likely be detected should also be studied. Any potential subject to whom the treatment is thought to be harmful or subjects likely to prematurely withdraw from the study should generally be excluded. To ensure comparability between groups, inclusion and exclusion criteria should be the same for the device and control groups.

The group of enrolled patients can either be homogeneous (patients with similar characteristics) or heterogeneous (subjects differ in identifiable character-istics) in composition. A homogeneous study population may make the assess-ment of efficacy more straightforward, because the similarity of patients within the study population may not require analysis of study data by distinct prognostic subgroups. If eligibility criteria are too narrowly defined, however, recruitment may be hampered and study results may not be readily generalized. Heteroge-neous populations may afford the opportunity to discover whether or not the device is effective in a separate subgroup of patients, but may necessitate a larger sample size if prognostically different subgroups are enrolled. A sponsor must carefully consider how homogeneous or heterogeneous the recruited patient pop-ulation should be. This decision may largely rest on an assessment based on preclinical information of the kinds of patients for whom the device will likely be safe and effective.

Typical inclusion and exclusion criteria relate to subject demographics such as age and sex, pregnancy status, projected life span, history of certain chronic diseases, use of concomitant medications, likelihood the patient will complete all follow-up, and the presence of other confounding factors. Once an investigator has determined that a particular patient is eligible to participate in the study, a mechanism should be put in place to ensure that all eligible patients are offered the opportunity to participate. The FDA wants to ensure that investigators do not select patients subjectively, limiting the applicability of the device or masking some unidentified exclusion criteria.

Marketing claims also should be considered in drafting eligibility criteria. If the company's marketing experts say that a specific target patient population is necessary for ultimate commercial success, that population must be represented in the study.

D. Assignment of Intervention

Different methods have been developed for assigning patients to the investigational device group and the control group in a systematic manner that avoids selection bias. Selection bias occurs when, intentionally or unintentionally, patients with certain characteristics are more readily assigned to one treatment group than another. The result of selection bias is that patients who have important prognostic factors may be disproportionately assigned to one group, thus obscuring the interpretation of any differences in outcome between the groups.

It is generally accepted that randomization is the preferred method for reducing selection bias. Randomization tends to guard against imbalances of baseline prognostic factors between groups, protects against conscious or subconscious actions of study investigators that could lead to biased assignment of patients, and provides the probabilistic basis for most statistical analyses.

Depending on the study, randomization procedures can be tailored to specific needs. For example, in block randomization, an equal number of patients is assigned to the various treatment groups from a specified number of enrollees (e.g., for every ''block'' of six patients randomizing three patients to the device group and three patients to the control group). Randomization can be carried out centrally by the sponsor or locally by each study investigator, especially if sizable variation is anticipated between centers. Stratification randomization (randomization of patients to study treatment groups within predefined strata) can also be used to achieve a balance of patients within prognostic subsets of patients across the study groups.

E. Double-Blind Trials

There are a number of techniques whereby two or more medical devices may be effectively tested and compared in a double-blind manner. Once process is to have two (or more) surgeons each implant or insert different devices and to have an independent surgeon (who is kept blind) review all patients. Each surgeon may implant only one type of device, or may be permitted to implant all of the devices being compared. In the latter situation, devices should be implanted in a random order. Since many surgeons will have preferences as to the devices they use and also will be more experienced in implanting certain devices, they will generally prefer being assigned to only one type of device. Since differences in surgical skills rather than the device implanted may influence patient outcome, it is preferable to have several (or many) different surgeons each implant one specific device and a different group of surgeons each implant the other device studied. Alternatively, all surgeons may be trained in the device's use so that they each achieve a minimal standard of technical competence. A third possibility is to measure and grade the skills of each surgeon and to consider this assessment in the evaluation of the results.

If multiple hospitals are involved in a trial of a medical device, it is often necessary to control for differences in hospital care. This may be done by having at least one surgeon at each hospital assigned to insert device number 1 and a different surgeon or group of surgeons at each hospital chosen to insert device number 2. It is also important to ensure that all patients meet standard criteria to enter the trial to eliminate the possibility that surgeons at one hospital select patients differently than surgeons at another hospital.

F. Sample Size

Because the number of patients to be recruited into a study is critical, the issue of how many patients to enroll must be considered early in the planning stage. As observed by the Temple committee, many clinical trials in which sample size requirements were not carefully considered lacked statistical power or the ability to detect device effects of clinical importance.

Computation of required sample size is based on testing the particular hypothesis stated by the sponsor. For example, the null hypothesis (the hypothesis to be tested) may be that the proportion of patients with a successful outcome in the investigational device group is the same as that in the control group. The alternative hypothesis may be that the proportion of successes is greater in the test device group. In testing the hypothesis, two types of errors can be made. A type I error occurs when the null hypothesis is incorrectly rejected (i.e., concluding that the test device is better than the control, when in reality it is no better). A type II error is made when the null hypothesis is incorrectly accepted (i.e., concluding that there is no difference when the test device is better). The probability of a type I error is referred to as alpha, and the probability of a type II error as beta. The power of a statistical test (1 minus beta) is the probability that the null hypothesis is rejected if truly false; that is, power is the ability to detect a real difference of a specified magnitude between treatments. Typically, ODE prefers to see hypotheses tested at a 5% level of significance with at least 80% power.

Factors that can affect the determination of sample size include the type of primary end point analyzed, the desired size of the type I and II errors, and assumptions about the anticipated success rates in the device and control groups. Planned subgroup analyses, anticipated significant between-center variation, prerandomization stratification, and anticipated dropouts may also affect the proposed sample size. Moreover, whether a study is designed to show a difference in effectiveness or equivalence to a predicate device will have a significant impact on sample size calculations.

Intuitively, the larger the anticipated clinically meaningful difference between patients treated with a new device and patients treated with a control, the smaller the number of patients that will be required to demonstrate differences in the treatments. Similarly, the smaller the anticipated difference, the larger the number of patients that will be required to detect whether or not there is, in fact, a difference. Intuition may be less helpful, however, in determining an adequate number of patients when a company is trying to design a study to show its device is equivalent to another product.

The FDA typically requires that sponsors fully justify their proposed sample size by providing the following information:

The hypothesis to be tested
The magnitude of a clinically meaningful difference between study groups
Assumptions about the anticipated performance of the device and control
The formula for computing sample size
The assumed size alpha and beta errors

Sample sizes for device clinical studies typically vary from less than 100 to nearly 300 patients for a therapeutic device. Several hundred to more than 1000 samples may be needed when studying a diagnostic device. The sample size for diagnostic studies is most often greater due to the need to establish the sensitivity and specificity of the diagnostic, which often cannot be done in an analysis of small numbers of samples that may or may not have the adequate number of positives to determine whether or not the diagnostic is efficacious.

G. End Points

End points, or response variables, should be as clearly and precisely defined as possible. The sponsor should select outcome variables that are the most informative, the most clinically relevant, and the least prone to bias. Stating the specific end points in advance facilitates planning of study design and calculation of sample size.

Primary end points, which are designed to address the primary objectives of the study, form the principal basis for determining whether or not the device is safe and effective, thus the number of primary end points should be kept low to minimize confusion about the trial outcome. An individual patient's outcome relative to a primary end point often results in the patient's treatment being denied as a success or failure. Accordingly, the calculation of sample size is based on an analysis of the primary end points. Primary end points should be distinguished from secondary end points, which are designed to address secondary study objectives.

End points can be objective or subjective, depending on the device and particular indications being studied, but should be capable of unbiased assessment. End points can be based on quantitative or categorical variables, thus an end point may show a change from one discrete state to another (e.g., living to dead), from one state to any of several others (e.g., from one disease stage to another), or from one level of a continuous variable to another (e.g., percentage graft assimilation). Sometimes response variables are combinations of variables, in which events are combined if any one event occurs too infrequently to observe in a reasonable number of patients or if a combination of responses is needed to determine if the patient has a successful outcome. A sponsor must also determine when during the course of the study the primary end point is to be measured (e.g., reduction in pain at 6 months after application of the device).

Because of a history of prior misadventure, the use of surrogate end points is often not well received by FDA. Surrogate end points are outcomes that are not themselves readily discernible as a clinical benefit to a patient, but that may be correlated with a clinical benefit. For example, an improvement in some hemodynamic parameter may show the device is working, but the improvement in this laboratory parameter may not be easily translated into a clinical benefit to the patient (i.e., mortality, morbidity). On the other hand, reduction in serum cholesterol may be an acceptable surrogate end point because its relation to a clinical benefit is well described in the scientific literature. Where a surrogate end point is to be relied upon, however, some clear consensus from FDA that the end point is appropriate is essential.

Examples of some broadly defined end points are 12-month patency rates for vascular grafts, 3-year rates of osseointegration for endosseous dental implants, and sensitivity and specificity of a device to diagnose cancer. The end points and success criteria should be discussed in detail with FDA prior to initiation of the study. Of course, it would be disastrous if the company were to choose end points, complete the study, and then have to start over again because FDA rejected the end points. Although FDA could reverse its judgment on the proper end points upon completion of the study, the sponsor should seek to reduce the risk of disagreement through careful planning and open and continuing communication with ODE.

H. Blinding (Masking)

Blinding (recently retitled masking) should be implemented to reduce several types of potential bias. If patients believe they are receiving a certain treatment, they may imagine certain beneficial or adverse effects resulting from the assigned treatment. If the investigators know the intervention assigned, controls may not be followed as closely, or concomitant therapy may be disproportionately applied to one group of patients to compensate for the investigator's potential bias. Bias can also occur when the person charged with evaluating response variables intentionally or inadvertently shades the outcome measures in favor of a particular treatment.

Masking can take various forms in clinical trials. In an unblinded trial, both the patient and study investigator know which treatment has been assigned. In a typical single-blind study, only the investigator, not the patient, knows which treatment has been assigned. In a double-blind study, neither the subject nor the clinical investigator knows the assignment of intervention. Sometimes modified double-blind studies are conducted, in which the study investigator responsible for implementing the device knows the treatment assignment, but the observer responsible for evaluating safety and effectiveness outcomes does not. Although double-blind device studies are usually more complex and more difficult to conduct than other clinical trials, they are usually preferred by FDA. Triple-blind studies include those in which, in addition to the patient and investigator being blinded, the committee monitoring or analyzing the study results does not know the identity of the groups.

I. Comparability of Patients in Study Groups

At baseline, before the investigational device is applied or the control is utilized, the control group should be similar in relevant respects to the device group, so that differences in outcome may be reasonably attributed to the action of the device being studied. If, for example, the treatment and control groups differ at baseline relative to factors that are known to affect outcome, it is often difficult to meaningfully compare the rates of therapeutic success in the two groups, even with statistical adjustment. Accordingly, it is essential that relevant factors be assessed at baseline to determine the comparability of the treatment and control groups, and to determine whether or not statistical adjustment is feasible if the groups are imbalanced. As noted previously, one of FDA's major concerns in utilizing historical controls is the fact that the control and device groups may not be comparable, and differences therefore may impact upon the safety and efficacy evaluation.

J. Other Design Considerations

Decisions regarding the study design parameters described above have clear statistical implications. Other aspects of study design are equally important, but may involve less obvious statistical considerations. A sponsor must, for example, take the following actions when planning a study:

It goes without saying that before any clinical study may be performed with a device, either the device must already be approved for such use in humans or an IDE must have been granted. There are very limited exceptions to this (primarily custom devices and veterinary devices).
Consider the number of investigational sites to be employed. (Multicenter

studies are essential. The number of centers should be large enough to recruit the required number of patients, but small enough to pool results.)

Anticipate the duration of the study, including length of follow-up and recruitment period.

Select study investigators who are sufficiently qualified to use the investigational device.

Ensure informed consent is obtained from all patients.

A sponsor should be prepared to specify each essential study design parameter *before* conducting a clinical trial of its device. This will demonstrate to CDRH that the sponsor knows the device and knows the expected results of the clinical trial, and as a result can confidently approach the agency. With today's environment at FDA, the sponsor that is not sure which claims are appropriate or what end points to select should seriously consider conducting a feasibility study before entering into clinical trials.

K. Adverse Reactions

When commonly expected types of complications from a medical device are known, the data collection forms may list these for the investigator to check off. Although this practice is not as common in clinical trials evaluating medicines, there are a number of advantages and justifications for its use in tallying "adverse reactions" due to medical devices. For example, the number of likely adverse reactions resulting from medical devices are usually fewer than for medicines and may be more precisely described.

Federal regulations in the United States require manufacturers and importers of medical devices to report serious device-related injuries and deaths to the FDA. Physicians and other health professionals are encouraged to report their experiences to the manufacturer, directly to the FDA Product Monitoring Branch, or indirectly to the FDA via the problem reporting program administered by the *United States Pharmacopoeia*. A newsletter of world medical device news (*Clinica*) is published by George Street Publications in Surrey, United Kingdom.

L. Study Contact

Appropriate conduct of the clinical study is essential to ensure uniform implementation of the protocol and to obtain meaningful study results. During the planning phase, the likelihood of obtaining a sufficient number of patients in a specified period of time and the development of specific recruitment techniques must be evaluated. Data collection should be structured so that all data necessary to evaluate baseline comparability and outcome measures are collected. Efforts should also be directed at ensuring that key data are of high quality, and that missing and inconsistent information is minimized. Quality control methods should include techniques for data measurement, recording, transfer to computer databases, editing, verification, and changing of incorrect or missing data.

Mechanisms should be put in place during the planning phase to ensure investigator compliance with the protocol and patient compliance with treatment and follow-up. Study monitoring, specifically required under the IDE regulations, is essential to ensure consistent implementation of the protocol and collection of quality data. Good clinical practice (GCP) regulations provide significant guidance on these issues, particularly the documentation aspects (FDA, 1981).

M. Study Data Analysis

The Temple report clearly recommended that the study protocol describe the methods of data analysis that are to be employed on the data collected in the study. The planned data analysis should include any plans to exclude certain treated patients from the analysis, any planned subgroup comparisons, the identification of the primary end point from the several response variables, any planned interim analyses, and the specific statistical tests to be used.

Because excluding randomized patients from analysis can lead to biased results, FDA prefers to see an intent-to-treat analysis; that is, an analysis of all randomized patients who received any treatment.

Subgrouping on the basis of outcome variable scan also leads to biased results, and any planned subgroup analyses should therefore be set forth in the analysis plan.

While it is desirable in a clinical trial to have groups of subjects that are comparable except for the treatment being studied, all prognostic factors may not be perfectly balanced. Covariate adjustment (a statistical method used to adjust outcome measures based on imbalances between groups at baseline) can be used to minimize the effect of such differences. Discussion of such adjustment and identification of potential covariates should be included in the analysis plan.

A data analysis plan may also discuss contemplated pooling of results across various types of patients; for example, pooling across investigational sites, pooling across certain subgroups of patients, and potential pooling of U.S. and European clinical results. Where several end points will be analyzed to determine if the clinical study is a success, the issue of multiple comparisons also needs to be addressed in the data analysis plan. If several statistical tests are performed, it is likely that some will be significant by chance alone. If multiple end points are evaluated, statistical adjustment or increased sample size should thus be contemplated by the analysis plan.

In the interest of simplicity, FDA prefers that sponsors wait until all patients have been recruited before analyzing study data. There are situations, however, in which sponsors may wish to analyze data in the middle of the clinical trial;

for example, where there is a significant possibility of a safety problem or the potential for an overwhelming beneficial treatment response. Such analyses, termed ''interim analyses,'' are thus used, especially when a clinical study could be terminated early for safety or efficacy reasons. Since the use of interim analyses can affect the statistical interpretation of outcome measure, sponsors should discuss the possible use of these analyses in the IDE data analysis plan.

One reason for FDA's requirement of a prospective data analysis plan is to ensure that the sponsor is sufficiently confident in the design of the clinical trial to specifically identify how the device will perform. The FDA frowns upon exploratory trials forming the pivotal basis for device approval, viewing such studies as ''fishing expeditions'' in which the study is conducted and the collected data are analyzed to find some result that can be presented as significant to the agency.

N. IRB

No matter how trivial, any studies conducted involving human subjects must be performed with the involvement and guidance of an institutional review board (IRB). The sponsor should have adequate preclinical safety data in hand and be organized in such a manner as to cause the IRB to be comfortable that there is no unwarranted risk to patients in the trial being proposed.

Because IRBs play such a pivotal role in the review process for medical devices, it is important to understand the requirements of IRBs. The FDA has delineated the requirements for IRB membership, qualifications, functions, and operation in 21 CFR Part 56. An IRB is defined in the regulations as ''any board, committee, or other group formally designated by an institution to review, to approve the initiation of, and to conduct periodic review of biomedical research involving human subjects'' [21 CFR § 56.102(g)]. The primary purpose of IRB review is to ensure the protection of the rights and welfare of the human research subjects. Highlights of the basic requirements for IRBs as outlined in the regulations include the following:

Membership. Each IRB must have at least five members, and they must have varying backgrounds. Detailed requirements with regard to membership are established to prevent discrimination and protect against bias.

Functions and operations. The IRB is required to follow written procedures with regard to conducting both its initial review (discussed in Chapter 5) and its continuing review of research. Written procedures are also required to ensure prompt reporting to the IRB and FDA of unanticipated problems that involve risks to human subjects or others.

Informed consent. IRBs are required to ensure that information given to subjects as part of the informed consent is in accordance with the requirements for such consent set out in 21 CFR § 50.25.

Continuing review. IRBs are required to conduct continuing review of research at intervals appropriate to the degree of risk, but not less than once per year. They have authority to observe, or have a third party observe, the consent process and the research.

Suspension of approval. If research is not being conducted in accordance with the IRB's requirements or if the study has been associated with unexpected serious harm to subjects, the IRB has the authority to suspend or terminate approval of the research. In this case, the IRB must report the suspension or termination to the investigator, institutional officials, and FDA. The report must include a statement of the reasons for the IRB's action.

The FDA has increasingly focused its attention on the activities of IRBs in the past few years, demonstrating its authority over these bodies by stepping up its inspection of IRBs. Observations of noncompliance have resulted in numerous warning letters pertaining to deficiencies found in record keeping, protocol changes, and patient informed consent. If an IRB or the institution in which a clinical investigation is being conducted fails to take adequate steps to correct deviations observed by FDA during such inspections, FDA may disqualify the IRB or parent institution if "The IRB has refused or repeatedly failed to comply with the applicable regulations. The noncompliance adversely affects the rights or welfare of the human subjects in a clinical investigation" [21 CFR § 56.121 (b)].

FDA has told some IRBs to discontinue the approval of new studies until certain corrective actions have been taken. In fiscal year 1994, five IRBs were disqualified by FDA for failure to comply with appropriate regulations. After being disqualified, an IRB can become requalified upon the correction of all deficiencies; however, reinstatement requires a finding by the Commissioner that the IRB can meet all applicable standards (21 CFR § 56.123).

O. Clinical Safety Studies

There are some specific clinical studies that are performed with the single objective of ensuring device (or device material) safety. Most of these, such as those performed for contact lenses, vascular graft materials, and tampons, are specific for a device type. The repeat insult patch test (RIPT), however, is used only to evaluate safety and is common to all devices with significant human exposure.

RIPT. The RIPT comes in several forms (Marzulli and Maibach, 1991), but as an example case the nine-patch test is presented here.

Induction phase. A sufficient amount of the test article (an amount to adequately cover the surface of the patch unit—approximately 0.1–0.15 grams was placed onto an occlusive patch, which was applied to the back of each subject between the scapulae and waist, adjacent to the spinal midline.

The subjects were instructed to remove the patch 24 hr after application. Twenty-four-hr rest periods followed the Tuesday and Thursday removals, and

48-hr rest periods followed each Saturday removal. The sites were scored by a trained examiner just prior to the next patch application. This procedure was repeated every Monday, Wednesday, and Friday until nine applications of the test article were made.

Procedurally, if a subject developed a positive reaction of a two-level erythema or greater during the induction phase, or at the discretion of the study director—if the skin response warranted a change in site, the patch would be applied to a previously unpatched, adjacent site for the next application. If a two-level reaction (or greater) occurred at the new site, no further applications would be made. Any reactive subjects would be subsequently challenge-patch tested, however.

Challenge phase. After a rest period of approximately 2 weeks (no applications of the test article), the challenge patches are applied to previously unpatched (virgin) test sites. The sites are scored 24 and 72 hr after application. All subjects are instructed to report any delayed skin reactivity that might occur after the final challenge-patch reading. When warranted, selected test subjects are called back to the investigators' facility for additional examinations and scoring to determine possible increases or decreases in challenge patch reactivity.

Skin responses for both the induction and challenge phases of the study are scored according to the following six-point scale:

0 = No evidence of any effect
+ = Barely perceptible (minimal, faint, uniform, or spotty erythema)
1 = Mild (pink, uniform erythema covering most of the contact site)
2 = Moderate (pink–red erythema uniform in the entire contact site)
3 = Marked (bright red erythema with or without petechiae or papules)
4 = Severe (deep red erythema with or without vesiculation or weeping)

All other observed dermal sequelae (e.g., edema, dryness, or hypo- or hyperpigmentation) are appropriately recorded and described as mild, moderate, or severe).

II. EPIDEMIOLOGY

Epidemiology looks at the association between adverse effects seen in humans and a selected potential "cause" of interest, such as use of or exposure to a medical device, device material, or contaminant. Those involved in the safety of medical devices must have a working knowledge of epidemiology, as it has been intimately involved in most of the major safety concerns (real and perceived) associated with medical devices during the last 20 years (as shall be reviewed in the last chapter of this book), and provides an essential tool for risk assessment (McMahon and Pugh, 1970; Gordis, 1988).

Epidemiology is sometimes simply defined as the study of patterns of health in groups of people (Paddle, 1988). Behind this deceptively simple definition is an incredibly complex and diverse science, rich in concepts and methodology. The group of people of interest can be very small, historically consisting of as few as two people (Goudie et al., 1985). At the opposite extreme, studies of the geographic distribution of diseases using national mortality and cancer incidence rates have provided clues about the etiology of several diseases, such as cardiovascular disease and stomach cancer. The patterns of health studied are also wideranging and may include the distribution, course, and spread of disease. The term disease also has a loose definition in the context of epidemiology and might include ill-defined conditions such as Ginger Jake and toxic shock syndromes or consist of an indirect measure of impairment such as biochemical and hematological parameters or liver function measurements.

Epidemiology and toxicology differ in many other ways, but principally in that epidemiology is essentially an observational science, in contrast to the generally experimental nature of toxicology. The opportunistic nature of epidemiology has been commented upon by several authors (e.g., Paddle, 1988; Utidjian, 1987). The epidemiologist often has to make do with historical data that have been collected for reasons that have nothing to do with epidemiology. Nevertheless, the availability of personnel records such as lists of new employees and terminations, payrolls and work rosters, and exposure-monitoring data collected for compliance purposes, has enabled many epidemiological studies to be conducted in the occupational setting. The epidemiologist thus has no control over who is exposed to an agent or device, the levels at which they are exposed to the agent of interest, or to what other agents they may be exposed. The epidemiologist has great difficulty in ascertaining what exposure has taken place and certainly has no control over lifestyle variables such as diet, exercise, and smoking.

Despite the lack of precise data, the epidemiologist has one major advantage over the toxicologist: an epidemiology study documents the actual health experiences of human beings subjected to real-life exposures in an occupational, environmental, or clinical use setting. Indeed, Smith (1988) has recently expressed the view that the uncertainty in epidemiology studies resulting from exposure estimation may be no greater than or less than the uncertainty associated with extrapolation of results from animals to man. Regulatory bodies such as the U.S. Environmental Protection Agency (EPA) are starting to change their attitudes toward epidemiology and to recognize that it has a role to play in the process of risk assessment (Greenland, 1987). There is a continuing need, however, for epidemiologists to introduce more rigor into the conduct of their studies and to introduce standards equivalent to the GLPs under which animal experiments are performed.

A. Measurement of Exposure

Wegman and Eisen (1988) made the point that epidemiologists place much greater emphasis on the measure of response than on the measure of exposure. They claim that this is because most epidemiologists have been trained as physicians and are consequently more oriented toward measuring health outcomes. It is certainly true that a modern textbook of epidemiology such as Rothman's (1986) provides minimal guidance about what the epidemiologist should do with exposure assessments. This is probably as much a reflection of the historical paucity of quantitative exposure information as a reflection on the background of epidemiologists, however. Nevertheless, it is surprising how many epidemiological studies do not contain even a basic qualitative assessment of exposure. The contrast between epidemiology and toxicology is never more marked than in the area of estimation of dose response. Not only can the toxicologist carefully control the conditions of the exposure to the agent of interest, but he can also generally be sure that his animals have not come into contact with any other toxic agents. The medical epidemiologist conducting a study of patients exposed to a hepatotoxin would certainly have to control for alcohol intake and possibly for exposure to other hepatotoxins in the clinical, work, and home environments. Nevertheless, it can be argued that epidemiology studies more accurately measure the effect on human health of real-life exposures. The epidemiologist must therefore frequently develop sampling strategies that generate exposure data suitable for both compliance and epidemiological purposes. For patients, of course, the situation is usually different. Quantitating exposures is generally straightforward.

If an exposure matrix has been constructed with quantitative estimates of the exposure in each device's use and time period, it is a simple matter to estimate cumulative exposure. It is a more difficult process when, as is commonly the case occupationally, only a qualitative measure of exposure is available (e.g., high, medium, or low). Even when exposure measurements are available, it may not be sensible to make an assumption that an exposure that occurred 20 years ago is equivalent to the same exposure yesterday. The use of average exposures may also be questionable, and peak exposures may be more relevant in the case of outcomes such as asthma and chronic bronchitis.

B. Epidemiological Study Designs

What follows is a brief introduction to the most important types of studies conducted by epidemiologists, with an attempt to briefly describe the principles of the major types of epidemiological studies in order to assist the toxicologist in understanding the reporting of epidemiological studies and the assumptions made by epidemiologists.

1. Cohort Studies

Historical Cohort Study. When the need arises to study the health status of a group of individuals, there is often a large body of historical data that can be utilized. If sufficient information exists on individuals exposed in the past to a potential hazardous device or material, it may be possible to undertake a retrospective cohort study. The historical data will have been collected for reasons that have nothing to do with epidemiology. Nevertheless, the availability of medical records and morbidity and mortality indices has enabled many epidemiological studies to be conducted (in particular, mortality studies).

The principles of a historical cohort study can also be applied to follow a cohort of patients prospectively. It should be emphasized that many historical data studies have a prospective element insofar as they are updated after a further period of follow-up. There is no reason why reproductive performance, incidence of serious bacterial infections, or almost any measure of health status of an individual should not be studied retrospectively if sufficient information is available.

Mortality and cancer incidence studies are unique among retrospective cohort studies in that they can be conducted using national cancer and mortality reports even if there has been no medical surveillance of the patient population of interest. A historical cohort study also has the advantages of being cheaper and providing estimates of the potential hazard much earlier than a prospective study. Historical cohort studies are beset by a variety of problems, however. Principal among these is the problem of determining which patients have been exposed to the exact device of interest, and if so, to what degree. In addition, it may be difficult to decide what is an appropriate comparison group. It should also be borne in mind that in epidemiology, unlike animal experimentation, random allocation is not possible and there is no control over the factors that may distort the effects of the exposure of interest, such as smoking, alcohol use, and standard of living.

Cohort Definition and Follow-Up Period. A variety of sources of information are used to identify patients exposed to a particular potential hazard, to construct a medical and occupational history, and to complete the collection of information necessary for follow-up. It is essential that the cohort be well defined and that criteria for eligibility be strictly followed. This requires that a clear statement be made about membership of the cohort so that it is easy to decide whether a patient is a member or not. It is also important that the follow-up period be carefully defined. For instance, it is readily apparent that the follow-up period should not start before exposure has occurred. Furthermore, it is uncommon for the health effect of interest to manifest itself immediately after the initiation of device use, and allowance for an appropriate biological induction (or latency) period may need to be made when interpreting the data.

Comparison Subjects. The usual comparison group for many studies is the appropriate portion of the national population. It is known, however, that there are marked regional differences in the mortality rates for many causes of death. Regional mortality rates exist in most industrialized countries, but have to be used with caution because they are based on small numbers of deaths and estimated population sizes. In some situations the local rates for certain causes may be highly influenced by the mortality of the patients being studied. Furthermore, it is not always easy to decide what the most appropriate regional rate of comparison is, as many employees may reside in a different region from the plant.

An alternative or additional approach is to establish a cohort of unexposed but otherwise comparable individuals for comparison purposes. For example, some studies of breast implant recipients have been restricted to female health care professionals and use others from this same group who have not received implants as a control group. Patients with very low exposures to the device type of interest can often provide similar information, however. A good discussion of the issues is found in the proceedings of a conference entirely devoted to the subject (MRC, 1984).

Analysis and Interpretation. The first stage in the analysis in a cohort study consists of calculating the number of deaths expected during the follow-up period. In order to calculate the expected deaths for the cohort, the survival experience of the cohort is broken down into individual years of survival, known as ''person-years.'' Each person-year is characterized by the age of the cohort member, the time period in which survival occurred, and the sex of the cohort member. The person-years are then multiplied by age, sex, and time-period-specific mortality rates to obtain the expected number of deaths. The ratio between observed and expected deaths is expressed as a standardized mortality ration (SMR) as follows:

$$\text{SMR} = 100 \times \frac{\text{Observed deaths}}{\text{Expected deaths}}$$

An SMR of 125 thus represents an excess mortality of 25%. An SMR can be calculated for different causes of death and for subdivision of the person-years by factors such as level of exposure and time since first exposure.

Interpretation of cohort studies is not always straightforward, and there are a number of selection efforts and biases that must be considered (Rothman, 1986). Occupational cohort studies routinely report that the mortality of active workers is less than that of the population as a whole. It is not an unexpected finding, since workers usually have to undergo some sort of selection process to become or remain workers. Nevertheless, this section effect, known as the ''healthy worker'' effect, can lead to considerable argument over the interpretation of study results, particularly if the cancer mortality is as expected but the all-cause mortality is much lower than expected. Similar possibilities must be considered for device recipient cohorts, who are likely to receive more medical services than the general population.

Proportional Mortality Study. There are often situations in which one has no accurate data on the composition of a cohort but does possess a set of death records (or cancer registrations). Under these circumstances a proportional mortality study may sometimes be substituted for a cohort study. In such a mortality study the proportions of deaths from a specific cause among the study deaths is compared with the proportion of deaths from that cause in a comparison population. The results of a proportional mortality study are expressed in an analogous way to those of the cohort study with follow-up. Corresponding to the observed deaths from a particular cause, it is possible to calculate an expected number of deaths based on mortality rates for that cause and all causes of death in a comparison group and the total number of deaths in the study. The ratio between observed and expected deaths from a certain cause is expressed as a proportional mortality ratio (PMR), as follows:

$$PMR = 100 \times \frac{\text{Observed deaths}}{\text{Expected deaths}}$$

A PMR of 125 for a particular cause of death thus represents a 25% increase in the proportion of deaths due to that cause. A proportional mortality study has the advantage of avoiding the expensive and time-consuming establishment and tracing of the cohort, but the disadvantage of little or no exposure information.

Prospective Cohort Study. Prospective cohort studies are no different in principle from historical cohort studies in terms of scientific logic, the major differences being timing and methodology. The study starts with a group of apparently healthy individuals whose health and exposure is studied over a period of time. As it is possible to define in advance the information that is to be collected, prospective studies are theoretically more reliable than retrospective ones. Long periods of observation may be required to obtain results, however.

Prospective cohort studies or longitudinal studies of continually changing health parameters such as lung function, incidence of inflammatory joint disease, blood biochemistry, and hematological measurements, pose different problems from those encountered in mortality and cancer incidence studies. The relationships between changes in the parameters of interest and device exposure measurements have to be estimated, and if necessary, a comparison made of changes in

the parameters between the groups. These relationships may be extremely complicated—compounded by factors such as aging—and difficult to estimate, as there
may be relatively few measurement points. Furthermore, large errors of measurement in the variables may be present because of factors such as within-laboratory
variation and temporal variation within individuals. Missing observations and
withdrawals may also cause problems, particularly if they are dependent on the
level and change of the parameter of interest. These problems may make it difficult to interpret and judge the validity of statistical conclusions. Nevertheless,
prospective cohort studies provide the best means of measuring changes in health
parameters and relating them to exposure.

2. Case-Control Study

In a case-control study (also known as a case-referent study), two groups of
individuals are selected for study, one of whom has the disease whose causation
is to be studied (the cases) and the other of whom does not (the control). In the
context of the chemical industry, the aim of a case-control study is to evaluate
the relevance of past exposure to the development of a disease. This is done by
obtaining an indirect estimate of the rate of occurrence of the disease in an exposed and unexposed group by comparing the frequency of exposure among cases
and controls.

Principal Features of Case-Control Studies.   Case-control and cohort
studies complement each other as types of epidemiological studies (Schlesselman, 1982). In a case-control study the groups are defined on the basis of the
presence or absence of a given disease, and hence only one disease can be studied
at a time. The case-control study compensates for this by providing information
on a wide range of exposures or other causes (background health problems of
patients, e.g.), which may play a role in the development of the disease. In contrast, a cohort study generally focuses on a single exposure but can be analyzed
for multiple disease outcomes. A case-control study is a better way of studying
rare diseases because a very large cohort would be required to demonstrate an
excess of rare diseases. In contrast, a case-control study is an inefficient way of
assessing the effect of an uncommon exposure, when it might be possible to
conduct a cohort study of all those exposed.

The complementary strengths and weaknesses of case-control and cohort
studies can be used to advantage. Increasingly mortality studies are being reported
that utilize "nested" case-control studies to investigate the association between
the exposures of interest and a cause of death for which an excess has been
discovered. Case-control studies have traditionally been held in low regard, however, largely because they are often badly conducted and interpreted. There is
also a tendency to overinterpret the data and misuse statistical procedures. In
addition, there is still considerable debate among leading epidemiologists them-

selves as to how controls should be selected (e.g. Poole, 1986; Schlesselman and Stadel, 1987).

Analysis and Interpretation.   In a case-control study it is possible to compare the frequencies of exposures in the cases (exposed) and controls (unexposed). What one is really interested in, however, is a comparison of the frequencies of the disease in the exposed and the unexposed. The latter comparison is usually expressed as a relative risk (RR), which is defined as

$$RR = \frac{\text{Rate of disease} \in \text{exposed group}}{\text{Rate of disease} \in \text{unexposed group}}$$

It is clearly not possible to calculate the RR directly in a case-control study, since exposed and unexposed groups have not been followed in order to determine the rates of occurrence of the disease in the two groups. Nevertheless, it is possible to calculate another statistic, the odds ratio (OR), which, if certain assumptions hold, is a good estimate of the RR. For cases and controls the exposure odds are simply the odds of being exposed, and the OR is defined as

$$OR = \frac{\text{Cases with exposure}}{\text{Controls with exposure}} \Big/ \frac{\text{Cases without exposure}}{\text{Controls without exposure}}$$

An OR of 1 indicates that the rate of disease is unaffected by the treatment being studied. An OR greater than 1 indicates an increase in the rate of disease in exposed workers.

Matching.   Matching is the selection of a comparison group that is, within stated limits, identical with the study group with respect to one or more factors, such as age, years of device use or treatment, and smoking history, which may distort the effect of the exposure of interest. The matching may be done on an individual or group basis. Although matching may be used in all types of studies, including follow-up and cross-sectional studies, it is more widely used in case-control studies. It is common to see a case-control study in which each case is matched to as many as three or four controls.

Nested Case-Control Study.   In a cohort study the assessment of exposure for all cohort members may be extremely time-consuming and demanding of resources. If an excess of incidence of death has been discovered for a small number of conditions, it may be much more efficient to conduct a case-control study to investigate the effect of exposure. Instead of all members being studied, only the cases and a sample of noncases would be compared with regard to treatment history. There is thus no need to investigate the exposure histories of all those who are neither cases nor controls. The nesting is only effective if there are a reasonable number of cases and sufficient variation in the treatment of the cohort members, however.

C. Other Study Designs

1. Descriptive Studies

There are large numbers of records in existence that document the health of various groups of people. Mortality statistics are available for many countries and even for certain devices and treatment types (e.g., Pell et al., 1978; Paddle, 1981). Similarly, there is a wide range of routine morbidity statistics, in particular those based on cancer registrations (Waterhouse et al., 1982). These health statistics can be used to study differences between geographic regions (e.g., maps of cancer mortality and incidence presented at a symposium) (Boyle et al., 1989), device use, and time periods. Investigations based on existing records of the distribution of disease and of possible causes are known as descriptive studies. It is sometimes possible to identify hazards associated with the development of rare conditions from observation of clustering in occupational groups, treatment groups, or geographical areas.

2. Cross-Sectional Studies

Cross-sectional studies measure the cause (treatment) and the effect (disease) at the same point in time. They compare the rates of diseases or symptoms of a treated group with an untreated group. Strictly speaking, the treatment information is ascertained simultaneously with the disease information. In practice, such studies are usually more meaningful from an etiological or causal point of view if the treatment assessment reflects treatment and past medical history. Current information is often all that is available, but it may still be meaningful because of the correlation between current treatment and relevant past treatments.

Cross-sectional studies are widely used to study the health of groups of patients who are exposed to possible hazards but do not undergo complete regular surveillance (asthmatics and diabetics, e.g.). They are particularly suited to the study of subclinical parameters such as blood biochemistry and hematological values. Cross-sectional studies are also relatively straightforward to conduct in comparison with prospective cohort studies and are generally simpler to interpret.

3. Intervention Studies

Not all epidemiology is observational, and experimental studies have a role to play in evaluating the efficiency of an intervention program to prevent disease (e.g., fluoridation of water). An intervention study at one extreme may closely resemble a clinical trial with individuals randomly selected to receive some form of intervention (e.g., use of latex gloves). In some instances, however, it may be a whole community that is selected to form the intervention group. The selection

TABLE 15.3 Differences Between Animal and Human Studies

Parameter	Animal study	Human study
Ethics	Provided that governmental animal cruelty/rights acts are not contravened, it is perfectly acceptable to knowingly expose the animal to carcinogens, mutagens, teratogens, etc.	It is unethical to knowingly and deliberately expose humans to carcinogens, mutagens, teratogens, etc.
Conduct	Good laboratory practice (strict adherence to GLP)	Protocol for study (protocol may change during study).
Subject observation	Monitored case histories (record of animal health throughout study)	Exhaustive follow-up. (Sometimes subjects are untraceable/disappear.)
Dose	Regulated exposure (defined dose at defined intervals)	Defined exposed group. (It may only be known whether there was a potential for exposure but not at what level.)
Length of exposure	Depending on the suspected effect of the chemical (generally lifetime for carcinogens, throughout organogenesis for teratogens, generations for reprotoxins)	Various (depending on whether chemical is an occupational, marketplace, or environmental hazard).
Pattern of exposure	Single chemicals at around the maximal tolerated does; dose levels constant	Mixed exposure at varied levels (usually "pulse" exposure).
Comparison groups	Randomized uniformity (control group known to have no exposure, otherwise identical with exposed group)	Valid exposed group. (It can only be assumed that the only different variable is exposure.)
Genetic homogeneity	Generally "inbred" strain used; hence, high degree of genetic homogeneity	High degree of heterogeneity.
Death	Standardized necropsy (every animal subject to pathological examination)	High degree of heterogeneity.
Relevance	Extremely relevant to the species in which data were generated (transspecies relevance unknown)	Extremely relevant to man.

may or may not be random. The toxicologist might argue that even if selection were random, such a study of two communities, each consisting of many individuals, was in a sense a study of only two subjects. He should ask himself first, however, whether the "three rats to a cage" design of many subacute toxicity studies really generates three independent responses per cage.

Finally, the reliability of the collected data in epidemiology studies is, as with toxicology studies, reflective of the effort and care put into collecting the data. In particular, it should be kept in mind that data arising from medical assessments is to be much preferred to that generated by patient self-reports.

III. CONCLUSION

There are fundamental differences between human and animal studies. Some of these are summarized in Table 15.3. In the end, however, it is of course the effects in humans that we are most concerned about. This gives the well-conducted and conclusive studies significantly greater weight than preclinical studies in assessing human risk (Brown and Paddle, 1988; Glocklin, 1987; Freireich et al., 1966; Davidson et al., 1986; Calabrese, 1986).

REFERENCES

Anon. (2000). FDA's BIMO programs are broken, OIG says, Guide Med. Dev. Reg. Monthly Bull., August.

Boyle, P., Muir, C. S., and Grundmann, E. (1989). Cancer Mapping, Springer-Verlag, Berlin.

Brown, L. P. and Paddle, G. M. (1988). Risk assessment: Animal or human model? Pharm. Med., 3: 361–374.

Calabrese, E. J. (1986). Animal extrapolation and the challenge of human heterogeneity, J. Pharm. Sci., 75: 1041–1046.

Davidson, I. W. F., Parker, J. C., and Beliles, R. P. (1986). Biological basis for extrapolation across mammalian species, Reg. Toxicol. Pharm., 6: 211–237.

FDA. (1981). Protection of human subjects informed consent standards for institutional review boards for clinical investigations, Fed. Reg., Jan. 27.

Freireich, E. J., Gehan, E. A., Rall, D. P., Schmidt, L. H., and Skipper, H. E. (1966). Quantitative comparison of toxicity of anticancer agents in the mouse, rat, hamster, dog, monkey, and man, Cancer Chemo. Rep., 80: 219–244.

Glocklin, V. C. (1987). Current FDA perspective on animal selection and extrapolation. In: Human Risk Assessment: The Role of Animal Selection and Extrapolation (M. V. Roloff, Ed.). Taylor and Francis, London, pp. 15–22.

Gordis, L., Ed. (1988). Epidemiology and Health Risk Assessment, Oxford University Press, New York.

Goudie, R. B., Jack, A. S., and Goudie, B. M. (1985). Genetic and developmental aspects of pathological pigmentation patterns, Curr. Top. Pathol., 74: 132–138.

Greenland, S., Ed. (1987). Evolution of Epidemiologic Ideas: Annotated Readings on Concepts and Methods, Epidemiology Resources, Chapel Hill, NC.

Kahan, J. S. (1994). Medical Devices: Obtaining FDA Market Clearance, Parevel International, Waltham, MA.

McMahon, B. and Pugh, T. F. (1970). Epidemiology, Principles and Methods, Little, Brown, Boston.

MRC. (1984). Expected Numbers in Cohort Studies, Medical Research Council Environmental Epidemiology Unit, scientific report no. 6, Southampton, UK.

Paddle, G. M. (1981). A strategy for the identification of carcinogens in a large, complex chemical company. In: Quantification of Occupational Cancer: Banbury Report 9 (R. Peto and M. Schneiderman, Eds.). Cold Spring Harbor Laboratory, Cold Spring Harbor, NY, pp. 177–186.

Paddle, G. M. (1988). Epidemiology. In: Experimental Toxicology: The Basic Principles (D. Anderson and D. M. Conning, Eds.). Royal Society of Chemistry, London, pp. 436–456.

Pell, S., O'Berg, M., and Karrh, B. (1978). Cancer epidemiologic surveillance in the Du Pont company, J. Occupa. Med., 20: 725–740.

Poole, C. (1986) Exposure opportunity in case-control studies, Amer. J. Epidem., 123: 352–358.

Rothman, K. J. (1986). Modern Epidemiology, Little, Brown, Boston.

Schlesselman, J. J. (1982). Case-Control Studies: Design, Conduct, Analysis, Oxford University Press, New York.

Schlesselman, J. J. and Stadel, B. V. (1987). Exposure opportunity in epidemiologic studies, Amer. J. Epidem., 125: 174–178.

Smith, A. H. (1988). Epidemiologic input to environmental risk assessment, Arch. Environ. Health, 43: 124–127.

Spilker, B. (1995). Guide to Clinical Trials, Raven, New York.

Utidjian, H. M. D. (1987). The interaction between epidemiology and animal studies in industrial toxicology. In: Perspectives in Basic and Applied Toxicology (B. Ballantyne, Ed.). John Wright, Bristol, UK., pp. 309–329.

Waterhouse, J. A. H., Muir, C. J., Shanmugaratnam, K., and Powell, J., eds. (1982). Cancer Incidence in Five Continents, vol. IV, International Agency for Research on Cancer, Lyon (IARC Scientific Publication no. 42).

Wegman, D. H. and Eisen, E. A. (1988). Epidemiology. In: Occupational Health: Recognizing and Preventing Work-Related Disease (B. S. Levy and D. H. Wegman, Eds.). Little, Brown, Boston, pp. 55–73.

16

Special Studies

The previous chapters in this book have primarily addressed the tests applicable to all or broad ranges of medical devices. Regulatory authorities (and responsible practice) have also, however, established some specific testing requirements for a number of broadly utilized but somewhat specialized devices, such as cardiovascular devices and prostheses (ISO, 1989a–1992; AAMI, 1996), contact lenses and their solutions (CRDH, 1985; 1995a), and tampons (CDRH, 1995b). These evaluations require some specialized tests. In addition, there is one promulgated (but now infrequently used) test, the ''mouse safety'' or systemic injection test, which fits none of the previous classifications and needs to be briefly considered here.

I. CARDIOVASCULAR DEVICES AND PROSTHESES

Interactions that mainly affect cardiovascular devices and that may or may not have an undesirable effect on the subject are as follows:

1. Adsorption of plasma proteins, lipids, calcium, or other substances from the blood onto the surface of the device or absorption of such substances into the device
2. Adhesion of platelets, leukocytes, or erythrocytes onto the surface of the device or absorption of their components into the device
3. Alterations in mechanical and other properties of the device

Interactions that have a potentially undesirable effect on the patient (animal or human) are as follows:

1. Activation of platelets, leukocytes, or other cells, or activation of the coagulation, fibrinolytic, complement, or other pathways, including immunotoxicity (immunosuppression, immunopotentiation, or immunomodulation)
2. Formation of thrombi on the device surface
3. Embolization of thrombotic or other material from the device's luminal surface to another site within the circulation
4. Injury to circulating blood cells resulting in anemia, hemolysis, leukopenia, thrombocytopenia, or altered function of blood cells
5. Injury to cells and tissues adjacent to the device
6. Intimal hyperplasia or accumulation of other tissue on or adjacent to the device, resulting in reduced flow or affecting other functions of the device
7. Adhesion and growth of bacteria or other infectious agents to or near the device.

Procedures used to evaluate cardiovascular devices in animals are essentially the same as those employed in the clinical setting. Animal models permit continuous device monitoring and systematic controlled study of important variables, however.

The test protocols recommended follow certain general guidelines. Thrombosis, thromboembolism, bleeding, and infection are the major deterrents to the use and further development of advanced cardiovascular prostheses. For devices with limited blood exposure (<24 hr), important measurements are related to the acute extent of variation of hematologic, hemodynamic, and performance variables, gross thrombus formation, and possible embolism. With prolonged or repeated exposure (>24 hr) or permanent contact, emphasis is placed on serial measurement techniques that may yield information regarding the time course of thrombosis and thromboembolism, the consumption of circulating blood components, the development of intimal hyperplasia, and infection. In both of the above exposure and contact categories, assessment of the hemolysis is important. Thrombus formation may be greatly influenced by surgical technique, variable time-dependent thrombolytic and embolic phenomena, superimposed device infections, and possible alterations in exposed surfaces; for example, intimal hyperplasia and entothelialization.

The consequences of the interaction of artificial surfaces with the blood may range from gross thrombosis and embolization to subtle effects such as accelerated consumption of hemostatic elements; the latter may be compensated or lead to depletion of platelets or plasma coagulation factors.

Disturbances of organ function may occur due to blood/device interaction. For instance, kidney function and pulmonary function may be affected by activated blood coagulation and platelet/leukocyte/complement interactions.

Platelet survival and plasma levels of the platelet-specific proteins PF-4 and β-TG may reflect the extent of platelet activation in vivo (and perhaps risk of thromboembolism), even in the absence of significantly elevated rates of platelet consumption. The template bleeding time is an index of in vivo platelet function; a prolonged value suggests thrombocytopenia or a qualitative platelet disorder, such as may occur during cardiopulmonary bypass. Measurements of platelet activating factor (PFA) may indicate activation of intrinsic coagulation.

Localization of thrombotic material by radionuclide imaging techniques using radiolabeled platelets has been demonstrated in studies of vascular grafts, valve prostheses, and other devices, both implants and externally communicating devices. In addition, duplex scanning and a careful examination of the explanted device can provide very useful information.

The choice of an animal model may be restricted by size requirements, the availability of certain species, and cost. It is critical that the investigators be mindful of the physiological differences and similarities of the species chosen with those of humans, particularly those relating to coagulation, platelet functions and fibrinolysis, and the response to pharmacological agents such as anesthetics, anticoagulants, thrombolytic and antiplatelet agents, and antibiotics. Because of species differences in reactivity and variable responses to different devices, data obtained from a single species should be interpreted with caution. Nonhuman primates such as baboons bear a close similarity in hematologic values, blood coagulation mechanism, and cardiovascular system to the human. An additional advantage of a nonhuman primate is that many of the immunologic probes for thrombosis developed for humans are suitable for use in other primates. These probes include PF-4, β-TG, FPA, TAT, and F_{1+2}. The dog is a commonly used species and has provided useful information; however, device-related thrombosis in the dog tends to occur more readily than in the human, a difference that can be viewed as an advantage when evaluating this complication. The pig is generally regarded as a suitable animal model because of its hematologic and cardiovascular similarities to the human. The effect of the surgical implant procedure on results should be kept in mind and appropriate controls included.

A. Cannulae

Cannulae are typically inserted into one or more major blood vessels to provide repeated blood access. They are also used during cardiopulmonary bypass and other procedures. They may be tested acutely or chronically and are commonly studied as arteriovenous (AV) shunts. The use of cannulae appears to induce little alteration in the levels of circulating blood cells or clotting factors. Like other indirect blood path devices, cannulae generally require less testing than devices in circulating blood.

B. Catheters and Guidewires

Most of the tests considered under cannulae are relevant to the study of catheters and guidewires. The location or placement of catheters in the arterial or venous system can have a major effect on blood/device interactions. It is advised that simultaneous control studies be performed using a contralateral artery or vein. Care should be taken not to strip off thrombus upon catheter withdrawal. In situ evaluation may permit assessment of the extent to which intimal or entrance site injuries contributed to the thrombotic process. Kinetic studies with radiolabeled blood constituents are recommended only with chronic catheters, but may be useful for imaging thrombus accumulation in vivo. Angiography and Doppler blood flow measurements may also be useful.

C. Anti-Infective Materials

Implantable medical devices such as cannulae, catheters, and stents are indispensable in the management of critically and chronically ill patients for the administration of electrolytes, drugs, parenteral nutrients, blood components, or drainage of secretions and pus. Artificial heart valves, prosthetics, ceramics, metals, and bone cements are now common implants or implant materials. All of these implants save human lives and enhance the quality of life. At the same time they are the leading cause for millions of primary nosocomial bloodstream infections with substantial morbidity and mortality (Bisno and Waldnagel, 1994). A property common to all these biomaterials is the ease by which they are colonized by pathogenic and nonpathogenic microorganisms, often requiring immediate removal.

Several methods have been devised to decrease the risk of foreign body-associated infections. These include the use of meticulous hygienic precautions, the development of hydrophillic materials to minimize bacterial adhesion, and impregnation with antiseptics, antibiotics, and a host of other pharmaceutical products. Silver—in particular free silver ions—is well known for its powerful and broad-spectrum antimicrobial activity, still allowing the independent use of therapeutic antibiotics. The investigation of the antimicrobial activity of implants containing silver as an antimicrobial agent is difficult because many silver compounds are poorly water-soluble, resulting in low concentrations of silver ions released into the surrounding medium. The antimicrobial efficacy of polymers impregnated with elementary silver therefore cannot be tested by routine agar diffusion measurements. Like other procedures, the agar diffusion technique was also inappropriate for a simultaneous high-throughput screening prototype devices. Bechert et al. (2000) have proposed a very promising microplate-based system for such evaluations.

D. Extracorporeal Oxygenators, Hemodialyzers, Therapeutic Apheresis Equipment, and Devices for Absorption of Specific Substances from Blood

The hemostatic response to cardiopulmonary bypass may be significant and acute. Many variables, such as use of blood suction, composition of blood pump priming fluid, hypothermia, blood contact with air, and time of exposure, influence test values. Emboli in outflow lines may be detected by the periodic placement of blood filters ex vivo or the use of ultrasonic radiation or other noninvasive techniques. Thrombus accumulation can be directly assessed during bypass by monitoring performance factors such as pressure drop across the oxygenator and oxygen transfer rate. An acquired transient platelet dysfunction associated with selective alpha granule release has been observed in patients on cardiopulmonary bypass; the template bleeding time and other tests of platelet function and release are particularly useful.

Complement activation is caused by both hemodialyzers and cardiopulmonary bypass apparatus. Clinically significant pulmonary leukostasis and lung injury with dysfunction may result. For these reasons it is useful to quantify complement activation with these devices.

Because of their high surface-to-volume ratio, therapeutic apheresis equipment and devices for absorption of specific substances from the blood can potentially activate complement, coagulation, platelet, and leukocyte pathways. Examination of blood/device interactions should follow the same principles as for extracorporeal oxygenators and hemodialyzers.

E. Ventricular-Assist Devices

These devices may induce considerable alteration in various blood components. Factors contributing to such effects include the large foreign surface area to which blood is exposed, the high flow regimes, and the regions of disturbed flow, such as turbulence or separated flow. Tests of such devices may include measurements of hemolysis; platelet and fibrinogen concentration; platelet survival; complement activation; and close monitoring of liver, renal, pulmonary, and central nervous system function. A detailed pathologic examination at surgical retrieval is an important component of the valuation.

F. Heart Valve Prostheses

Invasive, noninvasive, and in vitro hydrodynamic studies are important in the assessment of prosthetic valves.

2D and M mode echocardiography make use of ultrasonic radiation to form images of the heart. Reflection from materials with different acoustic impedances are received and processed to form an image. The structure of prosthetic valves can be examined. Mechanical prostheses emit strong echo signals, and the movement of the occluder can usually be clearly imaged. The quality of the image may depend upon the particular valve being examined, however. Echocardiography may also be useful in the assessment of the function of tissue-derived valve prostheses. Vegetations, clots, and evidence of thickening of the valve leaflets are elucidated. Using conventional and color flow Doppler echocardiography, blood flow regurgitation can be identified and semiquantified.

Measurements of platelet survival and aggregation, blood tests of thrombosis and hemolysis, pressure and flow measurements, and autopsy of the valve and adjacent tissues are also recommended.

G. Vascular Grafts

Both porous and nonporous materials can be implanted at various locations in the arterial or venous system. The choice of implantation site is determined largely by the intended use for the prosthesis. Patency of a given graft is enhanced by larger diameter and shorter length. A rule of thumb for grafts less than 4 mm ID is that the length should exceed the diameter by a factor of 10 (e.g., 40 mm for a 4-mm graft) for a valid model. Patency can be documented by palpation of distal pulses in some locations and by periodic angiography. Ultrasonic radiation, magnetic resonance imaging (MRI), and positron emission tomography (PET) may also be useful. Results of serial radiolabeled platelet imaging studies correlate with the area of nonendothelialized graft surface in baboons. Radiolabeled platelets facillitate noninvasive imaging of mural thrombotic accumulations. Serial measurements of platelet count, platelet release constituents, fibrinogen/fibrin degradation products, and activated coagulation species also are recommended. Autopsy of the graft and adjacent vascular segments for morphometric studies of endothelial integrity and proliferative response can provide valuable information.

H. IVC Filters and Stents

These devices can be studied by angiography and ultrasonic radiation. Other techniques useful for vascular graft evaluation are appropriate here as well.

II. TAMPONS

Tampons occupy a unique niche in both commerce and medical device regulation. They are sold freely at any commercial outlet (supermarket, drugstore, mini-market, etc.) without restriction or control, and they are used regularly by as many as 38 million women in the United States (and many more overseas), but do require premarket review and approval as a device by the FDA. As a result of the toxic shock syndrome (TSS) scare of the early 1980s (see Chapter 17 for details on this) and continuing concerns as to their potential effects on both vaginal microflora and the induction of TSS toxin, the obstetrics–gynecology devices branch of CDRH maintains separate testing requirements and guidelines for menstrual tampons (CDRH, 1995b). The unique aspects of these requirements from a safety point of view are that testing be performed to evaluate both the effects of new and revised products on vaginal microflora and to determine their potential to lead to the production of TSS toxin. These specific tests are presented later in this chapter.

Also of concern is the potential for any potentially hazardous materials to be leached from the tampon into the vaginal environment. Though this is a general concern, there has recently been imposed a specific requirement to evaluate dioxins in the absorbent fibers of the tampon.

III. CONTACT LENSES AND THEIR SOLUTIONS

Contact lenses also present a unique case for both medical device regulation and for safety assessment. Whether hard lenses or one of the varieties of disposable soft lenses, the device itself is provided by prescription from a licensed professional and is placed into intimate contact with the eyes of the user on a daily basis over a period of years. The solutions used to clean and disinfect the lenses, however, are bought as over-the-counter consumer products without control on their direct sale.

Such disinfecting and cleaning solutions are considered and regulated as devices (as they are not supposed to have any direct therapeutic effect on the body and are essential for the use of the lenses themselves). Such solutions also have direct daily contact with the eyes of millions of individuals on a daily basis over a period of years. As such, they must be evaluated for both their potential local and systemic effects, and they are regulated under specific guidelines from the contact lens branch of the CDRH (1985; 1995a). The specialized test specifically mandated for their evaluation is the 21-day eye irritancy test in rabbits, as described later in this chapter. The component materials in such solutions must be carefully considered, however (and potentially evaluated experimentally) for systemic effects as well (Hackett and Stern, 1991). Such systemic toxicity evaluations are not generally performed in the rabbit, but are conducted with ocular administration of test solutions.

IV. SPECIFIC TESTS

A. Embryotoxicity

Device and labware (primarily disposable syringes and culture dishes) utilized in in vitro fertilization (IVF) clinics are required to be screened for embryotoxicity. Both the *Guidelines for Human Embryology and Andrology Laboratories* (1992; promulgated by the American Fertility Society) and the regulations of the Commission on Laboratory Accreditation of the College of American Pathologists require the performance of such tests to assess the media, materials, and supplies that will be used during human in vitro fertilization procedures. Three different test systems currently see some use, two forms of the mouse embryo test (one form that starts with a one-cell embryo and another that uses a two-cell embryo as a starting point) and the hamster sperm motility test. These in vitro embryo assays have been found to be effectively predictive of in vivo results (Neubert et al., 1986).

The mouse embryo test has significant limitations as a predictive screen for assessing the quality of the culture conditions used in human in vitro fertilization (Brigin et al., 1986). Its use is required, however, by the minimal standards for IVF programs presented by the American College of Obstetrics and Gynecology (ACOG; 600 Maryland Ave., S.W., Washington, D.C. 20024). There are numerous considerations for quality control and maintaining assay performance (Quinn and Whittingham, 1982; Rinehart et al, 1988; Roblero and Riffo, 1986; Saito et al., 1984; Wiley et al., 1986).

1. Mouse Embryo Assay

Despite its limitations, mouse embryo culture is the only simple reproducible method available for testing the embryo toxicity of culture conditions used in human IVF. Until a more sensitive system is developed, therefore, this assay is an essential component of a quality control program in human IVF (Biggers et al., 1981; Gianaroli et al., 1986; Davidson et al., 1988). There are numerous basic technique manuals for this methodology (Gerrity, 1988), and what is described here is adapted from these.

Materials.   Chemicals and media include the following:

1. Pregnant mare serum gonadotropin (PMSG; Diosynth Corporation, Chicago; Gestyl)
2. Human chorionic gonadotropin (Sigma Chemical Company, St. Louis; #CG-10)
3. Dulbecco's phosphate buffered saline (Gibco Labs, Grand Island, NY; #450-1300)
4. Ham's F-10 culture media (Gibco Labs, Grand Island, NY; #450-1200)
5. BWW media (optional)
6. Human serum albumin (Fraction V, Sigman Chemical Company, St. Louis; #A-1653)

Animals. F_1 of C_3B_6 (Charles Riber, Wilmington, MA); male and female mice are used. This strain of mouse responds well to superovulation and will undergo embryo development from two-cell stage to blastocyst in culture in 72 hr.

In selecting a strain of animals for use in this bioassay, it is essential to determine whether or not development from two-cell to blastocyst does occur in the strain selected (i.e., Is there a two-cell block in the strain that is intended for use?). The presence of a two-cell block can be investigated by harvesting both two-cell and four- to eight-cell embryos from the strain of mouse in question by simply altering the embryo collection times. These embryos are then cultured under the usual conditions. If development of the four- to eight-cell embryos proceeds to the blastocyst stage while the two-cell embryos have stopped development, a two-cell block exists. If development is poor in both groups, a problem with the culture medium should be suspected. The response of the mouse strain to superovulation regimens is also important; a minimum of 30 to 40 embryos from each animal is the goal. Finally, expense and availability in each geographic area may be important (Pannaud et al., 1987). It may also be cost-effective to use a less expensive strain of male mice. For a summary of these characteristics in various strains of mice, see Ackerman et al. (1983; 1984; 1985).

Mice should be housed under a 12-hr light/dark cycle (lights on at 6:00), with standard laboratory chow and water available ad libitum. Female mice may be group-housed according to appropriate American Association for Accreditation of Laboratory Animal Care standards (usually 4 to 5 to a cage). Male mice must be individually housed. For best results in mating, always add female mice to the male cage, *not* the reverse. Use only sexually mature animals (6–8 weeks of age); avoid using female animals that are aged (over 3 months). Replace all males every 4 to 5 months. Female mice may be randomly selected for injection without attention to the stage of the estrus cycle. All animals must acclimate to their new environment for 1 week after shipping.

Gonadotropins (PMSG + hCG)

1. Prepare stock solutions at a concentration of 100 IU/ml in saline or distilled water.
2. Freeze in small aliquots convenient for a single use. Do not refreeze gonadotropin after thawing.
3. Store PMSG and hCG in a freezer at 70°C or in a freezer that is *not* self-defrosting or frost-free. The freeze/thaw cycle of a standard kitchen frost-free refrigerator will inactivate frozen gonadotropins rapidly.
4. Never filter sterilize gonadotropins; they bind tightly to filters, leaving a biologically inactive (though sterile) solution.

Animal Preparation

1. To superovulate female animals, inject intraperitoneally with 7 IU of PMSG. For best results, inject animals between 3 and 6 p.m.

2. 48 hr after PMSG injection, inject animals with 7 IU of hCG. For best results, inject animals between 3 and 6 p.m.

3. Immediately after giving the hCG injection, place one female mouse into the cage of one male mouse. For best results, do not exceed two female mice per male mouse.

4. *Time of sacrifice.* Approximately 24 hr after hCG injection for one-cell embryos; approximately 36 hr after hCG injection for two-cell embryos. These times will vary somewhat with the strain of mouse used.

5. For guidelines on how many female mice to use for each assay, see Section IV.B.5.

It should be noted that frozen embryos are commercially available and may be used, although their baseline viability levels are less than those of fresh embryos. See Table 16.1 for a schedule summary.

Setup and Preparation

1. Place 1 ml of prewarmed Dulbecco's PBS in each of several 35-mm petri dishes (one dish per mouse). Place on a slide warmer to maintain approximate 37°C before use. Prepare several extra dishes of PBS for filling the flush syringe.

2. Pre-equilibrate the media and sera to be tested in an incubator containing 5% CO_2 in air, preferably overnight.

3. When testing media or sera, the following guidelines are useful. (These guidelines are illustrated in Table 16.2.)

    a. A control medium that has been previously tested must be used in addition to the test medium. Some laboratories make use of a standard medium that is known to support mouse embryo development, such as BWW medium or Tyrode solution, for this purpose.

TABLE 16.1   Schedule for Superstimulation of $F_1C_3B_6$ Mice

PMSG injection (3–6 p.m.)	HCG injection (3–6 p.m.)	Recovery: 1-cell embryo (3–6 p.m.)	Recovery: 2-cell embryo (8–10 a.m.)
Monday	Wednesday	Thursday	Friday
Tuesday	Thursday	Friday	Saturday
Wednesday	Friday	Saturday	Sunday
Thursday	Saturday	Sunday	Monday
Friday	Sunday	Monday	Tuesday
Saturday	Monday	Tuesday	Wednesday
Sunday	Tuesday	Wednesday	Thursday

TABLE **16.2** Example of Typical Setup for a Falcon 3047 Microtiter Plate to Test Five Different Treatments with Four Different Mice

Mouse number[b]	Treatment[a]				
	1	2	3	4	5
1	0	0	0	0	0
2	0	0	0	0	0
3	0	0	0	0	0
4	0	0	0	0	0

Note: Sample 1-ml microtiter plate (Falcon 3047) for mouse embryo culture. [a] Treatments (sample to be tested): 1. control medium—either BWW containing 3 mg/ml of human serum albumin (HAS) or Ham's F-10 (previously tested batch 100) + 3 mg/ml HAS; 2. unknown batch Ham's F-10 (e.g., batch 101) + 3 mg/ml HAS; 3. unknown fetal cord serum (FCS) batch 001 in batch 100 Ham's f-10; 4. unknown FCS batch 002 in batch 100 Ham's F-10; 5. unknown FCS batch 003 in batch 100 Ham's F-10, where batch 100 = previously tested Ham's F-10, batch 101 = unknown new batch of Ham's F-10.
[b] All of the embryos from each mouse to be evenly split across the five treatments.

The author recommends use of a previously tested batch of Ham's F-10 medium that is less than 3 weeks old.

b. When testing unknown (untested) sera, always test in a culture medium that has been previously tested.

c. A protein source must be added to the control medium as well as to the medium to be tested (Caro and Trounson, 1984; Ogawa et al. 1987). The protein source must be a previously tested batch of serum or human serum albumin (fraction V); concentration 3 mg/ml. (This source of protein should not be included in medium that is used to screen untested sera.)

d. There is a high degree of mouse-to-mouse variability in the rate of fertilization of ova and in the rate and number of embryos to complete development, therefore all of the embryos from one mouse should be pooled and divided evenly among treatment conditions.

e. Do not pool all embryos from all mice and then divide because of the large interanimal variation in development. If all the poor embryos are not evenly distributed across treatments, it may bias interpretation of the test results. Mice that yield greater than 25% fragmented, unfertilized, or one-cell embryos or embryos that have developed beyond the two-cell stage should be excluded from the testing procedure.

    f. For a sample of assay setup, see Table 16.2. For convenience, 1-ml microtiter plates (Falcon 3047) containing 1 ml of test media in each well may be used. These trays have four rows (A-D) and five columns (1–5).

    g. The setup of the test wells (the bioassay scheme) may be recorded.

4. Guidelines for deciding on the number of mice to inject are as follows:

    a. Each mouse should yield 30 to 40 embryos.

    b. It is best to have at least five embryos per treatment; therefore, one mouse could test five treatments easily. Replicates are required, so additional mice must be injected.

    c. Not all mice will superovulate.

    d. For the sample given in Table 16.2, five mice would have to be injected. At least five embryos from mouse 1 would be placed in wells A_1 through A_6. This process would be repeated with mouse 2 in row B, and so on.

    e. When testing a new batch of plasticware to determine if it is embryotoxic, always be certain to use embryos obtained from the same mouse grown in the same medium but placed in previously tested plasticware as a control.

    f. Media and sera for in vitro fertilization (IVF) should be tested in the incubator used for IVF as a quality control measure to evaluate the entire embryo culture system (Arny et al., 1987; Barrach and Neubert, 1980).

Removal of Oviducts.

1. Sacrifice animals by cervical dislocation.

2. Soak the animal with 70% alcohol to minimize hair contamination when the abdomen is opened.

3. Use coarse instruments to open the abdomen. Pneumothorax the animal. To accomplish this, make a midline cut from the pubic symphysis through the diaphragm using coarse scissors and forceps. Extend the cuts laterally to flap the skin back.

4. Using fine instruments, isolate the reproductive tract and identify the oviducts. (Refer to Figure 16.1.)

5. When removing the oviduct, it is important to avoid handling or squeezing the oviduct itself. For ease of handling, first sever the uterine horn as shown in Figure 16.1, cut 1. Use this piece of tissue as a kind of handle for grasping the tissue. Next cut the oviduct between the ovary and the oviduct as shown in Figure 16.1, cut 2. At this point, the oviduct is free from the mouse and is held by a piece of uterine

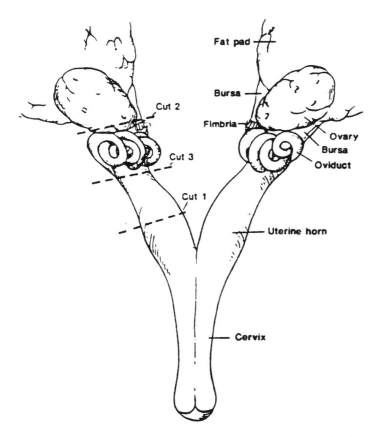

FIGURE 16.1   Schematic description of female mouse reproductive tract and surgical removal of oviducts.

horn. Hold this piece of tissue over a 30-mm petri dish containing
warm PBS. Holding the uterine horn, cut between the uterine horn and
the oviduct as in Figure 16.1, cut 3, allowing the oviduct to drop into
the warm PBS.

6.   Repeat with second oviduct.
7.   For best results, flush these two oviducts before proceeding to sacrifice
     the next mouse. Do not pool oviducts from several mice in the same dish.

Flushing the Oviducts

1.   Fill a 1-cc syringe with warm PBS and place a 30-gauge, 1-in. needle
     on the end. Sterile, disposable needles of this size are available from
     Becton Dickinson and are convenient and inexpensive to use. The

sharp end of this needle is a problem for some investigators, but practice can eliminate puncturing the sides of the oviduct. Some groups prefer to blunt the end of the needle using an emery board; these needles must be resterilized before use. Custom-made needles that have no bevel or point can also be ordered from several manufacturers, but these needles are expensive and are not disposable.

2. Place the 35-mm petri dish on the stage of the dissecting microscope and examine the oviduct grossly to identify the fimbria (refer to Figure 16.1) and the uterine end of the oviduct.

3. Carefully work the 30-gauge needle into the fimbriated end of the oviduct, using the forceps to grasp the oviduct. (Very fine watchmakers' forceps will make handling simpler.)

4. Gently press the plunger on the syringe and watch the embryos flush out of the uterine end of the oviduct. If the needle is properly placed, the injection of medium should partially distend the oviduct. Flushing should require no more than 0.1 ml of medium. The smaller the volume flushed, the easier the recovery of embryos once these have been flushed into the dish.

5. If the needle goes through the wall of the oviduct, withdraw it partially and attempt to pass the needle beyond the puncture site, grasping the oviduct distally. Flush again.

6. It is also possible to flush from the uterine end of the oviduct. This end has a more muscular wall and some will prefer to handle the oviduct at this end.

7. Check the dish to ensure that the embryos have been flushed.

8. If none of the above techniques work, it is also possible to use the needle and forceps to break the oviducts, allowing the embryos to spill out. This method is much more time-consuming, however, and the number of embryos obtained may be reduced.

9. Repeat the procedure with the second oviduct. Pool the embryos from both oviducts. Separate out all embryos that are not two-cell embryos (including fragmented embryos, one-cell embryos, and embryos at four cells or beyond). When collecting two-cell embryos, if more than 25% of the embryos recovered are unfertilized, fragmented, one-cell, or have developed beyond the two-cell stage, that mouse should not be used in testing and all of the embryos should be discarded. Place equal numbers of two-cell embryos in each treatment to be evaluated.

10. It is most convenient to handle the embryos using a Pasteur pipe pulled to a fine bore over a low flame and attached to a PiPump.

11. Place the microtiter plate containing the embryos in the incubator and repeat the procedures above with each mouse in sequence.

12. Record the total number of embryos in each well.

Monitoring and Analyzing Results

1. Mouse embryos should be observed at 24-hr intervals after placing in culture (i.e., 24, 48, and 72 hr after collection). Embryos may be examined directly under the dissecting microscope in the test wells of the microtiter plate or in petri dishes. The method used is a matter of personal preference. Petri dishes have a large surface area to scan in order to find and examine all of the embryos. While microtiter plates confine the embryos to a small area for observation, the optical properties of these dishes often make it difficult to see embryos that settle around the edges of the well. Flat-sided culture tubes have also been used for these purposes but necessitate a large volume of media and attention to adequate equilibration of the media. Finally, some investigators prefer to place the embryos on a slide with a coverslip; this method only permits observation of the embryos at the final observation time point.

2. The total number of embryos in each well should be verified and the state of development noted each day that the embryos are observed. Care must be taken to make these observations rapidly since the pH and temperature of the media will change while the embryos are outside the incubator. Such changes may retard embryonic development. For research applications, it is particularly useful to see if the rate of development is altered and at what stage development stopped. For the strain of mice used here ($F_1 C_3 B_6$), embryos should progress from two-cell to hatched blastocyst in 72 hr. Some labs prefer to make a single observation at 72 hr and record the percentage of total embryos that have progressed from two-cell to hatched blastocyst. If 75% of the embryos do not progress from two-cell to hatched blastocyst in 72 hr, the serum, media or other test substance should be considered less than optimal, and therefore discarded. Since mouse embryos are quite hardy when grown in culture, conditions that retard development should not be taken lightly. Media that "comes close to passing" should be retested before use. This would be reflected at 72 hr after embryo collection. Inspection of results at 24 and 48 hr will indicate when development stopped.

3. Timing of development

Stage of development	Time (hr)
1 cells	−12
2 cells	0 (time placed in culture)
4−8 cells	24
Morula	36
Early blastocyst	48
Hatched blastocyst	72

4. Returning to the example presented in Table 16.1, comparisons are within rows. (Control A_1 is compared to treatments A_2–A_6.) Comparisons between rows are an indication of the interanimal variation. From a statistical viewpoint, this interanimal variation must be taken into account before valid statistical comparisons using pooled date between mice can be made. If examination of results from mouse 1 indicate that in the control treatment (A1) only 50% of the embryos reached hatched blastocyst, this mouse should be dropped from the data set. (Please note that the purpose of this assay is to screen for embryo toxicity, so a good control group is essential. Use of this assay for a research application would not permit dropping of data.) If all controls A_1, B_1, C_1, and D_1 showed slowed development, however, the assay should be repeated.

5. The use of one-cell mouse embryos in addition to or even in place of two-cell embryos has been advocated (Quinn et al., 1984). These embryos are apparently more sensitive to adverse culture conditions than are two-cell embryos. There are also different requirements for embryo development from the one-cell to the two-cell stage than for two-cell and beyond, making their use a more rigorous quality control measure.

Uses of the Bioassay.   All new batches of media should be tested using the mouse embryo bioassay. Experience indicates that Ham's F-10 medium will support mouse embryo development for up to a month after preparation, but no conclusions can be drawn concerning effects on human embryo development. Furthermore, the purity of the water (the largest single component of the medium) will decline with time. As a precaution, the medium should be discarded 2 weeks after preparation. Gloves worn during any surgery or manipulation of the embryos may also be a source of problems (Naz et al., 1986).

All sera used in the IVF program should be tested in the mouse embryo bioassay after heat inactivation and filter sterilization. Experience indicates that far more sera than media will be rejected due to bioassay results. Although results vary from center to center (Condon–Mahoney et al., 1985), experience has demonstrated that less than 5% of media tested will be discarded based on results of mouse embryo culture. Careful screening of sera, however, leads to rejection of 25–30% of sera. Programs that do not test sera might inadvertently expose human embryos to embryo toxic serum and compromise success rates. The mouse embryo bioassay is not an all-or-nothing test; a test serum may permit growth to a four-cell, eight-cell, or even unhatched blastocyst stage. Obviously, the same sera used in the human IVF setting may yield seemingly normal embryonic development that actually halts after embryo transfer. The fact that human ova undergo fertilization and cleavage up to the point of transfer should not be taken as a sign that the sera are safe for embryos unless verified in the mouse serum.

Testing serum drawn using the IVF stimulation cycle is often not possible because of time constraints. In addition, if clomid is used during ovulation induction, it has a direct embryo toxic effect (Laufer et al., 1983). If maternal serum is to be used as a protein source, it must be drawn in a cycle prior to the IVF cycle to permit adequate testing. All sera used for IVF that are not actual matched patient sera should be screened for HTLV-III, hepatitis surface antigen, and core antibody. In cases in which IVF is used as a treatment of immunologic infertility or for infertility of unknown etiology, the patient's own serum should not be used. Alternatives include the use of fetal cord serum or appropriately screened donor serum.

The use of serum may not be necessary in human IVF. Caro and Trounson (1984) compared media without added protein or supplemented with albumin or fetal cord serum for the ability to sustain mouse embryo development in vitro. When the resultant embryos were transferred to pseudopregnant recipients, they produced pregnancy rates significantly higher than the group in which no protein supplementation was used. The same authors also did a similar study in a human IVF program (Caro and Trounson, 1986). In this report, 10% maternal serum in T6 culture medium was compared with T6 medium containing no protein. There was no significant difference in pregnancy rate in the group in which no protein was used to supplement the media. A similar result has been described by European investigators (Menezo et al., 1984; Feichtinger et al., 1986). Feichtinger's group made use of commercially available Menezo B-1 medium. Thus far these studies have not been done using Ham's F-10, the culture medium most widely used in the United States.

All new batches of plasticware, tubing, and so on, or any material that comes into contact with human eggs or embryos, should be tested for embryo toxicity. This is easily accomplished by placing known embryo-safe pretested medium in contact with the test surface (either by washing the medium or actually culturing embryos in it) and performing the assay as described. This is a useful method for testing the effectiveness of glassware-washing techniques, cleansing of surgical instruments (aspiration needle), transfer catheters, and any other item that comes in contact with the human eggs, sperm, or embryos. Adverse effects of plasticware on embryo development have also been described by Schiewe et al. (1984).

In summary, when using this strain of mice, any condition that does not result in mouse embryo development from the two-cell to hatched blastocyst in 72 hr should be discarded or re-evaluated.

The limitations of this assay are often overlooked. It can only detect conditions that are grossly and harshly embryonic. It cannot detect or differentiate growth-promoting factors. Perhaps pregnancies in IVF programs are associated with the coincidental use of serum containing a growth-promoting factor that cannot be discerned by the mouse embryo assay. The addition of protein to the medium may absorb toxic substances, as may the amino acids present in Ham's F-10 medium. The medium may therefore quench the system, dampening the sensitivity of the assay. It is therefore possible that mouse embryos will develop in conditions that might slow or stop human development. In the human RAF-ET procedure, embryos are transferred at an early stage of development. It is possible that these embryos stagger through one or two cleavage divisions, after which they cease development. This same phenomenon often occurs in the mouse embryo system in the presence of embryotoxic substances, but only longer periods of observation allow detection of the problem. Many labs have had experience with mouse embryos growing in a variety of conditions that are less than optimal. These embryos appear to be relatively indestructible when grown in Ham's F-10.

Some laboratories formerly made use of sperm viability assays for testing culture media, sera, and so on. Human spermatozoa from normal men, however, are even more resistant to adverse conditions than are mouse embryos. In addition, the end point of sperm viability is usually a subjective parameter (e.g., motility) (Gorrill et al., 1991). This method has therefore been largely abandoned. Perhaps this method of media evaluation will be resurrected when computer-assisted, objective methods of measurement of sperm motility, velocity, and even lateral head displacement are more widely available. Finally, a hamster sperm viability assay has recently been devised that purports even greater sensitivity to embryotoxic factors and is simpler, more chemically defined, and more economical than the mouse bioassay. A bioassay system for embryo-derived platelet-activating factor has been described for differentiating viable embryos. This assay may be useful for predicting the success of embryo transfer (O'Neill et al., 1985). Frozen mouse embryos are now available commercially for use in IVF quality control. Unfortunately, these embryos are frozen at the eight-cell stage and have therefore bypassed the more sensitive stages of development. Furthermore, to carry out adequate quality control testing weekly would be prohibitively expensive.

In conclusion, there is a need for objective, sensitive, and reproducible methods for testing materials used in human IVF for both embryotoxic and growth-promoting factors. The limitations of the mouse embryo bioassay are obvious; however, it is the standard of practice in the field and should be required in all settings. The hamster sperm motility assay should be considered as an alternative to the mouse embryo assay.

V. TWENTY-ONE-DAY EYE IRRITATION STUDY IN RABBITS

This study is intended to identify the irritation potential of a test contact lens or lens disinfectant solution compared to that caused by a control lens or disinfectant solution.

Sixteen young adult (2–3.5 kg) New Zealand white rabbits are randomized into two groups.

Test and control lenses (or lenses soaked in test and control disinfectants) are inserted into the right eyes of each rabbit in the appropriate group (control or test) once daily for 21 consecutive days. The test or control contact lens will be carefully placed over the cornea of each rabbit. The lens will remain in place for 24 hr. After 24 hr the contact lens will be removed, the eye examined, and a new lens placed on the cornea for 24 hr. This procedure will be repeated for 21 consecutive days. The treated eye of each animal is examined and scored for irritation of the cornea, iris, and conjunctiva pretest prior to each daily application of the contact lens and again 24 hr following the last application (day 22). A handheld source of illumination will be used to aid in examining the eyes. Ocular responses will be graded according to the scale in Table 16.3. Additional signs will be described.

A. Analysis of Data

Calculations. The primary eye irritation score for each rabbit is calculated from the weighted Draize scale. The method of calculation is indicated on the scale included herein.

Interpretation. The interpretation of the scores recorded is based on the number of rabbits with positive scores. A positive score is any score for opacity of units, or a score of 2 or more for redness or chemosis.

Irritant. An irritant is a test article that under the conditions of this study causes a positive score in four to six rabbits with unwashed eyes [16 CFR 1500.3(c)(4)].

Indeterminate. If positive scores are noted in two to three animals with unwashed eyes, irritation potential of the test article is not classified.

Nonirritant. If positive scores are recorded in no animals or one animal, the test article is classified as a nonirritant.

VI. SYSTEMIC INJECTION TEST

This test (USP, 1996) is designed to evaluate systemic responses to the extracts of materials under test following injection into mice. Long both an FDA requirement and mainstay for use in quality control of lots of devices, now it is not either because of careful consideration of the minimal benefit derived despite the significant use of animals involved.

A. Test Animal

Use healthy, not previously used albino mice weighing between 17 and 23 grams. For each test group use only mice of the same source. Allow water and food, commonly used for laboratory animals and of known composition, ad libitum.

TABLE 16.3 Scale for Scoring Ocular Lesions

1.	Cornea	
	a. Opacity: degree of density (area most dense taken for reading):	
	No ulceration or opacity	0
	Scattered or diffuse areas of opacity (other than slight dulling of normal luster), details of iris clearly visible	1
	Easily discernible translucent area, details of iris slightly obscured	2
	Opalescent areas, no details of iris visible, size of pupil barely discernible	3
	Opaque cornea, iris not discernible through the opacity	4
	b. Area of cornea involved:	
	One-quarter (or less), but not zero	1
	Greater than one-quarter, but less than one-half	2
	Greater than one-half, but less than three-quarters	3
	Greater than three-quarters up to whole area	4
	Score = A × B × 5	
	Maximum total	80

2.	Iris	
	a. Values:	
	Normal	0
	Folds above normal, congestion, swelling, circumcorneal injection (any or all of these or combination of any thereof), iris still reacting to light (sluggish reaction is positive)	1
	No reaction to light, hemorrhage, gross destruction (any or all of these)	2
	Score = A × 5	
	Maximum total	10

3.	Conjunctivae	
	a. Redness (refers to palpebral and bulbar conjunctivae excluding cornea and iris):	
	Blood vessels normal	0
	Some blood vessels definitely hyperemic (injected)	1
	More diffuse, deeper crimson red, individual vessels not easily discernible	2
	Diffuse beefy red	3
	b. Chemosis:	
	No swelling	0
	Any swelling above normal (includes nictating membranes)	1
	Obvious swelling with partial eversion of lids	2
	Swelling with lids about half closed	3
	Swelling with lids more than half closed	4
	c. Discharge:	
	No discharge	0
	Any amount different from normal (does not include small amounts observed in inner canthus of normal animals)	1
	Discharge with moistening of the lids and hairs just adjacent to lids	2
	Discharge with moistening of the lids and hairs and considerable area around the eye	3
	Score = (A + B + C) × 2	
	Maximum total	20

Source: Draize et al., 1944.

TABLE 16.4 Injection Procedure—Systemic Injection Test

Extract or blank	Dose/kg	Route[a]	Injection rate (μ1/sec)
Sodium chloride injection	50 ml	IV	100
1 in 20 solution of alcohol in sodium chloride injection	50 ml	IV	100
Polyethylene glycol 400	10 g	IP	—
Drug product vehicle (where applicable)	50 ml	IV	100
	50 ml	IP	—
Vegetable oil	50 ml	IP	—

[a] IV = intravenous (aqueous sample and blank); IP = intraperitoneal (oleaginous sample and blank).

B. Procedure

Agitate each extract vigorously prior to withdrawal of injection doses to ensure even distribution of the extracted matter. Visible particulates should not be injected intravenously, however. Inject each of the five mice in a test group with the test sample or the control blank as outlined in Table 16.4, except to dilute each gram of the extract of the test sample prepared with polyethylene glycol 400, and the corresponding blank with 4.1 volumes of sodium chloride injection to obtain a solution having a concentration of about 200 mg of polyethylene glycol per ml.

Observe the animals immediately after injection, again 4 hr after injection, and then at least 24, 48, and 72 h later. If during the observation period none of the animals treated with the extract of the test sample shows a significantly greater biological reactivity than the animals treated with the control blank, the test sample meets the requirements of this test. If any animals treated with the test sample show only slight signs of biological reactivity and not more than one animal shows gross symptoms of biological reactivity or dies, repeat the test using groups of 10 mice. On the repeat test, the material passes if all 10 animals treated with the test sample show no significant biological reactivity above that seen in the test blank animals.

VII. PRODUCTION OF TOXIC SHOCK SYNDROME TOXIN-1 (TSST-1)

Tampons that were found to be associated with the highest risk of TSS, including those made of polyester foam plus carboxymethylcellulose chips and polyacrylate rayon, differed from the other products principally in their chemical composition. A system has been developed for testing designed primarily to determine whether or not tampon fibers and other components have the propensity to increase production of TSST-1 (Parsonnet et al., 1996; Wong and Downs, 1989). Cultivation conditions and toxin analyses are such that small differences in TSST-1 can be detected—differences that may not be manifest under less hospitable conditions. All experiments are performed with the investigators blinded as to the nature of the test products in order to prevent bias in the interpretation of laboratory results. Codes are not broken until the results have been submitted to the manufacturer. All test products and controls are either cultivated simultaneously (in triplicate) or with one sample of each product (and control) represented in a series of consecutive experiments. Two types of controls are run with each experiment: culture medium alone, in order to determine whether or not the test products induce production of more TSST-1 than is made in the absence of a tampon, and incubation with tampons, that were associated with the highest risk of TSS and that have been shown to increase production of TSST-1 in a variety of test systems. This system is well suited to identify any adverse influence of tampon constituents on production of TSST-1 and accordingly, on risk of TSS.

A. Methods

1. Materials

Strain MN8, a TSST-1 producing strain of *Staphylococcus aureus* isolated from a patient with menstrual TSS, is used in these experiments. Bacteria are cultivated in medium consisting of 3% N-Z-amine A (Sheffield Products, Norwich, NY), a pancreatic digest of casein, plus 1% yeast extract (Difco Laboratories, Detroit), which is known to yield high levels of toxin (Wong and Downs, 1989).

    Tampons (with the investigators being blinded as to the chemical composition of constitutive fibers and additives) constitute the test material. Rely Regular tampons are used as controls. Each tampon is weighed and the mean weight of each type of tampon is calculated. As there was a narrow range of weights for each type of tampon, the mean weight of each type is used to calculate how much medium to use in cultivations. Tampons are sterilized by exposure to ethylene oxide using an Anprolene sterilizer.

2. Shake-Flask Cultivations

Tampons are placed in sterile fashion into 250-ml Erlenmeyer flasks, to which are added appropriate volumes of culture medium so as to yield a constant weight/volume ratio of tampon to medium of 4%. All tampons are tested in triplicate in a single experiment except for Rely, which is run in duplicate. Three flasks containing medium alone are inoculated as a control. Strain MN8 is suspended in medium to an optical density of 0.8 at 650 nm, which is intended to yield a bacterial concentration of approximately 1.0×10^9 cfu/ml at the start of incubation.

Flasks are incubated in a shaking water bath under the following conditions: 37.0°C, 90 revolutions per min, and gas mixture of 5% carbon dioxide, 20% oxygen, and 75% nitrogen. This set of conditions has been shown to yield high levels of TSST-1 in vitro. After 20 hr, culture fluids are decanted from the flasks in order to recover all fluid not retained by the tampons. Experiments have shown that the decantate is also representative of fluid retained by the tampon, in terms of both bacterial numbers and concentration of toxin. Culture fluids are streaked onto blood agar plates to check for purity, and aliquots are removed for determination of bacterial numbers. Bacteria are then removed by centrifugation and the resultant supernatants are harvested for testing for TSST-1, which is measured using a competitive ELISA, as described by Parsonnet et al. (1985).

3. Statistics

Results from replicate samples are pooled for statistical analysis. Results of test tampons and Rely are compared with those of medium along by ANOVA, with statistical significance determined by Fisher's protected least significant difference test (P,0.05). Two analyses are run, one including all samples and one excluding Rely regular tampons.

VIII. IN VITRO EVALUATION OF THE EFFECTS OF POTENTIAL TAMPON MATERIALS ON pH AND GROWTH OF VAGINAL MICROFLORA

The role of vaginal microflora both as a protective element against and as a possible catalyst for the development of TSS has received considerable attention during the last 5 years. The recognition that many cases of TSS are associated with menstruation, along with the widespread use of tampons in this country, has led to the proposal that this form of catamenial protection may alter the normal microflora during menstruation and thus potentiate the proliferation of *Staphylococcus aureus* and the production of TSST-1.

Bartlett et al. (1977) evaluated both the quantitative and qualitative composition of the vaginal microflora in a study of a small group of women. These volunteers submitted self-obtained swabs during a single menstrual cycle, including the menstrual period. The most noteworthy finding was that the number of anaerobes remained relatively constant during the entire cycle, although there was considerable variation from an additional group of volunteers whenever in the course of the menstrual cycle they appeared for a vaginal examination. A quantitative assessment of the microflora for both groups combined revealed a 100-fold decrease in the number of anaerobes in the last week of the menstrual cycle compared with the numbers obtained during menstrual flow.

These findings were confirmed by the observations of Sautter and Brown (1980), who obtained vaginal swabs for a small number of volunteers several times during 1 month. They found that the variety of bacterial phenotypes isolated from any individual remained relatively constant, but that the numbers of each microbial species changed at different times during the cycle.

In a more extensive study conducted by Johnson et al. (1985), samples were obtained from 34 women by a vaginal wash method during both the menstrual and intermenstrual phase of the cycle. Quantitative assessment of the microflora during the menstrual cycle revealed that the total number of bacteria did not change significantly from one sample interval to another. Qualitative evaluation in the microflora did show significant variations during the menstrual cycle.

A. Method

Six strains representative of bacterial species commonly isolated as part of the vaginal microflora of menstruating women are used to evaluate the effect of tampons on bacterial growth in vitro (Onderonk et al., 1977; 1987 a, b). Three strains (*Lactobacillus acidophilus, Prevotella bivia*, and *Peptostreptococcus anaerobius*) are included as representatives of the obligate anaerobes, and three strains (*Staphylococcus aureus, S. epidermidis*, and *E. coli*) are included as representatives of the facultative anaerobes present as part of the vaginal microflora. All six strains are grown in a defined medium simulating genital tract secretions under the anaerobic conditions associated with the human vagina. For each bacterial strain, two duplicate flasks containing approximately one-half of a tampon are inoculated and sampled as described previously. In addition, two control flasks containing defined medium and no tampon material are inoculated with the same bacterial strain for each strain. Each flask was sampled at time 0 and after 24 and 48 hr of incubation, and the aliquots of each sample were plated onto appropriate media for a determination of total counts. All counts are recorded as the $\log_{10}$ cfu/ml of medium. Differences between the broth control and any of the test tampons is noted after 24 and 48 hr of incubation. Differences of less than one log in counts are within the normal variability for this growth system and are considered to be random observations rather than specific trends.

One can also measure the effect on pH of the vaginal duplicating media (VDM) following addition of test materials. Each measurement is performed in triplicate and the mean value plotted. The medium is adjusted to have a starting pH of either 5.0 or 6.0 to assess the buffering ability of the test substance on the test broth.

One can also measure the effect that tampons containing various concentrations of new materials have on VDM broth pH when placed into the broth solutions. The pH is measured at 1, 2, and 3 hr after tampon addition and the results expressed as the change from the starting pH of the broth prior to addition of the tampon. Each tampon is tested in triplicate. In order to assess the maximal potential effect of tampon addition, the VDM is adjusted to a starting pH of 5.0.

IX. INFLAMMATORY RESPONSES TO BIOMATERIALS

To test the inflammatory responses induced by biomaterials, the cage implant system (Jurgenson et al., 1990) is most often used. This system allows the sequential examination of the exudate surrounding the implant without the need to sacrifice the animal. Utilizing this investigation, too, Merchant et al. (1984) have shown that monocytes and macrophages follow the appearance of neutrophils in the exudate and that macrophages have a preferential adsorption to the biomaterial. Neutrophils have a relatively shorter presence (hours to days,) and disappear from the exudate more rapidly than macrophages, which remain for days to weeks or longer in the presence of a foreign body or infection. Eventually macrophages become the predominant cell type in the exudate, resulting in a chronic inflammatory response.

REFERENCES

AAMI. (1996). Biological Evaluation of Medical Devices, 5th ed., AMI, Rockville, MD.

Ackerman, S. B., Swanson, F. J., Adams, P. J., and Wortham, J. W. E. Jr., (1983). Comparison of strains and culture media used for mouse in vitro fertilization, Gamete Res., 7: 103–109.

Ackerman, S. B., Swanson, F. J., Stokes, G. K., and Veeck, L. L. (1984). Culture of mouse preimplantation embryos as a quality control assay for human in vitro fertilization, Gamete Res., 9: 145–152.

Ackerman, S. B., Stokes, G. L., Swanson, R. J., Tailor, S. P., and Fenwick, L. (1985). Toxicity testing for human in vitro fertilization programs, J. in Vitro Fert. Embryo Transfer, 2: 132–137.

Arny, M., Nachtigall, L., and Quagliarello, J. (1987). The effect of preimplantation culture conditions on murine embryo implantation and fetal development, Fert. Ster., 48: 861.

Barrach, H. J. and Neubert, D. (1980). Significance of organ culture techniques for evaluation of prenatal toxicity, Arch. Toxicol., 45: 161–187.

Bartlett, J. G., Onderdonk A. B., Drude, E., et al. (1977). Quantitative bacteriology of the vaginal flora, J. Infec. Dis., 136: 271–277.

Bechert, T., Steinepicke, P., and Guggenbichler, J. (2000). A new method for screening anti-infective biomaterials, Nature Med., 6(8): 1053–1056.

Biggers, J. D., Whitten, W. K., and Whittingham, D. G. (1981). The culture of mouse embryos in vitro. In: Methods in Mammalian Embryology (J. C. Daniel Jr., Ed.). W. H. Freeman, San Francisco, pp. 86–116.

Bisno, A. L. and Waldnagel, F. A. (1994). Infections Associated with Indwelling Medical Devices, 2nd ed, American Society for Microbiology, Washington, DC.

Brigin, J., Hogan, B., et al. (1986). Manipulating the Mouse Embryo, Cold Spring Harbor Laboratory, Cold Spring Harbor, NY.

Caro, C. M. and Trounson, A. (1984). The effect of protein on preimplantation mouse embryo development in vitro, J. in Vitro Fert. Embryo Transfer, 1: 183–187.

Caro, C. M. and Trounson, A. (1986). Successful fertilization, embryo development, and pregnancy in human in vitro fertilization (IVF) using a chemically defined culture medium containing no protein, J. in Vitro Fert. Embryo Transfer, 3: 215–217.

CDRH. (1985). Testing Guidelines for Class III Soft (Hydrophillic) Contact Lens Solutions, Contact Lens Branch, ODE, CDRH, DFA, July.

CDRH. (1995a). Premarket Notification (510(k)) Guidance Document for Contact Lens Care Products, Contact Lens Branch, ODE, CDRH, U.S. Food and Drug Administration, June 7.

CDRH. (1995b). Draft Guidance for the Content of Premarket Notification for Menstrual Tampons, Obstetrics-Gynecology Devices Branch, ODE, CDRH, U.S. Food and Drug Administration, May 25.

Condon-Mahoney, M., Wortham, J. W. E. Jr., Bundren, J. C., Witmyer, J., and Shirley, B. (1985). Evaluation of human fetal cord sera, Ham's F-10 medium, and in vitro culture materials with a mouse in vivo fertilization system, Fert. Ster., 44: 521–525.

Davidson, A., Vermesh, M., Lobo, R. A., and Paulson, R. J. (1988). Mouse embryo culture as quality control for human in vitro fertilization: The one-cell versus the two-cell model, Fert. Ster., 49: 516.

Draize, J. H., Woodard, G., and Calvery, H. O. (1944). Methods for the study of irritation and toxicity of substances applied topically to the skin and mucous membrane, J. Pharm. Exp. Ther., 82: 377–390.

Feichtinger, W., Kemeter, P., and Menezo, Y. (1986). The use of synthetic culture medium and patient serum for human in vitro fertilization and embryo replacement, J. in Vitro Fert. Embryo Transfer, 3: 87–92.

Gerrity, M. (1988). Mouse embryo culture and bioassay. In: In Vitro Fertilization and Embryo Transfer: A Manual of Basic Techniques (E. P. Wolf, Ed.). Plenum, New York, pp. 57–76.

Gianaroli, L., Seracchioli, R., Ferraretti, A. P., Trounson, A., Flamigni, C., and Bovicelli, L. (1986). The successful use of human amniotic fluid for mouse embryo culture and human in vitro fertilization, embryo culture and transfer, Fert. Ster., 46: 907.

Gorrill, R., Rinehart, J., Tamhane, A. C., and Gerrity, M. (1991). Comparison of the hamster sperm motility assay to the mouse one-cell and two-cell embryo bioassays as quality control tests for in vitro fertilization, Fert. Ster., 55(2): 345–354.

Guidelines for Human Embryology and Andrology Laboratories (1992), Fert. Ster. supplement 1, 58: 4, pp. 1A–16S.

Hackett, D. W. and Stern, M. E. (1991). Preclinical toxicology/safety considerations in the development of opthalmic drugs and devices. In: Dermal and Ocular Toxicology (D. W. Hobson, Ed.). CRC Press, Boca Raton, FL.

ISO. (1989a). Cardiovascular implants—Cardiac valve prostheses. ISO 5840-1.

ISO. (1989b). Cardiac pacemakers—Part 1: Implantable pacemakers. ISO 5840-1.

ISO. (1989c). Cardiovascular Implants—Tubular Vascular Prostheses—Part 1: Synthetic Vascular Prostheses. ISO 7198-1.

ISO. (1989d). Cardiovascular Implants—Tubular Vascular Prostheses—Part 2: Sterile Vascular Prostheses of Biological Origin—Specification and Methods of Test. ISO 7198-2.

ISO. (1989e). Cardiovascular Implants and Artificial Organs—Blood–Gas Exchangers. ISO 7199.

Johnson, S. R., Petxold, C. R., and Galask, R. P., (1985). Qualitative and quantitative changes of the vaginal microbial flora during the menstrual cycle, Amer. J. Repro. Immunol. Microbio., 9: 1–5.

Jurgensen, C. H., Huber, C. H., Zimmerman, T. P., and Worlber, G. (1990). 3-Deazaadenosine inhibits leukocyte adhesion and ICAM-1 biosynthesis in tumor necrosis factor-stimulated human endothelial cells, J. Immunol., 144: 653.

Laufer, N., Pratt, B. M., DeCherney, A. H., Naftolin, F., Merino, M., and Merkert, C. L. (1983). The in vivo and in vitro effects of clomiphene citrate on ovulation, fertilization, and development of cultured mouse oocytes, Amer. J. Ob. Gyn., 147: 633–639.

Menezo, Y., Testart, J., and Perrone, D. (1984). Serum is not necessary in human in vitro fertilization, early embryo culture, and transfer, Fert. Ster., 42: 750–755.

Merchant, R., Anderson, J. M., Phua, K., and Hiltner, A. (1984). In vivo biocompatibility studies. II. Biomer: Preliminary cell adhesion and surface characterization studies, J. Biomed. Mat. Res., 18, 309.

Naz, R. K., Janousek, J. T., Moody, T., and Stillman, R. J. (1986). Factors influencing murine embryo bioassay: Effects of proteins, aging of medium, and surgical glove coatings, Fert. Ster., 46: 914.

Neubert, D., Blankenburg, G., Chahoud, I., et al. (1986). Results of in vivo and in vitro studies for assessing prenatal toxicity, Environ. Health Persp., 70: 89–103.

Ogawa, T. and Marrs, R. P. (1987). The effect of protein supplementation on single-cell mouse embryos in vitro, Fert. Ster., 47: 156.

Onderdonk, A. B., Zamarchi, G. R., Rodriguez, M. L., Hirsch, M. L., Munoz, A., and Kass, E. H. (1987a). Quantitative assessment of vaginal microflora during the use of tampons of various compositions, Appl. Environ. Microbio., 53: 2774–2778.

Onderdonk, A. B., Zemarchi, G. R., Rodriguez, M. L., Hirsch, M. L., Munoz, A. and Kass, E. H. (1987b). Qualitative assessment of vaginal microflora during use of tampons of various compositions, Appl. Environ. Microbio., 53: 2779–2784.

Onderdonk, A. B., Polk, B. F., Moon, N. E., Goren, B., and Bartlett, J. G. (1977). Methods for quantitative vaginal flora studies, Amer. J. Ob. Gyn., 122: 777–781.

O'Neill, C., Pike, I. L., Porter, R. N., Gidley-Baird, A. A., Sinosich, M. H., and Saunders, D. N. (1985). Maternal recognition of pregnancy prior to implantation: Methods of monitoring embryonic viability in vitro and in vivo, Ann. NY Acad. Sci., 442: 429–439.

Pannaud, J., Reme, J. M., Monrozies, X., Favrin, S., Sarramon, M. F., and Pontonnier, G. (1987). Mouse system quality control is necessary before the use of new material for in vitro fertilization and embryo transfer, J. in Vitro Fert. Embryo Transfer, 4: 56.

Parsonnet, J., Mills, J. T., Gillis, Z. A., and Pier, B. G. (1985). Competitive, enzyme-linked immunosorbent assay for toxic shock syndrome toxin-1, J. Clin. Microbio., 22: 26–31.

Parsonnet, J., Modern, P. A., and Giacobbe, K. D. (1996). Effect of tampon composition on the production of toxic shock syndrome toxin-1 by *Staphylococcus aureus* in vitro, J. Infect. Dis., 173.

Quinn, P. and Whittingham, D. G. (1982), Effect of fatty acids on fertilization and development of mouse embryos in vitro, J. Androl., 3: 440.

Quinn, P., Warners, G. N., Kerin, J. F., and Kirby, C. (1984). Culture factors in relation to the success of human in vitro fertilization and embryo transfer, Fert. Ster., 41: 202–209.

Rinehart, J. S., Bavister, B. D., and Gerrity, M. (1988). Quality control in the in vitro fertilization laboratory: Comparison of bioassay systems for water quality, J. in Vitro Fert. Embryo Transfer, 5: 335.

Roblero, L. S. and Riffo, M. D. (1986). High potassium concentration improves preimplantation development of mouse embryos in vitro, Fert. Ster., 45: 412.

Saito, H., Berger. T., Mishell, D. R., and Marrs, R. P. (1984). Effect of variable concentration of serum on mouse embryo development, Fert. Ster., 41: 460.

Sautter, R. L. and Brown, W. J. (1980). Sequential vaginal cultures from normal young woman, J. Clin. Microbio., 11: 479–484.

Schiewe, M. C., Schmidt, P. M., Bush, M., and Wildt, D. E. (1984) Effect of absorbed/retained ethylene oxide in plastic culture dishes on embryo development in vitro, Theriogenology, 21: 2160 (abstract).

USP. (1996). Systemic injection test. In: United States Pharmacopoeia XXIII, United States Pharmacopoeia Convention, Rockville, MD.

Wiley, L. M., Yamami, S., and Van Muyden, D. (1986). Effect of potassium concentration, type of protein supplement, and embryo density on mouse preimplantation development in vitro, Fert. Ster., 45: 111.

Wong, A. C. L. and Downs, S. A. (1989). Investigation by improved syringe method of effect of tampons on production in vitro of toxic shock syndrome toxin-1 by *Staphylococcus aureus*, J. Clin. Microbio., 27: 2482–2487.

17

Case Histories and Problem Resolution

Public and societal perceptions of the safety of medical devices (and therefore, to a large extent, regulatory requirements to establish safety prior to marketing) have been shaped by the "known" history of the issue. Unfortunately, the publicly known history is primarily based on what has appeared in the popular press, which continues to mean primarily a litany of problems.

The last 30 years have seen six cases of significance in the public mind. By examining these six cases, their causes, the regulatory responses to them, and solutions to the problems they revealed, the medical device researcher and developer can learn some valuable lessons. After reviewing these cases, biocompatability problem-solving approaches, and the means to place actual risks in context, risk assessment will be considered.

I. PHTHALATE AND OTHER RESIDUALS LEACHING FROM DEVICES

Since the Second World War, plastics have come to be used as the major material in the fabrication of disposable medical devices. Starting in the early 1960s, reports began to appear about the toxicity of various chemical additives used in plastic formulations (Guess and O'Leary, 1969; Autian, 1972; Mayer et al., 1972; Eckardt and Hinden, 1973), particularly those in polyvinylchloride (PVC), which were found to readily leach out into blood and IV solutions stored in or passing through them. Much of this attention came to focus on the phthalate plasticizers, particularly di-2-ethylbenzyl phthalate (DEHP).

Studies clearly established that there was a time-dependent leaching of DEHP from PVC bags into blood and blood components stored in such bags, even at refrigerator temperatures (4°C) used for prolonged storage of the blood materials (Peck et al., 1979; Sasakawa and Mitomi, 1978; Miripol and Stern, 1977; Jaeger and Rubin, 1973). Such migration also occurred from other PVC devices into blood, IV fluids, and dialysis fluids, which also had significant contact time with such plastics. The two populations with the greatest resulting exposures were hemophiliacs (who received frequent transfusions of blood) and kidney dialysis patients (who received treatment three or four times a week).

Studies in monkeys (Peck et al., 1979), rats (Daniel and Bratt, 1973; Carter et al., 1974), and stored human blood (Rock et al., 1978) also established that significant portions of the DEHP was hydrolyzed to mono-2-ethyl-hexylphthalate (MEHP). The amount of lipids in the blood strongly influenced the rate of leaching.

Both DEHP and MEHP at relatively low concentrations cause liver damage (Lake et al., 1976; Nikonorow et al., 1973), and both compounds accumulate in the fatty tissue of the liver. At high levels in the diet, DEHP causes liver cancer in rodents (Sheftel, 1994).

DEHP was subsequently discontinued as a plasticizer after a great deal of concern and study. Other additives (benzothiazoles and other vulcanization accelerators in rubbers, e.g.) and contaminants (e.g., nickel and chromium) have subsequently also been found to migrate into solutions in contact with them (Lazarus, 1980; Petersen et al., 1981; Meek and Pettit, 1985; Roster and Gruenwald, 1986).

It should be expected that there will be migration of some amount of any residual monomer, additive, or contaminant in a plastic or elastomer used in devices into any fluid (or mucous membrane tissue) with which there is contact. If any of these leachable materials is also toxic, there may be a risk to patients— real or perceived. It is essential to know the composition of materials used in devices at least qualitatively, and should one of the potentially leachable materials present a hazard, it becomes essential to know how much is present and (if the amount present is sufficient) how much is leached into solutions and the amount of time that the device will be in contact. The issue was given new life in the period from 1998 to 2001 due to our technological ability to measure increasingly small amounts of phthalates in human tissue.

II. DALKON SHIELD

Efforts to prevent pregnancy by placing a foreign object in a woman's uterus date back many centuries. Devices made of glass, ivory, wood, wool, silkworm gut, silver, gold, copper, zinc, and pewter in a variety of sizes and shapes have all been used for this purpose. The reason for the contraceptive effect of an intra-uterine device (IUD), that does not create a barrier to the entry of sperm into the uterus, has never been satisfactorily established. One theory is that in its reaction to the device the body produces white cells that destroy the sperm or the fertilized egg. Another is that the IUD somehow interferes with the ability of the fertilized egg to attach itself or to remain attached to the wall of the uterus.

Infection and injury have historically been associated with IUDs, and they were not widely used until the late 1960s. Then, growing dissatisfaction with the adverse effects of birth control pills, together with mounting concern over the "population explosion," caused renewed interest in the development of a safe IUD as a means of contraception. The possibility was enhanced by two scientific advances. One was the development of antibiotics that provided a method of treating those uterine infections that did occur. The other was the invention of malleable, inert plastic, which could be compressed during insertion and then regain its intended shape, and which would not break down or chemically interact with bodily fluids.

The Dalkon Shield intrauterine device was designed in 1968 by Hugh Davis, a gynecologist on the faculty of the Johns Hopkins Medical School, and Irwin Lerner, an electrical engineer and part-time inventor. In 1964 John Hopkins had opened a family planning clinic under Davis's supervision, and through this clinic Davis was able to test various newly developed IUDs, mostly on low-income, black women from Baltimore. A major design problem with most of these IUDs was the frequency with which they were expelled as a result of the body's natural efforts to rid itself of a foreign object.

The Dalkon Shield was specifically designed to control the problem of expulsion. It is a piece of flexible plastic, about ¾ in. across, shaped like a shield to approximate the shape of the uterine cavity. The device has four or five prongs jutting out of each side at a downward angle. Because of the direction of the prongs, the device resisted expulsion. The same prongs often made insertion or removal painful and difficult, however, and they were responsible for the tendency of the device to embed itself in the uterine wall or to perforate the uterus.

A more serious design problem of the Dalkon Shield related to its string. One end of the string was tied to the bottom of the plastic shield and the other end was tied in a knot. When the device was in the uterus, the string passed through the cervix into the vagina. Its purpose was to allow the woman to check that the device was in place and to assist in its removal.

"Tailstrings" designed to serve these purposes are found on all IUDs, but on IUDs other than the Dalkon Shield the tailstring is made of a single plastic filament—a "monofilament"—in order to avoid the absorption of moisture, and with it bacteria. The entry of bacteria from the vagina into the uterus is a major cause of dangerous and potentially life-threatening uterine infections, known as pelvic inflammatory disease (PID). Frequently, a hysterectomy must be performed to overcome PID, and even when a hysterectomy is not necessary, infertility can result.

Davis and Lerner did not use a monofilament string on their new Dalkon Shield. The monofilament strings they tested were either too weak and would break during removal because of the resistance offered by the prongs, or too stiff and would cause discomfort to the man during intercourse. Instead, Davis and Lerner used a multifilament string, named Supramid, which was composed of hundreds of tiny nylon strands encased in a nylon sheath. Supramid was made by a company in West Germany and used primarily in the repair of horse tendons. Davis and Lerner hoped that the sheath would prevent vaginal fluid from entering the spaces between the strands and moving up into the uterus, a phenomenon called "wicking" (Sobol, 1991).

For two reasons, the sheath did not do its job. First, Davis and Lerner inexplicably failed to seal its ends. Fluid from the vagina could enter into the open end at the bottom of the sheath and wick up past the knots to the open end at the top inside the uterus. Indeed, the nylon sheath made the problem of wicking worse because it shielded the bacteria inside the sheath from the antibacterial action of the mass of viscous fluid in the cervix known as the cervical plug. Second, the sheath developed holes either in the initial tying process or as a result of decomposition after the IUD was in place. These holes allowed the bacteria to escape into the uterus without even reaching the top of the string (Tatum et al., 1975).

The two men formed the Dalkon Corporation, which in February 1970 began commercial sales of the shield. Marketing rights were purchased by the A. H. Robins Company in June of 1970 (Sivin, 1993). Some 4.5 million of the devices were distributed throughout the world, mostly between 1971 and 1975 (Byrne, 1992).

In 1973, the U.S. Food and Drug Administration (FDA) conducted an inquiry into the Dalkon Shield device. In 1974 the company ceased manufacturing in the United States, but did not stop marketing elsewhere in the world until later. Stocks were still available outside the United States in the early 1980s.

People started taking legal action against the manufacturer soon after the Dalkon Shield was marketed, but Robins declared bankruptcy in 1985 to shield itself from the onslaught of litigation. A trust was set up, and with the publicity ordered by the bankruptcy court, claims flooded in from all around the world.

Fifteen thousand American women sued Robins before the company declared bankruptcy in August of 1985, and a $3.3 billion settlement was reached in 1988 (Nocera, 1995). These suits were due to unacceptable rates of pregnancy, PID, and death in women who used it. The manufacturer knew of these defects in March of 1972, but at least 1 million device insertions are believed to have occurred after that. Thousands of women have reportedly suffered severe and debilitating medical problems, including pain and bleeding, uterine perforations, PID, septic abortion, ectopic pregnancies, and unplanned pregnancy. Women have become sterile, many having hysterectomies in their twenties, and many spending the rest of their lives on hormonal replacement therapy. By 1976, 17 women were known to have died in the United States following the use of the shield.

A side effect of these events was a public belief that all IUDs were unsafe, and a business belief that all IUDs were litagens. As a result, this form of birth control largely disappeared from the marketplace (Mumford and Kessel, 1992), despite evidence that the Dalkon Shield may have been acceptable, safe, and effective when properly inserted, and no evidence that the other two significant forms of IUDs (Lippes Loop and the copper IUDs) were not effective or safe (Sivin, 1993).

Premarket clinical efficacy safety testing of the Dalkon Shield was insufficient, manufacturing quality control was poor, and once widely sold, clinical use was poorly controlled. Additionally, preclinical safety testing was almost nonexistent and did not reflect any consideration of device design, intended use, or probable misuse.

III. TALC ON GLOVES AND CONDOMS

Particles of talc have been identified on both the surface of surgeons' rubber gloves and on latex condoms, as well as in sections of tissue classified as "starch" or "foreign body" granulomas.

The use of gloves to prevent contamination of operative wounds was accidental. The first person to use them in the United States was the wife of Dr. W. S. Halstead, who used gloves in the operating room to protect her hands and arms from the carbolic acid (in which the instruments were kept), which caused her a severe dermatitis. Joseph Bloodgood has the distinction of being the first surgeon to wear gloves in every operation starting in 1896. Many years later Halstead commented on the usefulness of gloves and described how they were only a minimal hindrance (Singh et al., 1974).

The earlier preparation for dry lubrication of surgical gloves was Lycopodium spores, and later, talcum powder. These two agents fell into disrepute when it was reported that a definite foreign body reaction to talc occurred in numerous regions of the body. In 1947, Lee and Lehman demonstrated experimentally the advantages of a cornstarch derivative and its apparent safety in human tissues. It was widely accepted, and in the 1950s a cornstarch derivative (Biosorb) rapidly replaced talc as a surgical glove powder.

The adverse effects of cornstarch in patients were first recorded by Snierson and Woo (1955), who reported two cases with incisional granulomas. Since then, numerous reports of granuloma formation due to cornstarch have been recorded in various anatomic sites, such as the abdominal cavity, pulmonary parenchyma, pleura, paranasal sinuses, mastoid, testes, and biopsy scars. Granuloma formation has been reported following percutaneous absorption of cornstarch material up the female genital tract following a pelvic examination.

Numerous experimental studies using the abdominal cavity of mice, dogs, rabbits, and guinea pigs have been carried out to evaluate cornstarch as a glove powder lubricant. Injections into the soft tissues of the backs of hamsters and mice have produced cornstarch granulomas. Single reports have also been mentioned in experiments carried out on the brain, spinal cord, and peripheral nerves by Wise, as well as on lung, knee joint, and tendon (Postlethwaite et al., 1949). A single case report of synovial involvement has appeared in the literature, as a letter to the editor of the *Journal of the American Medical Association*. It involved a patient who developed a granuloma at the site of excision of a ganglion from the wrist.

Postlethwaite implanted a "pinch" of glove powder in the knee joints of six dogs, and found no gross changes in the synovium at the end of 14 and 28 days, but did find microscopic tissue reaction. Only rarely were starch granules seen, and there was no evidence of granuloma formation. The degree of intra-articular inflammation is directly related to the amount of powder per surface area of the joint. In an abdominal operation, the entire hand of the surgeon may be introduced into the body cavity.

The recognition that the use of talc as a surgical glove powder was responsible for the postoperative development of peritoneal adhesions and tissue granulomas at the site of operation (Lichtman et al., 1946; Eismann et al., 1947) stimulated the search for an inert absorbable substitute, and resulted in its eventual replacement by a starch powder (Lee and Lehman, 1947; Postlethwaite et al., 1949), which initially appeared to produce no ill effects within the peritoneal cavity. There have, however, been numerous reports over the past two decades suggesting that the use of starch powder could also result in a granulomatous reaction similar to that produced by talc (Snierson and Woo, 1955; McAdams, 1956; Nash, 1971; Neelly and Davis, 1971; Cohen and Safaie-Shirazi, 1973). Starch granuloma peritonitis secondary to the glove powder reaction has now become recognized as a clinical entity (Sobel et al., 1971), and Taft et al. (1970) suggested that the severity of the condition may be related to the type of starch used. The starch powder has also been shown to produce granulomas and adhesions in experimental animals (Lee et al., 1952; Perper et al., 1971; Ignatius and Hartmann, 1972).

Recent reports, however, indicate that starch particles may not always have been responsible for the development of the granuloma peritonitis and that contaminants of the dusting powder used in the surgeons' gloves must be taken into consideration (Henderson et al., 1975). Similar reports have appeared associating dry lubricants on condoms with adverse tissue responses.

Given the long-standing knowledge of the systemic effects of particulates introduced into the body cavities, it should have been clear that any solid, poorly soluble, or insoluble particle introduced into the body or a body cavity is likely to cause a foreign body response-mediated reaction in the body. Similar responses are seen to the wear particles produced from artificial joint implants.

IV. TOXIC SHOCK SYNDROME

The tampon was first introduced in 1936. Since then its use in menstruating women has expanded greatly, with an estimated 73 million women using it up to five times a day, five days a month for up to 38 years (Houppert, 1995). Although there were reports in the literature as early as 1966 (Maguire, 1966; Orem and Beck, 1981) that tampons were associated with vaginal infections ("tampon vaginitis"), the cases were generally mild and transitory. There was no history of serous medical problems (requiring hospitalization) or of deaths associated with tampon use until 1978, some three years after Procter & Gamble first test-marketed the Rely superabsorbent tampon in 1974.

The FDA began to monitor negative reaction to tampons in 1974 through the Device Experience Network (DEN). Complaints were registered by consumers as well as health professionals, complaints that described experiences with mucosal alterations in the vaginal area, drying, layering, lacerations, micro-ulcers, hemorrhaging, and dermatitis. In several instances doctors stated that they had reported these experiences to the manufacturers and had been ignored.

In 1977 four cases of tampon-induced vaginitis were described by Barrett, who wrote that these should "alert the clinician to consider the possibility of tampon-induced pressure or chemical irritation in the differential diagnosis of a vaginal ulceration . . . second, the patients could have manifested an idiosyncratic reaction to the chemicals in the deodorized tampon" (Schrock, 1980).

In November of 1978, toxic shock syndrome (TSS) was first described in *Lancet* (Todd et al., 1978). Toxic shock syndrome is an acute onset, multiorgan illness that resembles severe scarlet fever. The illness is caused by *Staphylococcus aureus* strains that express TSS toxin-1 (TSST-1), enterotoxin B, or enterotoxin C. TSST-1 is associated with menstrual TSS and approximately one-half of nonmenstrual cases; the other two toxins cause nonmenstrual cases, 47% and 3% respectively. The three toxins are expressed in culture media under similar environmental conditions. These conditions may explain the association of certain tampons with menstrual TSS. Biochemically, the toxins are all relatively low molecular weight and fairly heat- and protease-stable. Enterotoxins B and C share nearly 50% sequence homology with streptococcal scarlet fever toxin A; they share no homology with TSST-1 despite sharing numerous biological properties (Schlievert and Blomster, 1983; Thomas and Withington, 1985; Bohach et al., 1990). Numerous animal models for development of TSS have suggested mechanisms of toxin action, although the exact molecular action is not known. The toxins are all potent pyrogens, induce T lymphocyte proliferation, require interleukin-1 release from macrophages, suppress Ig production, enhance endotoxin shock, and enhance hypersensitivity skin reactions. The genetic control of the toxins has been studied and suggests the exotoxins are variable traits.

Toxic shock syndrome is a serious, potentially life-threatening condition resulting from an exotoxin of *S. aureus*. Presenting symptoms include high fever, diarrhea, nausea, and vomiting, progressing to hypotension, oliguria, conjunctival hyperemia, and an erythematous rash over the trunk, abdomen, and extremities. Most, but not all, cases of TSS have been associated with the use of tampons during menstruation, postsurgical infections, and stab wounds. It can occur in postrhinoplasty patients with and without nasal packing. There have been cases reported in the literature of TSS associated with suction-assisted lipectomy (SAL).

In 1978 Todd described seven children aged between 8 and 17 years who presented with a high fever, headache, confusion, diarrhea, and a scarlatiniform rash, some of whom developed prolonged shock, disseminated intravascular coagulation, renal failure, and hepatic abnormalities. One patient died and all suffered from fine desquamation of the skin of the hands and feet. A phase group I *S. aureus* was isolated from mucosal or sequestered (empyema, abscess) sites in five of the patients, and this was found to produce a previously unreported exotoxin which caused a positive Nikolsky sign in newborn mice (producing a cleavage in the basal layer of the skin as opposed to the granular layer cleavage seen with the exfoliation produced by the phase group II staphylococcus). Todd also commented on the similarity between his cases and cases of Kawasaki's disease, Rye's syndrome, and staphylococcal scalded skin syndrome, and it was later suggested that reported cases of "adult" Kawasaki's disease were probably cases of TSS. In 1980 Schrock was the first to describe an association between TSS and tampon usage in menstruating women. This association was confirmed by further studies. TSS was first linked (by the CDC) with menstruation in May 1980 and with Rely users in August and September of that same year. The manufacturer withdrew Rely from the market immediately. The first TSS sort trial was held in 1982.

In a Wisconsin study of 38 cases, it was found that 37 were women, 35 of these cases occurred during menses, and 97% of these patients used tampons. The overall incidence of TSS in this study was found to be 6.2 cases: 100,000 menstruating women with a mortality rate of 2.6% compared with the national figure of 8.4%. The first case reported in the United Kingdom was in November

1980. Since then there have been over 80 cases reported to the Public Health Laboratory at Colindale. The disease predominantly affects menstruating women in the 20-to-30-year age group and the incidence seems to be very low in non-Caucasians.

Before antibiotic treatment had been started, isolated *S. aureus* belonging to phase group II from 74% of vaginal and cervical culture had been obtained from TSS patients. In both these studies, blood cultures from TSS patients were negative. This finding is consistent with other reports suggesting, as Todd initially postulated, that the clinical features are due to the absorption of a toxin. There have been more recent reports, however, in which *S. aureus* has been isolated from blood cultures, although the incidence is very low. The strong association with tampon usage led to the investigation and comparison of brands, with a special interest in the "superabsorbent" tampons containing carboxymethylcellulose and polyester foam that were introduced in 1980. No significant difference was found between types, although the Rely tampon (Procter & Gamble) was withdrawn from the market in the United States. It was suggested that inherently contaminated tampons might be the cause, but the absence of positive cultures for *S. aureus* and the occurrence of TSS among users of all brands make this unlikely.

Most attention has been made to tampon, menses-related TSS, although the original description of TSS was in children, with *S. aureus* being isolated from various sites. Since then Reingold et al. (1982a,b) have made an extensive review of 130 cases of nonmenstrual TSS, with *S. aureus* being isolated from a variety of sites, including surgical wounds, adenitis, bursitis, postpartum infections, packed nasal cavities, and deep abscesses. Of the nonmenstrual TSS patients, the mortality rate was 9.2%, 68% were women, and the patients were significantly older. As with menses-related TSS, the incidence of bacteremia was low (3%)

Recurrence of TSS occurs in the menstruating group only, with the incidence as high as 28%. The second episode usually occurs during the first or second menstrual period after the initial episode, which is usually the most severe. The incidence of recurrences can be reduced following treatment with the appropriate antistaphylococcal antibiotics during the initial episode and cessation of tampon use in the subsequent periods.

There were reported to be 1,138 cases of TSS in 1980, with 38 deaths, and as many as 94 deaths overall. Whether due to a new, more pathogenic strain of bacteria or to more absorbent tampons or some contaminant in tampon materials (or some combination of these factors), the need to ensure that tampons neither seriously alter vaginal microflora nor promote production of TSST-1 was clear, and (as described in Chapter 16) such testing is now performed prior to device approval.

It is not clear what the relative contributing weights of the different compo-
nents of the TSS problem were. Swift and decisive action definitely served to
reduce the public's perception of the continuation of the problem.

V. LATEX ALLERGY

The advent of public awareness and concern about acquired immune deficiency
syndrome (AIDS) during the mid-1980s greatly increased the demand for condoms and gloves—of which the majority are made from latex. Protective gloves,
commonly associated with aseptic surgical technique, are now worn in virtually
all procedures involving exposure to blood, body fluids, or mucous membranes.
The AIDS epidemic and worry of infection transmittal have been an impetus for
the donning of latex gloves by health-care professionals, equipment sales and
service technicians, office cleaning staff, and individuals responsible for waste
removal. Approximately 20 billion latex gloves were used in 1991 alone (Fay
and Sullivan, 1992). As this utilization of gloves continues to escalate, increasing
numbers of physicians, nurses, dentists, laboratory technicians, and patients are
reporting latex hypersensitivity reactions in great frequency and severity.

Delayed hypersensitivity reactions in the form of allergic eczematic contact
dermatitis to natural rubber such as latex surgical gloves or other latex products
has been observed for many years. Since 1979, when the first case of immediate
hypersensitivity (contact urticaria) from latex was reported by J. K. Nutter (Gonzales,
1992) latex medical problems (Shumnes and Darby, 1984; Estlander et al., 1986)
have increased multifold. Between 1988 and 1992, the FDA received reports of
more than 1000 systemic type I allergic reactions to latex, of which at least 15 were
fatal (Scarbeck, 1993).

As a result of the regulatory requirements from the CDC, Occupational
Safety and Health Administration (OSHA), and state regulatory boards, the wearing of gloves is no longer limited to health-care facilities. Workers in nursing
homes, schools, law enforcement agencies, reference laboratories, emergency
medical services, and linen services, along with hospitals and funeral services,
have donned latex gloves. Due to the increased use of latex, latex hypersensitivity
affects not only the surgical team, but these high-risk groups as well.

Fisher (1992) reported 7% of physicians, nurses, and dentists now acquire a
delayed allergic, eczematous contact dermatitis, whereas 3% show an immediate
allergic urticarial reaction to the aqueous protein fraction of latex. This urticarial
reaction may be accompanied by anaphylaxis. Iatrogenic and intraoperative contact urticaria and anaphylaxis of patients contacting rubber gloves worn by physicians are being reported with more frequency. Due to the increase in these reports,
in March 1991 the FDA alerted health-care professionals about the potential of
severe allergic reactions to medial devices made of latex.

Presently the incidence of latex sensitization is unknown. Latex sensitivity has been reported in one of 800 patients (0.128%) prior to surgery (Turjanma, 1993). Latex allergy in children with spina bifida ranges from 28–67% (Kelly et al., 1994), however. Health-care workers with atopic allergy have been reported to have a 24% prevalence of a positive latex skin-prick test, while the overall prevalence in health-care workers is 7–10% (Arellano et al., 1992).

Latex is very widely used—not just in many medical devices (e.g., gloves, condoms, catheters, and the stoppers of syringes), but also in many everyday items (e.g., balloons and tires). Once an individual is sensitized, exposure to any of these can evoke a potentially deadly response. There are at least two operative mechanisms for the range of responses seen (Lang, 1996).

A. Delayed Hypersensitivity

Type IV delayed hypersensitivity is the predominant immunological response (82%) to natural rubber latex (Sussman, 1995). Although skin irritation may be due to friction, maceration, frequent hand washing, and antimicrobial soap, exposure to rubber gloves or glove powder should be considered a potential allergen. The usual delayed hypersensitivity reaction is induced by low-molecular-weight chemical additives: vulcanizers, stabilizers, accelerators (thiurams, mercaptobenzothiazole, carbamates), and antioxidants in *p*-paraphenylenediamine black-rubber mix (Fay and Sullivan, 1992; Sussman et al., 1991).

The immunologic pathways and mediators to delayed contact dermatitis include the development of immunized T lymphocytes able to recognize the antigen, which usually occurs in 7 days. It is believed that the Langerhans cell mediates this process by engulfing the antigen on primary exposure, migrating to lymph nodes, and then presenting the antigen to helper T cells. The sensitized helper T cell then re-enters the skin immunologically prepared for the next encounter with the antigen. Upon secondary exposure to the antigen, the lymphocytes release cytokines that recruit macrophages and other inflammatory cells to elicit the cutaneous reaction that will peak in approximately 48 hr (Gonzales, 1992).

B. Immediate Hypersensitivity

Immediate hypersensitivity reactions tend to be more serious because they involve not only the skin but also mucosal surfaces. These manifestations occur within minutes and may include contact urticaria, angioedema, rhinitis, and respiratory symptoms such as dyspnea and asthmatic attacks. Systemic reactions have been reported to occur in patients with latex protein allergies and are more likely to occur with prior mucosal exposure to gloves, balloons, or dental dams. Patients subject to immediate reactions are at risk of severe or fatal consequences if the hypersensitivity is unrecognized when they are examined or operated on by health-care professionals wearing latex gloves.

The immunological pathway or mechanism involved in immediate latex hypersensitivity is quite different from that of the delayed reactions. Immediate latex hypersensitivity reactions are believed to be mediated by immunoglobulin E (IgE) (Gonzales, 1992; Slater, 1992; Sussman et al., 1991). Interaction of IgE and antigen induces local release of histamine and arachidonic acid metabolites. The release of these agents results in increased vascular permeability to the antigen and systemic immediate reactions. It is believed that the antigen in the IgE-mediated response is a latex protein or polypeptide (Warpinski et al., 1991). It is not clear at all, however, that the increased incidence and severity of responses seen since the demand for gloves and condoms went up is due solely to there being increased numbers of people being exposed with increased frequency. Certainly such is not the case with the most sensitive population, children with spina bifida. A significant component in the causality may well be a change in either the sources of latex or the processing procedures (or both).

A spectrum of IgE-mediated allergic responses to latex was presented in an article by Sussman and co-workers (1991). They reported 14 patients sensitized by exposure to latex gloves. The manifestations in response to the latex exposure varied greatly according to the route of latex antigen presentation. The patients' symptoms often occurred immediately after exposure to latex, however. Skin contact usually elicited urticaria. Allergic rhinitis, conjunctivitis, and asthma were usually the result of exposure to airborne particles of latex. Systemic effects from latex occurred due to contact with surgeons' gloves intraoperatively. Anaphylactic shock included these symptoms plus tachycardia and hypotension.

Sussman et al. (1991) reported positive latex skin tests from all the patients. Serum IgE antibody to latex was found with latex radioallergosorbent test (RAST) in all patients tested except one. Other studies have shown immediate hypersensitivity reactions to latex to be IgE-mediated by skin testing, basophil histamine release, RAST, enzyme-linked immunosorbent assay (ELISA), and IgE immunoblots.

Though traditional in vivo delayed contact sensitization testing should have been sufficient to detect the increased delayed sensitization response potential of latex products, it did not. More important, such traditional sensitization tests cannot function to detect IgE-based responses (although the mouse PLNA would). More extensive immunotoxicity testing is clearly called for in the case of a natural product-based, high-exposure material used for devices, and careful attention must be paid to source materials provided by vendors for approved devices, particularly when demands for the material are sharply increased over a brief period of time.

VI. SILICONES IN DEVICES

As presented in Chapter 2, silicones have come into broad use in medical devices since the 1950s (McGregor, 1953). In various chemical and physical forms, they are present in syringes (as lubricants), in shunts and catheters (in tubing), and in implants (as films and gels).

Since 1964, silicone-filled breast implants have been put into an estimated 1 million women, with the average cost of the actual implant being $195 in 1990. Prior to this, there were some claims of association of breast cancer with implants and speculative reports of immunologically mediated health problems associated with exposure to silicone in implants and from kidney dialysis (Laohapand et al., 1982; Baldwin and Kaplan, 1983; Bommer et al., 1983), but these had neither been scientifically verified (Heggers et al., 1983) nor successful in litigation in court. A persistent problem was (and remains) a confusion on the part of some as to the difference between silica (of which some forms are immunotoxic) (Uber and McReynolds, 1982) and the silicones.

Starting in early 1991, there was an explosion in litigation over silicone breast implants with suits by women claiming harm from the implants. (To date, lawyers' attempts to mount class action suits among other categories of patients extensively exposed to silicones, such as diabetics, have failed despite extensive advertising.)

Small amounts of silicone fluid from the gel have leaked through the outer envelope of the implant. (This leakage was not noticeable to the woman and tended to be contained within the capsule of scar tissue that inevitably forms around the implants.) In some women, the capsule of scar tissue contracted excessively, distorting and hardening the breasts and often causing discomfort. In about 5% of women, an implant ruptured, releasing silicone gel into the surrounding tissues and flattening the breast, but these local complications, unpleasant as they were, were not the basis for most of the alarm about breast implants, nor were they the focus of the multimillion-dollar lawsuits.

Instead, a growing number of Americans had come to believe that breast implants could cause devastating effects on the rest of the body. In particular, silicone gel-filled implants were said to be responsible for an ill-defined constellation of disorders known as connective tissue diseases. These diseases—which include systemic lupus (SLE), rheumatoid arthritis, and scleroderma—are thought to involve a disturbance in the immune system that turns the body's protective defenses against itself. The result is an autoimmune disease that can produce profound weakness and fatigue along with variable damage to the joints, skin, and internal organs. The symptoms and ills identified have continued to shift, and such a poor definition of a syndrome has caused significant uncertainty as to mechanism (indeed, as to the actual existence of a silicone-related disease moiety at all). This makes performance of an epidemiological study capable of deciding the issue impossible. One theory was that silicone, leaking slowly from the implants, provokes an immune reaction that then somehow turns into an autoimmune process. It was the unproven theory (and variations on it) that served as the basis for the largest lawsuits, but the question of whether or not silicone gel-filled breast implants cause connective tissue disease is not ultimately a matter of opinion or legal argument; it is a matter of biological fact. Either they cause connective tissue disease (alone or in conjunction with other factors), or they do not, and the only way to answer the question is through epidemiologic studies.

To be sure, there are many individual stories (some medically proven, others not) of connective tissue disease developing after the placement of breast implants, but these anecdotal reports alone do not constitute evidence that the implants caused the disease. One such case is dramatically presented in the book *Informed Consent* (Byrne, 1996), though not in a scientifically critical or dispassionate manner. They could well represent pure coincidence. Each year, for example, about 100 women with breast implants can be expected to come down with lupus or scleroderma by chance alone. Since connective tissue disease can occur in women with or without implants, the only way to demonstrate that implants actually contribute to the disease is to show that the incidence is significantly higher in women with breast implants than in those without, yet it was not until June 16, 1994, 2 years after breast implants were taken off the market and 2 months after the class-action settlement was announced, that the first such study of the possible link between breast implants and connective tissue disease was published, and that study failed to find a link.

In the study, May Clinic researchers compared a group of 749 women who had received breast implant between 1964 and 1991 with 1498 of their neighbors, matched for age. The researchers found that the implant group was no more likely to develop connective tissue disease (or related symptoms and abnormal tests) than the group without implants. This was only one study, of course, and was not large enough to rule out some increase in risk, but it did cast doubt on the link between breast implants and connective tissue disease at a time when many people assumed the theory had been proven.

Meanwhile, at least four other well-designed epidemiologic studies were underway. The largest was a retrospective cohort study of about 450,000 American women in the health professions. Although they have not been published yet, interim results indicate no association between breast implants and connective tissue diseases, with the possible exception of rheumatoid arthritis. Another large retrospective cohort study, published in the *New England Journal of Medicine* in June 1995, also found no association between implants and connective tissue diseases, and so addressed the claim that disease caused by breast implants may not fulfill all the usual criteria for ''classic'' connective tissue disease.

The remaining two epidemiologic studies, published in 1994 and 1995, dealt just with scleroderma. Scleroderma, a disease characterized by extensive scarring of the skin and sometimes of internal organs, is the connective tissue disease most closely linked by anecdotal reports to silicone breast implants. Neither study could find an association. While all together these studies don't mean that there can be *no* link between connective tissue disease and breast implants, they do mean that any risk of connective tissue disease from implants is so small that it has been impossible to detect. The most recent epidemiology study (Hennepens et al., 1996, released in February), did find "a small but statistically significant increased risk" (one in 30,000 per year of implant exposure) of contracting immune-system illness. This small potential difference of risk, however, may only represent the well-recognized influence of self-reporting in a highly publicized situation. Wong (1996) subsequently overviewed and performed a meta-analysis on 15 epidemiology studies that he had identified on breast implants and connective tissue disease, and found that they "did not provide any evidence of a causal relationship between silicone breast implants and connective tissue disease."

The result of litigation to date, however, is sobering. Facing one product liability case after another, the breast implant manufacturer's, while maintaining that the implants were safe, eventually agreed to the largest class-action settlement in the annals of American law. In April 1994, the major manufacturers settled for $4.25 billion, a billion of which was explicitly set aside for the lawyers involved. Although nearly any woman with implants would be entitled to something under the terms of the settlement, women were permitted to opt out if they thought they could do better on their own. As of June 1, 1995, some 440,000 women (about a quarter of all women with breast implants in this country) had registered to participate in the class-action settlement, but with vigorous encouragement from plaintiffs' attorneys, about 15,000 (half of them foreigners, for whom the terms of the settlement are less generous) have opted to seek higher damages individually.

The terms of the class settlement were remarkably generous and broad. All women with breast implants were entitled to compensation if they had, or within the next 30 years developed, any of 10 connective tissue diseases or symptoms suggestive of such disease, provided the symptoms began or worsened after the implants were placed. Of the $4.25 billion, $1.2 billion was set aside for women claiming to have implant-related illnesses already—248,500 women of the 440,000 registered as of June 1. The amount of compensation was to be determined by the type of disorder, its severity, and the woman's age at onset. A chart or grid sent to all women with breast implants showed the exact amounts. For example, a woman over 56 with mild Sjögren's syndrome (dryness of the eyes and salivary glands) would receive $140,000. Claimants were not required to show that the implants were related to the illness. In addition, women who were not ill could receive lesser amounts for emotional distress. They would also be reimbursed for all uninsured medical costs related to breast implants, including evaluations, treatment of implant rupture, and removal of implants. Husbands, "significant others," and children born before April 1, 1994, were also entitled to make claims. Children, for example, could claim compensation for injuries caused by their mothers' implants (a particularly mysterious provision, since no such injury has ever been demonstrated).

Women claiming current illness were required to submit substantiating medical records. If these were not sufficient to place the woman in the appropriate category on the grid, the woman's doctor was to send the diagnosis, along with copies of relevant records. Beyond this, there would be no attempt to verify the woman's medical condition. A doctor's diagnosis or the medical records would be challenged only if they failed to meet the eligibility requirements (e.g., swollen joints or abnormal substances in the blood) that can be objectively measured; some (e.g., fatigue or muscle aches) cannot. In fact, it would be possible to qualify for compensation without any objective manifestations of illness whatsoever. For example, a woman could claim joint and muscle aches, disturbed sleep, fatigue, and burning pain in the chest, none of which can be objectively verified by her doctor or anyone else and collect up to $700,000.

In the end, the class-action settlement has seemingly unraveled. In early May of 1995, Judge Sam C. Pointer, the Alabama federal judge who is overseeing the settlement, announced that the size of the compensation for each woman would have to be revised downward. It was apparent that the $1.2 billion set aside for current claims would nowhere near cover them, and as it looked like each woman would receive less, more women have opted out of the settlement and gone for jury trials, leaving the manufacturers little reason to stay in. (Dow Corning, which had pledged to contribute half the amount of the settlement, has already filed for Chapter 11.) The company will now have all claims against it held up in bankruptcy court for years. A desperate Judge Pointer charged the attorneys representing both sides to try to negotiate a new agreement by August 30, 1995, presumably one involving increased contributions from the manufacturers. "There are just too many sick women," said Ralph Knowles one of the lawyers representing the plaintiffs. "I didn't think it was going to be anything like that. If I did, we would have never agreed to the $4.25 billion."

Whatever happens to this settlement, a great deal of damage has already been done. It did not take plaintiffs' attorneys long to realize that breast implants are not the only medical devices on the market that contain silicone. Several class actions have already been filed on behalf of the approximately 300,000 men with silicone-containing penile implants. Breast implant litigation has also contributed to new alarmism about Norplant, the highly reliable contraceptive that is placed under the skin of the arm in six very small, silicone-coated rods. The number of product liability lawsuits against Wyeth-Ayerst, the manufacturer of Norplant, and its parent company, American Home Products, has, according to a *New York Times* story, swelled from 20 in Norplant's first 3 years on the market to 180 in 1994. Forty-six class-action suits have been filed on behalf of

Norplant users, and implants of the contraceptive have fallen from 800 a day to 60. The illnesses attributed to it include autoimmune and connective tissue-like disorders, yet as with breast implants, there is no evidence to implicate Norplant in these disorders.

More worrisome still is the indirect threat to all medical devices, whether they contain silicone or not. Under our liability laws, plaintiffs can make claims against any party involved in the manufacture of an allegedly harmful product, no matter how remote the involvement. Suppliers of raw materials (or biomaterials) for medical devices can be sued, then, even if they have nothing to do with the design and manufacture of the product. The sale of biomaterials for medical devices is a small part of the business of most big suppliers, but the resulting revenues can quickly be offset by the legal liabilities.

Ostensibly because of such risks, three large suppliers of biomaterials have already pulled back from the market. Dow Corning, a supplier as well as a manufacturer, has drastically scaled back sales of silicone to other manufacturers of medical devices and may stop selling it altogether. The embargo will probably affect a wide variety of silicone-containing devices, ranging from the useful to the vital. Among them are cardiac pacemaker wires, artificial joints, mechanical heart valves, intraocular lenses (used after cataract surgery), implantable arteriovenous shunts for people on chronic dialysis, and shunts for people with hydrocephalus (a potentially lethal condition in which fluid accumulates in the brain). Dow Chemical Company has stopped supplying a material used in pacemaker components. DuPont announced in 1993 that it would sever connections with the permanent medical implant industry. It will no longer provide medical manufacturers with Dacron polyester, which is used in vascular grafts, or a number of other materials. In DuPont's calculus, what had happened with silicone could happen with any other constituent of medical devices.

Under these conditions, a large number of important medical products may become scarce or even unavailable. In May 1994, Senator Joseph Lieberman of Connecticut, then the chairman of the Governmental Affairs Subcommittee on Regulation and Government Information, held hearings on the impact of product liability suits on the availability of medical devices. Among those who testified was Elenor Gackstatter, president of Meadox Medicals, a manufacturer of vascular grafts and other devices. Gackstatter said that she had tried to contact 15 alternative suppliers of polyester yarn after DuPont announced it would no longer supply Dacron to her company. None of them—not even foreign suppliers—would deal with American manufacturers because of the liability risks. Many manufacturers have a 2 or 3 year supply of biomaterials on hand, but when that is depleted, there may be a serious shortage. Said Lieberman, ''This is a public health time bomb, and the lives of real people are going to be lost if it explodes.''

Meanwhile, an extensive battery of immune toxicity tests has been performed on the silicones that were used in implants. To date, none of these has established any immune system effects.

Any medical device or pharmaceutical with a sufficiently large and long patient exposure base will have the potential of evoking unforeseen adverse responses in one or more subpopulations of the exposed patient population, either in reality or in the perception of the public and civil legal system. Such devices or agents must be fully tested against the range of possible biologic effects, and mere adherence to existing guidelines (with careful and informed scientific consideration) is not adequate. Perceived subpopulation "risks" must be aggressively investigated to fully understand both mechanisms and the relative extent of the risk.

VII. PROBLEM SOLVING

When the biological evaluation of medical devices is approached as a routine function involving nothing more than successfully passing a series of biocompatibility tests, there is little opportunity for innovatively managing positive test results, which indicate that a material is toxic. Blind compliance is not the intent of the International Organization for Standardization (ISO) or FDA, however. Manufacturers have the freedom and the responsibility to apply the ISO biological evaluation standard in a way that ensures the biological safety of their devices while conservatively managing resources. Neither ISO 10993-1 nor the FDA memorandum on its use specify pass/fail criteria for biological testing, recognizing that it is almost impossible to set general criteria and that manufacturers are in the best position to determine what level of toxicity is acceptable for their products.

Based on careful comparisons of biocompatibility and clinical data, some companies have determined the highest safety test score relating to unacceptable performance for a specific class of products and use this value as the pass/fail criterion. At many companies, however, there is a tendency to panic when biological safety test results are positive. The possibility of a positive result can call into question carefully considered material choices, threaten costly delays in product development schedules, and raise doubts about test strategies. Manufacturers may hastily pursue many directions at once, ending with an array of conflicting information, or they may forget that the goal of biological safety testing is to determine whether or not a material or device is safe for its intended use, and not (necessarily) to determine the cause of toxicity.

The best approach to any situation in which the ideal may be unobtainable is to follow a planned course of action, first confirming the facts at hand, then considering the options for future actions. Applied to the problem of positive biocompatibility test results, this means methodically confirming that the test procedure was followed as intended and that the test result is reproducible, and then considering whether the toxicity can be eliminated or is acceptable. The steps in this procedure are (Stark, 1996) as follows:

1. Confirming the test procedure.
   a. Was the test performed and interpreted properly?
   b. Was the proper test article employed (and so identified)?
   c. Was the test article properly sampled and prepared (including storage, extraction, and any manipulation)?
   d. Was the test properly conducted?
2. Confirming that the proper material was supplied.
   a. Was the material properly manufactured?
   b. Sterilized?
   c. Cleaned?
3. Confirming the reproducibility of the test.
   a. Can the results be replicated?
4. Eliminating the source of toxicity. If all the above are confirmed, can the cause of test failure/toxicity be removed from the product?
   a. By using different materials of formulations?
   b. By washing, rinsing, or otherwise removing a process contaminant?
   c. By improving process or material quality control?

If all of these steps do not lead to a product that passes the required test paradigm, then one must consider whether the identified toxicity presents an unacceptable risk or whether the hazards are either justifiable or irrelevant to the actual use of the device.

While the ideal situation is eliminating any potential toxicity, this is not always possible. Toxicity may be intrinsic to the product and impossible to eliminate without compromising product function. One familiar example is the electronic componentry of pacemakers and cochlear implants. The toxic circuitry in these devices must be contained within a nontoxic case so it cannot leach out and injure the implant recipient. Another example is a simple product called an adhesive remover. No matter how it is formulated, the product is always a mixture of organic solvents that carry with them the possibility of systemic toxicity subsequent to skin absorption.

Medical devices that must cure in situ are also intrinsically toxic. The curing process of products such as casts, dental cements, and bone cements may involve the generation of free radicals or other reactive chemical moieties, or may be exothermic. In addition, implants made from nickel alloys carry an intrinsic level of toxicity. Nickel is a cardiac toxin, an oxytoxic agent, and a common sensitizing agent. (An estimated 5% of the population is allergic to nickel contact.) The possibility of nickel being released into the biological environment always poses the risk of toxic response.

There are also some devices whose functions result in injury; for example, a medical tape designed to hold an appliance onto the skin. If the appliance is life-supporting, the tape will be expected to adhere to the skin with some high degree of tenacity so that the device will not fall away. This high adhesion level is likely to result in skin injury when the tape is ultimately removed.

In each of these examples, the toxicity is intrinsic to the device; suitable (nontoxic) alternative materials do not exist, or the device will not function as intended if the injurious material is removed. The manufacturer is left with no alternative but to accept the toxic material. The strategy becomes one of justifying its use.

A. Justifying Use of the Material

There are three approaches to justifying the use of a toxic material in a medical device. The first is to compare the level of toxicity of the material to a comparable material that is currently being used by the manufacturer. If the new material has a lower level of toxicity than the current one and the current one has a safe history of use in the marketplace, the use of the new material may be justified because it is a move in the direction of decreased toxicity and increased biological safety.

The second approach is to compare the level of toxicity of the material to a comparable material that is currently being used in a competitive product. Again, if the new material has a lower level of toxicity than the competitive material in the same biological safety test, and the competitive material has a history of safe use in the marketplace, the use of the new material may be justified.

In the third approach the maximum dose and the no-observable-adverse-effect level (NOAEL) for the material are calculated and then compared. To determine the level at which no adverse effect occurs, the sample is titrated by using decreasing amounts in the test system. The highest concentration of sample at which no effect is observed is the NOAEL, which can be expressed in units, surface area, weight, or volume of material. The maximum dose of a material equals the units, surface area, weight, or volume of material to which a patient will be exposed during a typical course of therapy. If a material's maximum dose is 100-fold less than its NOAEL, the material is considered safe for use. (The 100-fold criterion is based on a 10-fold variation between species and a 10-fold variation within species.) The comparison must be repeated for each biological safety test giving a positive response.

The NOAEL approach has been employed to justify the use of nickel alloys in implants. The amount of nickel released by in situ corrosion is compared with the maximum permissible amount of nickel that can be given per day in IV fluids, which was determined from IV injection of nickel in dogs. If the release of nickel through corrosion is less than the amount that can be safely given in IV fluids, the alloy would be considered safe for implantation. For such situations, one must conduct (and provide to regulatory bodies) a risk assessment.

VIII. RISK ASSESSMENTS

ISO 14971-1 (1998) sets forth the requirements and means of conducting and presenting a risk assessment (analysis) for medical devices.

While every medical manufacturer desires to construct its devices from entirely safe materials, in reality not all materials are entirely safe. Generally, if one looks long enough at small enough quantities, some type of risk can be associated with every material.

Risk can be defined as the possibility of harm or loss. Health risk, of course, is the possibility of an adverse effect on one's health. Risk is sometimes quantified by multiplying the severity of an event times the probability the event will occur, so that

Risk = severity × probability

While this equation appears useful in theory, in practice it is difficult to apply to the biological safety of medical devices. The process known as health-based risk assessment attempts to provide an alternative strategy for placing health risks in perspective.

A structure for the risk assessment process has been detailed in a publication prepared by the U.S. National Academy of Sciences (NRC, 1983; Gad, 1999). Although devised primarily for cancer risk assessment, many of the provisions also apply to the assessment of other health effects. The major components of the paradigm are (1) hazard identification, (2) dosage-response assessment, (3) exposure assessment, and (4) risk characterization.

This general approach to risk assessment was adapted to medical devices via the draft CEN standard *Risk Analysis*, published in 1993, and more recently via the ISO standard, *ISO 14538-Method for the Establishment of Allowable Limits for Residues in Medical Devices Using Health-Based Risk Assessment* (ISO, 1998). At the present time, FDA is also working to develop a health-based risk assessment protocol adapted to medical devices. Informally called the medical device paradigm, the document is not yet generally available.

Some manufacturers may object that regulators are once again attempting to impose a "drug model" on medical devices. We shall see in the following pages, however, that judicious application of these risk assessment principles can provide a justification for using materials that carry with them some element of risk, and that may under traditional biocompatibility testing regimes be difficult to evaluate or be deemed unsuitable for medical device applications.

A. Method

Hazard Identification.   The first step in the risk assessment process is to identify the possible hazards that may be presented by a material. This is accomplished by determining whether a compound, an extract of the material, or the material itself produces adverse effects, and by identifying the nature of those effects. Adverse effects are identified either through a review of the literature or through actual biological safety testing.

Dose-Response Assessment.   The second step is to determine the dose response of the material; that is, what is the highest weight or concentration of the material that will not cause an effect. This upper limit is called the *allowable limit*. There are numerous sources in the literature from which to determine allowable limits. Some will be more applicable than others, and some may require correction factors.

Exposure Assessment.   The third step is to determine the exposure assessment by quantifying the *available dose* of the chemical residues that will be received by the patient. This is readily done by estimating the number of devices to which a patient is likely to be exposed in a sequential period of use (e.g., during a hospital stay) or over a lifetime. For example, a patient might be exposed to 100 skin staples following a surgical procedure, or to two heart valves in a lifetime; thus the amount of residue available on 100 skin staples or two heart valves would be determined.

Risk Characterization.   Characterizing the risk constitutes the final step of the process. The allowable limit is compared with the estimated exposure; if the allowable limit is greater than the estimated exposure by a comfortable safety margin, the likelihood of an adverse event occurring in an exposed population is small, and the material may be used.

B. Case Studies

We can best get a sense of how these standards work by looking at some actual case studies that illustrate the risk assessment process.

1. Nitinol Implant

Nitinol is an unusual alloy of nickel and titanium that features the useful property of "shape memory." A nitinol part can be given a particular shape at a high temperature, then cooled to a low temperature and compressed into some other shape. The compressed part will subsequently deploy to its original shape at a predetermined transition temperature. This device is particularly useful, since it gives a transition temperature at approximately the temperature of the body (37°C).

Hazard Identification. One concern with using nitinol in implant applica-tion is the potential release of nickel into the body. Although nickel is a dietary requirement, it is also highly toxic (it is a known cause of dermatitis, cancer subsequent to inhalation, and acute pneumonitis from inhalation of nickel car-bonyl), and to exert a toxic feature is particularly beneficial for vascular implant applications in which the shape of the device in its compressed state eases the insertion process. The nitinol deploys as it is warmed by the surrounding tissue, expanding to take on the desired shape of a stent, filter, or other device. The transition temperature depends on the alloy's relative concentrations of nickel and titanium; a typical nickel concentration of 55–60% is used in medical effect on cellular reproduction. It is a known sensitizer, with approximately 5% of the domestic population allergic to this common metal, probably through exposure from costume jewelry and clothing snaps. *The biocompatibility question at hand is whether or not in vivo corrosion of nitinol releases unsafe levels of nickel.*

Dose-Response Assessment. A search of the world medical literature re-vealed that the recommended safe level of exposure to nickel in IV fluids is a maximum of 35 µg/day. This value can be taken as an allowable limit of nickel exposure for a 70-kg (the 154-lb so-called standard male) adult.

The IV fluid data are based on subjects that are compatible to the patients who will be receiving nitinol implants. The data are for humans (not animals), for ill patients (not healthy workers or volunteers), and for similar routes of expo-sure (IV fluid and tissue contact). For these reasons, no safety correction factor need be applied to the allowable limit of exposure.

Exposure Assessment. The available dose of nickel from nitinol implants can be estimated from data found in the literature. In one study, dental arch wires of nitinol were extracted in artificial saliva, and the concentration of nickel measured in the supernatant. Corrosions reached a peak at day 7, then declined steadily there after. The average rate of corrosion under these conditions was 12.8 µg/day cm^2 over the first 28 days.

Risk Characterization. A comparison of the available dose with the al-lowable limit for IV fluid levels shows that there is approximately a threefold safety margin, assuming that the implanted device is a full 1 cm^2 in surface area. (Devices with less surface area will contribute even less to the nickel concentra-tion and have an even larger safety margin.) Considering the high quality of the data, a threefold safety margin is sufficient to justify using nitinol in vascular implants.

2. Wound-Dressing Formulation

Today's wound dressings are highly engineered products, designed to maintain the moisture content and osmotic balance of the wound bed so as to promote optimum conditions for wound healing. Complex constructions of hydrocolloids and superabsorbers, these dressings are sometimes used in direct tissue contact over full-thickness wounds that penetrate the skin layers.

Hazard Identification. There have been reports in the literature of patients succumbing to cardiac arrest from potassium overload, with the wound dressing as one of the important contributors of excess potassium in the bloodstream. The effects of potassium on cardiac function are well characterized. Normal serum levels of potassium are 3.8 to 4 milliequivalents (mEq) per liter. As the potassium concentration rises to 5 to 7 mEq/liter, a patient can undergo cardiac arrest and die. *The biocompatibility issue to be explored is whether or not a wound dressing formulation might release dangerous levels of potassium if used on full-thickness wounds.*

Dose-Response Assessment. An increase of approximately 1 mEq/liter of potassium is likely to provoke mild adverse events in most patients. Assuming that the average person's blood volume is 5 liters, a one-time dose of 5 mEq/liter of potassium may begin to cause adverse reactions. This value can be considered to be the allowable limit of potassium for most patients.

Exposure Assessment. Let us suppose that each dressing contains 2.5 grams of potassium bicarbonate. Since the molecular weight of potassium bicarbonate is 100 grams mole, each dressing contains 0.025 mole of sodium bicarbonate, or 0.025 mEq/liter of potassium. If a patient were to use four dressings in a day, the available dose of potassium would be 0.1 mEq/day.

Risk Characterization. Comparing the available dose of potassium (0.1 mEq) to the allowable limit (5 mEq) shows that there is a 50-fold safety margin. Considering that patients may be small in size or may receive potassium from additional sources, such as IV fluids, this safety margin is too small, and so the dressing should be reformulated.

3. Perchloroethylene Solvent

A manufacturer of metal fabricated parts uses perchloroethylene to clean the finished pieces. Perchloroethylene has many advantages as a cleaner and degreaser: it is highly volatile, does not damage the ozone layer, and is very effective as a precision cleaning solvent.

The most common use of perchloroethylene is in the dry cleaning industry, but it is also commonly used in the electronics industry to clean circuit boards.

Hazard Identification. The downside of perchloroethylene is that it is highly toxic, with a material safety data sheet several pages in length listing adverse effects ranging from dizziness to death. Biocompatibility testing on solvent-cleaned parts would be meaningless; the solvent concentration on the part is so small that any effects of the solvent would be masked by the natural biological process of the test animals. *The biocompatibility question that must be answered is whether or not sufficient residual perchloroethylene remains on the cleaned metal parts to pose a health hazard.*

Dose-Response Assessment. Threshold limit values (TLVs) are values that indicate the maximum level of a chemical that a healthy worker could take in on a daily basis over the course of his or her work life with out experiencing any adverse effects. The TLV for perchloroethylene is 50 ppm/day (50 ml of perchloroethylene per 10^3 liter of air) by inhalation. The average person inhales 12,960 liters of air per day, making this equivalent to 650 ml of perchloroethylene per day. Since the vapor density of perchloroethylene is 5.76 grams liter, the TLV is equal to 2.7 grams of perchloroethylene per day by inhalation. Because TLVs for inhalation—as opposed to direct tissue exposure—are determined based on healthy individuals (not ill patients), we will divide the TLV by an uncertainty factor of 100 (i.e., 10) to account for a different route of exposure and 10 to account for healthy-to-ill persons. By this method, we obtain an allowable perchloroethylene limit of 37 mg/day.

Exposure Assessment. To calculate an available dose of perchloroethylene, we need some additional information. In this case, the manufacturer brought a number of cleaned metal pieces into equilibrium within a closed jar then analyzed the headspace above the pieces by using high-pressure liquid chromatography to determine the concentration of perchloroethylene released. The concentration of perchloroethylene was undetectable by high-performance liquid chromatography. Since the limits of this analytical method are 2 ppb, this value was taken as the concentration of perchloroethylene in the headspace. Taking the weight of the metal pieces, the number of pieces tested, and the volume of the headspace, it was calculated that the amount of perchloroethylene per single piece was a maximum of 1.0 ng/piece. If we suppose that a patient might be exposed to a maximum of 50 pieces over a lifetime, then the maximum available dose of perchloroethylene from the pieces would be 50 ng.

Risk Characterization. A comparison of the available dose (50 ng) to the allowable limit (37 mg/day) indicates an ample safety margin.

4. Ligature Material

A manufacturer purchases commercial black fishing line to use as a ligature in a circumcision kit. Because the ligature is not "medical grade," a cytotoxicity test is routinely conducted as an incoming inspection test. It was assumed that a negative cytotoxicity test would be associated with an acceptable incidence of skin irritation.

Hazard Identification. A newly received lot of the fishing line failed the cytotoxicity test. The extraction ratio of this material—of indeterminate surface area—was 0.2 grams/ml, with a 0.1-ml aliquot of sample extract being applied to a culture dish; thus 0.2 grams/ml $\times$ 0.1 ml = 0.02 grams represents a toxic dose of fishing line.

Dose-Response Assessment. A titration curve was obtained on the sample extract. If the sample was diluted 1:2, the test was still positive; however, if the sample was diluted 1:4, the test was negative, thus 0.02 grams/4 = 0.005 grams of fishing line, the maximum dose that is not cytotoxic. This value was called the allowable limit of fishing line.

Exposure Assessment. Each circumcision kit contained about 12 in. of line, but only about 4 in. of the material was ever in contact with the patient. Since an 8-yard line was determined to weigh 5 grams, the available dose of fishing line was calculated to be 5 grams/288 in. $\times$ 4 in. = 0.07 grams.

Risk Characterization. A comparison of the available dose (0.07) with the allowable limit (0.005 grams) convinced the manufacturer to reject the lot of fishing line.

C. Sources of Data

Data for calculating the allowable limit of exposure to a material can come from many sources, most of them promulgated by industrial and environmental hygienists and related agencies. (Review Chapter 2 on data sources for a better understanding of this area.)

D. Uncertainty Factors

An uncertainty factor is a correction that is made to the value used to calculate an allowable limit. It is based on the uncertainty that exists in the applicability of the data to actual exposure conditions. Typically, uncertainty factors range in value from 1 to 10. For example, a correction factor of 10 might be applied for data obtained in animals rather than humans, or to allow for a different route of exposure. In other words, for every property of available data that is different from the actual application, a correction factor of between 1 and 10 is applied. In our first example, had a small amount of data been obtained in animals by a different route of exposure, an uncertainty factor of 1000 might be applied.

E. Safety Margins

A safety margin is the difference or ratio between the allowable limit (after correction by the uncertainty factor) and the available dose. How large does a safety margin need to be? Generally, a safety margin of 100$\times$ or more is desirable, but this can depend on the severity of the risk under consideration, the type of product, the business risk to the company, and the potential benefits of product use.

IX. CONCLUSION

Ensuring the safety of medical devices (both new and, as a quality control concern, established) is an ongoing challenge. Strict adherence to regulatory requirements in the intended markets is essential but not sufficient. Careful and continuous consideration must be given to both the ''known'' potential problems (as presented in this text, e.g.) and also to those new areas of concern made visible by the continued advancement of science and extension of human experience. Immunotoxicity is currently the most apparent area of real and new but ill-defined concern.

Medical device manufacturers have two predominant questions when it comes to material biocompatibility. The first is: ''We have a material that we absolutely must use in our device, but it fails a biocompatibility test. Can we justify using the material anyway?'' The second is: ''We have a material that we absolutely must use in our device, but carcinogenicity and/or chronic toxicity testing is required. Can we justify omitting these tests?'' Judicious application of health-based risk assessments can help with both these issues, often providing a fast, cost-effective answer to both questions.

Additionally, the seemingly safe and fixed field of regulatory safety assessment for devices is (and will remain through the current decade) in flux. The author believes that FDA (and other regulatory) requirements will continue to become more stringent until they are indistinguishable from those for pharmaceuticals, and the economic forces causing companies to have to compete in a worldwide market will only intensify, making the regulatory standards for device approval confused (although harmonization under ICH and ISO will continue to make progress) and equivalent to the highest national standard in which companies intend to compete.

REFERENCES

Arellano, R., Bradley, J., and Sussman, F. (1992). Prevalence of latex sensitization among hospital physicians occupationally exposed to latex gloves, Anesthesiology, 77: 905–908.

Autian, J. (1972). Toxicity and health threats of phthalate esters: Review of the literature. Toxicology Information Response Center, article no. ORNC-TRIC-72-2, Oak Ridge National Laboratory, Oak Ridge, TN.

Baldwin, C. M. Jr. and Kaplan, E. N. (1983). Silicone-induced human adjuvant disease, Ann. Plast. Surg., 10: 270–273.

Bohach, G. A., Fast, D. J., Nelson, R. D., and Schlievert, P. M. (1990). Staphylococcal and streptococcal pyrogenic toxins involved in toxic shock syndrome and related illnesses, Crit. Rev. Microbio., 17: 251–272.

Bommer, J., Waldher, R., and Ritz, E. (1983). Silicone storage disease in long-term hemodialysis patients, Contr. Nephrol., 36: 115–126.

Byrne, J. (1996). Informed Consent, McGraw-Hill, New York.

Byrne, K. (1992). Medical records in litigation: The Dalkon shield story, AMRO, 2: 11–14.

Carter, J. E., Roll, D. B., and Petersen, R. V. (1974). The in vitro hydrolysis of di(2-ethylhexy)phthalate by rat tissues, Drug Metab. Dispos., 2: 341.

Cohen, W. N. and Safaie-Shirazi, S. (1973). Starch granulomatous peritonitis, Amer. J. Roentgenol. Radium Ther. Nucl. Med., 117: 334–339.

Daniel, J. W. and Bratt, H. (1973). The absorption, metabolism and tissue distribution of di(2-ethyl-hexyl)phthalate in rats, Toxicology, 2: 51.

Eckhardt, R. E. and Hindin, R. (1973). The health hazards of plastics, J. Occupa. Med., 15: 809.

Eismann, B., Seeling, M. G., and Womack, N. A. (1947). Talcum granuloma: Frequent and serious complication, Ann. Surg., 126: 820–832.

Estlander, T., Jolanski, R., and Kanerva, L. (1986). Dermatitis and urticaria from rubber and plastic gloves, Cont. Dermatitis, 14: 20–25.

Fay, M. F. and Sullivan, R. W. (1992). Changing requirements for glove selection and hand protection, Biomed. Instr. Tech., 26: 227–232.

Fisher, A. A. (1991). Management of allergic contact dermatitis due to rubber gloves in health and hospital personnel, Cutis, 47: 301–302.

Gad, S. C. (1999) Product Safety Assessment, Shared Dehper, New York.

Gonzales, E. (1992). Latex hypersensitivity: A new and unexpected problem, Hosp. Prac., 15: 137–151.

Guess, W. L., and O'Leary, R. K. (1969). Toxicity of a rubber accelerator, Toxicol. Appl. Pharm., 14: 221–231.

Heggers, J. P., Kassovsky, N., Parsons, R. W., Rosbon, M. C., Pelley, R. P., and Raine, T. J. (1983). Biocompatibility of silicone implants, Ann. Plast. Surg., 11: 38–45.

Henderson, W. J., Melville-Jones, C., Barr, W. T., and Griffiths, K. (1975). Identification of talc on surgeons' gloves and in tissue from starch granulomas, Brit. J. Surg., 62: 941–944.

Hennepens, C. H., Lee, I., Cook, N. R., et al. (1996). Self-reported breast implants and connective tissue diseases in female health professionals, JAMA, 275: 616–621.

Houppert, K. (1995). Embarrassed to death, Village Voice, Feb. 7.

Ignatius, J. D. and Hartman, W. M. (1972). The glove starch peritonitis syndrome, Ann. Surg., 175: 388–397.

ISO. (1998). Medical Devices—Risk Management—Application of Risk Analysis, ISO 14971-1.

Jaeger, R. J. and Rubin, R. J. (1973). Extraction, localization and metabolism of di-2-ethylhexyl phthalate from PVC plastic medical devices, Environ. Health Persp., 3: 95.

Kelly, K. J., Kurp, V. P., Reijula, K. E., and Fink, J. N. (1994). The diagnosis of natural rubber latex allergy, J. Allergy Clin. Immunol., 93: 813–816.

Lake, B. G., Branton, P. J., Gangoli, S. D., Butterworth, K. R., and Grasso, P. (1976). Studies on the effects of orally administered di(2-ethylhexyl) phthalate in the ferret, Toxicology, 6: 341.

Lang, L. D. (1996). A review of latex hypersensitivity, Toxic Sub. Mech., 15: 1–11.

Laohapand, T., Osman, E. M., Morley, A. R., Ward, M. K., and Kerr, D. N. S. (1982). Accumulation of silicone elastomers in regular dialysis, Proc. EDTA, 19: 143–152.

Lazarus, J. M. (1980). Complications in hemodialysis: An overview, Kidney Int., 18: 783–796.

Lee, C. M., Collins, W. T., and Largen, T. L. (1952). Reappraisal of absorbable glove powder, Surg. Gyn. Ob., 95: 725–737.

Lee, C. M. and Lehman, E. P. (1947). Experiment with non-irritating glove powder, Surg. Gyn. Ob., 84: 689.

Lichtman, A. L., McDonald, J. R., Dixon, C. F., and Mann, F. C. (1946). Talc granuloma, Surg. Gyn. Ob., 83: 531–546.

Maguire, D. (1966). Tampon vaginitis, J. S. C. Med. Assoc., 62: 432.

Mayer, F. L. Jr., Stalling, D. L., and Johnson, J. L. (1972). Phthalate esters as environmental contaminants, Nature, 238: 411.

McAdams, G. B. (1956). Granuloma caused by absorbable starch glove powder, Surgery, 39: 329–336.

McGregor, R. R. (1953). Silicones in pharmacy, Pharm. Int., Jan.: 24–26, 63.

Meek, J. H. and Pettit, B. R. (1985). Avoidable accumulation of potentially toxic levels of bevothiazoles in babies receiving intravenous therapy, Lancet, 2: 1090–1092.

Miripol, J. E. and Stern, I. J. (1977). Decreased accumulation of phthalate plasticizer during storage of blood as packed cells, Transfusion, 17: 71–72.

Mumford, S. D. and Kessel, E. (1992). Was the Dalkon shield a safe and effective intrauterine device? The conflict between case-control and clinical trial findings. Fert. Ster., 57: 1151–1176.

Nash, D. F. E. (1971). Glove powder, Brit. Med. J., 3: 329–336.

Neelly, J. and Davies, J. D. (1971). Starch granulomatosis of peritoneum, Brit. Med. J., 3: 625–629.

Nikonorow, M., Mazur, H., and Piekacy, H. (1973). Effect of orally administered plasticizers and polyvinylchloride stabilizers in the rat, Toxicol. Appl. Pharm., 26: 253–259.

Nocera, J. (1995). Fatal litigation, Fortune, Oct. 16: 60–82.

NRC. (1983). Risk Assessment in the Federal Government: Managing the Process, National Research Council, Washington DC.

Orem, C. and Beck, J. (1981). The tampon: Investigated and challenged, Women Sci. Health, 6: 105–122.

Peck, C. C., Odom, D. G, Friedman, H. I., et al. (1979). Di-2-ethylhexyl phthalate (DEHP), and mono-2-ethylhexyl phthalate (MEHP): Accumulation in whole blood and red cell concentrates, Transfusion, 19: 137–146.

Perper, J. A., Pidlaon, A., and Fisher, R. S. (1971). Granulomatous peritonitis induced by rice starch, Amer. J. Surg., 122: 812–817.

Peterson, M. C., Vine, J., Ashley, J. J., and Nation, R. L. (1981). Leaching of 2-(2-hydroxyethylmercapto-)benzothiazole into contents of disposable syringes, J. Pharm. Sci., 70: 1139–1143.

Postlethwaite, R. W., Howard, H. L., and Schanher, W. P. (1949). Comparison of tissue reaction to talc and modified starch glove powder, Surgery, 25: 22.

Reingold, A. L., Hargrett, N. T., Shands, K. N., et al. (1982a). Toxic shock syndrome surveillance in the United States: 1980 to 1981, Ann. Intern. Med., 96 (part 2): 875–880.

Reingold, A. L., Hargrett, N. T., Dan, B. B., Shands, K. N., Strickland, B. Y., and Broome, C. V. (1982b). Nonmenstrual toxic shock syndrome: A review of 130 cases, Ann. Intern. Med., 96: 871–874.

Rock, G., Secours, V. E., Franklin, C. A., Chu, I., and Villeneuve, D. C. (1978). The accumulation of mono-2-ethylhexylphthalate (MEHP) during storage of whole blood and plasma, Transfusion, 18: 553–558.

Roster, F. and Gruenwald, H. W. (1986). Contaminants in blood of infants on prolonged intravenous therapy, Lancet, 1: 380–381.

Sasakawa, S. and Mitomi, Y. (1978). Di-2-ethylhexylphthalate (DEMP) content of blood or blood components stored in plastic bags, Vox Sansg, 34: 81–86.

Scarbeck, K. (1993). Latex: Is it safe?, Acad. Gen. Dent., 21: 2–6.

Schlievert, P. M. and Blomster, D. A. (1983). Production of staphylococcal pyrogenic exotoxin type C: Influence of physical and chemical factors, J. Infec. Dis., 147: 236–242.

Schrock, C. G. (1980). Disease alert, JAMA, 243:1231.

Sheftel, V. O. (1994). Handbook of Toxic Properties of Monomers and Additives, CRC Press, Boca Raton, FL.

Shumnes, E. and Darby, T (1984). Contact dermatitis due to endotoxin in irradiated latex gloves, Cont. Dermatitis, 10(4): 240–244.

Singh, I., Chow, W. L., and Charlani, I. V. (1974) Synovial reaction to glove powder, Clin. Orthoped., 99: 285.

Sivin, I. (1993) Another look at the Dalkon shield: Meta-analysis underscores its problems, Contraception, 48: 1–12.

Slater, J. E. (1992). Allergic reactions to natural rubber, Ann. Allergy, 68: 203–209.

Snierson, H. and Woo, Z. P. (1955). Starch powder granulomata: A report of 2 cases, Ann. Surg., 142:1045.

Sobel, H. J. Schiffman, R. J., Camden, N. J., Schwarz, R., and Albert, W. S. (1971). Granulomas and peritonitis due to starch glove powder, Arch. Pathol., 91: 559–568.

Sobol, R. B. (1991). Bending the Law: The Story of the Dalkon Shield Bankruptcy, University of Chicago Press, Chicago.

Stark, N. J. (1996). Managing positive biocompatibility test results, Med. Dev. Diag. Ind., Oct.: 148–163.

Sussman, G. L. (1995). Allergy to latex rubber, Ann. Intern. Med., 122: 43–44.

Sussman, G. L., Taro, S., and Dolovich, J. (1991). The spectrum of IgE-mediated responses to latex, JAMA, 265: 2844–2847.

Taft, D. A., Lasersohn, J. T., and Hill, L. D. (1970). Glove starch granulomatous peritonitis, Amer. J. Surg., 120: 231–236.

Tatum, H. J., Schmidt, F. H., Phillips, D., McCarty, M., and O'Leary, W. M. (1975). The Dalkon shield controversy: Structural and bacteriological studies of IUD tails, JAMA, 231: 711–717.

Thomas, D. and Withington, P. S. (1985). Toxic shock syndrome: A review of the litera-
    ture, Ann. Royal Coll. Surg., 67: 156–158.

Todd, J., Fishaut, M., Kapral, F., and Welch, T. (1978). Toxic shock syndrome associated
    with phage group 1 staphylococci, Lancet, 1: 16–18.

Turjama, K. (1993). European medical experiences from latex protein allergy: The present
    position, Proceedings International Conference of Rubber Consultants and the Euro-
    pean Rubber Journal, pp. 17–19.

Uber, C. L. and McReynolds, R. A. (1982). Immunotoxicology of silica, CRC Rev. Tox-
    icol., 10: 303–320.

Warpinski, J. R., Folgert, J., Cohen, M., and Bush, R. K. (1991). Allergic reaction to latex:
    A risk factor for unsuspected anaphylaxis, Allergy Proc., 12: 95–102.

Wong, O. (1996). A critical assessment of the relationship between silicone breast implants
    and connective tissue diseases, Reg. Toxicol. Pharm., 23: 74–85.

Appendix A: Selected Regulatory and Toxicological Acronyms and Abbreviations

510(k)	Premarket notification for change in a device
AALAS	American Association Laboratory Animal Science
AAMI	Association for the Advancement of Medical Instrumentation
ABT	American Board of Toxicology
ACGIH	American Conference of Governmental Industrial Hygienists
ACT	American College of Toxicology
ADI	Allowable daily intake
AIDS	Acquired immune deficiency syndrome
AIMD	Active implantable medical device
ANSI	American National Standards Institute
APHIS	Animal and Plant Health Inspection Service
ASTM	American Society for Testing and Materials
CAS	Chemical Abstract Service
CBER	Center for Biologic Evaluation and Research (FDA)
CDER	Center for Drug Evaluation and Research (FDA)
CDRH	Center for Devices and Radiological Health (FDA)
CFR	Code of Federal Regulations
CFAN	Center for Food and Distribution (FDA)
CIIT	Chemical Industries Institute of Toxicology
CPMP	Committee on Proprietary Medicinal Products (U.K.)
CPSC	Consumer Product Safety Commission
CRF	Code of Federal Regulations
CSE	Control standard endotoxin
CSM	Committee on Safety of Medicines (U.K.)
CTC	Clinical trial certificate (U.K.)

CTX	Clinical trial certificate exemption (U.K.)
CVM	Center for Veterinary Medicine (FDA)
DART	Development and Reproduction Toxicology
DHHS	Department of Health and Human Services
DIA	Drug Information Associates
DMF	Device (or drug) master file
DOE	Department of Energy
DOT	Department of Transportation
DSHEA	Dietrary Supplement Health and Education Act
EEC	European Economic Community
EM	Electron microscopy
EPA	Environmental Protection Agency
EU	European Union
FCA	Freund's complete adjuvant
FDA	Food and Drug Administration
FDC	Food Drug and Cosmetic
FDCA	Food, Drug and Cosmetic Act
FDLI	Food and Drug Law Institute
FHSA	Federal Hazardous Substances Act
FIFRA	Federal Insecticides, Fungicides and Rodenticides Act
GCP	Good clinical practices
GLP	Good laboratory practices
GMP	Good manufacturing practices
GPMT	Guinea pig maximization test
HEW	Department of Health, Education and Welfare (no longer in existence)
HIMA	Health Industry Manufacturer's Association
HSDB	Hazardous substances databank
IARC	International Agency for Research on Cancer
ICH	International Conference on Harmonization
id	Intradermal
IDE	Investigational device exemption
IND(A)	Investigational new drug application
ip	Intraperitoneal
IRAG	Interagency Regulatory Alternatives Group
IRB	Institutional review board
IRLG	Interagency regulatory liaison group
ISO	International Standards Organization
IUD	Intrauterine device
iv	Intravenous
JECFA	Joint Expert Committee for Food Additives
JMAFF	Japanese Ministry of Agriculture, Forestry, and Fishery
LA	Licensing Authority (U.K.)
LAL	*Limulus* amebocyte lysate
LD_{50}	Lethal dose 50: The dose calculated to kill 50% of a subject population, median lethal dose

LOEL	Lowest observed effect level
MAA	Marketing Authorization Application (EEC)
MD	Medical device
MHW	Ministry of Health & Welfare (Japan)
MID	Maximum implantable dose
MOE	Margin of exposure
MOU	Memorandum of understanding
MRL	Maximum residue limits
MSDS	Material safety data sheet
MTD	Maximum tolerated dose
NAS	National Academy of Science
NCTR	National Center for Toxicological Research
NDA	New drug application
NIH	National Institutes of Health
NIOSH	National Institute of Occupational Safety and Health
NK	Natural killer
NLM	National Library of Medicine
NOEL	No-observable-effect level
NTP	National Toxicology Program
ODE	Office of Device Evaluation
OECD	Organization for Economic Cooperation and Development
PDI	Primary dermal irritancy
PDN	Product development notification
PEL	Permissible exposure limit
PhRMA	Pharmaceutical Research and Manufacturers Association
PL	Produce license (U.K.)
PLA	Produce license application
PMA	Premarket approval applications
PMN	Premanufacturing notice
po	Per os (orally)
PTC	Points to consider
QAU	Quality assurance unit
RAC	Recombinant DNA Advisory Committee
RCRA	Resources Conservation and Recovery Act
RTECS	Registry of Toxic Effects of Chemical Substances
SARA	Superfund/Amendments and Reauthorization Act
sc	Subcutaneous
SCE	Sister chromatic exchange
SNUR	Significant new use regulations
SOP	Standard operating procedure
SOT	Society of Toxicology
SRM	Standard reference materials (Japan)
STEL	Short-term exposure limit
TLV	Threshold limit value
TSCA	Toxic Substances Control Act

USAN	United States Adopted Name Council
USDA	United States Department of Agriculture
USEPA	United States Environmental Protection Agency
USP	United States Pharmacopoeia
WHO	World Health Organization

Appendix B: Contract Testing Laboratories

Laboratory	Address	Phone number
Consumer Product Testing Company	70 New Dutch Lane Fairfield, NJ 07004	(973) 808-7111
MB Research Laboratories, Inc.	P.O. Box 178 Spinnertown, PA 18968	(215) 536-4110
Micro Test Laboratories, Inc.	P.O. Box 848 Agawam, MA 01001	(413) 789-4334
Nelson Laboratories	6280 South Redwood Road Salt Lake City, UT 841123-6600	(800) 826-2088
North American Science Associates, Inc.	2261 Tracy Road Toledo, OH 43619	(419) 227-6882
Northview Pacific Laboratories, Inc.	2800 Seventh Street Berkeley, CA 94710	(510) 548-8440
SGS U.S. Testing Company, Inc.	291 Fairfield Avenue Fairfield, NJ 07004	(201) 575-5252
STS duo TEK, Inc.	7500 W. Henrietta Road Rush, NY 14543	(716) 533-1672
TOXIKON	15 Wiggins Avenue Bedford, MA 01730	(617) 275-3330
Viromed Biosafety Laboratories	6101 Blue Circle Drive Minneapolis, MN 55343	(800) 582-0077 (952) 563-3926

Appendix C: Notable Regulatory Internet Addresses

Organization or publication	Web address (URL)	Sample main topics
Agency for Toxic Substances and Disease Registry	www.atsdr.cdc.gov	
Australian Therapeutic Goods Administration	http://www.health.gov.au/tga	Medical devices; GMP codes; Parliamentary Secretary's Working; Status Document; Party on Complementary Medicines; medical releases; publications; site map; related sites
Canadian Health Protection Branch	http://www.hc-sc.gc.ca/hpb	Medical devices; chemical hazards; food; product safety; science advisory board; diseases; radiation protection; drugs; HPB transition policy, planning and coordination
ChemInfo	www.indiana.edu/~cheminfo/ca_csti.html	SirCH: Chemical Safety or Toxicology Information
Code of Federal Regulations	http://www.access.gpo.gov/nara/cfr/cfr-table-search.html	NARA Code Sections
Cornell Legal Library	http://www.law.cornell.edu	Code of Federal Regulations; Supreme Court decisions; U.S. Code; Circuit Courts of Appeal
EPA	www.epa.gov	
European Agency for the Evaluation of Medicinal Products	http://www.eudra.org/en_home.htm	What's new; documents forum; other sites
European sites	http://www.eucomed.be/eucomed/links/links.htm	European institutions; related sites
Food and Drug Administration (FDA)	www.fda.gov	Foods; human drugs; biologics; animal drugs; cosmetics; medical devices/radiological health

Item	Address	Notes
FDA—CDRH	www.fda.gov/cdrh/index.html	Home page
Search site	www.fda.gov/cdrh/search.html	Search CDRH site
Comment	www.fda.gov/cdrh/comment4.html	Comment on CDRH site
Device Advice	www.fda.gov/cdrh/devadvice/32.html	
PDF Reader	www.fda.gov/cdrh/acrobat.html	
General Principles of Software Validation (draft) Guidance for Industry	www.fda.gov/cdrh/comp/swareval.html	Text
Division of Small Manufacturers Assistance	www.fda.gov/cdrh/dsma/dsmamain.html	
	www.fda.gov/cdrh/dsma/cgmphome.htm	
	www.fda.gov/cdrh/humfac/frqar.html	Good manufacturing practice (GMP; also known as the quality system regulation); final rule text as published in the *Federal Register*
	www.fda.gov/cdrh/fr1007ap.pdf	
	www.fda.gov/cdrh/gmpasci.zip	
	www.fda.gov/cdrh/comp/designed.pdf	PDF version of Design Control Report and Guidance
Design Control Guidance for Medical Device Manufacturers	www.fda.gov/cdrh/comp/designgd.html	Text
Design Control Guidance for Medical Device Manufacturers	www.fda.gov/cdrh/comp/designgd.pdf	PDF version
Design Control Inspection Results	www.fda.gov/cdrh/dsma/dcisresults.html	First year rollout final design control inspection results and presentation text
Do it by Design: An Introduction to Human Factors in Medical Devices	www.fda.gov/cdrh/humfac/doit.html	By Dick Sawyer, Office of Health and Industry Programs
	www.fda.gov/cdrh/humfac/doitpdf.pdf	PDF version of *Do It by Design: An Introduction to Human Factors in Medical Devices* by Dick Sawyer
Human Factors Implications of the New GMP Rule	www.fda.gov/cdrh/humfac/hufacimp.html	Text

Organization or publication	Web address (URL)	Sample main topics
Medical Device Quality Systems Manual: A Small Entity Compliance Guide (document withdrawn)	www.fda.gov/cdrh/dsmzza/gmpman.html	Text
	www.fda.gov/cdrh/comp/ghtfproc.html	Draft Global Harmonization Task Force (GHTF) process validation guidance text
Guidance on Information Disclosure by Manufacturers to Assemblers for Diagnostic X-ray Systems	www.fda.gov/cdrh/comp/ghtfproc.pdf www.fda.gov/cdrh/comp/2619.html	PDF version
Guidance on quality system regulation information for various premarket submissions text	www.fda.gov/cdrh/comp/2619.pdf www.fda.gov/cdrh/comp/qsrpma.html	PDF version
CDRH letter to manufacturers	www.fda.gov/cdrh/yr2000/cdrh/letters/980921/y2kcompltr.html	Letter to manufacturers—Y2K issue for production processes and quality system software text
CDRH letter to manufacturers	www.fda.gov/cdrh/yr2000/cdrh/letters/980921/y2kcompltr.pdf	PDF version of letter to manufacturers
GMP/QS workshops with CDRH participation	www.fda.gov/cdrh/dsma/workshop.html	
FDA/Industry Exchange workshops on medical device quality systems inspection techniques	www.fda.gov/cdrh/meetings/qsitmeet.html	
Quality system inspections reengineering	www.fda.gov/cdrh/gmp/gmp.html	

FDA—field operations	www.fda.gov/ora/	What's new; import program; inspectional, science and compliance references; federal/state relations
Design controls	www.fda.gov/ora/inspect_ref/qsreq/ dcrpgd.html	Design control report and guidance text
	www.fda.gov/ora/inspect_ref/igs/ elec_med_dev/emcl.html	Guide to inspections of electromagnetic compatibility aspects of medical device quality systems text
Guide to Inspections of Quality Systems	www.fda.gov/ora/inspect_ref/igs/qsit/ qsitguide.htm	QSIT inspection handbook text
Guide to Inspections of Quality Systems	www.fda.gov/ora/inspect_ref/igs/qsit/ QSITGUIDE.PDF	PDF version of QSIT inspection handbook text
Food and Drug Law Institute	http://www.fdli.org	Special interest; publications; multimedia; order products; academic programs; directory of lawyers and consultants; contact us
Health Industry and Manufacturers Association (HIMA)	http://www.himanet.com	About HIMA; newsletter; HIMA calendar; industry resources; business opportunities; FDA/EPA/OSHA; reimbursement/ payment; global year 2000; government relations; public relations; small company; diagnostics
International Regulatory Monitor (monitor)	http://www.go-nsi.com/pubs	Editorial portion of newsletter
Internet Grateful Med	www.igm.nlm.nih.gov	
Japanese Ministry of Health and Welfare	http://www.mhw.go.ip/english/index.html	Organization; Y2K problem; statistics; white paper; related sites
Library of Congress	http://thomas.loc.gov	Searchable database of federal legislation, *Congressional Record* and committee information

Organization or publication	Web address (URL)	Sample main topics
Medical Device Link	http://www.devicelink.com	News; consultants; bookstore; links; discussion; magazines (MDDI; MPMN; IVD Technology)
National Archives and Public Records Administration	http://www.access.gpo.gov/su_ docs/aces/aces140.html	Code of Federal Regulations; *Federal Register*; laws; U.S. Congress information
National Library Network	www.toxnet.nlm.nih.gov	TOXNET: Toxicology Data Network, a cluster of databases on toxicology, hazardous chemicals, and related areas
National Toxicology Program	http://ntp-server.niehs.nih.gov/	
New quality system (QS) regulation	www.fda.gov/bbs/topics/ANSWERS/ ANS00763.html	FDA talk paper announcing the GMP final rule text
Regulatory Affairs Professionals Society (RAPS)	http://www.raps.org	Certificates; resource center; publications; chapters; related links; contacting RAPS
U.S. Department of Commerce	http://204.193.246.62	Bureau of Export Administration; International Trade Association; Patent & Trademark; National Institute of Standards and Technology
University of Pittsburgh	www.pitt.edu	
World Health Organization	http://www.who.int	Governance; health topics; information sources; reports; Director-General; About WHO; International Digest of Health; Legislation (http://www.who.int/pub/dig.html)

Appendix D: Non-U.S. Medical Device Regulators

Organization or publication	Web address (URL)	Sample main topics
CE Marketing	www.sos.se/sose/nt/medtekn/cemark.htm	This is a Swedish government site that provides specific information regarding CE marking, which is necessary to market medical devices in the European Community member nations.
European Union (EU)	http://europa.eu.int/	This is a multilingual gateway to information about all activities of the EU.
Health Canada	www.hc-sc.gc.ca	Provides useful information about the regulation of all medical products in Canada, and other Canadian government health programs.
Medical Device Agency	www.medical-devices.gov.uk	Provides useful information about the regulation of medical devices in the United Kingdom.
National Institute of Health Sciences—Japan	www.nihs.go.jp	Provides useful information about the regulation of medical devices and pharmaceutical products in Japan.
Therapeutic Goods Administration	www.health.gov.au/tga	Provides useful information about the regulation of medical devices and pharmaceutical products in Australia.

Index

551